D0848102

Biological Weapons Defense

Infectious Disease

SERIES EDITOR: *Vassil St. Georgiev*
National Institute of Allergy and Infectious Diseases
National Institutes of Health

Biological Weapons Defense: *Infectious Diseases and Counterbioterrorism,* edited by *Luther E. Lindler,* PhD, *Frank J. Lebeda,* PhD, *and George W. Korch,* PhD, 2005

Microbial Genomes, edited by *Claire M. Fraser,* PhD, *Timothy D. Read,* PhD, *and Karen E. Nelson,* PhD, 2004

Management of Multiple Drug-Resistant Infections, edited by *Stephen H. Gillespie,* MD, 2004

Aging, Immunity, and Infection, by *Joseph F. Albright,* PhD, *and Julia W. Albright,* PhD, 2003

Handbook of Cytokines and Chemokines in Infectious Diseases, edited by *Malak Kotb,* PhD, *and Thierry Calandra,* MD, PhD, 2003

Opportunistic Infections: *Treatment and Prophylaxis,* by *Vassil St. Georgiev,* PhD, 2003

Innate Immunity, edited by *R. Alan B. Ezekowitz,* MBChB, DPhil, FAAP, *and Jules A. Hoffmann,* PhD, 2003

Pathogen Genomics: *Impact on Human Health,* edited by *Karen Joy Shaw,* PhD, 2002

Immunotherapy for Infectious Diseases, edited by *Jeffrey M. Jacobson,* MD, 2002

Retroviral Immunology: *Immune Response and Restoration,* edited by *Giuseppe Pantaleo,* MD, and *Bruce D. Walker,* MD, 2001

Antimalarial Chemotherapy: *Mechanisms of Action, Resistance, and New Directions in Drug Discovery,* edited by *Philip J. Rosenthal,* MD, 2001

Drug Interactions in Infectious Diseases, edited by *Stephen C. Piscitelli,* PharmD, and *Keith A. Rodvold,* PharmD, 2001

Management of Antimicrobials in Infectious Diseases: *Impact of Antibiotic Resistance,* edited by *Arch G. Mainous III,* PhD, and *Claire Pomeroy,* MD, 2001

Infectious Disease in the Aging: *A Clinical Handbook,* edited by *Thomas T. Yoshikawa,* MD, and *Dean C. Norman,* MD, 2001

Infectious Causes of Cancer: *Targets for Intervention,* edited by *James J. Goedert,* MD, 2000

Biological Weapons Defense

Infectious Diseases and Counterbioterrorism

Edited by

Luther E. Lindler, PhD

*National Biodefense Analysis and Countermeasures Center, Fort Detrick, MD,
and Department of Bacterial Diseases, Walter Reed Army Institute of Research,
Silver Spring, MD*

Frank J. Lebeda, PhD

*Department of Cell Biology and Biochemistry,
US Army Medical Research Institute of Infectious Diseases,
Fort Detrick, MD*

George W. Korch, PhD

*Director, National Biodefense Analysis and Countermeasures Center
Fort Detrick, MD*

Forewords by

David R. Franz, COL (RET.), DVM, PhD
*Florida Division, Midwest Research Institute,
Palm Bay, FL*

Matthew Meselson, PhD
*Belfer Center for Science and International Affairs,
Department of Molecular and Cellular Biology, Harvard University,
Boston, MA*

HUMANA PRESS ✳ TOTOWA, NEW JERSEY

Production Editor: Angela L. Burkey and Amy Thau

Cover design by : Patricia F. Cleary

Cover Illustration: Images of macrophages infected with *Bacillus anthracis* spores. $DiIC_{16}$(3) labeled RAW264.7 macrophages (red) were infected with Green Fluorescent Protein-expressing spores of *B. anthracis* (Sterne strain) and repeatedly imaged by confocal microscopy. Multiple separate focal planes were collapsed into a single fluorescence images that were then overlayed into corresponding brightfield images. The frames shown here represent 5 h postinfection. The green-colored spores develop into bacilli over the course of the infection. Image courtesy of Gordon Ruthel, Wilson Ribot, and Timothy Hoover (United States Army Medical Research Institute of Infectious Diseases).

For additional copies, pricing for bulk purchases, and/or information about other Humana titles, contact Humana at the above address or at any of the following numbers: Tel: 973-256-1699; Fax: 973-256-8341; E-mail: humana@humanapr.com, or visit our Website: www.humanapress.com

Photocopy Authorization Policy: Authorization to photocopy items for internal or personal use, or the internal or personal use of specific clients, is granted by Humana Press Inc., provided that the base fee of US $25.00 per copy is paid directly to the Copyright Clearance Center at 222 Rosewood Drive, Danvers, MA 01923. For those organizations that have been granted a photocopy license from the CCC, a separate system of payment has been arranged and is acceptable to Humana Press Inc. The fee code for users of the Transactional Reporting Service is: [1-58829-184-7/05 $25.00].

Printed in the United States of America. 10 9 8 7 6 5 4 3 2 1

e-ISBN: 1-59259-764-5

Library of Congress Cataloging-in-Publication Data

Biological weapons defense : infectious disease counterbioterrorism / edited by Luther E. Lindler, Frank J. Lebeda, George Korch.
   p. ; cm. -- (Infectious disease)
   Includes bibliographical references and index.
   ISBN 1-58829-184-7 (alk. paper)
   1. Bioterrorism. I. Lindler, Luther E. II. Lebeda, Frank J.
III. Korch, George. IV. Series: Infectious disease (Totowa, N.J.)
   [DNLM: 1. Bioterrorism--prevention & control. 2. Communicable Disease Control--methods. 3. Disaster Planning.   WA 295
B615
 2004] RC88.9.T47B544 2004
 303.6'25--dc22

                                                                                                   2004004125

Foreword

In 2003, the President's budget for bioterrorism defense totalled more than $5 billion. Today, the nation's top academic scientists are scrambling to begin work to understand *Bacillus anthracis* and develop new vaccines and drugs. However, just five years ago, only the US Department of Defense (DOD) seemed concerned about these "exotic" agents. In 1997, the DOD spent approximately $137 million on biodefense to protect the deployed force, while academe, industry, local governments, and most of our federal leadership was oblivious to, and in some cases doubtful of, the seriousness of the threat.

The National Institutes of Health (NIH) received the largest budget increase in the organization's history. Fortunately, during this time of national urgency, a sound base exists on which to build our defenses against this new threat. A relatively small cadre of dedicated scientists within the US Army Medical Research and Materiel Command (USAMRMC) laid this foundation over the past 20 years.

While the nation as a whole slept, bacteriologists, virologists, immunologists, and clinicians—both military and civilian—were busy studying the pathogenesis of "exotic" organisms; developed vaccines, drugs, and diagnostics; educating health care providers; supporting state and federal law enforcement in the development of bioforensics; and contributing technical expertise to international arms control and national defense policy. During the 1990s, as the nation's military forces were being downsized, the US Army Medical Research Institute of Infectious Diseases, the DOD's lead laboratory for medical biodefense, lost approximately 30% of its personnel authorizations. Yet, the scientists within the command developed new vaccine candidates and recombinant delivery systems for anthrax, smallpox, plague, brucellosis, the botulium neurotoxins, and staphylococcal toxins along with the viral encephalitides. They established the nation's finest biological forensic diagnostics capability, demonstrated the efficacy of an antiviral drug against smallpox, and led the nation in medical biodefense education.

The dedicated scientists of the USAMRMC and the several other outstanding contributors from the Centers for Disease Control and Prevention, academia, and international organizations to this volume are recognized worldwide as experts in biological weapons defense. They were hard at work in the laboratory before the public even realized there was such a threat, and they stood in the gap for all of us after October 4, 2001, when the United States experienced its first biological terrorism attack in modern history. It was an honor for me to serve with them.

David R. Franz, COL (RET.), DVM, PhD
Florida Division
Midwest Research Institute
Palm Bay, FL

Foreword

Biological Weapons Defense: Infectious Disease and Counterbioterrorism focuses on measures for dealing with the possible deliberate causation of disease and on the underlying science. The fundamental advances in molecular biology of the last several decades are only beginning to find relevant application in the development of effective sensors, rapid early diagnostics, vaccines, antimicrobials, antitoxins, and other relevant prophylactic, therapeutic, and supportive measures. Advances will also come with the increased understanding of pathogenesis and of the mechanisms by which contagious diseases spread from person to person, leading to improved practical measures to limit outbreaks, including measures that can be taken by an informed public.

Such advances will certainly be useful against naturally occurring diseases, including those that are newly emerging or re-emerging and, in the eventuality, against deliberately caused disease as well. Still, experience suggests that practical applications available to the public, although sure to come, will most likely come at a slower pace and at greater cost than legislators and the general public may expect. Unlike the conquest of certain naturally occurring communicable diseases, effective protection against deliberately caused disease will remain problematic.

All of the agents or groups of agents to which specific chapters in *Biological Weapons Defense: Infectious Disease and Counterbioterrorism* are devoted were selected as candidate biological weapons in the old offensive biological warfare (BW) programs of the United Kingdom, the United States, and the Soviet Union. Some of these agents were brought to the stage of mass production, were field-tested, and then stockpiled in bulk and in munitions. It is remarkable how much of the technical base was foreseen even before the big BW programs got underway, as exemplified, for example, in the 1942 report of Theodor Rosebury and Elvin Kabat, declassified in 1947 and published that year in the *Journal of Immunology (1)*. By 1960, much of the technology of selecting, producing, and disseminating disease agents as weapons could be found in the open literature. Aside from the novel and modified agents that can be imagined, all of the "select agents" (except for smallpox) designated by the Centers for Disease Control and Prevention remain accessible from clinics or natural foci. Even so, despite the industrial-scale preparations that have come and gone and the hundreds of wars and bitter insurgencies that have transpired in the past half-century, there has been no BW, and only a few small-scale acts of bioterrorism or, more accurately, biocrime.

Prudent measures to prepare for a major biological attack and to limit its consequences are certainly in order. However, undisciplined speculation that a major biological attack is inevitable risks distracting us from measures intended to keep biological weapons from coming into use in the first place. Inadequate attention is being given to measures to sustain and reinforce the constraints that protect our species from exploiting biotechnology for hostile purposes, as it has exploited other major technologies *(2)*. Whatever the underlying reasons that have averted BW and bioterrorism, and whatever the factors that might disrupt this desirable state of affairs, they deserve closer and more disinterested study and attention than they have received so far.

As the old Western and Soviet programs recede into the past, the number of persons with the specific knowledge and skills required to create devastating biological weapons was rapidly declining. But some biodefense activities, especially secret ones, have begun to reverse this trend by causing a new generation of scientists, engineers, and others to turn their attention to vulnerabilities and conceivable future threat agents, and hence to technologies with offensive potential. The expanded number of facilities and individuals working with dangerous pathogens also makes access to these agents easier, and the number of individuals who may become motivated to make hostile use of them greater.

Beyond that, the impression of extensive secret work risks motivating other states to initiate or expand secret programs of their own, further multiplying the pool of potential security risks and perhaps verging into offensively oriented activities. Closer to home, a further risk of secrecy in biodefense work is that it risks losing the confidence of the public, essential to the actual implementation of protective measures. The practice of public health traditionally rests on open discussion and public understanding in order to gain the acceptance and trust of those it is intended to benefit.

Considering the great and growing pervasiveness of biotechnology, the key element in averting bioterrorism and biowarfare is not access but intent, whether on the part of individuals, groups, or national governments. At the level of the individual scientist and through our institutions and professional societies there is a modest but easily practiced way in which we can address the element of intent. That is the customary openness and professional amicability to which scientists are traditionally accustomed. Scientific visits, exchanges, joint projects, studies abroad, development of personal friendships across cultures and across national frontiers are intellectually and professionally beneficial, as well as personally rewarding. Beyond that, the more openness within a society as a whole, the more likely it is that improper activities within it will come to light or, better, be discouraged in the first place.

Matthew Meselson, PhD
Belfer Center for Science and International Affairs
Department of Molecular and Cellular Biology
Harvard University
Boston, MA

REFERENCES

1. Rosebury, T. and Kabat, E. A. (1947) Bacterial Warfare. J. Immunol. 56, 7–96.
2. Meselson, M. (2002) Bioterror: What Can Be Done? In: *Striking Terror.* (Silvers, R. and Epstein, B., eds.) New York Review Books, New York, NY, pp. 259–276.

Preface

The attacks on the World Trade Center (WTC) and the Pentagon and the first major use of bioterrorism that coincided in the fall of 2001 are now infamous. The Al Qaeda perpetrators of the horrible attacks on the WTC and Pentagon were clear in their intent. However, to date we have not achieved a similar clear understanding regarding the distribution of anthrax spores in the US postal system. We know neither exactly who perpetrated this crime, nor the perpetrators' exact intent. What is known is that the anthrax letter attacks cost billions of dollars to clean up, caused major disruptions in the everyday lives of countless citizens, undermined the trust and confidence that citizens have long held in this bastion of everyday life, and resulted in the deaths of innocent citizens. The impact was felt not only in the United States but also in countries around the world, as panic was precipitated by the possibility of innocuous "white powder" being an infectious agent.

The scientists and leadership within the US Department of Defense (DOD) played a unique role in mitigating this event by performing the initial identification of the infectious material (anthrax) as well as advising and participating in the decontamination process in the Hart Senate office building. Indeed, it can be argued that the DOD was the only federal agency capable of fully responding to this threat at that time because of its long-standing mission to provide the means to defend against a biological weapons attack. This critical mission has now transitioned into the newly established Department of Homeland Security (DHS).

The DOD biological defense program and similar defense programs in other countries have long involved research aimed at countering the use of biological and chemical weapons. The United States also had an active offensive biological program from the 1950s until 1969, when it was terminated by President Nixon.

Given the experience and history of the defense-associated programs in the development of countermeasures and in planning for future research in this area, *Biological Weapons Defense: Infectious Disease and Counterbioterrorism* is heavily represented by researchers who work within the biological defense community. However, we have also included contributors from other communities, including academia, the Centers for Disease Control and Prevention, the Department of Energy (DOE), and the Department of Health and Human Services (DHHS). Most of these groups have been working with various aspects of bioterrorism for the past four years. The intensity and urgency of those efforts have increased since the 2001 attacks. Also, within the DHHS, funding has been greatly increased for bioterrorism research and for the development of medical countermeasures. It is anticipated that this increase in funding will yield further discoveries that will enhance national defense.

Even with the warnings of experts and the years of funding and preparation for an act of bioterrorism, the United States was not fully prepared for the anthrax attacks. Because of the decades of research and development that DOD scientists and physicians had accomplished in the treatment, prevention, and diagnosis of these rare diseases, many individuals and research centers within the DOD were asked to "step up" in that time

ix

of national crisis. This is an indication of the professionalism and capabilities of this relatively small group of people. It was against this backdrop that *Biological Weapons Defense: Infectious Disease and Counterbioterrorism* was written. The purpose of this volume is to cover many aspects of the defense against biological agents that we, as members of the human community, must address on a continuing basis. We have divided this volume into four parts that concentrate on the major areas of interest and research.

Part I, "Preparation and Military Support for a Possible Bioterrorism Incident," provides the reader with a view into the behind-the-scenes efforts that many people might not be aware of because they are outside the government network. This includes the policy and laws that govern the DOD and its programs. We have also included aspects of event modeling as well as a general description of the diseases of greatest concern.

Part II, "Medical Countermeasures and Decontamination," gives an account of general knowledge of these particular diseases including pathogenesis, treatment, and the unique aspect of studying the aerosol route of infection.

Part III, "Emerging Threats and Future Preparation," could have easily been titled "future directions." The number of nefarious manipulations or discovery of previously unknown threats that might be developed into biological weapons is almost unlimited. This section informs readers of these threats and describes some of the ongoing research that attempts to counter these unknown agents. This section includes genomic efforts, which describe the current rapid pace of information that is gleaned from analysis of the genomes and proteomes of these agents. Following the anthrax letters, there has been a continuing effort by the National Institutes of Health, DOD, and DOE in the area of biodefense genomics. This research has the potential to accelerate many aspects of preparation against the use of biological weapons, including future threats, diagnostics, therapeutics, vaccinations, pathogenesis, genotyping, and forensics.

Finally, Part IV, "Diagnostic Development for Biowarfare Agents," discusses the many aspects of the development and use of our current technology to identify and characterize these infectious organisms.

Although it was not possible to cover every aspect of biodefense in this volume, we hope readers will gain a greater understanding of the diseases caused by these organisms and develop a sense of the scope of issues that must be overcome to develop necessary medical countermeasures to bioterrorism. Readers should also understand the status of current programs and future plans regarding specific diseases as well as future technology or future threats.

A quote from retired US Army Major General Phillip K. Russell could be considered a theme for this book: "Deficiencies in our scientific knowledge and a paucity of experts will ultimately limit our capability to rapidly and precisely identify agents and respond effectively in a crisis" *(1)*. *Biological Weapons Defense: Infectious Disease and Counterbioterrorism* is intended to give readers a sense of where we are on this issue and where we are moving in the future. We hope that you will find our book informative.

Luther E. Lindler, PhD
Frank J. Lebeda, PhD
George W. Korch, PhD

REFERENCES

Russell, P. K. (1997) Biologic terrorism—responding to the threat. *Emerg Infect. Dis.* **3,** 203–204.

Disclaimer for US Department of Defense Authors

The opinions, interpretations, conclusions, and recommendations are those of the authors and are not necessarily endorsed by the US Army. All research was conducted in compliance with the Animal Welfare Act and other federal statutes and regulations relating to animals and experiments involving animals and adheres to principles stated in the *Guide for the Care and Use of Laboratory Animals*, National Research Council, 1996. The facilities where the research described herein was conducted is fully accredited by the Association for Assessment and Accreditation of Laboratory Animal Care International. The research by these authors was funded either entirely or partially by the Medical Biological Defense Research Program, US Army Medical Research and Materiel Command.

Contents

Contributors

JEFFREY J. ADAMOVICZ, PhD, LTC, USA • *Bacteriology Division, US Army Medical Research Institute of Infectious Diseases, Fort Detrick, MD*

SIV G. E. ANDERSSON, PhD • *Department of Molecular Evolution, University of Uppsala, Sweden*

GERARD P. ANDREWS, PhD, LTC, USA • *Bacteriology Division, US Army Medical Research Institute of Infectious Diseases, Fort Detrick, MD*

ROBERT S. BOROWSKI, PhD • *Homeland Security Institute-ANSER Corporation, Arlington, VA*

RICHARD H. BORSCHEL, PhD • *Department of Bacterial Diseases, Walter Reed Army Institute of Research, Silver Spring, MD*

ROBERT L. BULL, PhD • *Navy Biological Defense Research Directorate, Naval Medical Research Center, Silver Spring, MD*

TIMOTHY H. BURGESS, MD, MPH, LCDR, MC, USNR • *Immunology Section, Viral Diseases Department, Naval Medical Research Center, and Assistant Professor, Department of Medicine, Uniformed Services University of the Health Sciences, Bethesda, MD*

EILEEN CHOFFNES, PhD • *Policy and Global Affairs Division, The National Academies, Washington, DC*

MAY CHU, PhD • *Division of Vector-Borne Infectious Diseases, National Center for Infectious Diseases, Centers for Disease Control and Prevention, Ft. Collins, CO*

ROBERT G. DARLING, MD, CAPT, MC, USN • *Navy Medicine Office of Homeland Security, Bureau of Medicine and Surgery, Washington, DC, and US Army Medical Research Institute of Infectious Diseases, Fort Detrick, MD, and Department of Military and Emergency Medicine, Uniformed Services University of the Health Sciences, Bethesda, MD*

ZYGMUNT F. DEMBEK, PhD, LTC, MS, USAR • *Epidemiology Program, Connecticut Department of Public Health, Hartford, CT and Assistant Clinical Professor, Department of Community Medicine and Health Care, Graduate Program in Public Health, University of Connecticut Health Center, Farmington, CT*

DAVID DESHAZER, PhD • *Bacteriology Division, US Army Medical Research Institute of Infectious Diseases, Fort Detrick, MD*

MICHAEL DOBSON, PhD • *Department of Infectious and Parasitic Diseases, Armed Forces Institute of Pathology, Washington, DC*

TIMOTHY P. ENDY, MD, MPH, COL, MC, USA • *Division of Communicable Diseases and Immunology, Walter Reed Army Institute of Research, Silver Spring, MD, and Department of Medicine Uniformed Services University of the Health Sciences, Bethesda, MD*

MATT EUSSEN, MD • *Field Office, US Foreign Service, Katmandu, Nepal*

MATS FORSMAN, PhD • *National Defence Research Establishment, Umeå, Sweden*

DAVID R. FRANZ, COL (RET.), DVM, PhD • *Frederick Division, Midwest Research Institute, Frederick, MD*

TED L. HADFIELD, PhD • *Chief BioScience Advisor, Florida Division, Midwest Research Institute, Palm Bay, FL*

ROBERT J. HAWLEY, PhD, CBSP • *Safety and Radiation Protection, US Army Medical Research Institute of Infectious Diseases, Fort Detrick, MD*

ERIK A. HENCHAL, PhD • *Diagnostic Systems Division, US Army Medical Research Institute of Infectious Diseases, Fort Detrick, MD*

MICHAEL HEVEY, PhD • *Virology Division, US Army Medical Research Institute of Infectious Diseases, Fort Detrick, MD*

DAVID L. HOOVER, MD • *Department of Bacterial Diseases, Walter Reed Army Institute of Research, Silver Spring, MD*

XIAO-ZHE HUANG, PhD • *Department of Bacterial Diseases, Walter Reed Army Institute of Research, Silver Spring, MD*

ANNA JOHNSON-WINEGAR, PhD • *Office of the Secretary of Defense, Deputy Assistant Secretary for Chemical and Biological Defense, Washington, DC*

PATRICK W. KELLEY, MD, DrPH, COL (RET.), MC, USA • *Director, Board of Public Health, Institute of Medicine at the National Academies of Science, Washington, DC*

GEORGE W. KORCH, PhD • *Deputy Director, National Biodefense Analysis and Countermeasures Center, Fort Detrick, MD*

JOSEPH P. KOZLOVAC, MS, CBSP • *Environment, Health, and Safety, SAIC-Frederick, National Cancer Institute at Frederick, Fort Detrick, MD*

ARTHUR M. KRIEG, MD • *Department of Internal Medicine, University of Iowa College of Medicine, Iowa City, IA,* and *Coley Pharmaceutical Group, Wellesley, MA*

JAMES V. LAWLER, MD, LCDR, MC, UCDR • *Infectious Diseases Service, National Naval Medical Center, Bethesda, MD*

FRANK J. LEBEDA, PhD • *Department of Cell Biology and Biochemistry, US Army Medical Research Institute of Infectious Diseases, Fort Detrick, MD*

ROSS D. LECLAIRE, DVM, PhD • *Chief, Toxinology and Aerobiology Division, US Army Medical Research Institute of Infectious Diseases, Frederick, MD,* and *US Army Center for Health Promotion and Preventive Medicine, Camp Zama, Japan*

ELLIOT J. LEFKOWITZ, PhD • *Molecular and Genetic Bioinformatics Facility, University of Alabama at Birmingham, Birmingham, AL*

LUTHER E. LINDLER, PhD • *Science and Technology Directorate, National Biodefense Analysis and Countermeasures Center, Department of Homeland Security, Fort Detrick, MD,* and *Department of Bacterial Diseases, Walter Reed Army Institute of Research, Silver Spring, MD*

GEORGE V. LUDWIG, PhD • *Diagnostic Systems Division, US Army Medical Research Institute of Infectious Diseases, Fort Detrick, MD*

MATTHEW MESELSON, PhD • *Belfer Center for Science and International Affairs, Department of Molecular and Cellular Biology, Harvard University, Boston, MA*

CHARLES B. MILLARD, PhD, LTC, USA• *Chief of Toxinology and Aerobiology Division, US Army Medical Research Institute of Infectious Diseases, Fort Detrick, MD*

Dominique M. Missiakas, PhD • *Committee on Microbiology, University of Chicago, Chicago, IL*

William C. Nierman, PhD • *The Institute for Genomic Research, Rockville, MD*

David Norwood, PhD • *Diagnostic Systems Division, US Army Medical Research Institute of Infectious Diseases, Fort Detrick, MD*

Petra C. F. Oyston, PhD • *Defence Science and Technology Laboratory, CBS Porton Down, Salisbury, Wilts, UK*

Ian T. Paulsen, PhD • *The Institute for Genomic Research, Rockville, MD*

Julie Pavlin, MD, MPH, LTC, MC, USA • *Department of Field Studies, Walter Reed Army Institute of Research, Silver Spring, MD*

M. Louise M. Pitt, PhD • *Department of Aerobiology and Product Evaluation, Toxinology and Aerobiology Division, US Army Medical Research Institute of Infectious Diseases, Fort Detrick, MD*

Timothy D. Read, PhD • *The Institute for Genomic Research, Rockville, MD*

D. G. Cerys Rees, PhD • *Biomedical Sciences, Defence Science and Technology Laboratory, CBS Porton Down, Salisbury, Wilts, UK*

Cynthia A. Rossi, MS • *Diagnostic Systems Division, US Army Medical Research Institute of Infectious Diseases, Fort Detrick, MD*

Alan Schmaljohn, PhD • *Virology Division, US Army Medical Research Institute of Infectious Diseases, Fort Detrick, MD*

Olaf Schneewind, MD, PhD • *Committee on Microbiology, University of Chicago, Chicago, IL*

Karl Semancik, COL (RET.) BS, MBA • *Raytheon, Arlington, VA*

Rekha Seshadri, PhD • *The Institute for Genomic Research, Rockville, MD*

Herbert A. Thompson, PhD • *Rickettsial Section, Viral and Rickettsial Zoonoses Branch, Division of Viral and Rickettsial Diseases, National Center for Rickettsial Diseases, Centers for Disease Control and Prevention, Atlanta, GA*

Richard W. Titball, PhD • *Defence Science and Technology Laboratory, CBS Porton Down, Salisbury, Wilts, UK,* and *Department of Infectious and Tropical Diseases, London School of Hygiene and Tropical Medicine, London, UK*

Keith R. Vesely, PhD • *Chemical and Biological Defense Directorate, Defense Threat Reduction Agency, Alexandria, VA*

David M. Waag, PhD • *Bacteriology Division, US Army Medical Research Institute of Infectious Diseases, Fort Detrick, MD*

John V. Wade, DVM, PhD • *Battelle Memorial Institute, Biodefense Medical Systems, Columbus, OH*

Murray Wolinsky, PhD • *Bioscience Division, Los Alamos National Laboratory, Los Alamos, NM*

Jon Woods, MD • *Operational Medicine Division, US Army Medical Research Institute of Infectious Diseases, Fort Detrick, MD*

Brenda Wyler, BS, MBA • *Headquarters, Department of the Army, Washington, DC*

This book is accompanied by a value-added CD-ROM that contains an eBook version of the volume you have just purchased. This eBook can be viewed on your computer, and you can synchronize it to your PDA for viewing on your handheld device. The eBook enables you to view this volume on only one computer and PDA. Once the eBook is installed on your computer, you cannot download, install, or e-mail it to another computer; it resides solely with the computer to which it is installed. The license provided is for only one computer. The eBook can only be read using Adobe® Reader® 6.0 software, which is available free from Adobe Systems Incorporated at www.Adobe.com. You may also view the eBook on your PDA using the Adobe® PDA Reader® software that is also available free from Adobe.com.

You must follow a simple procedure when you install the eBook/PDA that will require you to connect to the Humana Press website in order to receive your license. Please read and follow the instructions below:

1. Download and install Adobe® Reader® 6.0 software

    You can obtain a free copy of the Adobe® Reader® 6.0 software at www.adobe.com

Note: If you already have the Adobe® Reader® 6.0 software installed, you do not need to reinstall it.

2. Launch Adobe® Reader® 6.0 software

3. Install eBook: Insert your eBook CD into your CD-ROM drive

    PC: Click on the "Start" button, then click on "Run"

    At the prompt, type "d:\ebookinstall.pdf" and click "OK"

Note: If your CD-ROM drive letter is something other than d: change the above command accordingly.

    MAC: Double click on the "eBook CD" that you will see mounted on your desktop.

    Double click "ebookinstall.pdf"

4. Adobe® Reader® 6.0 software will open and you will receive the message:

"This document is protected by Adobe DRM" Click "OK"

Note: If you have not already activated the Adobe® Reader® 6.0 software, you will be prompted to do so. Simply follow the directions to activate and continue installation.

Your web browser will open and you will be taken to the Humana Press eBook registration page. Follow the instructions on that page to complete installation. You will need the serial number located on the sticker sealing the envelope containing the CD-ROM.

If you require assistance during the installation, or you would like more information regarding your eBook and PDA installation, please refer to the eBookManual.pdf located on your CD. If you need further assistance, contact Humana Press eBook Support by e-mail at ebooksupport@humanapr.com or by phone at 973-256-1699.

*Adobe and Reader are either registered trademarks or trademarks of Adobe Systems Incorporated in the United States and/or other countries.

PART I

PREPARATION AND MILITARY SUPPORT FOR A POSSIBLE BIOTERRORISM INCIDENT

Department of Defense Capabilities Supporting Bioterrorism Response

Anna Johnson-Winegar, Karl Semancik, Robert S. Borowski, Keith R. Vesely, Brenda Wyler, Matt Eussen, and John V. Wade

1. INTRODUCTION

As the 20th century drew to a close, most biological defense professionals, both military and civilian, were in agreement that the probability of a bioterrorist event occurring in the United States was not a matter of *if*, but *when*. However, few expected to be engaged in countering the effects of a bioterrorist attack in October 2001. Although it is still unclear whether the anthrax letters were directly related to the more dramatic terrorist events of September 11 or merely took advantage of the "opportunity" they presented, the line has been crossed and there is no turning back. *"If"* is now behind us, and we are left with the burning issues of *"who, where, when next, and why"* (personal observation).

Fall 2001 pointed out both the possibilities and vulnerabilities of bioterrorism in a manner that virtually no one had predicted. Until that point a majority of the speculation, discussion, planning, training, and preparation for a bioterrorism event had focused on the use of a biological agent as a weapon of mass destruction (WMD). Whereas Department of Defense (DOD) personnel participated, and continue to contribute extensively in such discussions, other departments of the government have taken the lead for both planning and responding to a bioterrorist attack. Most working "definitions" of a biological WMD event were based on at least 1000 casualties; if an agent didn't meet that minimum criterion, it was often deemed inconsequential for planning purposes. The emphasis was focused more on the biological consequences of bioterrorism rather than on an act of terrorism using a biological agent. This is not a trivial distinction—four envelopes containing a highly virulent and extremely potent formulation of anthrax spores resulted in enormous fear, panic, disruption of the mail service, distrust in the US government's ability to protect its citizens, and hundreds of millions of dollars in remediation expenses by producing fewer than 22 cases of clinical anthrax and only 5 deaths.

The DOD Chemical and Biological Defense Research Program (CBDP) was designed to counter the threat of biological warfare (BW) agents employed against our military forces in a battlefield environment. Although many of the biological agents available for use by a terrorist are the same as those our potential adversaries have

From: *Infectious Diseases: Biological Weapons Defense: Infectious Diseases and Counterterrorism*
Edited by: L. E. Lindler, F. J. Lebeda, and G. W. Korch © Humana Press Inc., Totowa, NJ

perfected for the battlefield, the circumstances surrounding their use renders many of the military approaches to the problem impractical, inappropriate, or impossible to implement in a widespread manner in a civilian scenario. However, many of the technologies are readily applicable, as we have seen during this, our first major bioterrorism event.

2. THE BIOLOGICAL TIMELINE

Intentional dissemination of a biological agent (bacteria, virus, or toxin) for the purpose of producing casualties follows the same sequence of events whether it is BW or bioterrorism. In many instances, it is a matter of scale, depending on the quantity of material prepared and disseminated, the area affected, and thus, the number of potential casualties expected. There are seven phases common to both (*see* Fig. 1). The earlier in this timeline that one intervenes, the greater the likelihood of minimizing the total number of casualties and reducing further spread of the agent. A comprehensive biological defense strategy, whether to counter BW or bioterrorism, must address multiple points along this continuum. The response measures for bioterrorism differ from those currently employed for BW defense primarily in terms of their applicability and relative emphasis along this timeline.

3. BW DEFENSE

The battlefield BW threat has been well-characterized based on the ability of specific agents to be mass produced and weaponized. From a military perspective, the emphasis remains on countering BW agents delivered as an aerosol to produce mass casualties as a result of inhalation exposure. The Chairman of the Joint Chiefs of Staff (CJCS) validates a consolidated BW threat list annually. This list, with input from the Regional Combatant Commanders, prioritizes the BW threat based on the presence and maturity of a potential adversary's offensive BW capability within a given theater of operations. DOD's current biological defense strategy relies primarily on individual protection, starting with immunization against specific BW agents using US Food and Drug Administration (FDA) licensed vaccines and early, rapid biodetection. Immunization provides the greatest degree of protection in the event that an attack goes undetected. Rapid detection provides individuals with the necessary warning to don protective equipment and commanders with the information necessary to avoid contamination, anticipate and treat casualties, and initiate decontamination procedures. Currently, fielded chemical defense protective equipment (e.g., masks, suits, and gloves) provides adequate protection against all known BW agents delivered by an aerosol route; therefore, fielding a combination of immunization plus biodetection assures the greatest certainty of maintaining an effective fighting force in the face of a BW attack. Unfortunately FDA-licensed vaccines are not yet available for every BW threat agent and biodetection technology is limited to point-source biodetectors. With current biodetectors, both personnel and the detector must "breathe" the same BW agent "cloud" for some interval (seconds to minutes) before a positive alarm and subsequent agent identification (10–15 min). Recognizing this, the DOD also emphasizes R&D on rapid diagnostics, effective postexposure therapeutics, and efficient decontamination countermeasures. A fully integrated biological defense doctrine, supported by approved training, ties all of these countermeasures together. The collective goal of

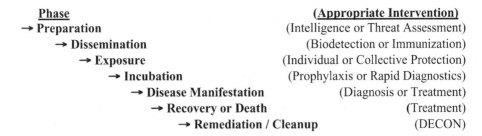

Phase	(Appropriate Intervention)
→ **Preparation**	(Intelligence or Threat Assessment)
→ **Dissemination**	(Biodetection or Immunization)
→ **Exposure**	(Individual or Collective Protection)
→ **Incubation**	(Prophylaxis or Rapid Diagnostics)
→ **Disease Manifestation**	(Diagnosis or Treatment)
→ **Recovery or Death**	(Treatment)
→ **Remediation / Cleanup**	(DECON)

Fig. 1. Seven phases of a biological "attack."

these countermeasures is to *maintain a fighting force capable of accomplishing its assigned mission* while *minimizing casualties to the greatest extent possible.*

4. THE BIOTERRORISM EVENT

The Department of Health and Human Services (DHHS) and Centers for Disease Control and Prevention (CDC) have developed a list of high priority biological agents that is similar to the DOD threat list. Most of the biological agents are zoonotic animal diseases that can also affect humans, particularly by the inhalation route (such as anthrax, plague, tularemia, brucellosis, and so on), rather than by typical human pathogens—the smallpox virus being a notable exception. The potential number of bioterrorism scenarios may only be limited by one's imagination; a bioterrorist is not constrained by the requirement to predictably produce a "significant" number of casualties at a specific time and place to achieve an operational goal. This expands the potential number of biological agents to choose from, as well as the route or means of dissemination. The location of the attack does not have to correlate with any larger concept of operations, and the bioterrorist is free to act on their own terms and timeline. Following the terrorist nerve agent attack in the Tokyo subway by Aum Shinrikio, it was learned that they had also attempted to release anthrax spores on at least three separate occasions. These events went undetected because no one was suspecting them, and no anthrax casualties occurred. The same could be said about any future bioterrorism event occurring in the United States. Unless the Homeland Security Advisory System alert status is high and biodetectors are set up around obvious high-value targets (e.g., government buildings) or high-profile events (e.g., the Olympics), the attack will likely go unnoticed unless it produces a "significant" number of recognizable casualties.

Most biological agent casualties following inhalation of an aerosol will initially present with nonspecific flu-like symptoms such as fever, malaise, muscle aches, and respiratory distress. These indications might easily be dismissed, particularly if an attack occurs during the season for their natural occurrence. The greatest tool to the civilian sector will be a robust and vigilant public health system that facilitates early recognition that a disease outbreak is abnormal and provides for a rapid, definitive diagnosis of the specific agent. Thus, the primary goal in countering bioterrorism is identifying and treating those individuals suspected of or known to be exposed to the agent to minimize casualties. Aside from a return to normalcy, there is no mission to accomplish. However, what may represent the greatest challenge as demonstrated by the anthrax letters, is to assure individuals that they have not been infected and can return to reside or work in a previously contaminated area. With these differences in mind, the following sections examine how biological defense countermeasures developed by the DOD for the battlefield can be applied to a bioterrorism event.

5. DOD BW COUNTERMEASURES

5.1. Biological Defense Vaccines

Preexposure immunization with FDA-approved vaccines remains the cornerstone of the DOD's medical force protection strategy; yet even within a military population, further analysis of "when" to immunize against "which" agent(s) is ongoing. The DOD's current BW defense vaccine acquisition strategy acknowledges the need to develop and license effective vaccines against all known BW threats, with stockpiles sufficient to support service members deployed in support of between half and two military theaters of war.

If one examines the current Anthrax Vaccine Immunization Program, the Secretary of Defense's decision to immunize the total force was based on three factors: the BW threat of anthrax warranted immunization of personnel at high risk (e.g., assigned or deployed to Southwest Asia or Korea); there was an available stockpile of FDA-licensed anthrax vaccine; and the "label" use of that product required six doses of vaccine given over 18 mo. Given the rapid turnover of personnel assigned to Southwest Asia or Korea, the short tour lengths, and the time necessary to receive the full immunization series, it was clear that the entire force would ultimately have to be immunized to provide adequate protection from anthrax. These conditions might not ubiquitously apply to all of the BW vaccines currently under development. It may be inappropriate to simply consider total force immunization as each new BW vaccine becomes licensed and available for use, depending on the nature of the threat and the immunization schedule required for each specific vaccine. Table 1 is a notional risk assessment matrix that might serve as one basis for a flexible immunization policy. It is based on the assumption that the decision of who needs to be immunized and at what time could be based on the magnitude of risk versus the time necessary to achieve protective immunity. It intentionally does not address specific BW agents by name so that it may focus attention on the operational use of the vaccines based upon these characteristics of both the agent and vaccine (*see* Table 1). In this example, if a BW agent was usually nonfatal, responded to available therapeutics (e.g., antibiotics), and a vaccine was available that afforded protection within 30 d after receiving two doses (14 d apart), then the decision might be to only stockpile that vaccine in limited quantities (Category D).

Although this is only one way of addressing the issues of whom to immunize and when (which, at the time of this writing, have not been approved or formally adopted by the DOD), it demonstrates the difficulties in identifying who is at risk and who should be vaccinated in a civilian population in anticipation of a bioterrorism event.

Vaccines have a long history of being safe and effective in preventing disease in individuals and being capable of eliminating disease in a population. However, when given to large numbers of people even the safest vaccine product has a likelihood of producing unwanted or unexpected side effects or adverse event in a small percentage of that population. The decision to vaccinate is always based on a benefit-to-risk (or a risk-reduction) analysis—does the benefit derived from immunization outweigh any

Table 1
Notional Risk Assessment Matrix for Developing
Immunization Schedules and Vaccine Stockpile Strategies

Time to immunity	Fatal no therapy	Fatal treatable	Nonfatal no therapy	Nonfatal treatable
>90 d	A*	A	B	B
<60 d	A	B	C	C
<30 d	B	B	C	D

Category A: Immunize the total force.
Category B: Immunize forward deployed and deployable forces.
Category C: Develop vaccine stockpile and immunize deploying forces.
Category D: Develop vaccine stockpile for contingency use.
*Note: Contagious and Communicable BW agents are considered in "Category A" by default.

potential untoward effects of the vaccine? The use of BW defense vaccines by the military relies on an intelligence estimate of the probability and the consequence of BW agent use as the risk part of this equation, with the desire to maintain an effective fighting force as the benefit. If one knew when and where a civilian bioterrorist attack was to occur, the benefit of immunization against the agent used would be clear. Unfortunately, the uncertainty of this risk for any given group of citizens in the United States makes the benefit-to-risk analysis very difficult.

Civilian use of vaccines as a means of countering bioterrorism falls into three possible categories: pre-exposure immunization of individuals suspected of being at high risk; immunization immediately following exposure (or suspected exposure), given in addition to therapy; and immunization of a larger segment of the population following bioterrorist use of a highly contagious agent to prevent epidemic spread. This analysis limits civilian BW defense vaccine use to three agents: anthrax, smallpox, and (perhaps, when an effective vaccine is licensed) plague. These three BW agents, discussed briefly here, will be covered in more depth in other chapters.

5.2. Biodetection

Rapid detection of biological agent aerosols remains a considerable challenge. Unlike volatile toxic chemicals or chemical warfare agents, biological agents exist as a particulate aerosol rather than as a vapor. A biological agent "cloud" behaves more like smoke than fog and biological agent "concentrations" are expressed in terms of particle counts rather than conventional measures of vapor, such as parts per million or milligrams per cubic meter. Because spores or bacteria or virus particles are rarely monodispersed but occur clumped together or adhering to dust particles, the unit of measure agent-containing particle per liter of air (ACPLA) has been adopted. It is this difference in physical characteristics that presents the greatest difficulty in biodetection. Given the potency of the agents in question, we are concerned with aerosols containing as few as 1–10 ACPLA.

Because these particles do not exert any vapor pressure, they are not amenable to the same types of detection technology used for volatile chemicals. The first step in aerosol biodetection involves actively drawing a fairly sizeable air sample through a collector–concentrator to trap the particles, which are usually then suspended in a buffered fluid sample. This sample is then applied to an identifier to determine the presence of a biological agent and its presumptive identity. For field detection, this is usually achieved using specific antibody binding in an enzyme-linked immunosorbant antibody (ELISA) assay or polymerase chain reaction (PCR) technology. Therefore, specific identification is limited to those agents for which there are handheld antibody assays or the necessary DNA probes and primers for PCR in field devices. Handheld assays are very similar in operation to a home pregnancy test kit: the liquid sample is applied, allowed to react for a set interval of time, and a "positive" test results in a visible color change on the antibody test strip that is detectible by the naked eye or an optical reader (usually with a laser). The PCR devices also result in a color change that is detected by the device. With proper sampling procedures, both handheld assays and PCR devices can also be used to presumptively identify biological agents from contaminated surfaces.

The sensitivity of handheld assays is a function of the purity and affinity of the antibodies used, but in any case, it will require a minimum number of organisms to register as positive. Use of automated ticket readers, rather than visual inspection for a color change, enhances sensitivity and reproducibility; however, the technology still has its limitations. PCR amplifies the agent's DNA, greatly enhancing sensitivity without loss of agent specificity. Field-portable devices are now available (*see* Subheading 5.3.). In addition to field identification, a confirmatory sample is usually collected and sent to a reference laboratory for definitive identification (which also answers the question of whether the biological agent is viable).

The first biodetector system was fielded in 1992, following Operation Desert Storm. The Biological Integrated Detection System (BIDS) was manned by two personnel who had to manually transfer suspected samples from the collector–concentrator to handheld assays and visually look for this color change. The Navy had a similar shipboard device called the Interim Biological Agent Detector (IBAD). Both BIDS and IBAD relied heavily on available commercial off-the-shelf technology.

Since fielding of the BIDS and IBAD, the process has been significantly automated, first in a device developed through the Advanced Concept Technology Demonstration process for Air Base/Port Biological Detection (known as Portal Shield) and more recently in the Joint Biological Point Detection System (JBPDS). Portal Shield was developed for fixed-site installation and achieved significant reductions in false-positive alarm rates by being arrayed as a sensor network in which more than one device had to give a positive reading for an alarm to be sounded. JBPDS can be configured for either fixed or mobile applications and is programmed to replace the BIDS and IBAD systems.

Both the Portal Shield device and JBPDS have a trigger associated with the collector–concentrator that senses an increase in the number of aerosol particles above the normal background levels, automatically sending a sample to the identifier only when there is a suspicious increase in particle count. This has two advantages: it takes humans out of the loop as far as sample collection, preparation, and transfer; and it reduces the enormous cost and logistics burden of consumables (buffer solutions and antibody tickets) that would be associated with continuous real-time monitoring if samples were analyzed simply at fixed intervals. The JBPDS is capable of identifying multiple agents in less than 15 min, unattended for missions up to 12 h between consumable replenishment. This tiered approach also allows quick, generic detection, followed by slightly longer, specific identification.

Both handheld assays and field-potable PCR were used to determine anthrax contamination of environmental surfaces as a result of the anthrax letters. The limiting factor in their utility for this purpose was not the devices themselves, but the heretofore untested swabbing and sampling techniques and procedures and their correlation with reference laboratory results. It should be noted that these devices, as described, were developed for environmental samples, not clinical specimens, and given the paucity of information regarding re-aerosolization or spread of anthrax spores under these circumstances, interpretation of results should be limited to presence/absence of spores or relative contamination.

Automated biodetectors developed for BW defense use, such as Portal Shield and JBPDS, have been deployed in support of high-visibility events (e.g., the Presidential Inauguration, G7-Summit, and the Olympics). However, their current cost ($300–$500K per device, depending on the numbers required and thus the size of the production base) limits their routine application in the civilian community. Many of their inherent technologies, particularly given the improvements in sensitivity, specificity, and decreased consumable burdens achieved in recent years, might one day find their way into simpler monitoring devices. Routine use of biodetectors in public areas (such as the ubiquitous smoke detector) is probably unrealistic until a significant technological breakthrough results in a solid-state (nonfluidic) identifier mechanism.

Broad-based employment of biodetectors in a civilian community may be limited more by questions of policy than technology. By their design and nature, they provide information that is far more applicable to a population than to any given individual, and in a civilian bioterrorism scenario, the response to an alarm might be quite different than on the battlefield. As previously stated, in a battlefield BW defense scenario, biodetection is just one part of an integrated biodefense system. Their deployment will be predicated on an intelligence assessment of the threat (thus dictating which agents the device must be capable of identifying and how the agent might be offensively deployed), where possible service members will be immunized against those threat agents. In either case, they will be equipped with (and most likely will carry with them) effective individual protective measures (e.g., protective masks) and/or medical countermeasures (such as packets of the antibiotic ciprofloxacin for anthrax postexposure treatment). Further, they have been trained as to the appropriate immediate response to take when an alarm is sounded.

The appropriate civilian response to an automated biodetector's alarm is less clear. Unlike a smoke detector, which sounds an alarm long before most individuals can actually smell the smoke and causes the unquestionable response to leave the building or be burned, the nature of the biological agent threat makes the response less clear. Depending on the biodetector's sensitivity and the interval of time required for it to alarm and/or identify the agent, individuals in the vicinity may have already breathed in a casualty-producing dose. Whereas limiting further exposure to those individuals is desirable, their dispersal as a group may be contraindicated from an epidemiological perspective. A single point-source device is insufficient to identify the extent of the attack or area of agent contamination; however, if deployed in the right place at the right time, it would provide information that a bioterrorism event has occurred and could identify which biological agent was used. Such early warning information would allow execution of plans to rapidly conduct active environmental sampling and, perhaps more importantly, to implement the diagnostic methods described here.

5.3. Diagnostics

The DOD has a very aggressive program to develop an FDA-approved diagnostic device capable of identifying at least eight specific BW agents of operational significance in numerous types of clinical samples and specimens. This program is in the process of downselecting from several of competing PCR-based technologies to develop and field a device known as the Joint Biological Agent Identification and Diagnosis System (JBAIDS). It will develop, validate, and field 8–10 gene probes and primers for PCR diagnosis of biological threat agents. JBAIDS will provide US forces with a reusable, portable, and modifiable diagnostic device capable of simultaneous, reliable identification of multiple biological organisms from appropriate clinical samples. JBAIDS will be operated by DOD medical laboratory personnel who are qualified in compliance with the Clinical Laboratory Improvement Act. FDA approval is critical, because the results of JBAIDS will be used to make diagnostic and therapeutic decisions about individual patients.

One enormous challenge facing clinicians trying to manage those individuals who either came in contact with, or were in the vicinity of, the anthrax letters was rapid and reliable identification of those who had in fact, been exposed. There were no validated field methods for such things as identifying anthrax spores in nasal swabs. It is unclear whether the techniques implemented would have yielded as comparable results with live bacteria or viruses. For a device such as JBAIDS to be effective, it will need to be validated with numerous types of clinical specimens (using research animals as surrogates for humans) to establish the timecourse of the agent's appearance in, or disappearance from, those various clinical specimens following an inhalation exposure. There are likely to be significant differences from one agent to another, based on the pathophysiology of the disease following exposure by inhalation.

This is an area that represents both the greatest opportunity for collaboration between the DOD and civilian medical research communities and the most significant potential return on investment. In an unanticipated, unannounced bioterrorism event, with a large number of exposed civilians, the first indication may be an increase in patients presenting with nonspecific respiratory illness accompanied by fever and malaise. Suspicions that it is not a naturally occurring disease outbreak will most likely be triggered by either the unexpected numbers of cases, the rapidity with which the symptoms progress, or the lack of responsiveness to conventional therapy. The ready availability of specific diagnostic devices such as JBAIDS, particularly if there is a parallel effort to develop diagnostic gene probes and primers for more common ailments, will significantly increase the likelihood of early definitive diagnosis of the first index case. As was seen with the first gentleman from Florida, once a diagnosis of inhalation anthrax had been made (and some degree of consensus was achieved that it was not a natural occurrence) the medical community at large became far more vigilant. Readily available, validated diagnostic methods also serve a secondary (but perhaps nearly as important) function: the ability to determine that a suspected casualty has not been exposed, thus allaying fear and concern in the individual and conserving precious, limited medical care facilities and services for those who actually need them.

5.4. Therapeutics

The DOD strategy of BW immunization, detection, individual protection, and diagnosis, although not ignoring therapeutics, has historically given it a lower priority. From the perspective of mission accomplishment, it is far preferable to prevent casualties than it is to treat them. By the time an individual is exhibiting symptoms following inhalation exposure with most BW agents, therapy is extremely difficult. For the bacterial agents, numerous broad-spectrum antibiotics (ciprofloxacin, doxycycline, penicillin, and derivatives or penicillin) have been shown to be effective in vitro. Most microbiology or pharmacology texts list suggested drugs or drug combinations shown to be effective in treating the naturally occurring disease, but their efficacy against an inhalation challenge can only be inferred from animal studies. For example, over half of the inhalational anthrax cases observed following exposure to the anthrax letters died in spite of very aggressive multidrug treatment regimens. Anthrax therapy represents the most challenging of the bacterial agents because of the uncertainty as to how long ungerminated spores can remain viable in the pulmonary lymph nodes following inhalation. Given the limited number of FDA-licensed antiviral agents, postexposure therapy for viral BW reagents remains primarily supportive in nature. Scientists at the US Army Medical Research Institute of Infectious Diseases (USAMRIID) continue to test the efficacy of these and other compounds being developed by various pharmaceutical manufacturers against the viral BW threat agents. Many of the toxin agents could be treated therapeutically with antitoxins; however, the only clinically available product at this time is for botulinum toxin, and it is in limited supply and for use only under an investigational new drug protocol.

The administration of hyperimmune globulin or antibodies against specific proteins is a therapeutic concept that has been known for many years. It has been used in the treatment and prevention of various diverse infections such as diphtheria, tetanus, botulism, and snake venom intoxication. The pathophysiology of many bacterial illnesses involves production and/or release of various of protein toxins. In theory, specific hyperimmune globulin could be used to circumvent or block these toxin activities. This could represent a final or prophylactic line of defense for patients potentially infected with drug- or vaccine-resistant strains of the pathogen. The use of hyperimmune globulin as an adjunct to antibiotics or vaccines in the treatment of anthrax in experimental animals has been demonstrated. These studies also serve to demonstrate that these antibodies might be used as an effective postexposure treatment for anthrax.

5.5. Individual and Collective Protection

DOD has fielded a diverse array of individual and collective protection countermeasures—from the individual service member's protective suit, gloves, and mask to combat vehicles or shelters equipped with high-efficiency filtration and providing an overpressure environment to prevent entry of contamination. Few of these items or systems have widespread, direct applicability to a civilian setting. None of the biological agents poses a percutaneous hazard; in most instances, the intact skin provides us with the first barrier to infection. Protective suits are limited in their applicability to those involved in sampling or clean-up of a biologically contaminated area and are already commercially available. In the absence of an indication to put them on (e.g., alarm by a Biodetector) protective masks for civilians are simply not practical. Once it is specifically known that a bioterrorist attack has occurred, the civilian responder community is already equipped with masks that are more appropriate to the threat than the military protective mask which is designed to protect against specific chemical as well as biological agents and is not suitable or approved for indiscriminant entry into an unknown noxious environment. Integration of biological filtration or pressure gradients into existing buildings (or new construction) is costly and maximally effective in either keeping contamination in or out of the structure, not necessarily both.

5.6. Decontamination

The goal of decontamination is to provide a capability for force restoration after a WMD attack. In the traditional sense, the DOD has pursued this area through development of systems that rely on the physical application and rinse of decontaminants on contaminated systems. Current systems are effective against a wide array of threat agents, including biologicals, but are logistical burdens with regard to time, labor, and material resources. Additionally, decontamination techniques and procedures present a significant safety burden.

The DOD has expended considerable developmental resources to improve our ability to decontaminate. However, there are significant technical challenges in this area. The first challenge is the development of decontaminants that are reactive, nonaqueous, noncorrosive, safe for use on sensitive equipment, environmentally safe, able to decontaminate a broad spectrum of biological agents, and that pose no unacceptable health hazards. The second challenge is the development of systems that effectively clean all surfaces while reducing the manpower and logistics burden.

The DOD has programs in place to develop systems and technologies to address these challenges. These programs include advances in sorbents, coatings, catalysis, and physical removal. This area has the potential for significant impact on restoration operations within the civilian community after a biological attack. Since September 11, the DOD has been instrumental in the application of technologies to restore entire buildings contaminated with biological spores and to ensure safe maintenance of the nation's postal system.

5.7. Modeling and Simulation

The understanding of the effects of biological agents is critical to an appropriate response that will protect the individual members of the nation's armed forces. This understanding is facilitated by the utilization of effective models and simulations that portray the physical effects and dispersion of biological agents after a release or attack. The DOD has expanded its efforts in this area through the establishment of a Chemical Biological Modeling and Simulation Advisory Council to examine and validate all models of chemical biological effects within the department.

The three models currently in use or under development within the DOD (Vapor, Liquid, Solid Tracking; Hazard Prediction and Assessment Capability, and Second Order Closure Integrated Puff) include advanced dispersion models that take into account real-time weather and complex terrain effects. Efforts are currently underway to integrate a functional combination of the "best of the best" capabilities from these three models into an interoperable architecture and a user-friendly interface resulting in the development of a Joint Effects Model (JEM). These advanced models will provide near instantaneous predictions of the effects of a biological release on the environment and the military force. JEM will be capable of modeling hazards in various scenarios including counterforce; passive defense; accidents and/or incidents; high altitude releases; urban nuclear, biological, and chemical (NBC) environments; building interiors; and human performance degradation.

Many of the algorithms used by the DOD, and in fact the models themselves, are being transferred for use in the civilian community by the DOD's consequence management forces and state and local first responders. The major challenge faced by the civilian community in using these models will continue to be the estimation of the source term used—the actual amount of biological agent released—which may differ substantially from DOD estimates based on weaponization.

6. DOD SUPPORT

The DOD is not a lead federal agency for response to terrorist incidents, but it provides significant and unique capabilities to support other agencies in conducting their responsibilities. Military support is provided to civil authorities under the auspices of the Federal Response Plan (FRP) and is governed by policies that distinguish between natural disasters and acts of terrorism. Requests for military support to natural disasters and accidents are approved by the Secretary of the Army (as DOD Executive Agent) and coordinated in advance with the Chairman of the Joint Chiefs of Staff. Requests for military support to civil authorities for terrorist incidents must be approved by the Secretary of Defense. On a case-by-case basis, the Secretary will decide whether to assign responsibility for the requested support to the DOD Executive Agent for Civil Support or to the Combatant Commander of the US Joint Forces Command (JFCOM). Missions assigned to JFCOM may be executed by its standing Joint Task Force for Civil Support (JTF-CS) or by the Response Task Force (RTF). When deployed for domestic operations, the JTF-CS and RTF report to the Secretary of Defense through their respective chains of command. In all cases, legal constraints bind military response. Doctrinally, military commanders are never in charge at a crisis response, but, rather, are supporting members of the Federal team.

6.1. Military Support Units

The DOD encompasses a wide range of special rapidly deployable organizations staffed by trained personnel and equipped with unique hardware. The Secretary of Defense has tasked JFCOM to establish a standing JTF-CS to lead DODs response efforts. The JTF-CS is commanded by a general/flag officer and includes an 8-person advance survey party and an 80-person headquarters staff (30 permanent personnel and 50 augmentees). Depending on the nature of the event, the JTF-CS is augmented by various agencies and operational units (medical, transportation, supply, and so on) that may be required in the crisis area. The RTF was established to maintain a military WMD consequence management response capability for the Atlanta Olympic Games. US Forces Command assigns missions east and west of the Mississippi River to the First and Fifth US Armies, respectively.

The US Army Soldier, Biological and Chemical Command (SBCCOM) Chemical-Biological Rapid Response Team (CB-RRT) is a Congressionally mandated, one-of-a-kind national asset that is capable of coordinating and synchronizing DODs technical assistance support (medical and nonmedical) for crisis response and consequence management operations involving WMD. Located at the Edgewood Area of Aberdeen Proving Ground in Maryland, the CB-RRT provides a technical support package specifically tailored for WMD incident response. The CB-RRT is composed of members of the Armed Forces and employees of the DOD with specialized chemical, biological, medical, and explosive ordnance disposal expertise who are capable of providing technical assistance to aid federal, state, and local officials in the response to and mitigation of incidents involving WMDs containing chemical or biological materials (or related hazardous materials). The CB-RRT can be under the operational control of a geographic CINC, JSOTF, or other designated JTF or can be in direct support of a lead Federal Agency. The unit is colocated with the SBCCOM 24-h operations center. The CB-RRT is designed to provide forward elements to assist the lead Federal Agencies (the Federal Bureau of Investigation [FBI], Federal Emergency Management Agency [FEMA], Environmental Protection Agency [EPA], United States Secret Service, United States Public Health Service, and others) with technical expertise and contingency development options during times of crisis. In addition, through the state-of-the-art SBCCOM operations center, the CB-RRT brings together some of the nation's leading chemical and biological technical experts without the need for the experts to be deployed to an incident site. Technical elements that are managed and coordinated by the CB-RRT include, but are not limited to, the US Army Technical Escort Unit; the US Army Edgewood Chemical and Biological Center; the US Army Edgewood Chemical and Biological Center Forensic Analytical Center (FAC); the US Army MEDCOM Special Medical Augmentation Response Teams (SMART) and Regional Medical Commands (RMC); the US Army Medical Research Institute of Chemical Defense (USAMRICD); the USAMRIID; the US Army Center for Health Promotion and Preventative Medicine; the US Navy Medical Research Center; the US Navy Environmental Health Center; the US Navy Environmental and Preventive Medicine Units; and the US Naval Research Laboratory.

USAMRIID plays a key role in national defense and in infectious disease research as the only maximum containment biological laboratory in the DOD for the study of highly hazardous diseases. USAMRIID collaborates with the World Health Organization in Geneva and the CDC in Atlanta in helping to diagnose and treat unusual diseases wherever they occur. USAMRIID has the unique capability of deploying up to two Aeromedical Isolation Teams (AITs), each composed of physicians, nurses, medical assistants, and laboratory technicians. These personnel are specially trained to care for and to transport patients with diseases caused by either BW agents or infectious diseases requiring high containment. The teams are deployable worldwide on a 12-h notice using US Air Force airlift. The AIT uses specialized isolation that maintains a contained environment under negative pressure and HEPA filtration to safely transport patients or to care for them in place for limited periods of time. This capability is limited to two patients at a time, based on the number of trained personnel and equipment on hand.

The US Marine Corps Chemical/Biological Incident Response Force (CBIRF) can respond to biological or chemical incidents to assist the on-the-scene commander in providing initial postincident consequence management. The CBIRF provides a standing, highly trained consequence management and force protection package tailored for short-notice response to terrorist-initiated chemical, biological, and/or radiological incidents and for credible threats.

State National Guard units form key elements of each state governor's emergency capability. As such, their role is generally performed at the direction of state authorities. The National Guard Civil Support Team (CST) WMD requirement came from the principle that domestic disaster relief is fundamentally a state mission. The units are deployed at the discretion of the state governor, unless they are federalized. The CST focus is on filling a void in the state's initial assessment capability and initiating requests for additional state or federal response assets. Each CST unit consists of 22 full-time National Guard personnel.

7. DOD CRISIS MANAGEMENT POLICY AND PRACTICE

In the event of a WMD incident, crisis and consequence management occur simultaneously, but there is only one on-the-scene commander. Local law enforcement establishes the perimeter, controls access to scene, and may begin interviews with witnesses; the FBI can take control of any WMD scene. The special agent in charge will call FBI assets to the scene, including the Hazardous Materials Response Unit and the Hostage Rescue Team. The special agent in charge may also request other federal assistance through the Attorney General. If the DOD is requested to provide assistance, Joint Special Task Forces are established, tailored to the mission profile. Usually, but not always, these units consist of explosive ordinance disposal technicians, DOD animal handlers, and/or Special Forces personnel. National Guard personnel, acting under the authority of the state governor, also are often utilized for area searches.

8. DOD CONSEQUENCE MANAGEMENT POLICY AND PRACTICE

The DOD is a signatory to the FRP. That plan, coordinated by the FEMA, takes an all-hazards approach to addressing actions to mitigate an incident. As with any emergency, the first line of response is the local first responder community, including police, fire, and emergency medical services. They also employ any mutual aid compacts they have with the surrounding area. When local resources are exhausted or overwhelmed or a critical capability is not available in the immediate area, the local authorities request assistance from the state. This is usually done through emergency management offices but can also flow through functional areas (i.e., local medical officials to state medical officials) or political channels (i.e., the mayor or county officials requesting help from the governor). The state can bring substantial resources to bear, including the National Guard. Many states are also members of emergency support compacts that permit one state's resources to be used in support of another member state.

When state resources are exhausted or overwhelmed or there is a need for a capability that is not available, the state goes to the federal government. This is accomplished when the governor declares a state of emergency or designates a specific disaster area. The governor then requests a presidential emergency declaration or a presidential disaster declaration. Once there is a presidential declaration, FEMA coordinates the federal response.

9. FEDERAL MEDICAL CONSEQUENCE MANAGEMENT POLICY AND PRACTICE

In accordance with the FRP, the DHHS is responsible for providing health and medical services, including those incidents of bioterrorism. DHHS has established the National Disaster Medical System (NDMS) to satisfy this responsibility. It must be noted that although DHHS exercises the consequence management responsibilities, the FBI continues to execute their crisis management responsibilities in parallel. The purpose of the NDMS is to supplement state and local medical resources during disasters or major emergencies and provide backup medical support to the DOD/DVA medical care systems during an overseas conflict. To that end, the NDMS provides medical response, patient evacuation, and definitive medical care. The NDMS, like the FRP, is an all-hazards response plan and addresses all aspects of consequence management medical care including:

- Assessment of health and medical needs
- Health surveillance
- Medical care personnel
- Health/medical equipment and supplies
- Patient evacuation
- In-hospital care
- Food, drug, and medical device safety
- Worker health/safety
- Radiological, chemical, and biological hazards
- Mental health
- Public health information
- Vector control
- Potable water, wastewater, and solid waste disposal
- Victim identification and mortuary services
- Veterinary services

The DHHS, recognizing the need to provide additional training and support for WMD incidents, developed WMD-specific national medical response teams within its disaster medical assistance teams. These teams provide triage, austere medical care, and casualty clearing/staging at disaster sites and patient reception at the local disaster reception areas. Each team is composed of roughly 100 personnel drawn from volunteers and in major metropolitan areas may be augmented by a Metropolitan Medical Response System grant and plan from DHHS, which provides additional resources for WMD incident planning, equipping, and training.

The DOD may be requested to assist at any stage of the NDMS and has some specific responsibilities in conjunction with the Department of Veterans Affairs to provide definitive medical care at existing facilities should an incident overwhelm hospital care facilities. During the incidents occurring in Fall 2001, the DOD provided assistance across the full spectrum of response. It deployed hospital ships to New York harbor in the aftermath of the September 11 attacks on the World Trade Center; it provided laboratory facilities and personnel to determine the nature and source of anthrax, the provision of environmental sampling systems for the detection and characterization of anthrax, and expertise on the decontamination of civilian facilities.

10. BIOLOGICAL EXERCISES AND LESSONS LEARNED

Preparations for terrorist incidents involving NBC/WMD have been ongoing since the Gulf War and the breakup of the Soviet Union. Early focus centered on fears that terrorists could obtain nuclear weapons as a result of profiteering by the former Soviets. However, the attacks on the Murrah Federal Building and the Tokyo subway system in 1995 added emphasis to the potential of high-yield explosives and chemical attacks. In the wake of the September 11 attacks and the mailing of the anthrax-contaminated letters, concern for bioterrorist incidents has caused officials at all levels of government to re-elevate both the threat and the governmental structures and resources to deal with such a threat. DOD support and cooperative efforts are vital to facilitating federal agency cooperation and resource sharing. Federal agencies have enhanced their ability to respond to terrorist incidents by conducting exercises that train key personnel and test response plans. Presidential Decision Directive 39, issued in June 1995, requires key federal agencies to ensure that their counterterrorism capabilities are well exercised.

Exercises fall into two general categories: tabletop and field exercises. Tabletop exercises are performed around a table, a classroom, or a simulated command post as the players progress through a scenario or series of scenarios and discuss how their agency or unit might react to different situations. Field exercises are performed in the field under simulated operational conditions. Such exercises focus on performing tasks at the operational and tactical levels and typically include the tactics, techniques, and procedures that would be used in a real incident. Field exercises test agency and interagency capabilities to actually deploy personnel and their equipment and coordinate them as they perform their tasks in a realistic setting. Numerous of key exercises held prior to the anthrax letters were beneficial in guiding response.

10.1. Biological Warfare Improved Response Program

The Biological Warfare Improved Response Program (BW-IRP), a multiyear program under the auspices of the DOD, developed two primary products: a BW response template and a prioritized list of response gaps and improvements. To help facilitate the template's use, a BW Decision Tree was developed. To validate the BW Response Decision Tree, a tabletop exercise of an unannounced anthrax attack on Baltimore City was conducted in April 1999. The participants concluded that the BW Decision Tree was extremely helpful in providing a quick overview of the BW Response Template, facilitating its use, and understanding the rationale for why it is needed.

In July 1999, a workshop was conducted in Wichita, Kansas, for the purpose of testing the scalability of the template to different geographic and demographic locations in the United States. The workshop concluded with relatively minor modifications to the template, thereby suggesting the template is scalable. Participants were concerned with issues of medical surveillance and handling or remains, which were areas where technology and/or procedural gaps existed.

The FBI National Domestic Preparedness Office/DOD Workshop conducted in January 2000 brought together the law enforcement and public health communities for the first time. Roles that each organization would assume during a biological incident were discussed and a joint questionnaire was developed to facilitate information sharing. The workshop results showed that it is necessary for all agencies to coordinate all public information releases so that mixed or conflicting information is not released. In addition, emergency management personnel realized that in an unannounced biological attack, management forces could not take action until indicators triggered an awareness that an unusual medical event had occurred.

The CDC/DOD Smallpox Workshop, held in April 2000, evaluated the application of the response template to a contagious disease. Results concluded that the areas of medical surveillance, vaccination/prophylaxis, and isolation/quarantine should be added to the template. The timely exchange of information once it has been obtained was an issue of concern. A recommendation was made that the National Guard WMD Civil Support Teams be trained and available to work medical surveillance. Training must include basic, multilingual presentations, instruction in the software that will be used for record keeping (such as tracking databases) electronic data transit, and system setup and maintenance. Surveillance personnel should be familiar with agent characteristics such as how to distinguish smallpox from chicken pox, modes of transmission, and appropriate methods of control.

In July 2000, a workshop with Dover, Delaware, and the Dover Air Force Base (AFB) was conducted to determine how a city and a military base could work together. Results showed that with minimal implementation, Dover AFB could rapidly monitor over-the-counter medication sales. The need to use pre-established protocols for communications and reporting was identified. A need for cooperative interhospital collaborative agreements was recognized, especially with respect to transfer of potential victims and the availability and use of isolation beds. During the workshop that USAMRIID, it was discovered does not have an established policy and procedure for communications with authorities located outside the air base. From this tabletop, emergency management personnel realized that in an unannounced biological attack, management forces could not take action until indicators triggered an awareness that an unusual medical event was occurring.

10.2. The Dark Winter Exercise

In June 2000, a senior-level war game called "Dark Winter," looked at the national security, intergovernmental, and information challenges of a biological attack in the United States homeland. During the 13 d of the war game, smallpox spread to 25 states and 15 other countries. Discussions, debates, and decisions focused on the public health response, an inadequate supply of smallpox vaccine, roles and missions of federal and state governments, civil liberties associated with quarantine and isolation, the role of the DOD, and potential military responses to the anonymous attack. One conclusion of the war-game was that a BW attack on the United States could threaten vital national security interests. Massive civilian casualties, breakdown in essential institutions, violation of democratic processes, civil disorder, loss of confidence in government, and reduced US strategic flexibility abroad are among the ways a biological attack might compromise US security. Dark Winter identified several key findings:

- Leaders are unfamiliar with the character of bioterrorist attacks, available policy options, and their consequences. These key decisions and their implications were dependent on public health strategies and the possible mechanisms to care for large numbers of sick people—issues not typically briefed or studied in the national security or defense community.
- Following a bioterrorist attack, leaders' key decisions would depend on data and expertise from the medical and public health sectors. The government lacks adequate strategies, plans, and information systems for the rapid flow and magnitude of data.
- The lack of sufficient vaccine or drugs to prevent the spread of disease severely limited management options. This includes vaccines and antibiotics and a means of effective distribution.
- The US healthcare system lacks the surge capacity to deal with mass casualties. The exercise found that a huge burden was placed on the medical system with the challenges of distinguishing the sick from the well; rationing scarce resources; and shortages of healthcare staff who were worried about becoming infected or bringing the infection home to their families.
- To end a disease outbreak after a bioterrorist attack, decision-makers will require ongoing expert advice from senior public health and medical leaders. As the smallpox epidemic grew and the number of available vaccines decreased, forcible constraints on citizens were the only tools available. But, the group discovered that a complete quarantine was not a logical solution. A complete quarantine would isolate people so that they would not be fed and they would not receive medical care.
- Federal and state priorities may be unclear, differ, or conflict, authorities may be uncertain, and constitutional issues may arise. State leaders were opposed to federalizing the National Guard because they were supporting the logistical and public supply needs.
- The individual actions of US citizens will be critical in ending the spread of contagious disease—leaders must gain the trust and sustained cooperation of the American people. The less prepared we are, the more threats there will be to civil liberties.

10.3. The TOPOFF 2000 Exercise

TOPOFF was a Congressionally mandated domestic counterterrorism exercise that included the participation of top-level officials, first responders, and law enforcement personnel engaging in the crisis and consequence management. The exercise took place in the Denver, Colorado metropolitan area and Portsmouth, New Hampshire, in May 2000. This marked the first time that a no-notice event included three simulated terrorism scenarios: a chemical weapons incident on Portsmouth, a bioterrorism/medical crime (plaque outbreak) in Denver, and a concurrent event involving nuclear devices in Washington, D.C. In essence, the exercise had one agency leading the crisis management and another for consequence management. The FBI, acting for the Department of Justice, was the lead federal agency for the crisis management response to a domestic WMD incident owing to its investigative and law enforcement role in bringing to justice any terrorists involved in such an incident. FEMA, acting in accordance with the Stafford Act, was the lead agency for consequence management and implemented the FRP in support of state and local officials.

The real-time deployment of assets and real-resource limitation in handling mass fatalities and casualties provided a vast amount of lessons learned. For example:

- Mobile satellite communications that are independent of military switches proved critical to WMD technical response support. The CB-RRT deployed with the Deployed Communications System (DCS) and established command and control within a 2-h period. DCS provided the Commander of the JTF-CS with eight separate telephone lines and allowed command and control to be exercised internal and external to the headquarters. In addition, the DCS provided area coverage with 120 cell phones and proved to be the only system available with this area coverage capability. The DCS allowed immediate technical response support, as well as reachback linkage to DOD labs and agencies.

- If multiple incident sites occur and 24-h operations are required, then manpower needs to be increased accordingly. A thorough manpower and mission analysis should occur in all units to ensure adequate staffing at all deployment sites.
- Several different emergency operations centers (EOCs) were set up by various state and federal and emergency management agencies. The EOCs were intended to help coordinate management of the crisis, but it was unclear to some observers how a number of distinct EOCs would be able to coordinate management, make decisions or communicate information to medical and public health stakeholders, such as hospitals. Although lines of authority were clear, much time was spent in consultation and debate through scheduled teleconferencing.
- Problems existed in moving antibiotics from the stockpile delivery point to the persons who need it for treatment and prophylaxis. The local capability to rapidly distribute antibiotics and other resources in an efficient manner was limited to a nurse and two technicians. The DOD Medical Logistics, with their expertise in moving from bulk to push packages, could have provided tremendous help in this area.
- Antibiotic distribution plans should be able to support additional centers of antibiotic distribution, thereby drawing crowds away from besieged hospitals and ensuring the ability to reach all segments of the population. This lesson learned was incorporated into responses to the recent anthrax bioterrorist attacks.
- A consensus needs to be made quickly about which groups should be assigned priority to receive antibiotics. This decision allows critical responders to remain healthy while managing the disaster. As the epidemic spreads, distribution decisions would quickly become more complicated, and the decision whether prophylaxis should be limited to demonstrated contacts or be given to the general populace will become a political rather than a medical decision.

10.4. Other Exercise Findings

DOD units have participated in various tabletop and training exercises conducted to help officials prepare for future bioterrorist attacks. The findings from these exercises have been consistent and progress has been made toward developing strategies to ensure that DOD capabilities will be maximally utilized.

Participants in various exercises felt that the reporting process for military medical assets was fragmented. For example, the Army reports of hospital activity are gathered on a monthly basis. This long timeframe is not helpful for emergency events. Emergency reporting systems that can be implemented quickly to get current status information on military medical resources are needed.

Participants felt that state labs have limited CB capabilities, which will lead to greater reliance on DOD mobile labs to analyze samples. Sampling procedures are unclear and a standard needs to be developed. Developing a gold standard for sampling procedures and agreed protocols for state and federal laboratories allows consistent analysis to be conducted from the beginning of an event.

Decontamination standards guidelines should be developed by the federal agencies in conjunction with states. A threshold for the decontamination of contaminated emergency equipment is essential to guide the establishment of local procedures.

A common theme from participants is that DOD units will face a logistical battle. Coordination of medical assets to include personnel and equipment will be their primary task during the initial stages. Life support issues will soon follow. The questions on who will provide food, water, and shelter for victims and other displaced personnel will have to be addressed. Force protection is an issue that has been rarely addressed in exercises.

Various exercises have expressed significant needs in developing early-warning biodetectors, advanced diagnostic kits, an integrated public health surveillance system, interoperable robust communications, and advanced incident management tools.

11. CONCLUSION

The DOD has the greatest capabilities in biological defense, but the responsibility for dealing with the domestic threat of biological weapons by a terrorist falls on multiple federal, state, and municipal agencies and the civilian healthcare community. DOD units do not come to an incident unless they are requested. Even then, the units come under very definitive guidelines. They are not in charge and never will be. The military has no legal authority to simply appear if an incident occurs. In domestic disasters, the local authorities—law enforcement, firefighters, and rescue workers—would respond first. If the incident grew to the point that the local authorities could not handle the situation, then the governor would be contacted and state organizations would enter the picture. If the state's emergency management group could not handle the situation, federal agencies would enter to provide support.

Despite all the shortcomings, officials state that the nation is far better equipped to deal with biological terror today than a decade ago. Extensive exercises and analytic efforts at the federal, state, and local levels will be essential over the coming years to improve US preparedness in the face of a biological weapons attack.

Numerous of the technologies and procedures developed by the DOD for BW defense can be applied in one form or another to a civilian bioterrorism event. Probably the most readily transferable and immediately valuable is the wealth of data and experience, both medical and nonmedical, developed for military application. The DOD is in the process of strengthening its links to the civilian community through interagency coordination and groups such as the Inter-Agency Board for Equipment Standardization.

KEY REFERENCES AND SELECTED READING

US Code
- Robert T. Stafford Act, 48 USC 5121
- Economy Act, 31 USC 1535
- Comprehensive Terrorism Prevention Act of 1995, 18 USC 2332

Federal Response Plan and Terrorism Incident Annex
- http://www.fema.gov/rrr/frp/
- http://www.rand.org/publications/MR/MR1251/MR1251.AppG.pdf

DOD Directives
- DODD 3525.1, Military Support to Civil Authorities (MSCA)
- DODD 3025.15,Military Assistance to Civil Authorities (MACA)
- DOD's Manual for Civil Emergencies (DOD 3025.1M)

DOD Doctrine
- JP 3-07.2, "Joint Tactics Techniques and Procedures for Antiterrorism"
- JP 3-11, "Joint Doctrine for Operations in NBC Environments"
- FM 3-11.21 "Multiservice TTPs on NBC Consequence Management"

SBCCOM CB-RTT
- http://www2.sbccom.army.mil/cbrrt/fs_cbrrt.htm

Biological Warfare Improved Response Program (BW-IRP)
- http://www2.sbccom.army.mil/hld/bwirp/

Dark Winter Exercise
- http://www.homelandsecurity.org/darkwinter/index.cfm

TOPOFF Exercise
- Biodefense Quarterly, September 2000, Volume 2, Number 2, *A Plague on Your City*
- http://www.state.gov/s/ct/rls/fs/2002/12129.htm

2

Modeling for Bioterrorism Incidents

Zygmunt F. Dembek

1. INTRODUCTION

A training gap exists in the preparation necessary for first responders, hospital, health department, and law enforcement personnel from local, state, and federal agencies should a bioterrorism event occur. Because of the unique nature of a bioterrorism event, the definition of a "first responder" has evolved to include hospital and public health personnel *(1)*, who may lack an understanding of the overall incident command structure, in general, and the hospital emergency incident command structure, specifically. Additionally, agencies that traditionally rely on their own infrastructure (e.g., public health, law enforcement) to perform their normal functions must rely on new partners to respond to a bioterrorism event. Intensive coordinated planning and training efforts that bring all participant agencies together to understand each other's roles and responsibilities in a disaster can remedy these disparities.

Irrespective of the current level of preparedness of municipal, state, or federal agencies, the same methods that are used to assist coordinated planning and training for other catastrophic events can be used to plan for bioterrorism. These techniques include the composition of an agency- or government-specific disaster response plans, conducting tabletop exercises, and holding a live drill exercise. Realistic disaster scenarios should be incorporated into each of these training techniques to familiarize participants with each others' roles and responsibilities and to plan for the unique nature of a bioterrorism event. The primary emphasis herein is on the tabletop exercise, which can be conducted by a municipality, state, or federal entity even in the absence of a formalized response plan and without the resources and expenses required for a live drill exercise. A bioterrorism scenario used in statewide training will be examined, along with the participant's response to that scenario. Actual bioterrorism incidents will be considered, as will the various essential components of the public health response to bioterrorism.

2. PREDICTING FUTURE BIOTERRORISM EVENTS

The ability to predict a future terrorist attack with a biological weapon against a civilian population presents an enormous, if not impossible, challenge. When designing bioterrorism scenarios, planners must think "out of the box" in addition to using knowledge of prior biological attacks and natural disease outbreaks. The anthrax cases caused by contaminated letters that occurred in late 2001 clearly demonstrated

From: *Infectious Diseases: Biological Weapons Defense: Infectious Diseases and Counterterrorism*
Edited by: L. E. Lindler, F. J. Lebeda, and G. W. Korch © Humana Press Inc., Totowa, NJ

the ability of small amounts of a finely milled biological agent to cause disease. Those mailings, directed at political and media targets, also demonstrated the potential extensive repercussions that can result even with a small-scale attack. Importantly, extensive media coverage can amplify terrorist objectives. Large-scale anxiety, fear of contamination, economic loss, exhaustion of antibiotic supplies for prophylaxis (necessary and unnecessary), and extensive (and expensive) decontamination efforts were just some of the ripple effects from the anthrax mailings.

The release of a biological agent by aerosol is among the most effective methods a terrorist could employ to expose large numbers of individuals *(2)*. The simultaneous infection of those exposed to an infective agent dose would be the primary result, with potential reaerosolization of a persistent biological agent possibly leading to more exposures and infections. A recent example of the potential for a biological agent to become a persistent health threat occurred when anthrax spore-laden envelopes passed through postal service mail sorter machinery in Washington, DC. The pressure on the envelopes from the mail handling processors forced anthrax spores through unsealed portions of the envelope and resulted in numerous of infections in postal workers at the facility *(3)*.

A highly concentrated aerosolized cloud of a biological agent could more readily be achieved in an enclosed space, such as a building, rather than in open-air dispersal outdoors. By way of example, when the Aum Shinrikyo released chemical agents that became entrained in an office building in Matsumoto in 1994, they caused about 200 persons to be hospitalized and 7 deaths *(4)*. The Aum Shinrikyo also attempted several releases of botulinum toxin in an outdoor environment in Yokosuka and Yokohama in 1990 and in Tokyo in 1993. These attempts failed to cause any recognized cases of illness, perhaps as a result of several factors, including the dilution effect by the environment on a small amount of agent *(5)*.

Another potential vehicle for the future use of a pathogen for bioterrorism is through the contamination of the food supply. In American society, the farm-to-table continuum, which includes growing, processing, distribution, and preparation, has a myriad of potential vulnerabilities for contamination *(6)*. One wake-up call to purposeful food contamination with an infectious disease pathogen occurred in 1984 in The Dalles, Oregon. The perpetrators of this crime sprayed *Salmonella typhimurium* in salad bars *(7)*. The desired outcome was to influence an election by causing illness among voters, thereby causing them not to vote. This clearly meets the definition of a bioterrorist's objectives *(5)*. A second example occurred in Texas in 1996, when another food-borne pathogen, *Shigella dysenterae*, was used in the contamination of pastries given to coworkers at a laboratory *(8)*. This incident is considered a biocrime, because the motivation behind this activity lacked political, ideological, or religious underpinnings *(5)*.

One can also study the many nonpurposeful food-borne pathogen contaminations to determine avenues for potential purposeful outbreak scenarios. An outbreak in Minnesota in 1985 affecting more than 16,000 persons with antimicrobial-resistant salmonellosis was eventually hypothesized to have been caused by cross-contamination of raw milk into a pasteurized milk product sold to the public *(9)*. Although this outbreak had occurred unintentionally, a significant criminal investigation occurred simultaneously with the epidemiological investigation because of the size of the outbreak and the associated deaths of 14 individuals who consumed the milk product *(9)*. This outbreak and many others *(10–12)* demonstrate that food-borne bioterrorism has perhaps greater chances of success the closer to the table that contamination occurs, thus circumventing issues of dilution of the pathogen and destruction by cooking/pasteurization.

Water-borne contamination is perhaps more difficult for a terrorist to achieve, because the large volumes and the extensive water purification process in use in industrialized countries should tend to negate a biological contaminant. However, a determined enemy could overcome the purification process. Deleterious effects could also result from purposeful biological contamination of the water supply distribution system after the purification process. A private well-water supply system may be more vulnerable to attack because a private well may have a smaller volume of water and may not have as an extensive water purification process as a public water supply. One example of an extensive water-borne disease outbreak resulting from contaminated well-water is the *Escherichia coli* O157:H7 and *Campylobacter sp.* outbreak that occurred in 1999 at a New York State county fair *(13)*. More than 900 illnesses and 2 deaths resulted from this bacterial contamination of well water. Although this event was not a planned terrorist event, the potential for a terrorist to purposefully contaminate a well is apparent. The possibility of a purposeful contamination of a public water fountain should also be considered. A recent natural outbreak of gastroenteritis was associated with an interactive water fountain at a Florida beachside park *(14)*. One can imagine the effect of, for example, a large amount of botulinum toxin surreptitiously added to a public water fountain in a similar manner.

Infected vectors, such as plague-infected fleas or encephalitis-infected mosquitoes, can also be used to transmit disease. During the Japanese occupation of China during World War II, fleas were used in some of the horrific biological weapons experiments conducted by Japanese Military Unit 731 *(15)*. According to Alibek *(2)*, the release of infected vectors is not particularly effective for military or terrorist purposes because of the high probability of affecting those producing the weapons or in proximity to the site of release.

2.1. Probable Scenarios for a Bioterrorism Attack

The terrorist use of a pathogen that is normally endemic or periodically epidemic in a certain population would be more difficult to detect as an unusual event than an exotic pathogen. Therefore, a bioterrorism attack could be masked as a naturally occurring outbreak. This kind of covert attack might be detected initially in numerous ways, such as by an astute clinician or by laboratory identification. However, epidemiological surveillance and investigation will ultimately determine whether an attack is intentionally induced. Certain indicators, or red flags, could point toward an intentional event, for example, changes in the normally occurring season of illness (e.g., influenza in the summer), host illness patterns (i.e., ill animals in conjunction with ill persons, both infected with a similar zoonotic illness), or unusual geographical patterns of illness (e.g., many outbreaks of the same bacterial illness occurring simultaneously).

A terrorist attack might have special features associated with it that would not be expected in the course of a natural outbreak. These could include the use of a combination of agents, either different pathogens mixed together or a biological pathogen in combination with a chemical or radiological one. Attacks may occur in multiple locations (yielding multiple point-source outbreaks), such as the anthrax mail outbreak during fall 2001 or the *Salmonella typhimurium* outbreak caused by contamination of multiple salad bars throughout The Dalles, Oregon, in 1984 *(7)*. Additionally, the presentation of the disease may be unusual (e.g., multiple cases of pneumonic tularemia rather than the more common ulceroglandular presentation).

A potential terrorist might choose to use a pathogen not usually considered to be a biological threat, and perhaps not even monitored by public health agencies, such as the West Nile virus, which was responsible for a natural outbreak in New York in 1999 *(16)*. The introduction and establishment of West Nile virus in the United States was considered by some to have been a purposeful event *(17)*. Finally, the use of novel or genetically engineered strains of agents by terrorists could be particularly insidious. The development of antibiotic-resistant and novel chimeras has been claimed of the former Soviet biological weapons program by one of its past directors, Dr. Ken Alibek *(18)*.

Large-scale bioterrorism attack scenarios with agents such as smallpox and anthrax have been published in civilian theoretical exercises *(19,20)*. It has been suggested that a large-scale biological attack against a civilian population is much less likely than a small-scale attack *(21)*. According to Leitenberg *(21)*, a small-scale biological attack through crude dispersal of a biological agent in an enclosed area is the most likely mode of attack. One benchmark of a successful exercise is to have the participants respond to an unanticipated event followed by participation in a lessons learned summary that will enable them to learn from their mistakes. Exercises that involve as many of the various local, state, and federal emergency response partners as possible will greatly foster the development of a team response approach *(22)*. This type of exercise will also enable each participant group to discover their weaknesses and strengths (and each others') in response to a disaster.

Finally, it should also be noted that synergistic effects have been demonstrated in animal models for combined radiation and biological pathogen exposure *(23,24)*. As horrible as the consequences may be to consider, it will behoove the biological disaster planner to consider similar worst-case scenarios when designing exercises.

2.2. Modeling of Probable Scenarios: Response Plan, Tabletop Exercise, and Live Drill

An important component of training for a bioterrorism event is to involve participants in a progression of planning steps from a theoretical response to prepare for an actual event. The sequence usually used by hazardous materials trainers for modeling an incident response among participants is to develop a response plan, conduct tabletop exercises, and then to engage participants in a live drill.

2.2.1. Response Plan

A comprehensive plan of incident response is created with each participating agency contributing a description of their resources, capabilities, and roles in an emergency incident. The final plan describes the interactive roles of each agency, their responsibilities, and how they work together and communicate with each other as a cohesive whole in response to an incident. This plan is then reviewed and accepted by each agency and is revised annually with any changes in personnel, resources, and responsibilities.

2.2.2. Tabletop Exercise

The response plan is vetted through an exercise involving all of the primary incident response players. The exercise is designed to task the response plan and study a coordinated response using the incident command system (ICS) and hospital emergency incident command system (HEICS), communications, and lines of control between the players, which are vital components required in response to a bioterrorism event *(25,26)*. At the conclusion of the tabletop exercise, a thorough lessons learned review is conducted to examine how the players responded to the incident. A tabletop exercise can vary in length from an hour or two to several days, depending on the resources to be tested by the drill. Finally, a report should be written to summarize the exercise, response, and observations and should be distributed to all participants.

Several bioterrorism tabletop scenarios have used a combination of weapons of mass destruction (WMD) events: either a fire or a hazardous materials (hazmat) scenario along with the surreptitious release of a biological agent. Examples include two tabletop exercises that were used at the Connecticut Fire Academy during 2001 and the tabletop exercise used in the November 2001 US Army Medical Research Institute of Infectious Diseases (USAMRIID)/VA *(27)* satellite broadcast. The use of a combined WMD scenario in a tabletop exercise permits the involvement of the various first responders (fire, police, EMS) and hospital personnel in the exercise and also presents the most challenging model for a bioterrorism event. The events of late 2001 presented an unexpected and unmodeled scenario: the use of the postal system to deliver anthrax spore-containing envelopes to media and political targets. The demands of this unexpected bioterrorism event on the public health resources would have been overwhelming in the absence of a coordinated preparation. The tabletop exercise serves as a good starting point for training to achieve a better-coordinated response.

2.2.3. Live Drill

Perhaps the most thorough way to test an emergency response plan is to conduct a live drill incorporating all of the players in their real-life roles using their actual equipment and resources. This is the most resource-intensive way to test an emergency response plan *(28)*, and would best be undertaken in the presence of an existing plan in which the players are already familiar with their response roles. A live drill is normally conducted when most of the players are unaware of the timing of the event *(28)*. This type of exercise is best followed by an extensive evaluation incorporating comments from participants and a final written report that incorporates the participant's comments as well as those of the official observers. Any necessary changes discovered through this exercise should be made to the appropriate emergency response plans.

3. THE IMPORTANCE OF THE TABLETOP EXERCISE AS A BIOTERRORISM TRAINING TOOL

At the time of this writing, few state public health agencies had developed a comprehensive bioterrorism or WMD response plan. Prior federal funding specifically targeted for statewide bioterrorism plan development has funded few states to develop these plans. In the absence of a written response plan, a bioterrorism tabletop exercise can be successfully conducted with the participants following their standard protocol for emergency disaster events. An exercise conducted in this manner can be viewed as an important source of information for the development of a bioterrorism response plan, because unprepared-for deficiencies will quickly become evident during the tabletop exercise.

Two bioterrorism tabletop exercises were conducted in Connecticut in 2001 at the State Fire Academy located in Windsor Locks. For training, this Fire Academy has available a ping-pong table-sized model of a hypothetical city, "Peterboro," with HO-scale (1:87) model buildings, vehicles, and paraphernalia. Peterboro's hypothetical population of 14,593 is spread over 43 square miles, with two fire stations (three fire engines, and ladder, command, utility, rescue, and ambulance vehicles; all staffed by fire and EMS personnel); a police department (three cars available per shift, with off-duty officers subject to recall); and a small community hospital with a 10-bed emergency department. Altogether, 40 buildings are present on the tabletop, located on six main highways, and a railroad spur is present in the northern section of the town. Any city or town could inexpensively duplicate this ingenious model to train first responders and hospital personnel to learn to work together in an emergency situation.

Participants in these tabletop exercises have included federal (e.g., USPHS, Federal Bureau of Investigation [FBI], FEMA, CT and MA ARNG WMD-CST teams, and the US Army Soldier and Biological Chemical Command [SBCCOM]), state (e.g., state police bomb squad, Department of Environmental Protection Haz-Mat team, and Office of Emergency Management) and local (e.g., police, fire, EMS, and physicians) responders. Although this is a good representation of first responders, a thorough exercise would also include other potential participants (e.g., morticians, medical examiners, media representatives) and key elected officials.

When players participated in a tabletop exercise at the fire academy, they were identified by reflective vests clearly marked with their role, i.e., Fire Department, Police Department, EMS, Public Safety, and so on. Some of the past tabletop exercise drills at the fire academy have also been "facilitated" by providing the participants' with walkie talkies all set to the same frequency. This scenario tests the ability of the participants to create and adhere to an ICS disaster response model.

Our tabletop exercise began with the participants introducing themselves to each other and observers, followed by a general situational briefing to set the groundwork for the scenario. The briefing explained the layout and logistics of the community of Peterboro and the resources in the town available for fire, police, EMS, and hospital personnel. Participants were then sequentially handed a preprinted timed situation card. The participant read the card aloud, and then decided on an appropriate response to the situation and whether to include other participants in the decision as required. The exercise lasted about 60–90 min, followed by at least 60 min for a public debriefing, discussion, and analysis of the response by participants.

3.1. Bioterrorism Model Scenario

For these drills, the scenario consisted of a fire in Peterboro, with concurrent inhalational smoke injuries, the need for building evacuation, victim rescue, and some minor injuries among the emergency responders. Twenty minutes into the incident, participants heard a loud bang. The noise hypothetically originated about a block away from the fire. Five minutes later, a pesticide truck was found near the incident site, which was then turned away from the site by law enforcement personnel directing traffic.

After the first responders and hospital personnel described their actions to participants and observers, the scenario was fastforwarded for two follow-up scenarios, where victims present with plague (24 h) and tularemia (48 h). The tularemia scenario that was used is described here:

- On days 2 and 3, both domestic and wild dead animals were noted around Peterboro. Hordes of deerflies were also noted in certain areas of the town. Early on day 3, six patients (three of whom were pediatric) presented to the hospital emergency room (ER): all had fever, headache, malaise, and three had a nonproductive cough. By that afternoon, four additional patients presented at the hospital ER with similar symptoms.
- Early on day 4, 10 additional patients (6 pediatric) presented to the ER with similar symptoms, although a few of the patients also presented with substernal chest discomfort and loss of appetite. Later that morning, 25 patients (10 pediatric) presented with similar symptoms, and an additional nine arrived who had nonspecific findings such as fever and complaints of malaise. By midday, about 100 patients presented at the ER; roughly half were ill with the same symptoms seen in earlier patients. Two of the patients had painful purulent conjunctivitis with cervical lymphadenopathy. Chest X-rays revealed pleural effusions in some of the ill patients. By the early evening of day 4, 30 additional patients presented to the ER; 10 of these had no obvious disease manifestations but were worried. Three of the patients seen at the ER the previous day suffered respiratory arrest. The supplies of antibiotics at the hospital had been exhausted. Laboratory results on the patients have proved inconclusive to date. None of the patients who had evidence of pneumonia with sepsis responded to streptomycin therapy.
- By day 5, 35 more ill patients with similar symptoms presented to the ER, as well as 15 who had no obvious physical findings but were concerned. Also on day 5, an anonymous phone call to a local radio station claimed that "all unbelievers will soon perish in an apocalypse." One patient's chest X-ray revealed mediastinal lymphadenopathy. A lab technician who has handled some clinical samples developed pneumonia. During this day, a Gram-negative coccobacilli was identified from blood cultures and an immunofluoresence assay of a patient sputum sample revealed the presence of *Francisella tularensis*.
- On day 6, 10 of the patients seen in the past 3 d suffered respiratory arrest. Before the end of the day, more than 200 additional patients presented to the hospital ER, the majority of whom had a pneumonic process.
- On day 8, a serum sample rushed to Centers for Disease Control and Prevention (CDC) was determined to have an elevated titer for *Francisella tularensis*. There were 23 fatalities on this day, all from patients who had been ill since day 3 and had either self-medicated at home or had delayed antibiotic treatment.

3.2. Exercise Review and Lessons Learned

Immediately after the exercise was conducted, all participants and observers participated in an open forum to evaluate the response to the scenario. Among the lessons learned through evaluations from this tabletop exercise were:

- The initial presentation of nonspecific flu-like symptoms that were caused by a bioterrorism agent was not likely to alarm hospital emergency physicians in the initial stages of the outbreak. In this type of event, concern that a bioterrorism event had occurred would only come after a certain critical mass of patients presented for care. Astute emergency department staff may observe an additional patient influx and report this directly to state health authorities. Daily reporting to the state health authorities from a hospital-based syndromic surveillance system should have detected an increase in cases of a nondescript illness. This type of reporting is important to public health bioterrorism disease detection. The system should be sensitive enough to detect cases spread throughout a state's hospital system when sick individuals present to at different healthcare facilities.

Although syndromic surveillance models have been developed *(29)*, public health agencies have been left to construct their own unique models for syndromic surveillance of biological terrorism (BT)-associated diseases to meet their own needs.

- Hospital antibiotic stores can be exhausted rapidly. A system designed to alert state health authorities when unusually large amounts of antibiotics are used by hospitals should be put in place.
- All aspects of the hospital emergency response plan must be activated immediately once it is recognized that resources have become overwhelmed. Rapid establishment of hospital crowd control measures and of a public information office need to be in the plan.
- Chaos can evolve quickly and is best controlled by participant adherence to the ICS *(30)* and the HEICS *(31)*. These systems provide the framework for an organized response to a disaster by first responders and medical personnel. Both the public health and emergency management participants in a BT response have much to learn from these emergency response models.
- Should a large bioterrorism incident occur, the hospital personnel and materiel resources could be rapidly overwhelmed. Both the hospital and state contingency plans should plan for this.
- All first responders and medical personnel need to be attuned to unusual events, potential exposures, and patient symptoms. For example, inadvertent exposure to droplets and respiratory secretions from individuals with pneumonic plague may result in cases among healthcare providers and hospital personnel.
- Healthcare personnel must immediately notify the FBI when exposure to or use of a bioterrorism agent is suspected. This is of vital importance for the criminal and epidemiological investigations that must occur when there is a the purposeful use of a deadly pathogen. Coordinated criminal and epidemiological investigations are of vital importance and should occur simultaneously to identify ill and exposed individuals as well as to assist in the identification of those responsible for a BT event *(32)*.
- Local logistic expertise is vital to incident response. When logistics support fails, all aspects of the response fail, including the EMS system *(33)*.
- The state emergency operations center should be able to be activated at short notice. This is essential for the statewide coordination of emergency, medical, logistic, and other resources as needed by response personnel.

4. LESSONS LEARNED FROM A RECENT INTENTIONALLY SPREAD EPIDEMIC

A surreptitious small-scale biological attack occurred in the United States from September through November 2001, when spore-laden envelopes of *Bacillus anthracis* were sent to persons in the media and to the offices of two US Senators *(34)*. As a consequence, at least 23 individuals became ill from the handling of anthrax-tainted letters. Of those exposed, seven were confirmed (four others were suspected, but not confirmed) as having cutaneous anthrax, and 11 were confirmed as having developed inhalational anthrax. Five deaths occurred among those with inhalational anthrax *(35–37)*.

This act of bioterrorism created huge media interest *(34)*, perhaps in part because of the difficulties in responding to a bioterrorism scenario that was not previously anticipated. Among the misunderstandings about the bioterrorism use of anthrax were *(38)*:

- The historical death rate of virtually 100% among those having inhalational anthrax may be overestimated should extraordinary modern medical care be available.
- The lower limit of spores necessary to cause illness was (and is) not well-understood and may depend on other factors such as age, immunity status, and/or the presence of comorbid conditions.

- Public health authorities and government officials attempted to allay the fears of the public but messages were inconsistent, did not occur in real-time, and were sometimes contradictory.
- Medical and criminal investigations were not well-coordinated.
- Laboratories were rapidly overwhelmed with samples to rule out anthrax.

Many of these deficiencies have been identified previously through bioterrorism exercises *(20,39)* or predicted by modeling *(40)*. A study of anthrax dissemination from envelopes containing *Bacillus globigii* determined that significant amounts of respirable aerosol particles are released when an envelope is opened that contains as little as 0.1–1.0 g of bacterial spores *(41)*. Deficiencies in the governmental response to an unanticipated bioterrorism event may be addressed through the development of comprehensive response plans and an increase in public health response capacities.

Although no one (except perhaps a future perpetrator) can predict what biological pathogen(s) will be used against an unsuspecting target and how it will be used, the public has been sensitized to the intentional use of infectious disease agents as weapons following the events of late 2001.

5. COMPONENTS OF AN EFFECTIVE BIOTERRORISM RESPONSE: DEVELOPMENT OF BIOTERRORISM RESPONSE PLANS

The most comprehensive response plans developed to date to prepare for the use of biological weapons against a civilian population has been the Biological Weapons Improved Response Project (BW-IRP) as developed by the SBCCOM *(42)*. This program was developed to provide enhanced support to improve the capabilities of state and local emergency response agencies to prevent and respond to terrorist incidents involving WMDs at both the national and local levels *(42)*. BW-IRP publications include assessments of hospital resources and preparedness *(43)*, government preparedness for a smallpox outbreak *(44)*, the integration of public health and law enforcement in a bioterrorism investigation *(45)*, and an integrated approach to emergency medical response *(46)*.

Although this work has been transitioned to the US Department of Homeland Security, the templates that have been developed are invaluable for state and local biological weapons preparedness planning *(47)*. These outstanding templates should be more widely distributed to federal, state, and local government personnel to prepare for a BT event. For example, the BW-IRP's Criminal and Epidemiological Investigation Report *(45)* demonstrates how to improve coordination of an investigation between public health and law enforcement personnel, which is one of the key problems mentioned by Altman and Kolata in their article describing miscalculations that occurred with the anthrax letter investigations *(38)*.

An uneasy association exists at times between public health and law enforcement. Law enforcement (especially the FBI) has the lead role in bioterrorism crisis management and criminal investigation. Public health and law enforcement personnel must learn to work together and to appreciate each other as vital components of the investigative team for a bioterrorism event. Law enforcement personnel can gather much case-specific information for an epidemiological investigation and public health personnel can obtain information of use to the criminal investigation. Information of mutual interest to public health and law enforcement includes obtaining personal historical activities data from those who are ill and uncovering the nature of the incident or exposure that caused the illness *(45)*. Both the epidemiological and criminal investigation represent unique opportunities to obtain information that may be relevant to discovering the cause and source of a bioterrorism event and could also lead to early identification of those potentially exposed to a biological agent.

5.1. Pharmaceutical Supplies for Bioterrorism

Pretreatment (e.g., vaccination, chemoprophylaxis) is of limited use for many of the primary threat agents when used in a bioterrorism event *(2)*. Medications and medical supplies to be used in the response to biological attack need to be available for rapid deployment to any part of the United States. Therefore, the prepositioned Strategic National (pharmaceutical) Stockpile (SNS) is of primary importance in the medical response to a bioterrorist attack *(48)*. Delivery and distribution of the SNS should be part of the scenario response evaluation for a bioterrorism tabletop exercise. State medical authorities and civil defense, emergency preparedness, and pharmaceutical authorities need to work together for the SNS acceptance at the point of delivery. These agencies also need to designate responsibility for the pharmaceutical and patient monitoring process, as well as the delivery of medication where it is most needed. The SNS initially was deployed in response to the events of September 11, 2001, in New York City subsequent to activation of the Federal Response Plan *(49)*.

Mass prophylaxis must be preplanned, and needs to include *(48)*:

* Identification of responsibility for receipt of SNS.
* Designation of licensed health professionals to receive the controlled substance portion of the SNS.
* Identification of an appropriate airfield for incoming pharmaceutical and medical supplies.
* Acquisition of cargo handling equipment.
* Acquisition of secure storage facilities for breakdown and repackaging supplies.
* A tracking system that will enable SNS asset deployment.
* Logistics determinations including who will supply trucks and provide personnel to move supplies to distribution sites.
* Establishment of communication links between all key personnel/facilities dealing with SNS distribution and identifying contact personnel.
* Acquisition of baseline patient data and tracking of patients who receive chemoprophylaxis.

5.2. Veterinary Disease Surveillance

Veterinary and food surveillance for zoonotic pathogens is important for bioterrorism preparedness. Participants from the State Veterinarian's and Public Health Veterinarian's agency should be included in bioterrorism planning and training exercises. Some of the diseases associated with bioterrorism are endemic in the United States. Recently, both the ingestion of anthrax-contaminated meat *(50)* and a case of cutaneous anthrax *(51)* have occurred because of nonpurposeful naturally occurring anthrax exposures of animal origin. Anthrax, tularemia, Q fever, brucellosis, and pneumonic plague all can be acquired from wild or domestic animals. It is important to rapidly determine whether a disease is naturally acquired or the result of purposeful events caused by potential biological warfare agents. With the heightened awareness of bioterrorism, the recent naturally occurring incidents of brucellosis *(52)* and tularemia *(53,54)* have also been intimately examined for the potential of having been purposeful events.

5.3. Epidemiological Surveillance

Epidemiological surveillance for bioterrorism must operate continuously to be effective and should be sensitive enough to detect abnormal disease activity in a population, whether from a nonendemic disease (e.g., anthrax in postal workers) or an increase in a naturally occurring disease that has been purposefully introduced (e.g., hundreds of salmonellosis cases in Oregon) *(7)*. Databases that may be monitored include hospital admissions, 911 calls, unexplained deaths, use of over-the-counter medications, emergency department volume, and selected emergency department discharge diagnoses. The surveillance system must also possess the specificity to detect *any* of the reportable bioterrorism diseases. Although it is possible to construct a passive disease monitoring system to detect disease levels above those anticipated, it is exceedingly difficult to construct a passive surveillance system with specificity for bioterrorism diseases that identifies patients exposed to life-threatening illnesses with rapid symptom onset in time to administer potentially life-saving treatment or prophylaxis. The recent cases from exposure to anthrax-contaminated mail demonstrate this point *(35,36)*. Only an extremely rapid response can diagnose and identify cases of inhalational anthrax and pneumonic plague; however, this still may not be possible, even under the best of circumstances.

Initial disease detection, investigation and response usually occur at the local health department level *(55)*. An active epidemiological bioterrorism surveillance system includes the intense search for new or nonreported cases. An enhanced regional or statewide epidemiological surveillance system should be instituted following the report of any bioterrorism-related illness. Enhanced surveillance may uncover cases in areas where they have not yet been identified. To accomplish this, public health personnel must communicate with hospital infectious disease specialists; infection control managers; emergency, pharmacy, and laboratory departments; and nontraditional investigative partners such as veterinarians, medical examiners, funeral directors, law enforcement personnel, and others. Any profession that can contribute information toward the identification of new cases, those exposed to an infectious agent, and the origin of the disease are important allies in the public health investigation of a bioterrorism event.

5.4. Coordinate and Track Clinical and Laboratory Surveillance Activities

Laboratory capacity is a vital part of the public health network and is necessary to discover and respond to the occurrence of a bioterrorism event *(56)*. Electronic laboratory-based reporting is currently being developed and integrated into the public health infrastructure of seven states through CDC grant funding *(57)*. Perhaps the most important surveillance activity within the acute care hospital is the interaction between the hospital-based clinician and the clinical laboratory. However, even the best-designed reporting system can produce erroneous results. Misidentification errors, reporting errors, and lack of laboratory or clinical understanding or ability to characterize the pathogen all can contribute to pathogen misidentification or mischaracterization and have severe consequences for the patient *(58,59)*. In November 2001, although 10 inhalational anthrax cases had already occurred nationally in a 2-mo period *(35)*, a Connecticut hospital laboratory with a finding of Gram-positive rods isolated from a blood culture of a seriously ill patient did not report this discovery to state health authorities until 2 d later *(37)*. This laboratory finding was in fact from the 11th national case of inhalational anthrax. The nonreporting of this isolate to state authorities is perhaps not surprising, given that the finding of Gram-positive rods in a bacterial culture from a clinical specimen is routinely considered a contaminant. To be successful, active syndromic surveillance must incorporate laboratory reporting and seek to inculcate timely and accurate laboratory identification of bioterrorism pathogens. In the case of bioterrorism, the fear of reporting a false-positive should be overweighed by the necessity for enhanced alertness by other clinical laboratories in the reporting state.

5.5. Use of Quarantine

Certain highly contagious infectious diseases on the bioterrorism threat list (e.g., pneumonic plague, smallpox) necessitate the use of isolation and possibly quarantine measures and travel restrictions. The issues surrounding these extreme public health measures should be considered if these diseases are modeled in a tabletop or field exercise. A rapid response is of utmost importance. Should a highly contagious disease be released on a civilian population, a very small amount of time exists in which to detect and verify the infection, locate the time and place of attack, identify the affected population, and begin intervention *(40)*.

Rapid evaluation of the outbreak can determine the extent of exposure and help develop the most effective disease containment strategies. Public health authorities must conduct a thorough search for those exposed and for close contacts of those infected (e.g., immediate household members). Other important tasks include the identification and/or estimation of the population at risk and the development, in advance, of protocols for isolation and surveillance of cases. Hospital and public health authorities need to maintain case ascertainment surveillance data and conduct active prospective disease surveillance.

5.6. Psychosocial Effects

The importance of psychosocial effects was driven home by the horrific events of September 11, 2001. The entire nation felt the impact of the terrorist attacks. The psychosocial effects of an infectious disease outbreak on a large population was demonstrated during the 1994 pneumonic plague outbreak in Surat, India *(60)*. This outbreak caused an exodus of 600,000 people from the city of Surat, followed by a mass anxiety in the city of Delhi, about 600 miles away *(60)*. Hospitals in Delhi became flooded, and "chaos reigned supreme, rumor was the ruler" *(60)*. One important effect of fear and uncertainty was the purchase and hoarding of tetracycline. Similarly, there was a substantial increase in ciprofloxacin use in the United States following the anthrax spore mailings in 2001, and a resulting shortage in certain areas.

It is probable that for every person seeking care in a hospital for physical injuries or infection following a biological or chemical terrorist incident, at least 6–10 will present with psychological concerns *(61)*. Therefore, management of psychological casualties following a WMD incident must be incorporated into a tabletop exercise or live disaster drill. The use of bioterrorism in particular presents complex psychosocial challenges for a civilian population *(62)*. Features of bioterrorism may make group panic more likely *(62)*. Importantly, a lack of realistic training increases the possibility of a disorganized, ineffective response that will heighten the public's fear and break down trust in public institutions *(62)*. Even in the recent anthrax scare, some in the postal system were questioning the recommendations of the federal public health authorities.

5.7. Media Relations

Closely tied to psychosocial effects are the methods used by government officials when dealing with the media. Both the style and content of the news that people receive will influence how they react to news of a WMD event *(63)*. Some of the potential problems are illustrated by the response to media coverage of the Chernobyl accident *(64)*. Those who generate or transmit news should be intimately familiar with and use sound principles of risk communication. One useful source is an emergency response communications plan for bioterrorist events that has been written with input from the principal US public health and emergency response organizations and subsequently distributed to all state health department communications offices *(65)*.

A website for effective risk communication is maintained by the CDC's Agency for Toxic Substances and Disease Registry (ATSDR) at http://www.atsdr.cdc.gov/HEC/primer.html., and other websites have been specifically designed to provide information on bioterrorism-related issues (e.g., http://www.psandman.com/col/part1.htm). Government officials need to express empathy to the affected communities and not merely provide facts; they must also appreciate that the public's desire for risk knowledge may be different from an expert's opinion *(63)*. Information provided to the media by official sources should be accurate, honest, and timely *(63)*.

Given the impact that the media has on any disaster event, it would behoove tabletop or field exercise participants to include media representatives. Any fear of dealing with the media should be negated by the fact that the media is also the vehicle through which large numbers of people can be spoken to on an immediate basis *(66)*.

5.8. Hospital Needs

Community hospitals are a vital partner in the identification, triage, and treatment of those affected by bioterrorism. Rapid casualty care is of utmost importance immediately subsequent to a mass casualty incident. Patient transportation needs will increase greatly and the local EMS may become readily overwhelmed. Any bioterrorism exercise should consider auxiliary replacement of casualty transport through the use of state military or other resources. A statewide communications network should be in place to provide advance notification and coordinate movement to hospitals of incoming casualties *(43)*.

Hospitals should take the following initiatives to best prepare for a bioterrorism event *(43)*.

- Address casualty admission until maximum capacity is reached.
- Be able to redirect noncritical admissions.
- Conduct patient screening, triaging, and release of asymptomatic individuals, based on potential for exposure and illness.
- Obtain pertinent information for public health personnel.
- Establish contacts and agreements in advance with law enforcement so that information can be shared in a crisis situation.
- Identify a backup or overflow emergency evaluation and triage facility.
- Establish alternate care.

- Identify infection control capabilities.
- Establish training programs to decrease the potential that hospital personnel might also panic or fear their own safety from patient contact.

5.9. Mortuary Concerns

Fatality management is an important concern associated with the use of a bioterrorism agent. Disaster planning should always incorporate the state mortician's associations and the state medical examiner's office. During a catastrophic disaster, it is important to maintain a mortuary registry of similar deaths, manage familial visits, use morgues to provide central processing, establish long-term fatality storage facilities, determine final disposition for fatalities, establish family assistance centers, implement mass cremation if necessary, coordinate release of remains to families, and establish temporary internment options as appropriate *(43)*.

6. RECOMMENDATIONS FOR THE FUTURE

According to Congressional Subcommittee testimony given in July 2001: "We're much more likely to have low-consequence scenarios—the kind of thing that the guy down the street will do if he's mad at his neighbors or the IRS, and that won't be anthrax. You can't do smallpox or weaponized anthrax in your garage" *(67)*. Following the events of purposeful release of anthrax from September through November 2001, this statement may demonstrate the difficulty of predicting with any certainty a future terrorist scenario. However, those tabletop exercises that involve as many of the various local, state, and federal emergency response partners as possible should promote understanding between participants and help them to acquire the skills necessary to develop a team response approach to a WMD event.

It would be especially useful at this time to establish a national WMD bioterrorism gaming/exercise think-tank. This type of group could develop reasonable scenarios that could be used by state and local offices of emergency preparedness and health departments to consider likely resource-demanding events. The military model for these activities has been incorporated into war gaming training curricula with great success *(68)*. Incredibly, the collapse of World Trade Center by a terrorist group was predicted during a 2000 scientific symposium: "…not just disruption and some damage to the World Trade Center towers in Manhattan but the total destruction of both buildings and the surrounding area" *(69)*. However, this advice was not published until after the events of September 11, 2001.

7. CONCLUSION

First responders, hospital, health department, and law enforcement personnel from local, state, and federal agencies need enhanced training for bioterrorism events. Unique challenges are presented by the purposeful use of a biological pathogen on an unprotected and unsuspecting population. The training gap must be addressed at the local, state, and federal response level. This can be best accomplished if comprehensive bioterrorism response plans are developed and regular mutual training exercises occur. One productive format for mutual training in anticipation of a bioterrorism event is the use of a tabletop exercise. This scenario-driven training is quite flexible and can incorporate the training goals of the participating agencies. Importantly, a scenario can be devised to reflect the difficulties that will be encountered during a bioterrorism event, including laboratory and clinical identification of the disease, abnormal case-patient load, acceptance and distribution of the national pharmaceutical stockpile, monitoring the spread of disease, and a host of other community, state, or areawide problems. Once a comprehensive bioterrorism plan has been developed and training and resource gaps have been identified through conducting multiple tabletop exercises, one or more field exercises should be conducted to assess the ability of all participating agencies to respond in person to a bioterrorism event. Through plan development and training by use of comprehensive tabletop and field exercises, the various agencies involved will come to understand each others' organizational abilities and roles in response to these events. Although predicting the next bioterrorism event is difficult, if not impossible, there is no excuse why the organizations that are responsible for responding to such a crisis can not now develop and practice plans and response.

ACKNOWLEDGMENTS

The author is grateful for the review and comments by James L. Hadler, MD, MPH, Connecticut Department of Public Health; LTC Mark G. Kortepeter, MD, MPH, Medical Division, USAMRIID; CAPT. Robert G. Darling, MD, FACEP, and LTC Ross H. Pastel, PhD, Operational Medicine Divison, USAMRIID.

REFERENCES

1. Glass, A. T. and Schoch-Spana, M. (2002) Bioterrorism and the people: how to vaccinate a city against panic. *Clin. Infect. Dis.* **34,** 217–223.
2. Alibek, K. (2001) *Biological weapons: past, present, and future. Firepower in the lab: automation in the fight against infectious diseases and terrorism.* Joseph Henry, Washington, D.C., pp. xv, 177.
3. CDC. (2001) Evaluation of *Bacillus anthracis* contamination inside the Brentwood mail processing and distribution center—District of Columbia, October, 2001. *MMWR* **50,** pp. 1129–1133.
4. Olson, K. B. (1999) Aum Shinrikyo: once and future threat. *Emerg. Infect. Dis.* **5,** 513–516.
5. Carus, W. S. (1998) Working Paper. Bioterrorism and biocrimes: the illicit use of biological agents since 1990. Washington, D.C., Center for Counterproliferation Research, National Defense Univ. (Feb. 2001 Rev.).
6. Khan, A. S., Swerdlow, D. L., and Juranek, D. D. (2001) Precautions against biological and chemical terrorism directed at food and water supplies. *Public Health Rep.* **116,** 3–13.
7. Torok, T. J., Tauxe, R. V., Wise, R. P., et al. (1997) A large community outbreak of salmonellosis caused by intentional contamination of restaurant salad bars. *JAMA* **278,** 389–395.
8 Kolavic, S. A., Kimura, A., Simons, S. L., et al. (1997) An outbreak of *Shigella dysenteriae* Type 2 among laboratory workers due to intentional food contamination. *JAMA* **278,** 396–398.
9. Ryan, C. A., Nickels, M. K., Hargrett-Brean, N. T., et al. (1987) Massive outbreak of antimicrobial-resistant salmonellosis traced to pasteurized milk. *JAMA* **258,** 3269–3274.
10. CDC. (1998) Outbreaks of *Shigella sonnei* infection associated with eating fresh parsley—United States and Canada, July-August, 1998. *MMWR* **48,** 285–289.
11. CDC. (1998) Outbreak of *Escherichia coli* O157:H7 infection associated with eating fresh cheese curds—Wisconsin, June 1998. *MMWR* **49,** 911–913.
12. CDC. (2002) Outbreak of Salmonella serotype Kotbus infections associated with eating alfalfa sprouts—Arizona, California, Colorado and New Mexico, February–April, 2001. *MMWR* **51,** 7–9.
13. CDC. (1999) Public health dispatch: Outbreak of *Escherichia coli* O157:H7 and Campylobacter among attendees of the Washington County fair—New York, 1999. *MMWR* **48,** 803.

14. CDC. (2000) Outbreak of gastroenteritis associated with an interactive water fountain at a beachside park—Florida, 1999. *MMWR* **49,** 565–568.
15. Gold, H. (1995) Unit 731 Testimony. Tokyo: Yenbooks.
16. CDC. (1999) Outbreak of West Nile-like virus encephalitis—New York, 1999. *MMWR* **l48,** 845–849.
17. Preston, R. (1999) *Dispatch: West Nile Mystery.* The New Yorker, October 18,25.
18. Alibek, K. and Handelman, S. (1999) *Biohazard: The Chilling True Story of the Largest Covert Biological Weapons Program in the World- Told from the Inside by the Man Who Ran It.* Random House, New York.
19. O'Toole, T. (1999) Smallpox: an attack scenario. *Emerg. Infect. Dis.* **5,** 540–546.
20. Inglesby, T. V. (1999) Anthrax: a possible case history. *Emerg. Infect. Dis.* **5,** 556–560.
21. Leitenberg, M. (2001) Biological weapons in the twentieth century: a review and analysis. *Crit. Rev. Microbiol.* **27,** 267–320.
22. Tyre, T. E. (2001) Wake-up call: a bioterrorism exercise. *Mil. Med.* **166(Suppl. 2),** 90,91.
23. Landauer, M. R., Elliott, T. B., King, G. L., et al. (2001) Performance decrement after combined exposure to ionizing radiation and *Shigella sonnei. Mil. Med.* **166(Suppl. 2),** 71–73.
24. Shoemaker, M. O. (2001) Combined effects of Venezuelan equine encephalitis IIIA virus and gamma irradiation in mice. *Mil. Med.* **166(Suppl. 2),** 88,89.
25. Cook, L. (2001) The world trade center attack: the paramedic response: an insider's view. *Crit. Care* **5,** 301–303.
26. Cook, L. (2001) Use this proven system for disaster communications. *Emerg. Dept. Manag.* **13,** 136–138.
27. http://www.usamriid.army.mil/education/index.html#satellite
28. Hoffman, R. E. and Norton, J. E. (2000) Lessons learned from a full-scale bioterrorism exercise. *Emerg. Infec. Dis.* **6,** 652,653.
29. Canas, L. C., Lohman, K., Pavlin, J. A., et al. (2000) The Department of Defense laboratory-based global influenza surveillance system. *Mil. Med.* **165,** 52–56.
30. Stratton, S. J., Hastings, V. P., Isbell, D., et al. (1996) The 1994 Northridge earthquake disaster response: the local emergency medical services agency experience. *Prehospital Disaster Med.* **11,** 172–179.
31. Stratton, S. J., Hastings, V. P., Isbell, D., et al. (2001) Use this proven system for disaster communications. *Emerg. Dept. Manag.* **13,** 136–138.
32. Final report of the Biological Warfare Improved response Program (BW-IRP) NDPO/DoD Criminal and Epidemiological Investigation Workshop January 19-21, 2000 to U.S. Army Soldier and Biological Chemical Command (SBCCOM), December 2000.
33. Maniscalco, P. M. and Christen, H. T. (1999) EMS incident management: emergency medical logistics. *Emerg. Med. Serv.* **28,** 49–52.
34. Lipton, E. and Johnson, K. (2001) *A Nation Challenged: The Anthrax Trail; Tracking Bioterror's Tangled Course.* The New York Times, December 26.
35. Jernigan, J. A., Stephens, D. S., Ashford, D. A., et al. (2001) Bioterrorism-related inhalational anthrax: the first 10 cases reported in the United States. *Emerg. Infect. Dis.* **7,** 933–944.
36. CDC. (2001) Update: investigation of bioterrorism-related anthrax and interim guidelines for exposure management and antimicrobial therapy, October, 2001. *MMWR* **50,** 909–919.
37. CDC. (2001) Update: investigation of bioterrorism-related inhalational anthrax—Connecticut, 2001. *MMWR* **50,** 1049–1051.
38. Altman, L. K. and Kolata, G. (2002) *Anthrax Missteps Offer Guide to Fight Next Bioterror Battle.* The New York Times, January 6.
39. Inglesby, T. V., Grossman, R., O'Toole, T. (2001) A plague on your city: observations from TOPOFF. *Clin. Infect. Dis.* **32,** 436–445.
40. Giovachino, M. and Carey, N. (2001) Modeling the consequences of bioterrorism response. *Mil. Med.* **166,** 925–930.

41. Kournikakis, B., Armour, S. J., Boulet, C. A., et al. (2001) Risk Assessment of Anthrax Threat Letters. Tech. Rep. DRES TR-2001-048, Suffield, Ontario, Canada: Defense Research Establishment Suffield.

42. http://www.dtic.mil/ndia/2001wmd/mughal2.pdf

43. http://hld.sbccom.army.mil/downloads/bwirp/bwirp_executive_summary.pdf

44. http://hld.sbccom.army.mil/downloads/bwirp/bwirp_cdc_dod_smallpox_workshop.pdf

45. http://hld.sbccom.army.mil/downloads/bwirp/bwirp_npdo_dod_ceir.pdf

46. http://hld.sbccom.army.mil/bwirp/bwirp_acc_blue_book_download.htm

47. http://hld.sbccom.army.mil/downloads/bwirp/bwirp_updated_decision_tree_report.pdf

48. http://www.bt.cdc.gov/stockpile/index.asp

49. CDC. (2001) New York City department of health response to terrorist attack, September 11, 2001. *MMWR* **50,** 821,822.

50. CDC. (2000) Human ingestion of Bacillus anthracis-contaminated meat—Minnesota, August, 2000. *MMWR* **49,** 813–816.

51. CDC. (2001) Human anthrax associated with an epizootic among livestock—North Dakota, 2000. *MMWR* **50,** 677–680.

52. CDC. (2000) Suspected brucellosis case prompts investigation of possible bioterrorism-related activity—New Hampshire and Massachusetts, 1999. *MMWR* **49,** 509–512.

53. CDC. (2001) Tularemia—Oklahoma 2000. *MMWR* **50,** 704–706.

54. Feldman, K. A., Enscore, R. E., Lathrop, S. L., et al. (2001) An outbreak of primary pneumonic tularemia on Martha's Vineyard. *N. Engl. J. Med.* **345,** 1601–1606.

55. Hughes, J. M. (2001) Addressing emerging infectious diseases, food safety, and bioterrorism: common themes. Firepower in the lab: automation in the fight against infectious diseases and terrorism. Joseph Henry, Washington, D.C., v, pp. 55.

56. Skeels, M. R. (2001) Laboratories and disease surveillance *Mil. Med.* **165(Suppl. 2),** 16–19.

57. Pinner, R. W., Jernigan, D. B., and Sutliff, S. M. (2000) Electronic Laboratory-Based Reporting for Public Health. *Mil. Med.* **165(Suppl. 2),** 20–24.

58. Dembek, Z. F., Kellerman, S. E., Ganley, L., et al. (1999) Reporting of vancomycin-resistant enterococci in Connecticut: implementation and validation of a state-based surveillance system. *Infect. Control Hospital Epidemiol.* **20,** 671–675.

59. Tenover, F. C. (2001) Development and spread of bacterial resistance to antimicrobial agents: an overview. *Clin. Infect. Dis.* **33,** S108–S115.

60. Ramalingaswami, V. (2001) Psychosocial effects of the 1994 plague outbreak in Surat, India. *Mil. Med.* **166(Suppl. 2),** 29,30.

61. Lord, E. J. (2001) Exercises involving an act of biological or chemical terrorism: what are the psychological consequences? *Mil. Med.* **166(Suppl. 2),** 34,35.

62. Norwood, A. N. (2001 Psychological effects of biological warfare. *Mil. Med.* **166(Suppl. 2),** 27,28.

63. DiGiovanni, C. (2001) Pertinent psychological issues in the immediate management of a weapons of mass destruction event. *Mil. Med.* **166(Suppl. 2),** 59,60.

64. Revel, J. R. (2001) Meeting psychological needs after Chernobyl: the Red Cross experience. *Mil. Med.* **166(Suppl. 2),** 19,20.

65. Model emergency communications plan for infectious disease outbreaks and bioterrorist events. Washington, D.C.: ASTDHPPHE, May 2000.

66. Quigley, C. (2001) Dual-edged sword: dealing with the media before, during and after a weapon of mass destruction event. *Mil. Med.* **166(Suppl. 2),** 56–58.

67. Bioterrorism Testimony: Statement of Dr. Patricia Quinlisk before the Congressional Subcommittee on National Security, Veterans Affairs and International Relations in July, 2001. CSTE Update, Atlanta, No. 3, 2001.

68. Perla, P. P. (1986) A guide to navy wargaming. Alexandria, VA: Center for Naval Analyses.

69. Carter, C. (2001) National innovation to combat catastrophic terrorism. Firepower in the lab: automation in the fight against infectious diseases and terrorism. Joseph Henry, Washington, D.C., xvi, **187,** 1242–1248.

3

Biological Weapons Defense

Effect Levels

Ross D. LeClaire and M. Louise M. Pitt

1. INTRODUCTION

Many toxins and replicating agents have the potential for malevolent use. Of prime concern is the use of agents or toxins that would affect large populations. Delivery of these agents through food or water is of concern but is restricted by the quantity of agent required, thus limiting use to objectives where less than mass morbidity is intended. Contrary to popular perception, dilution factors and modern food supply refinement (to include water purification) significantly limit the efficient use of biological agents by the oral route of exposure *(1)*. Biological threat agents are most likely to be effectively delivered covertly and by aerosol in a biological warfare or terrorism scenario. Estimations of potential exposure levels have been derived to assist medical planners, logisticians, and field officers in predicting biological warfare contingency requirements.

The potential threat agents have been designated as either lethal or incapacitating; these terms are not absolute but imply statistical probabilities of response. Median lethal or median effective/infectious doses are presented when available for the following potential threat agents: ricin; botulinum neurtoxins; staphylococcal enterotoxin B (SEB); *Clostridium perfringens* epsilon toxin; T-2 toxin; *Francisella tularensis*; *Brucella melitensis /abortus/suis*; *Bacillus anthracis*; *Yersinia pestis*; *Coxiella burnettii*; *variola majo, Venezuelan equine encephalitis* (VEE), *eastern equine encephalitis* (EEE), and *western equine encephalitis* (WEE) viruses; and *filoviruses*. In addition, the potential implications of emerging and future technologies are discussed.

2. RESPIRABLE AEROSOL THREAT

Biological threat agents can be disseminated in an aerosol through the use of a broad range of delivery platforms, including conventional systems such as bombs and missiles and unconventional systems such as modified agricultural sprayers. Respirable aerosols represent the most significant threat of effectively exposing large numbers of personnel. Aerosol delivery of a few kilograms of infective or toxic agent can potentially affect personnel over tens or even hundreds of square kilometers. An event may occur without warning and may not be detected until the first casualties develop symp-

From: *Infectious Diseases: Biological Weapons Defense: Infectious Diseases and Counterterrorism*
Edited by: L. E. Lindler, F. J. Lebeda, and G. W. Korch © Humana Press Inc., Totowa, NJ

toms of illness. Because of the extent of potential casualties, estimations have been derived to assist medical planners, logisticians, and staff officers in predicting biological warfare contingency requirements *(2)*. Preparation of countermeasures for potential threats has necessitated prioritization to allocate limited resources *(3)*. Domestic preparedness for events involving weapons of mass destruction is a growing concern and a formidable task *(4,5)*.

2.1. Estimations and Assumptions

Estimations of exposure levels are complicated by aerosol dissemination and stability assumptions. Under ideal conditions, once an agent is disseminated, there is a short equilibration period before the aerosol is fully formed. Larger particles (>15 μm) do not remain suspended and tend to fall out in a short period of time. Within several minutes, the stable aerosol is composed largely of particles in the 1- to 5-μm range that remain suspended for long periods of time allowing for distribution over large areas. Individuals are infected at this point by breathing the air. In addition to not being maintained in the primary aerosol, larger particles (10–20 μm) and particles smaller than 0.5 μm are not retained well in the human respiratory track and are either exhaled or diffuse. Once the aerosol cloud has stabilized, its integrity is dependent on atmospheric stability (e.g., wind speed, thermal inversions, precipitation). Exposure estimates are frequently based on optimal combinations of temperatures, wind speeds, prevailing wind direction, cloud cover, and sunrise/sunset times. The effects of topography and vegetation are not often modeled.

Climatic conditions, such as ultraviolet light, humidity, and temperature affect agent viability in the aerosol cloud. Agents may have sufficient innate stability to remain viable or may be artificially stabilized. The spores produced by the genus Bacillus are extremely stable. Although exposure to spores at levels that cause disease from an inhalation route is not natural, dry spore preparations are extremely stable in bioaerosols. The rickettsia *C. burnetii* also develop an extremely stable spore-like state. *C. burnetii* infects many different animals and has been shown to survive in dry dust generated from contaminated afterbirth for months. Humans can become infected naturally through inhalation of contaminated dust. Factors affecting the viability of airborne organisms have been investigated as a matter of environmental and public health concern *(6–8)*. Examination of persistent aerosols has permitted evaluation of the conditions allowing resistance to aerosolization *(9)*. Numerous organisms could be stabilized in liquid or dry conditions and maintain viability in an aerosol but decay rapidly when exposed to ultraviolet light. This is typical for vegetative organisms such as the *Brucella sp.*, *F. tularensis*, and *Y. pestis*.

Estimations of infective or toxic exposure levels based on biological responses should also be viewed with caution. They are often based on extrapolations from epidemiological investigations. In some cases, they are based on human studies in healthy, young adult volunteers. In others, estimates are based on cross-species extrapolations. Animal to human extrapolations require dosimetric/allometric adjustment and assume effects in the experimental model are relevant to humans *(10)*. Relationships derived from comparative physiology and toxicology for required parameters are not always available from direct measurement and thereby require inference.

2.2. Variability in the Exposed Population

The physical and physiological condition of the population exposed will have a significant impact on the outcome of inhalation exposure to biological agent. General health, stress status (e.g., respiratory rate), medications, metabolic disorders, nutritional status, immune competence, operational scenarios, and the mission all are individual or unit factors that will impact the outcome. Additionally, agents are designated either as lethal agents (intended to kill) or as incapacitating agents (intended to cause disability). Not all individuals will die from an attack with a given lethal agent, and some (e.g., infants and people weakened by malnutrition, disease, or old age) might succumb to an attack with incapacitating agents. In addition, a specific agent can be both an incapacitating and a lethal agent depending on the dose delivered.

2.3. Biological and Toxin Threat Agent Factors

Features of biological agents that influence their potential for use as aerosol weapons include infectivity, virulence, toxicity, pathogenicity, incubation period, transmissibility, lethality, and stability. Agents may be replicating or nonreplicating. Factors related to their potential use are described in the North Atlantic Treaty Organization (NATO) Handbook on the Medical Aspects of NBC Defensive Operations *(11)* as described here.

2.3.1. Infectivity

The capability of microorganisms to establish themselves in a host species is variable. Pathogens with high infectivity cause disease with relatively few organisms, whereas those with low infectivity require a larger number. High infectivity does not necessarily mean that the symptoms and signs of disease appear more quickly or that the illness is more severe.

2.3.2. Virulence

The propensity of an agent for causing severity of disease is dependent on a diverse combination of agent and host factors. These factors are dynamic and often malleable. Different strains of the same microorganism often cause diseases of different severity.

2.3.3. Toxicity

The toxicity relates to the severity of illness (toxicosis) elicited by a toxin.

2.3.4. Pathogenicity

The ability of an agent to initiate a set of events (e.g., propagate attachment and penetration) that culminate in disease or abnormality defines its pathogenicity. A sufficient number of microorganisms or quantity of toxin must penetrate the body to initiate infection (the infective dose) or intoxication (the intoxicating dose). Infectious agents must then multiply (replicate) to produce disease.

2.3.5. Incubation Period

The time between exposure and the appearance of symptoms is known as the incubation period. This period is governed by many variables, including the initial dose, virulence, route of entry, rate of replication, and host immunological factors.

2.3.6. Transmissibility

Some biological agents can be transmitted from person-to-person directly. Indirect transmission (e.g., by arthropod vectors) may be a significant means of spread as well. In the context of biological warfare casualty management, the relative ease with which an agent is passed from person-to-person (that is, its transmissibility) constitutes the principal concern.

2.3.7. Lethality

Lethality reflects the relative ease with which an agent causes death in a susceptible population.

2.3.8. Stability

The viability of an agent is affected by various environmental factors, including temperature, relative humidity, atmospheric pollution, and sunlight. A quantitative measure of stability is an agent's decay rate (e.g., "aerosol decay rate").

2.3.9. Additional Factors

Additional factors that may influence the suitability of a microorganism or toxin as a biological weapon include ease of production, stability when stored or transported, and ease of dissemination.

In April of 1997, the US Department of Health and Human Services and Centers for Disease Control and Prevention (CDC) set forth regulations governing hazardous biological agents *(12)*. The intent was to accomplish four major goals: (a) identify biological agents potentially hazardous to the public health; (b) establish procedures for monitoring the acquisition of restricted agents; (c) provide safeguards for agent transport; and (d) create an alert system for improper attempts at acquiring restricted agents. The CDC identified 24 biological agents and 12 toxins that are listed in Table 1. The CDC maintains an active, categorized biological terrorism threat agent listing posted on their Internet site (http://www.bt.cdc.gov/Agent/agentlist.asp). Agents are tiered as A (highest priority), B (second-highest priority), and C (third-highest priority). There are several of similar threat agent lists categorized on different assessment factors. Although priority categorizations differ, the agent contents are similar. Based on assumptions and estimations discussed in Subheading 2.3., agents that possess the attributes that make them candidates for biological aerosol weapons are underlined in Table 1.

2.4. Delivery Platforms

Although agents such as ricin may have limited utility for open-air delivery, they are widely available. The relationship between aerosol infectivity and toxicity and the quantity of agent required to produce equivalent effects limit the number of agents that could be used to cause large numbers of causalities. The amount of ricin (highly toxic) needed to cover a 100-km^2 area and cause 50% lethality would be approx 8 metric tons, whereas only kilogram quantities of refined *B. anthracis* would be needed to achieve the same effect *(13)*. Dissemination of an agent such as ricin over a large area becomes logistically impractical. Others agents such as saxitoxin are difficult to produce in quantity and are not considered a practical threat. An exception to the toxicity and the quantity of agent required to produce equivalent effects are the trichothecenes (T-2 toxin).

Table 1
The Centers for Disease Control and Prevention List of Restricted Agents, 1997

Viral	Bacterial	Toxins	Rickettsial	Fungal
Crimean-Congo hemorrhagic fever	*Bacillus anthracis***	Abrin	*Coxiella burnetii***	Coccidioides immitis
Eastern equine encephalitis virus	*Brucella abortus, melitensis, and suis***	Aflatoxins	*Rickettsia prowazekii*	
Ebola virus*	*Burkholderia (Pseudomonas) mallei***	Botulinum neurotoxins*	*Rickettsia rickettsii*	
Equine morbillivirus	*Burkholderia (Pseudomonas) pseudomallei***	*Clostridium perfringens* epsilon toxin*		
Lassa fever virus	*Clostridium botulinum*	Conotoxins		
Marburg virus*	*Francisella tularensis***	Diacetoxyscirpenol		
Rift Valley fever virus	*Yersinia pestis***	Ricin*		
South American hemorrhagic fever viruses		Saxitoxin		
Tick-borne encephalitis complex viruses		Shigatoxin		
Variola major virus (smallpox virus)*		Staphylococcal enterotoxins*		
Venezuelan equine encephalitis virus*		Tetrodotoxin		
Hantavirus pulmonary syndrome		T-2 toxin (trichothecene)*		
Yellow fever virus				

*Based on assumptions and estimations discussed in Subheading 2.3., agents that possess the attributes that make them candidates for biological aerosol weapons affecting large populations are underlined.

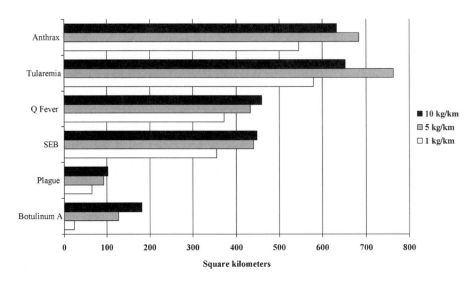

Fig. 1. Estimated agent cloud coverage at greater than or equal to the ED_{50} resulting from a 10-km ground line source. The ED_{50} represents the median dose estimated to affect 50% of a population. This is represented as lethality for anthrax, plague, and botulinum neurotoxin (serotype A), and incapacitation for tularemia, Q fever, and SEB. Area coverage estimates are based on the default values contained in the US Navy's Vapor, Liquid, and Solid Tracking (VLSTRACK) computer model. The model is used to simulate the spread of agent.

Their acute toxicity by the inhalation route is similar to that of Lewisite (circa 10^3 mg-minutes per cubic meter [mg: min/m^3]) but with dermal exposure T-2 is about 10 times more potent than liquid mustard [*bis*-(2-chloroethyl) sulfide] *(14)*. The trichothecenes are considered to be primarily blister agents that cause severe skin and eye irritation at low-exposure doses.

Many nations spent years determining which biological agents had the greatest strategic and tactical potential. Properties considered included level of infectivity/toxicity; ease of production in large quantities; and stability during storage, dissemination, and in aerosol. Stability is a major concern. For example, although extremely potent, botulinum neurotoxin may be a less effective agent because of its lower stability in the environment that limits area coverage *(15)*. Compared to botulinum neurotoxin serotype A, SEB is estimated to be less potent but is relatively stable and may produce significant lethal and incapacitating effects over large areas. The estimated comparative area coverage of several threat agents is shown in Fig. 1 *(16)*. *Variola major*, *Y. pestis*, *B. anthracis*, and botulinum neurotoxin have been cited as the top four most likely agents. Additional attributes that make an agent even more dangerous include being communicable from person-to-person and having no treatment or vaccine. After factoring in these characteristics, anthrax (although not communicable) and smallpox are the two diseases with greatest potential for mass casualties and civil disruption.

3. PROBABLE RESPIRABLE BIOLOGICAL AND TOXIN THREATS

Tables 2–5 shows selected diseases whose causative organisms are considered as potential biological agents. Unless otherwise noted, these results represent data based on dynamic aerosols generated by a nebulizer. Infectious agents were in medium or

Table 2
Viral Agents

Agent	Aerosol LD$_{50}$[a]	Incubation period	Fatality rate
Variola major	Unknown	7–17 d	20–40%
Venezuelan, eastern, and western equine encephalitis virus	**VEE**: mouse LD$_{50}$ = 2.8 PFU[b] **EEE**: guinea pig LD$_{50}$ = 1210 PFU[c]; mouse LD$_{50}$ = 540 PFU	1–5 d **EEE**: 50–75%	**VEE** and **WEE**: uncommon (<1%)
Filovirus (Ebola and Marburg viruses)	Unknown	6–7 d	50–90%

[a]The LD$_{50}$ and ID50 are the dose of agent expected to cause death or incapacitation, respectively, to 50% of those exposed.
[b]PFU (plaque forming unit; mouse LD$_{50}$ = 540 PFU).
[c]US Army Research Institute of Infectious Diseases, unpublished data.

Table 3
Lethal Bacterial Agents

Agent	Aerosol LD$_{50}$	Incubation period	Disease severity (untreated)
Bacillus anthracis (inhalational anthrax)	55,000[a]	1–7 d	>90% death
Yersinia pestis (pneumonic plague)	343[b,c]	1–6 d	100% death

[a]U.S. Army Research Institute of Infectious Diseases, unpublished data (1991): *Macaca mulatta,* Ames strain.
[b]LD$_{50}$ determined as a delivered dose—no assumption about retention.
[c]US Army Research Institute of Infectious Diseases, unpublished data (1994): *Cercopithecus aethiops,* CO92 strain.

Table 4
Incapacitating Bacterial and Rickettsial Agents

Agent	ID$_{50}$ and ED$_{50}$	Incubation period	Fatality rate
Franciscella tularensis (tularemia)	10[a] (LD$_{50}$ <1000)	1–10 d	Type A: 40%[b] Type B: 5%[b]
Brucella melitensis/ suis/abortus (brucellosis)	ID$_{50}$ = 10–100	Variable 7–21 d to several mo	2%[b]
Coxiella burnetii[c]	30[a]	4–21 days (dose-dependent)	Rare

[a]Derived from human data.
[b]Fatality when untreated.
[c]*Rickettsia.*

Table 5
Select Toxin Agents

Agent	ED$_{50}$ and LD$_{50}$	Time of onset	Disease
Staphylococcal enterotoxin B	ED$_{50}$ = 0.0004 µg[a] LD$_{50}$ >0.02 µg/kg	1–12 h	Moderate: fever 38.3–40.6°C (101–105°F), incidence of fever is 50%. Severe: acute respiratory distress, shock, and death.
Botulinum toxins Serotype A (B–G discussed in text)	Estimated illness is 50% at about 0.00024 µg inhaled. LD$_{50}$ = 0.003 µg/kg	5 h to 7 d	Moderate exposure: abnormal vision, ptosis. Respiratory failure; 5 h to 2 d to onset; general muscular; incidence of mortality is 90%.
Ricin	LD$_{50}$ = 15 µg/kg[b]	15–20 h[a]	Target organ is the lung with death occurring between 36–48 h (massive pulmonary edema).
Clostridium perfringens epsilon toxin	ED$_{50}$ = 0.025 mg/kg[a] LD$_{50}$ unknown		Labored respiration, general malaise, massive hemorrhagic edema, and death in 4–24 h.
T-2 toxin (trichothecene)	LD$_{50}$ = 0.025–0.24, mg/kg[b]		

[a]Derived from human data
[b]US Army Research Institute of Infectious Diseases, unpublished data (1992), *Macaca mulata.*

water while toxins were in water and may have a carrier protein. Aerosol particle size ranged from 0.8 to 1.4 µm and exposures were 10 min. Rhesus macaques were anesthetized and respiratory parameters (minute volume [MV], and respiratory rate [RR]) were measured by whole-body plethysmograph. Rodents were awake and respiratory parameters were calculated from published formulas *(17)*. In all cases, no assumptions were made about retention. The inhaled-doses-delivered estimation is based on aerosol concentration, MV, and time. Total calculated dose is the product of aerosol concentration and exposure time.

3.1. Viral Agents

Potential viral biological weapon agents as shown in Table 2 include *Variola major*; the causative agent of smallpox, equine encephalitis viruses, including VEE, EEE, and WEE; and the filoviruses.

3.1.1. Variola Major

The concept of using variola virus in warfare is an old one. British colonial commanders considered distributing blankets from smallpox victims among Native Americans as a biological weapon. During the American Civil War, there were allegations about the use of smallpox as a biological weapon, although there is no evidence to support such allegations. In 1980, the World Health Organization (WHO) declared endemic smallpox eradicated. Although two WHO-approved repositories of variola virus remain at the CDC in Atlanta, GA, and at Vector in Novosibirsk, Russia, the extent of concealed stockpiles in other parts of the world remains unknown. The former Soviet Union has admitted to weaponizing *Variola major (18)*.

Because the host range of this virus is confined to humans, aggressive case identification and contact vaccination were ultimately successful in controlling the disease. *Variola virus* is highly stable and retains its infectivity for long periods outside the host. It is infectious by aerosol, but natural spread to other than close contacts is controversial. Approximately 30% of susceptible contacts became infected during the era of endemic smallpox. Major knowledge gaps exist regarding the adequacy of available animal models. Current models include monkeypox, cowpox, and rabbitpox. The ID_{50}/LD_{50} has not been established. No qualified model exists for the evaluation of the efficacy of antiviral therapy.

3.1.2. Equine Encephalitis Viruses

The characteristics of the equine encephalitis viruses (VEE, EEE, and WEE) lend themselves well to weaponization. This fact was recognized and these agents were included in offensive biological warfare programs that were initiated before or during World War II.

VEE virus is an arthropod-borne alphavirus endemic in northern South America, Trinidad, Central America, Mexico, and Florida. Eight serologically distinct viruses belonging to the VEE complex are associated with human disease; the two most important of these pathogens are designated subtype I, variants A/B and C. These agents also cause severe disease in horses, mules, burros, and donkeys (Equidae). Natural infections are acquired by the bites of a wide variety of mosquitoes. Equidae serve as amplifying hosts and sources of mosquito infection. In natural human epidemics, severe and often fatal encephalitis in Equidae always precedes disease in humans. Aerosol transmission has occurred in laboratory settings but is not known to occur naturally. There are approx 150 documented adult human accidental VEE exposures in laboratory settings. There was only one fatality. EEE is the most severe of the encephalitides, with high mortality and severe neurological sequelae. During outbreaks, the attack, morbidity, and mortality rates are highest among children and the elderly. Case fatality rates are estimated to be from 50 to 75%, but asymptomatic infections and milder clinical illness are certainly underreported.

The few published studies of EEE neuropathology *(19)* have used intracerebral, subcutaneous, and intraperitoneal (IP) inoculation of young chicks, hamsters, and mice *(12)*. Hamsters are 1000 times more susceptible to EEE infection than mice (one hamster IP LD_{50} = 1 PFU; one mouse IP LD_{50} = 1000 PFU). There are no published investigations in the open literature for aerosol infections and resultant neuropathology.

3.1.3. Filoviridae *(Ebola and Marburg)*

These viral hemorrhagic fever agents appear to be highly infectious by aerosol, and are quite stable *(20)*. Their existence as endemic disease threats and as potential biological warfare weapons suggests a formidable potential impact on military readiness. The incubation period is about 6–7 d in *Macaca mulatta* infected by aerosol. The initial sign is an increase in temperature (40–40.5°C) accompanied by loss of appetite, exhaustion, and recumbence. Animals die on days 10–11.

The *Filoviridae* include the causative agents of Ebola and Marburg hemorrhagic fevers. Marburg was first recognized in 1967 in Marburg, Germany, among laboratory workers exposed to the blood and tissues of African green monkeys that had been transported from Uganda. Ebola viruses are taxonomically related to Marburg viruses; they were first recognized in association with outbreaks that occurred in 1976 in small communities in Zaire and Sudan *(21)*. Secondary transmission occurred through reuse of unsterilized needles and syringes and nosocomial contacts.

3.2. Lethal Bacterial Agents

Bacterial organisms represent the greatest number of replicating agent pathogens presenting a potential biological warfare threat (*see* Table 3). Many produce exotoxins that damage cell membranes; inhibit protein synthesis, and are immune modulators, proteases, or activate secondary message pathways. The disease can be predominately lethal as with anthrax from *B. anthracis* or pneumonic plague from *Y. pestis*. A predominantly incapacitating disease may also occur from exposure to agents as *F. tularensis*, *B. melitensis/ suis/ abortus,* or *C. burnetii*.

3.2.1. B. anthracis

Because of the infectivity of *B. anthracis* spores by the respiratory route and the high mortality of inhalational anthrax, the military is concerned with its potential use as a biological weapon *(22)*. This concern was heightened by the revelation that the largest epidemic of inhalational anthrax in the 20th century, which occurred in Sverdlovsk, Russia, in 1979, occurred after *B. anthracis* spores were released from a military research facility located upwind from where the cases occurred *(23,24)*. Cases were also reported in animals located more than 50 km from the site. In addition, Iraq produced and fielded *B. anthracis* spores for use in the Gulf War *(25)*. In 2001, letters containing *B. anthracis* were distributed in the United States causing both inhalational and cutaneous anthrax in postal workers and others who either opened or came in contact with the letters. In October 2001, 4 workers died from inhalation anthrax and an additional 13 people developed cutaneous or inhalational disease as a result of intentional terrorist activity. These cases were associated with exposures to anthrax spores contained in letters mailed through the US Postal Service. This has led to a critical review and update of recommendations for medical and public health management following civilian population exposures *(26)*.

Anthrax is caused by *B. anthracis*, a large rod-shaped, Gram-positive, sporulating organism, the spores being the usual infective form. Anthrax is a zoonotic disease, primarily infecting cattle, sheep, and horses, although other animals may be infected as well. Humans may contract the disease, typically in its cutaneous or gastrointestinal forms, by handling contaminated hair, wool, hides, flesh, blood, and excreta of infected animals and from manufactured products such as bone meal. The inhalational form of anthrax is caused by the purposeful dissemination of aerosols containing spores. All human populations are susceptible. The spores are very stable and may remain viable for many years in soil and water. They will resist sunlight for varying periods. The risk of person-to-person transmission of the disease is very low. Handling corpses, particularly during autopsies, may pose a risk of cutaneous anthrax or even of secondary inhalation anthrax through inhalation of aerosolized blood droplets containing spores. There is limited information on field data for extrapolation in anthrax *(27)*.

3.2.2. Y. pestis

Plague has been associated with three pandemics in the 6th, 14th, and 20th centuries. During World War II, the Japanese army apparently used plague as a biological warfare agent in China several times. There is information available that suggests the former Soviet Union created a genetically engineered dry antibiotic-resistant form of plague, and during the Korean War, allied forces were accused of dropping it on North Korea insects that were capable of spreading plague and other infectious agents. No evidence exists to support this claim.

Plague is caused by a Gram-negative, nonacid-fast, nonmotile, nonsporulating, nonlactose-fermenting, bipolar coccobacillus. The naturally occurring disease in humans is transmitted from rodents by fleas. The most common form is bubonic plague (about 90%). Secondary septicemic plague occurs in about one-fifth of patients and secondary pneumonic plague in about 10%. If *Y. pestis* were used as a biological warfare agent, the primary manifestation would be epidemic pneumonia. The transmissibility of pneumonic plague from person to person is extremely high. Well-characterized model systems that emulate human exposure, pathogenesis, and resulting disease do not yet exist. Battlefield relevant levels of exposure are ill defined.

3.3. Bacterial and Rickettsial Incapacitants

Causality assessment must include agents that deprive individuals of the capacity to perform normally. In most cases, the dose of an agent will determine the response in an individual with regards to death or incapacitation. The limits of practical exposure to several bacterial and rickettsial agents result in responses that primarily incapacitate (*see* Table 4). With biological agents these are often related to febrile illnesses. Generally, performance impact in adults may be limited to decreased short-term endurance with body temperatures less than 101.5°F, whereas strength and cognitive ability are generally impaired with higher temperatures.

3.3.1. F. Tularensis

Tularemia is a zoonotic disease caused by the Gram-negative, facultative intracellular bacterium, *F. tularensis*. The disease is characterized by fever, localized skin or mucous membrane ulceration, regional lymphadenopathy, and, occasionally, pneumonia. *F. tularensis* is considered an important biological warfare threat because of its very high infectivity after aerosolization (Table 4).

F. tularensis is a small, aerobic, Gram-negative coccobacillus, often varying in size and shape. It is nonmotile and nonsporulating. Tularemia, also known as rabbit fever and deerfly fever, is a zoonotic disease that humans acquire under natural conditions through inoculation of skin or mucous membranes with blood or tissue fluids of infected animals or bites of infected deerflies, mosquitoes, or ticks. Less commonly, inhalation of contaminated dusts or ingestion of contaminated foods or water may produce clinical disease. Respiratory exposure by aerosol would cause typhoidal tularemia, often having a pneumonic component. Pneumonia occurs in 80% of patients with typhoidal pneumonia. The mortality rate with the untreated disease is roughly 40% for tularemia type A and 5% for tularemia type B. The organism can remain viable for weeks in water, soil, carcasses, and hides and for years in frozen rabbit meat. It is resistant for months to temperatures of freezing and below. Heat and disinfectants kill it rather easily.

3.3.2. B. melitensis/abortus/suis

The United States began development of *B. suis* as a biological weapon in 1942. The agent was formulated to maintain long-term viability, placed into bombs, and tested in field trials during 1944–1945 using animal targets. By 1969, the United States terminated its offensive program. Although munitions were never used in combat, the studies reinforced the concern that these organisms might be used as a biological warfare agent *(28)* (Table 4).

Brucellosis is a zoonotic infection of domesticated and wild animals caused by organisms of the genus *Brucella*. Brucellae are small, nonmotile, nonsporulating, nontoxigenic, aerobic, Gram-negative coccobacilli that may, based on DNA homology, represent a single species. Humans become infected by eating animal food products, directly contacting animals, or inhaling infectious aerosols. Symptoms after aerosol exposure are indistinguishable from those infected by other routes. When left untreated, the mortality rate is approx 2%. There is no direct evidence for an infectious dose, however, Brucellae are thought to be highly infectious with an ID_{50} of 10–100 organisms.

3.3.3. C. Burnetii

C. burnetii, the causative agent of Q fever, is a rickettsial organism. Mainly inhaling infected aerosols transmits the disease. Humans are the only hosts susceptible to infection by *C. burnetii* that develop an illness as a result of infection. The disease is distributed worldwide. The primary reservoir for human infection is livestock, particularly sheep, goats, and cattle. The organism is very resistant to pressure and desiccation, and may persist in a spore-like form in the environment for months. A biological warfare attack with Q fever would cause a disease similar to that occurring naturally. Such an attack may also create a reservoir of insects and mammals that could be a source of considerable secondary infection. Although some human exposure data are available, well-characterized model systems that emulate human exposure, pathogenesis, and resulting disease are not qualified (Table 4).

3.4. Toxins

True toxins are poisons of a biogenic origin, usually from microbial, marine, animal, or plant sources (Table 5). They are often proteinaceous and induce an antitoxin response in exposed vertebrate animals. True toxins may also be low-molecular organic compounds several of which can be synthesized. Numerous organisms (e.g., bacteria, fungi, algae, and plants) produce toxins. Many of the toxin agents are extremely poisonous, with a toxicity that is several orders of magnitude greater than the chemical nerve agents. Toxins were among the first biological agents employed. As early as 600 BC, Athens used the roots of the hellebore plant and the Assyrians used rye ergot to poison enemy drinking water wells.

3.4.1. Staphylococcal enterotoxin B

During the 1960s, when the United States had an offensive biological warfare program, SEB was studied extensively as a biological incapacitant. It was attractive as a weapon because it requires such a minute quantity to cause incapacitation. Although quoted as an incapacitant, SEB is lethal at very low concentrations and, therefore, should be considered as both an incapacitating and a lethal biological threat.

Staphylococcus aureus produces numerous exotoxins, one of which is SEB. Such toxins are referred to as exotoxins because they are excreted from the organism; however, they normally exert their effects on the intestines and thereby are called enterotoxins. SEB is one of the pyrogenic toxins that commonly causes food poisoning in humans after the toxin is produced in improperly handled foodstuffs and is subsequently ingested. SEB has a very broad spectrum of biological activity. This toxin causes a markedly different clinical syndrome when inhaled than it characteristically produces when ingested. Humans exposed to SEB by inhalation predominately become febrile and anorexic and develop a cough. The vomiting and diarrhea commonly associated with ingestion of the toxin (food poisoning) is not common. Significant morbidity is produced in individuals who are exposed to SEB by either portal of entry to the body. The mechanism of intoxication is thought to be from massive release of cytokines.

3.4.2. Botulinum Neurotoxins

Because of the extreme toxicity of botulinum neurotoxins, they were one of the first agents to be considered as a biological weapons agent. Before "offensive" research on biological warfare agents was renounced, researchers in the United States worked on the weaponization of botulinum neurotoxin; efforts began early during the World War II. Strains that produced the five serotypes known at that time were investigated and the serotype producing the most toxin, serotype A, was chosen for further study.

The botulinum neurotoxins are a group of seven related neurotoxins produced by the bacillus *C. botulinum*. These toxins, types A–G, could be delivered by aerosol over concentrations of troops. When inhaled, these toxins produce a clinical picture very similar to food-borne intoxication. In both cases, it produces a blood-borne toxicisis with the protein neurotoxin, binds to presynaptic membranes of neurons at peripheral synapses, and is internalized. The catalytic domain eventually is released into the cytosol, where it mediates a zinc-dependent proteolysis of key vesicular cytosolic docking proteins necessary for neurotransmitter release. This results in a characteristic descending flaccid paralysis beginning with cranial nerve dysfunction and progressing to peripheral nerve weakness and eventual respiratory distress. The time to onset of paralytic symptoms may actually be no longer than for food-borne cases, and may vary by type and dose of toxin. The clinical syndrome produced by one or more of these toxins are known as botulism. Toxin type A is the type most commonly associated with biological warfare. Table 6 gives comparative lethality data (where known) in rhesus macaques for serotypes A–G. The only human data available for inhalational exposure to botulinum toxin are from a laboratory accident where individuals were exposed to a sublethal dose of serotype A *(29)*.

3.4.3. Ricin

Because of its relatively high toxicity and ease of production, the United States considered ricin for weaponization during its offensive biological warfare program. The US Chemical Warfare Service began studying ricin as a weapon toward the end of World War I and continued through World War II. It is still a threat biological agent of great concern to date.

Ricin is a potent cytotoxin derived from the beans of the castor plant *(Ricinus communis)*. Over 1 million tons of castor beans are processed annually in the production of castor oil, which is used for medicinal and industrial purposes including the production

Table 6
Botulinum Toxin, Rhesus Macaque Model

Serotype	Inhalational LD$_{50}$ (MIPLD$_{50}$/kg)^{a,b}
A	350
B	7500
C	331
D	1585
E	Inhalation lethality in nonhuman primates unknown
F	135
G	Inhalation lethality in nonhuman primates unknown

[a]MIPLD$_{50}$: Mouse intraperitoneal LD$_{50}$.
[b]US Army Research Institute of Infectious Diseases, unpublished data.

of aircraft and marine engine lubricants, dyes, and paints. The waste mash from this process is approx 5% ricin by weight. Consequently, large quantities of ricin are easily and inexpensively produced. The beans of *Ricinus communis* consists of two hemagglutinins and two toxins. These toxins are heterodimers consisting of a cytotoxic A chain and a B-chain that binds to externally located cellular membrane receptors and serves to transport the A-chain intracellularly. Ricin toxins are potent site-specific *N*-glycosidases that cleave A4324 of rRNA, which results in the inhibition of protein synthesis. Other reported enzymatic activities of this toxin may represent differences in experimental procedures or the presence of additional, contaminating enzymes. The toxin can be transmitted through contaminated food and water, percutaneously via small pellets/projectiles designed to carry toxins, or as a biological warfare aerosol.

3.4.4. C. perfringens

C. perfringens is an anaerobic Gram-positive spore-forming bacillus that produces at least 15 toxins. Virulence factors of the organism are responsible for various diseases to include gas gangrene, food poisoning, necrotic enteritis, and enterotoxemia *(30)*. Spores germinate after warming slowly at ambient temperature. The reservoir is soil and the gastrointestinal tract of healthy persons and animals. Gas gangrene results from wound contamination spores of *C. perfringen*s. Unlike *B. anthracis* spores, there is no apparent disease caused by inhaling spores. There have been rare case reports of pulmonary infections associated with *C. perfringens (31,32)*.

Aerosol challenges of *C. perfringens* toxin have been reported to produce lethal pulmonary disease in laboratory animals. The *C. perfringens* toxins are highly toxic phospholipases. The spores or vegetative organisms have not been shown to produce disease in healthy individuals after inhalation. The infective dose is unknown. Although wound gangrene is a concern, there is not an established threat from aerosol exposure and inhalation of these toxins.

3.4.5. T-2 Toxin (Trichothecene)

Acute toxicity by the inhalation route is similar to Lewisite (c.a. 10^3 mg-min/m^3), but T-2 is about 10 times more potent than liquid mustard [*bis*-(2-chloroethyl) sulfide] with dermal exposure *(14)*. The trichothecenes are considered primarily blister agents that cause severe skin and eye irritation at low exposure doses. The LD$_{50}$ for the mouse is estimated to be 0.24 mg/kg for the guinea pig and 0.05 mg/kg for the rat. Subacute exposure reduces host resistance to bacterial or parasitic infections. The mycotoxins are not considered established threat agents by aerosol exposure. Evaluation of this agent as potential threat blister agents is limited.

3.4.6. Bioregulators

Bioregulators are agents closely related to substances normally found in the body. They may be active at very low doses and frequently have rapid effects. Recombinant technology has been employed by the pharmaceutical industry to produce several of these agents in quantity. Bioregulators may pose a threat if employed alone or physically combined with other agents. As biological response modifiers, bioregulators also have been used to modify responses to other agents. An experimental example was the insertion of the gene for interleukin-4 into a mousepox virus to enhance the response to vaccines. The result was a virus that was far more deadly than the wild type *(33)*. Altering the human smallpox virus in the same manner may increase the lethality radically *(34)*. Two of the obstacles to the use of these agents have been the ability to produce them in large quantities and to stabilize them for weaponization. If these barriers are overcome, these agents may become a significant threat. Unlike many other biological agents, they often have immediate biological effects and are more potent than traditional chemical agents. The complexity of production and dissemination of these agents currently limits their application as weapons.

3.5. Contamination and Reaerosolization (Persistence of Agents)

Long-term survival of infectious agents, preservation of toxin activity, and the protective influence of dust particles onto which microorganisms adsorb when spread by aerosols have all been documented. The potential exists for the delayed generation of secondary aerosols from previously contaminated surfaces. This is particularly worrisome from casualties recently exposed near the dissemination source where high levels of contamination may occur. The data from the field trials with the BG stimulant (Bacillus subtilis var. niger, formerly *Bacillus globigii* or BG simulant) were also used to model the re-aerosolization hazard posed by *C. burnetii*. The two biological agents considered in this document that pose a significant threat hazardous re-aerosolization are *B. anthracis* dry spores and *C. burnetii*. Inhaled spores of *B. anthracis* (LD_{50} 55,000) are highly virulent although the infectivity is moderate to high. Viable spores can persist in the environment for decades under ideal soil conditions. Only when the organism is exposed to oxygen does sporulation occur, and the pathogenic bacillus is produced. *C. burnetii* (ID_{50} c.a. 30) is a rickettsia-like organism with low virulence but remarkable infectivity. It forms a spore-like organism that is extremely heat-, pressure-, desiccation-, and antiseptic-resistant and can persist in the environment for weeks to months under harsh conditions. The primary mode of transmission is inhalation.

3.6. Cutaneous and Percutaneous Threat

With the exception of the trichothecenes, biological agents do not pose a threat because of percutaneous exposure. Dermal manifestations may be useful in the diagnosis and recognition of potential mass threat agent exposure *(35)*. To a lesser extent, particles may adhere to an individual or to clothing creating additional but less significant exposure hazards.

3.7. Person-to-Person (Communicable) Spread

Numerous agents may be transmitted through contact with biological material (e.g., tissue, blood, urine, and placentas) or resuspension of the agent in an aerosol. Kruse *(36)* reviewed cross-infection with various pathogens. *Brucella* and *C. burnetii* are two agents frequently spread by inhalation of resuspended organisms. Person-to-person aerosol spread represents the greatest communicable disease threat. Exposed hosts could readily become a secondary source of dissemination for some agents such as plague or smallpox. As recently as 1979 a case of smallpox contracted through aerosol exposure was reported *(37)*. Henderson *(38)* has reviewed smallpox as a biological weapon. Because of the aerosol threat, specific recommendations regarding smallpox include postexposure isolation and infection control, hospital epidemiology, and decontamination of the environment. Similarly, Inglesby has reviewed the medical and public health management concerns if *Y. pestis* (plague) were used as a biological weapon *(39)*. Again, because of the threat of aerosol spread, safety precautions to limit exposure from plague-infected patients include postexposure isolation and infection control, hospital epidemiology, and decontamination of the environment *(40)*. Although little is known regarding the filovirus aerosol infection risk for humans, there seems to be little risk for filovirus infections after an adequate quarantine period. There are indications that Ebola can be transmitted through aerosol exposure *(41,42)*. There are also indications that Marburg may be spread by aerosol in laboratory animals *(20,43)*.

3.8. Infection of Indigenous Vectors

Indigenous hosts and vectors for certain agents may result in increased occurrences of endemic disease. The required natural expansion of the host and vector populations would limit occurrences of epidemic disease. Examples include the release of agents such as the encephalitis viruses (VEE, EEE, and WEE) or *Y. pestis* in areas supporting their natural disease cycle.

4. FUTURE IMPLICATIONS OF NEAR-TERM ADVANCES IN BIOTECHNOLOGY

Naturally occurring biological agents are the best starting point for credible biological weapons. Advances in aerosol technology that may impact the future of biological threat agents center around the stabilization of biological aerosols, genetic alteration to stabilize threat agents, and the availability of threat agents. The first two areas impact on agent stability during storage, dissemination, and in the environment. Some organisms such as anthrax naturally form infectious spores, allowing the organism to survive in the environment under certain conditions for decades. The spores can be lyophilized, milled into a powder of 1–5 μm particles, and stored for many years. Few other agents can withstand this process. Lyophilized *Brucella* bacteria have been stored for several years and remained active; similar results have been obtained with *C. burnetii*. SEB has retained activity in the lyophilized state for decades. Many agents cannot withstand the process or lose potency quickly thereafter.

4.1. Stabilization of Aerosols

Microencapsulation is a current commercial process that has been employed to coat and stabilize many biologics for therapeutic application. This is a concept that may be subject to adversarial misuse with biological warfare agents. Other possible abuses of current technology may include such approaches as the genomic alteration of *B. anthracis* or another *Bacillus* spore former and *Variola major*, allowing the spore to serve as a vector for other agents. This could stabilize storage and delivery and allow for the incorporation of a multitude of agents. Other aspects of genetics that are subject to abuse include increasing agent infectivity/toxicity, genetic stabilization of replicating or nonreplicating agents, or the production of chimeric toxins.

4.2. Availability, Infectivity, Virulence, and Toxicity

Natural selection or advances in our understanding of biological processes may lead to new threats. If the speculative bacterial origin of agents such as tetrodotoxin and saxitoxin is definitively identified, then means of production in large quantities may become practical *(44,45)*. Emerging technologies may also pose the threat of increased biological agent availability. Genetic alteration to animals, bacteria, yeast, or plants to expression of proteins in large quantities are such technologies. In recent years, there has been great interest by the pharmaceutical industry in transgenic plants as photosynthetic bioreactors for large-scale production of quality bioactive proteins *(46)*. This has allowed for the production of large quantities of materials with potential clinical application but is also subject to misuse. Recombinant technology also allows for alteration of the threat agent in numerous ways that make it more infective, virulent, or toxic as with the case of mousepox mentioned earlier in the discussion of bioregulators.

5. CONCLUSIONS

Many agents, including bacteria, viruses, and toxins, can be used as biological weapons, but they do not necessarily need to be highly lethal to be effective. For practical, political, and moral reasons, incapacitation may be all that is necessary to cause the intended effect. The fact that biological weapons may also be used in combination with other types of weapons or to add to the disruption they produce cannot be underestimated. The inhalation of biological aerosols is by far the most important consideration when planning defenses against biological warfare attacks. Emerging capabilities that increase the threat from aerosol exposure include enhancements in agent transmissibility (packaging and delivery vehicles) and environmental stability. With the advent of genetic engineering, the ability to hide and transmit pathogens inside other organisms represents a modern technological threat.

Knowledge gaps are common where there are breaches in information regarding exposure levels among the biological agents and may include the following. The following areas hold the greatest potential for productive collaborative efforts resulting in information with long-term benefits in the development of medical countermeasures.

5.1. Detection and Diagnostics, Sensitivity, and Specificity

Field-portable systems that can detect all biological agents of interest are not available. For toxins, current deployable methods are effective at detecting in the nanogram/milliliter levels. Potentially lethal and low-level exposures could be missed. Gene amplification and detection have now been integrated portable nucleic acid analysis system and are sensitive when used for replicating agents but have limited value for toxins. Early warning capabilities will further strain the sensitivity requirements of field-portable systems.

Applied systems must also have low false-positive rates (high specificity). In contrast to sensitivity, biological agents at low levels are difficult to measure and discriminate from naturally occurring background materials. Detection of biological agents in the environment is the complicated by the myriad of similar organisms or material that are a presence.

5.2. Battlefield-Relevant Levels of Exposure

As discussed in this chapter, effect exposure levels may be estimated experimentally in various biologic models. The relevance to levels that may be attained on a battlefield has not been thoroughly investigated. It is for these levels that medical countermeasures must be developed. This has necessitated estimates of levels of exposure on the battlefield over a wide range of scenarios to include exposures that individuals are unlikely to exceed *(16)*. These estimated values then have been used to assess the potential health risks to exposed individuals *(11)*. With some important exceptions already mentioned, most biological agents decay rapidly once dispersed and exposed to the environment (e.g., dehydration, ambient ultraviolet [UV] light).

5.3. Low-Level Acute Exposure Effect (Near- and Long-Term)

The near- or long-term effects of nonlethal or low-level exposure to biological agents have been given little attention. For example, the effects that SEB has on the immune system have been systematically investigated. Low-level exposure may incapacitate to varying levels. The effect this has on susceptibility to endemic disease or amplification of the effects of other biological threats has not been sufficiently addressed. Another example is the toxin, ricin were the effects of acute lethal aerosol exposure to have been reported in several animal models *(47,48)*. With aerosol exposure the lung is the target organ for this toxin. Sublethal exposure causes pulmonary pathology (unreported data, US Army Medical Research Institute of Infectious Diseases). The acute incapacitating effects or long-term resolution of pathology are not known.

5.4. Model Systems That Emulate Human Exposure, Pathogenesis, and Resulting Disease

Limited human data exists for human aerosol exposure to potential biological agents (e.g., anthrax, plague, VEE) and may be used for comparison. When developing comparative animal models, considerations must be given to an agent's pathophysiologic mechanism and how well the substitute model predicts disease or toxicosis in humans. Modeling the human respiratory system is of particular importance with aerosol exposures *(49,50)*.

5.5. Exposure Levels for Treatment (Pre- or Postexposure) Breakthrough

As relevant battlefield exposure levels are determined, the efficacy of pre- and postexposure medical countermeasures must be resolved to include the limitation of protection or treatment provided. This has been done to a limited degree for vaccine candidates to protect against some agents such as the botulinum neurotoxin *(51–53)* and SEB *(54,55)*. For most proposed vaccines and treatments, this has not been comprehensively examined. As model systems that emulate human exposure become available, passive transfer of protection will provide one means of evaluation, particularly in vaccine candidates for medical countermeasures in which the importance of antibodies for protection has been established. With agents such as anthrax, this is of particular importance as predicted aerosol exposure levels may be hundreds or thousands of LD_{50}. In cases such as this, human challenge protection studies and field efficacy trials are not feasible in studying vaccine candidates. Comparisons of immune responses in human cohorts receiving vaccines using animal challenge and protection studies against spores will be important for new vaccines based on protein antigens inducing protective antibodies.

ACKNOWLEDGMENTS

The information contained in this chapter was, in large part, extracted from contributions by the authors to a NATO Long-Term Strategic Study on Defense Aspects of Chemical and Biological Warfare.

REFERENCES

1. Burrows, W. D. and Renner, S. E. (1999) Biological warfare agents as threats to potable water. *Environ. Health Perspect.* **107,** 975–984.
2. NATO. (1999) *Medical Planning Guide for the Estimation of NBC Battle Casualties, Biological AMed P-8(A)*, Volume II, Ratification Draft 1. North Atlantic Treaty Organization (NATO).
3. Macintyre, A. G., Christopher, G. W., Eitzen, E., Jr., et al. (2000) Weapons of mass destruction events with contaminated casualties: effective planning for health care facilities. *JAMA* **283,** 242–249.
4. Voelker, R. (2002) Bioweapons preparedness chief discusses priorities in world of 21st-century biology. *JAMA* **287,** 573–576.
5. Waeckerle, J. F. (2002) Domestic preparedness for events involving weapons of mass destruction. *JAMA* **283,** 252–254.
6. Webb, S. J. (1963) Factors affecting the viability of air-borne bacteria. *Can. J. Biochem.* **41,** 867–873.
7. Stephenson, E. H., Larson, E. W., and Dominik, J. W. (1984) Effect of environmental factors on aerosol-induced lassa virus infection. *J. Med. Virol.* **14,** 295–303.
8. Harper, G. J. (1961) Airborne micro-organisms: survival tests with four viruses. *J. Hyg. Cambridge* **59,** 479–486.
9. Goldberg, L. J., Watkins, H. M. S., Boerke, E. E., and Chatgny, M. A. (1958) The use of a rotating drum for the study of aerosols over extended periods of time. *Am. J. Hyg.* **68,** 85–93.
10. Bide, R. W., Armour, S. J., (2000) Yee, E. Allometric respiration/body mass data for animals to be used for estimates of inhalation toxicity to young adult humans. *J. Appl. Toxicol.* **20,** 273–290.
11. FM 8-9, *NATO handbook on the medical aspects of NBC defensive operations AMedP-6(B)*, Part II Biological. Dept. Army, 1996.
12. Ferguson, J. R. (1997) Biological weapons and US law. *JAMA* **278,** 357–360.
13. Spertzel, R. O., Wannemacher, R. W., Patrick, W. C., Linden, C. D., and Franz, D. R. (1992) *Technical ramifications of inclusion of toxins in the chemical weapons convention (CWC)*. Frederick: US Army Medical Research Institute of Infectious Diseases.
14. Wannemacher, R. W. and Wiener, S. L. (1997) Trichothecene mycotoxins, in: *Textbook of Military Medicine: Medical Aspects of Chemical and Biological Warfare*. (Zatjchuk, R., ed.), Borden Institute, Washington, D.C., pp. 658.

15. Henderson, D. A. (1999) The looming threat of bioterrorism. *Science* **283,** 1279–1282.
16. Bauer, T. J. and Gibbs, R. L. (1994) *Software users manual for the chemical/biological agent vapor, liquid, and solid tracking (VLSTRACK) computer model.* 2.0 ed. Dahlgren, VA: Naval Surface Weapons Center.
17. Guyton, A. C. (1947) Measurement of the respiratory volumes of laboratory animals. *Am. J. Physiol.* **150,** 70–77.
18. Tucker, J. B. (1999) Historical trends related to bioterrorism: an empirical analysis. *Emerg. Infect. Dis.* **5,** 498–504.
19. Hurst, E. W. (1936) Infection of Rhesus monkey (*Macaca mulatta*) and the guinea-pig with the virus equine encephalomyelitis. *J. Pathol. Bacteriol.* **42,** 271–302.
20. Lub, M., Sergeev, A. N., P'yankova, O. G., P'yankov, O. V., Petrishchenko, V. A., and Kotyarov, L. A. (1996) Clinical and virological characterization of the disease in guinea pigs aerogenically infected with marburg virus. *Russian Prog. Virol.* **3,** 34–37.
21. Jahrling, P. J. (1997) Viral hemorrhagic fevers, in: *Textbook of Military Medicine: Medical Aspects of Chemical and Biological Warfare.* (Zatjchuk, R., ed.), Borden Institute, Washington, D.C., pp. 591–602.
22. Friedlander, A. M. (1997) Anthraxin, in: *Textbook of Military Medicine: Medical Aspects of Chemical and Biological Warfare.* (Zatjchuk, R., ed.), Borden Institute, Washington, D.C., pp. 467–478.
23. Abramova, F. A., Grinberg, L. M., Yampolskaya, O. V., and Walker, D. H. (1993) Pathology of inhalational anthrax in 42 cases from the Sverdlovsk outbreak of 1979. *Proc. Natl. Acad. Sci. USA* **90,** 2291–2294.
24. Grinberg, L. M., Abramova, F. A., Yampolskaya, O. V., Walker, D. H., and Smith, J. H. (2001) Quantitative pathology of inhalational anthrax I: quantitative microscopic findings. *Mod. Pathol.* **14,** 482–495.
25. Franz, D. R. and Zajtchuk, R. (2000) Biological terrorism: understanding the threat, preparation, and medical response. *Disease-a-month* **46,** 129–192.
26. Inglesby, T. V., O'Toole, T., Henderson, D. A., et al. (2002) Anthrax as a biological weapon, 2002; updated recommendation for management. *JAMA* **287,** 2236–2252.
27. Lincoln, R. E., Walker, J. S., Klein, F., Rosenwald, A. J., and Jones, W. I. J. (1967) Value of field data or extrapolation in anthrax. *Fed. Proc.* **26,** 1558–1562.
28. Lebeda, F. J. (1997) Deterrence of biological and chemical warfare: a review of policy options. *Mil. Med.* **162,** 156–161.
29. Holzer, E. (1962) Botulism caused by inhalation. *Med. Klin.* **41,** 1735–1740.
30. Rood, J. I., McClane, B. A., Songer, J. G., and Titball, R. W. (1997) *The Clostridia. Molecular Biology and Pathogenesis of the Clostridia.* Academic, London.
31. Baldwin, L., Henderson, A., Wright, M., and Whitby, M. (1993) Spontaneous *Clostridium perfringens* lung abscess unresponsive to penicillin. *Anaesth. Intensive Care* **21,** 117–119.
32. Kwan, W. C., Lam, S. C., Chow, A. W., Lepawski, M., and Glanzberg, M. M. (1983) Empyema caused by *Clostridium perfringens. Can. Med. Assoc. J.* **128,** 1420–1422.
33. Jackson, R. J., Ramsay, A. J., Christensen, C. D., Beaton, S., Hall, D. F., and Ramshaw, I. A. (2001) Expression of mouse interleukin-4 by a recombinant ectromelia virus suppresses cytolytic lymphocyte responses and overcomes genetic resistance to mousepox. *J. Virol.* **75,** 1205–1210.
34. Stephenson, J. (2001) Biowarfare warning. *JAMA* **285,** 725.
35. Cross, J. T. and Altemeier, W. A. (2000) Skin manifestations of bioterrorism. *Pediatr. Ann.* **29,** 7–9.
36. Kruse, R. H. and Wedum, A. G. (1970) Cross infection with eighteen pathogens among caged laboratory animals. *Lab. Anim. Care* **20,** 541–558.
37. Hawkes, N. (1979) Science in Europe: smallpox death in Britain challenges presumptions of laboratory safety. *Science* **203,** 855,856.

38. Henderson, D. A., Inglesby, T. V., Bartlett, J. G., et al. (1999)Smallpox as a biological weapon: medical and public health management. Working Group on Civilian Biodefense. *JAMA* **281,** 2127–2137.
39. Inglesby, T. V., Dennis, D. T., Henderson, D. A., et al. (2000) Plague as a biological weapon: medical and public health management. Working Group on Civilian Biodefense. *JAMA* **283,** 2281–2290.
40. Inglesby, T. V., Henderson, D. A., O'Toole, T., and Dennis, D. T. (2000) Safety precautions to limit exposure from plague-infected patients. *JAMA* **284,** 1648,1649.
41. Jaax, N., Jahrling, P., Geisbert, T., et al. (1995) Transmission of Ebola virus (Zaire strain) to uninfected control monkeys in a biocontainment laboratory. *Lancet* **346,** 1669–1671.
42. Johnson, E., Jaax, N., White, J., and Jahrling, P. (1995) Lethal experimental infections of rhesus monkeys by aerosolized Ebola virus. *Int. J. Exp. Pathol.* **76,** 227–236.
43. Bazhutin, N. B., Belanov, E. F., Spirdonov, V. A., et al. (1992) The influence of the methods of experimental infection with marburg virus on the course of illness in green monkeys. *Vopr. Virusol.* **3,** 153–156.
44. Kodama, M., Ogata, T., and Sato, S. (1988) Bacterial production of saxitoxin. *Agric. Biol. Chem.* **52,** 1075–1077.
45. Kodama, M., Ogata, T., Sakamoto, S., Honda, T., and Miwatani, T. (1990) Production of paralytic shellfish toxins by a bacterium *Moraxella sp.* isolated from *Protogonyaulax tamarensis. Toxicon* **28,** 707–714.
46. Finer, J. J. (1999) Plant protein secretion on tap. *Nat. Biotechnol.* **17,** 427.
47. Wilhelmsen, C. L. and Pitt, M. L. (1996) Lesions of acute inhaled lethal ricin intoxication in rhesus monkeys. *Vet. Pathol.* **33,** 296–302.
48. Brown, R. F. and White, D. E. Ultrastructure of rat lung following inhalation of ricin aerosol. *Int. J. Exp. Pathol.* **78,** 267–276.
49. Zhang, Z. and Kleinstreuer, C. Effect of particle inlet distributions on deposition in a triple bifurcation lung airway model. *J. Aerosol Med.* **14,** 13–29.
50. Zhang, Z., Kleinstreuer, C., and Kim, C. S. (2000) Effects of asymmetric branch flow rates on aerosol deposition in bifurcating airways. *J. Med. Eng. Technol.* **24,** 192–202.
51. Gelzleichter, T. R., Myers, M. A., Menton, R. G., Niemuth, N. A., Matthews, M. C., and Langford, M. J. (1999) Protection against botulinum toxins provided by passive immunization with botulinum human immune globulin: evaluation using an inhalation model. *J. Appl. Toxicol.* **19(Suppl 1),** S35–38.
52. Byrne, M. P. and Smith, L. A. (2000) Development of vaccines for prevention of botulism. *Biochimie* **82,** 955–966.
53. Byrne, M. P., Titball, R. W., Holley, J., and Smith, L. A. (2000) Fermentation, purification, and efficacy of a recombinant vaccine candidate against botulinum neurotoxin type F from *Pichia pastoris. Protein Expr. Purif.* **18,** 327–337.
54. LeClaire, R. D., Hunt, R. E., and Bavari, S. (2002) Protection against bacterial superantigen staphylococcal enterotoxin B by passive vaccination. *Infect. Immun.* **70,** 2278–2281.
55. Bavari, S., Ulrich, R. G., and LeClaire, R. D. (1999) Cross-reactive antibodies prevent the lethal effects of *Staphylococcus aureus* superantigens. *J. Infect. Dis.* **180,** 1365–1369.

PART II

MEDICAL COUNTERMEASURES AND DECONTAMINATION

4

Pathogenesis by Aerosol

M. Louise M. Pitt and Ross D. LeClaire

1. INTRODUCTION

Aerosols are the most likely and effective mode of dissemination of a bioterrorist agent whether it is a toxin or a bacterial or viral agent. The ideal biological threat agent would be delivered in a particle size that would allow it to persist suspended in the air for long periods of time and be inhaled deeply into the lungs of unsuspecting victims. The size range of particles that meet both of these criteria is 1–5 µm in diameter.

The diseases and toxicities associated with biological threat agents are usually either extremely rare (inhalational anthrax or pneumonic plague) or do not exist outside of the threat. In addition, the aerosol route is not the natural route of infection or intoxication (staphylococcal enterotoxin B and botulinum neurotoxins). Consequently, data from human cases are usually very scarce, and knowledge of human susceptibility and the pathogenesis of the human disease are minimal. The ability to evaluate the efficacy of potential medical countermeasures in the human population is rarely possible because of all these circumstances. Thus, we are dependent on animal models of disease for elucidating the pathogenesis and for both developing and testing medical countermeasures.

The choice of the appropriate animal model for each specific threat agent is extremely important but very difficult. Ideally, the disease process in the animal should be identical to that in humans. However, the susceptibility of animals to specific threat agents may vary several orders of magnitude across species and strains. Additionally, we must consider certain medical implications of aerosol exposure. The disease or toxicity is highly dependent on the aerosol characteristics, namely particle size. The deposition distribution of the agent in the respiratory tract affects the disease process; transport and clearance mechanisms differ in the various regions of the respiratory tract and, thus, impact the resultant pathogenesis or toxicity *(1)*.

Determining the appropriate basis on which to extrapolate dose across species presents a significant challenge. Animal-to-human extrapolations require dosimetric adjustment. An assumption is made that the effects in the experimental model are relevant to humans and that a common biological metric exists to allow equating biological effects across species *(2,3)*. Prediction of medical exposure risk based on experimental animal models is often extremely imprecise and difficult to validate.

From: *Infectious Diseases: Biological Weapons Defense: Infectious Diseases and Counterterrorism*
Edited by: L. E. Lindler, F. J. Lebeda, and G. W. Korch © Humana Press Inc., Totowa, NJ

This chapter discusses disease models for specific bioterrorist threat agents delivered by aerosol, in terms of deposition in the lung, particle size inhaled, whether route of infection/intoxication changes disease pathogenesis, and development of immunity.

2. INHALED AEROSOLS

The aerosol threat associated with inhalation of various biological agents is dependent on the characteristics of the aerosol, the physical and physiological characteristics of the individual, and the response by the individual to the aerosol exposure.

During inhalation (and exhalation) a portion of the inhaled aerosols may deposit on airway surfaces or be transferred to unexhaled air. The remainder is exhaled. The portion transferred to unexhaled air may, in turn, either be deposited in the airways or later exhaled *(4)*. These phenomena are complicated by interactions that may occur between possible deliquescent or hygroscopic particles and the water vapor present in the humid airways. Deposition can be defined as the quantity of inhaled airborne particles that are never exhaled but are deposited on surfaces in the respiratory airways *(5,6)*. Once deposited, clearance mechanisms are initiated. During clearance, inhaled particles can be translocated, transformed, and removed from the respiratory tract and then from the body *(7,8)*. Some particles are not cleared and, thus, are retained with-in the lungs *(9,10)*.

Therefore, the behavior and fate of inhaled airborne particles depends on not only the physical characteristics of the particles themselves but also on the nature of the airflow within the respiratory tract *(11,12)*. Knowledge of the anatomy of the respiratory tract is important in the consideration of the fate of inhaled particles.

2.1. The Human Respiratory Tract

The respiratory tract can be subdivided conveniently into three main regions called the nasopharyngeal (NP), the tracheobronchial (TB), and the pulmonary *(13)*. Figure 1 shows a general diagram of the human respiratory tract.

2.1.1. Nasopharyngeal Region

The NP region extends from the nostrils through the nasal passages, nasopharynx and hypopharynx to the larynx. The nasal passages are lined, except at the anterior end, with a vascular mucous membrane characterized by ciliated columnar epithelium and scattered mucous glands. In addition to warming and humidifying the incoming air, these nasal passages act as a filter for removing larger particles whose inertial properties cause impaction in the nasal passages or entrapment by the nasal hairs *(14)*. Experimental data indicate that the anterior one-third of the nose, where 80% of 7-μm diameter particles deposit, does not clear except by blowing, wiping, or other extrinsic means *(15)* and effective removal of insoluble particles may require 1–2 d. The posterior portions of the nose have mucociliary clearance, with half-times of about 6–7 h *(11,16)*.

2.1.2. Tracheobronchial Region

The TB region consists of the trachea and the ciliated bronchial airways down to and including the terminal bronchioles. A relatively small portion of all sizes of particles that pass through the NP region will deposit in the TB region *(17,18)*. Inertial impaction at bifurcations, sedimentation, and, for some small particles, Brownian movement

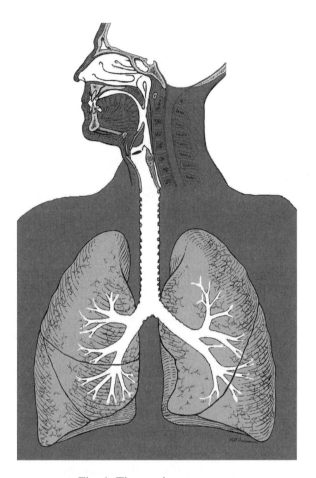

Fig. 1. The respiratory tract.

cause TB deposition *(19)*. Relatively soluble material may rapidly enter the blood circulation. The TB region is both ciliated and equipped with mucous-secreting elements so that clearance of deposited particles occurs rapidly by mucociliary action upward to the throat for swallowing. Particles depositing in the TB tree are probably distributed differently with respect to size, with smaller particles depositing deeper in the lungs. Thus, the clearance of particles from this region will vary, half-times being of the order of 0.5–5 h, with very little persisting for longer than 24 h *(18,20,21)*.

2.1.3. Pulmonary Region

The pulmonary region includes the respiratory bronchioles, alveolar ducts, alveolar sacs, atria, and alveoli, all the functional gas exchange sites of the lungs. Its surface consists of nonciliated epithelium with different secretory elements to those found in the TB region *(22)*. For particles to reach and deposit in this region, they must penetrate the NP and TB regions on inspiration and come into contact with pulmonary surfaces either by settling, diffusion, or interception. Smaller particles are of primary importance in pulmonary deposition *(23,24)*. Clearance for this region involves several mechanisms, including (a) dissolution of soluble material with absorption into the systemic circulation; (b) direct passage of particle into blood; (c) phagocytosis of particles by macrophages with translocation to the ciliated airways; and (d) transfer of particles to the lymphatic system including lymph nodes *(25–28)*.

2.2. Immunological Structure of Respiratory Tract

Immunologically, the respiratory system may be divided into two main compartments, the upper and lower respiratory tract. The upper region includes the NP and TB regions. These airways are covered predominantly by a ciliated epithelium, which overlies organized structures within the submucosa, including secretory glands and collections of lymphoid cells.

In this upper region, the majority of lymphoid tissue is most often associated with the large- and medium-sized airways. This tissue is organized into nodules and follicles, similar to those found in lymph nodes; however, it lacks a surrounding capsule *(29)*. This airway-associated lymphoid tissue is known as bronchus-associated lymphoid tissue *(30–32)*.

The lower respiratory tract (pulmonary region) is devoid of any organized lymphoid tissue. At the transition from the TB region to the pulmonary region, the mucosal surface gives way to a single layer of nonciliated epithelium overlying an interstitium composed of loose connective tissue, pulmonary capillaries, lymphatic vessels, and scattered lymphoid cells. Lymphoid cells are found in interstitial tissues or as free cells in the alveoli. These cells are capable of participating in specific and nonspecific immune responses and may form transient lymphoid aggregates upon stimulation from foreign antigenic material *(33)*.

2.3. Immunology of the Respiratory Tract

The nasopharyngeal mucous membranes, which comprise the largest mucosal epithelial surface of the body, line the entry of the respiratory tract and are in continual contact with the external environment. Pathogens and toxins encounter this thin, specialized mucosal epithelium upon inhalation, and this epithelium is the site of initial host–pathogen interactions with cellular and secretory components of the respiratory system *(34)*. Adequate surface protection, (prevention of invasion), depends on intimate cooperation between natural nonspecific defense mechanisms and acquired specific immunity *(35,36)*.

Nonspecific and specific immune responses provide important mechanisms for host resistance to pathogens in the lungs *(37)*. These responses occur largely within the airways, in relation to mucosal surfaces of the airways, adluminally in the pulmonary parenchyma, or in discrete lymph nodes associated with the respiratory tract *(29,33)*.

Immunological mechanisms of host resistance may be associated with cells or their secretory products. Various enzymes, cytokines, or antibodies may alter the pathogenesis of and/or provide nonspecific resistance to an agent introduced through the respiratory tract. Nonspecific cellular resistance is often mediated by neutrophil or macrophage phagocytosis of a pathogen. Macrophages previously activated because of a specific or nonspecific stimulus can protect against an unrelated foreign agent.

Specific immune responses either induced by prior vaccination or after challenge with foreign materials can result in antibody production and cell-mediated immunity *(38,39)*. In contrast to nonspecific immunity, specific immune responses require a longer time to develop fully, however, they can provide effective and longlasting protection *(40)*. Specific immunity in the respiratory tract to a specific foreign antigen may result either from introduction of antigen into an immunocompetent host at sites distal to the lungs (parenteral delivery) or from direct delivery of antigen to the respiratory tract (mucosal/deep lung targeting via intranasal or aerosol delivery).

3. PROTECTION BY VACCINATION

Parenteral inoculation is the most common route of vaccination, but it is an ineffective method of eliciting immunity at mucosal surfaces. Most biological agents of concern as bioterrorist threats utilize the mucosa as the portal of entry or as the initial site of colonization. Once agents penetrate the mucosal barrier, they are disseminated throughout the systemic circulation. This is especially true for aerosol-delivered threat agents.

3.1. Advantages of Local Immunity in Lungs for Bioterrorist Threats

The majority of biological threat agents do not require mucosal immunity to convey protection. However, local immune responses in the lungs, either mucosal in the upper respiratory region or a combination of mucosal and systemic in the lower region, could potentially neutralize the agent at the site of entry into the body before invasion and prevent disease.

However, there are some threat agents that appear to require mucosal immunity for protection. Although parenterally administered staphylococcal enterotoxin (SE) vaccine candidates protected rhesus monkeys from lethal SE type B (SEB) challenges, several animals experienced incapacitating signs after toxin challenge *(41,42)*. Existing data suggest mucosal and systemic immunity are required to prevent lethality as well as incapacitation caused by SE exposure. Mice vaccinated intranasally with SE vaccines were protected from inhalation and intraperitoneal toxin challenges and demonstrated levels of mucosal antibodies significantly higher than levels in mice vaccinated intramuscularly *(43)*. A mucosal respiratory immune response may improve vaccine efficacy by providing immunity at the portal of agent entry.

Protection from alphaviruses naturally transmitted from mosquitoes is believed to be primarily antibody-mediated. However, the association between circulating neutralizing antibody titers and protection from aerosol exposures has not been consistent. After exposure to infectious Venezuelan equine encephalitis (VEE) virus aerosols, the nasal epithelium, nasal-associated lymphoid tissue, and olfactory regions of mice are rapidly infected and viral antigens are found in the brain within 24 h *(44)*. Protection from VEE virus aerosols may be mediated by antibodies, virus-specific IgA, along the respiratory tract *(45,46)*.

Aerosols greater than 5 μm will deposit deep in the lungs where antigen is taken up by dendritic cells and macrophages resident in the interstitium or free in the alveolar spaces. Some will be transported by the draining lymphatics to the bloodstream and thus to the spleen, whereas some will remain in the lung interstitium and initiate local immunity. Thus, both a local and a systemic immune response will be produced.

There is a definite need for vaccination strategies that minimize and simplify dosing and scheduling, utilize multivalent vaccines, and employ inoculation methods other than the conventional needle delivery. Inhalation and intranasal strategies may provide more rapid protective immunity both locally in the lung and systemically. Indeed, transdermal or oral vaccination strategies may provide safer and more efficacious methods for stimulating both mucosal and systemic immunity.

4. DEPOSITION: HUMANS VS LABORATORY ANIMALS

Our reliance on data collected from animal experiments is essential for understanding the pathogenesis of diseases caused by biological threat agents. Thus, it is important to recognize the limitations of the animal model. Deposition and clearance of inhaled particles are likely to differ when comparing humans to laboratory animals. One of the major factors controlling the net dose delivered is the minute ventilation; therefore, small animals will receive a higher total dose because of their higher ventilation-to-body-weight ratios. In addition, there is variation even between animals of the same species, and deposition sites will vary despite similar particle size being used *(19)*. Smaller animals have a greater probability of retaining inhaled particles. For example, a 2-µm particle has the same probability of being retained in the mouse nose as an 8-µm particle in humans. The larger the particles are above 3 µm, the more chance of difference in regional deposition with humans. Total net dose may be the same, but biological effects may be different because the deposition sites and clearance rates are different. Clearance rates vary widely between species, in general, clearance in rats and mice is faster than in humans, monkeys, or guinea pigs *(3)*.

4.1. Effects of Particle Size on Infection

The disease or toxicity resulting from exposure to a biological threat agent delivered by aerosol is highly dependent on the particle size. Particle size impacts on the site of deposition in the respiratory tract. The deposition distribution dictates which transport and clearance mechanisms go into play and thus has a major effect on the pathogenesis or toxicity of the agent.

The importance of the site of deposition of inhaled particles in relation to infectivity is shown by the following examples: The dose of *Yersinia pestis*, the causative agent of plague, required to produce 50% lethality increases 2.5 times when the particle size increases from 1 to 12 µm; the dose of *Bacillus anthracis*, the causative agent of anthrax, increase 17 times; and dose of *Brucella suis* increases 600 times *(47–49)*.

In addition, disease caused by inhalation of a 1-µm particle size aerosol containing *B. anthracis*, is a systemic disease with mediastinal lymph node involvement, whereas inhaling 12 µm results in a localized infection with massive edema of the face and head. With *Y. pestis*, a 1-µm particle inhalation leads to primary pneumonic plague but 12 µm results in septicemia with hemorrhagic infarction in the lung.

Particle size also affects the toxicity of inhaled toxins. The toxicity of ricin increases as the mass median aerosol diameter of the particle diminishes. This is emphasized by the fact that intratracheal delivery of ricin is highly toxic whereas intranasal delivery has very low toxicity *(50)*.

5. ANIMAL-TO-HUMAN EXTRAPOLATION

The aerosol route of exposure to biological threat agents is often unnatural, the disease or intoxication is frequently life-threatening with no available licensed treatment, and the incidence of the naturally occurring disease is rare. Therefore, in the development of countermeasures, we commonly rely on animal models for the human disease. Determining the appropriate basis on which to extrapolate dose across species presents a significant challenge. Ideally, the pathogenesis of disease mimics that seen in humans, however, lack of human data often makes comparison with the animal model speculative. Additionally, anatomical differences (e.g., respiratory tract deposition distribution) and agent potency may vary several orders of magnitude across species and strains.

Nevertheless, we have to demonstrate efficacy of either a prophylactic or a therapeutic in appropriate animal models for the human disease against a relevant aerosol challenge and identify surrogate markers of efficacy that can be measured in humans. These data will then be used to license products to protect humans in the absence of human efficacy.

Aerosol studies performed in a laboratory have very stringent parameters in place to control the exposures. Temperature, humidity, and particle size are tightly controlled and the agent is freshly prepared. This is required for good scientific studies but complicates extrapolation to a field setting.

The following examples demonstrate not only the problems associated with the enormous challenge of using surrogate endpoints in animal models to show product efficacy but also the limitations of aerosol data generated in a well-defined environment.

5.1. Bacillus anthracis

Anthrax, the disease caused by *B. anthracis*, is an ancient disease of animals and humans that has been extensively studied over several decades. Despite this, the animal model most appropriate for extrapolation to humans remains uncertain for various of reasons. The limited available information on inhalational anthrax in humans makes a comparison with animal model data difficult. In addition, animal species differ in their natural resistance to the disease and a precise mechanism of death has yet to be established. However, the majority of knowledge of the pathogenesis of this disease comes from animal studies. Inhaled spores are phagocytosed by macrophages and carried in lymphatics to the draining tracheobronchial lymph nodes. The spores germinate and bacilli grow and spread to the mediastinal nodes, surrounding tissue, and systemic circulation thus seeding multiple organs.

The principal animal models used in laboratory investigations of experimental anthrax have been mice, rats, guinea pigs, rabbits, and rhesus macaques. The rhesus macaque has been considered an appropriate model for testing vaccine efficacy against inhalational anthrax *(51)*. The disease induced by respiratory exposure to spores of a virulent strain of *B. anthracis* is a rapidly fatal illness, with death occurring between days 2 and 7 postexposure. In addition, rhesus macaques inoculated with two doses of the licensed vaccine anthrax vaccine adsorbed (BioThrax) were protected against a lethal aerosol challenge of anthrax spores for up to 2 yr *(52)*.

Mouse strains differ significantly in their innate susceptibility to lethal infection by both a fully virulent strain and the nonencapsulated Sterne vaccine strain. The capsule appears to be of extraordinary importance as a virulence factor. Although capsule positive toxin minus strains are avirulent in guinea pigs, they are virulent for mice *(53)*. After vaccination with the licensed anthrax vaccine, AVA, mice are not protected against fully virulent organisms *(54)*.

Rats are resistant to *B. anthracis* infection but sensitive to toxin *(55)*. Vaccinating the naturally resistant rat results in only a slight increase in resistance to spore challenge *(56)*. Guinea pigs have been used extensively to test the immunogenicity of anthrax vaccines. AVA protects guinea pigs against a parenteral spore challenge but only partially protects them against a lethal aerosol spore challenge. The guinea pig is not a good predictor of vaccine efficacy compared to the rhesus macaque *(57)*.

Rabbits also have been used historically for anthrax research. These animals are sensitive to anthrax and are a good comparative predictor for vaccine efficacy in the rhesus monkey. AVA is efficacious in rabbits given two doses of the vaccine *(58)*.

The pathology of anthrax infection in nonhuman primates and lagomorphs was compared with that in humans. The predominant lesions observed in rabbits after aerosol exposures were comparable to those seen in humans and rhesus macaques (specifically hemorrhage, edema, and necrosis). Differences in inhalational anthrax among species may be attributed to varying susceptibility, resulting in more rapid progression to death in rabbits, compared to the slower course of the disease in humans *(59)*.

Therefore, based on the similarity of the pathology of the disease and the similar immune response to vaccination, rabbits and rhesus macaques have been chosen as the two most appropriate animal models for inhalational anthrax. Studies have been performed using the rabbit model of inhalational anthrax to demonstrate that antibodies to protective antigen, the main component of the licensed vaccine, are a surrogate marker of efficacy *(60)*.

5.2. Yersinia pestis

Plague has been known as a deadly and terrifying disease for at least 2200 yr. Pneumonic plague may occur secondary to septicemia spread after the bite of an infected flea or directly from aerosol exposure. Unlike inhalational anthrax, which is a systemic disease, pneumonic plague is a primary pneumonia. In humans, the disease begins as a bronchopneumonia characterized by numerous bacteria and a proteinaneous effusion in the alveoli.

Animals have played an essential role in studies on *Y. pestis*. Animal species and strains differ in susceptibility to *Y. pestis* and in response to vaccines. It is not known which animal model and set of responses most closely simulates the human disease. Guinea pigs respond differently from other model species to certain plague vaccines. Some mouse responses are also unique, in that some attenuated variants of *Y. pestis* have been reported to cause lethal disease in mice only. Thus, more than one animal species has to be used to characterize the in vivo responses to *Y. pestis* and vaccines.

Macaques have been used in plague research since 1898, when they were used by the discoverer of the plague bacilli, Yersin *(61)*. Investigations over the last 100 yr have shown that the disease in monkeys resembles that of humans. However, different species of monkeys vary in their susceptibility to *Y. pestis*. Both rhesus macaques and cynomolgus macaques are reported to be more resistant to *Y. pestis* infection that the African green monkey (AGM) whereas langurs are more susceptible, but data in the literature vary widely and aerosol studies are very limited.

In more recent studies, AGMs were chosen for vaccine studies because of their susceptibility to *Y. pestis* infection and the uniformity of the model. On exposure by aerosol to a lethal dose of both F1+ and F1– *Y. pestis* strains, they develop primary pneumonic plague. The disease course follows the same time frame as human disease with animals succumbing to the pneumonic plague within 24 h of clinical signs. The pathology of the disease very closely resembles that reported for the human disease *(62)*. However, when the onset of disease and mortality is compared with documented human cases, AGMs may be more susceptible than humans. Attenuated strains of *Y. pestis* that have been used safely as vaccines in humans have been shown to cause illness and death in AGMs. Additionally, a pilot study undertaken to assess the relative resistance of cynomolgus macaques to inhaled *Y. pestis* has shown that under similar laboratory conditions, the susceptibility of the macaques is similar to that of the AGM, thus questioning the older published information regarding their resistance. Thus, based on the information available to date, it is not apparent which nonhuman primate is the best model for the human disease.

5.3. Botulinum Toxin (BoNT)

Botulism is an uncommon but frequently fatal neuroparalytic disease caused by the action of a group of seven antigenically distinct neurotoxic (A–G) proteins (BoNT) produced by *Clostridium botulinum*. The protein neurotoxin binds at the presynaptic membrane of neurons at peripheral synapses and is internalized into an endosome through receptor-mediated endocytosis. The catalytic domain of BoNT mediates a zinc-dependent proteolysis of key vesicular cytosolic docking proteins necessary for neurotransmitter release. This inhibition of acetylcholine release at the neuromuscular junction results in a characteristic descending flaccid paralysis beginning with cranial nerve dysfunction and progressing to peripheral nerve weakness and eventual respiratory distress *(63)*.

Susceptibility of animals to different serotypes varies considerably across species. Botulism in humans from natural exposure is caused predominantly by serotypes A, B, E, and, rarely, F. Serotypes A and B are potent toxins that resist degradation in the gastrointestinal tract. Botulism may be caused by ingesting the toxin (food-borne) or growth of the organism in anaerobic environments such as closed lacerations (wound botulism) or the immature gastrointestinal tract (infant botulism). Aerosol exposure does not occur in nature. Although serotypes C and D have not been reported to cause naturally occurring human disease, serotype C has been shown to have potential clinical application and is toxic in other species, including primates. Serotype D causes disease in wildlife and domestic animals, but has not been reported to cause human food-borne disease. Serotype G has rarely been reported to cause disease. Types D and G are far less toxic in nonhuman primates. All seven serotypes are toxic by injection or aerosol exposure in guinea pigs and mice. Although the potency rank order differs among the species tested, serotypes A, C, and F appear to be the most toxic in terms of dose on onset of toxicity in nonhuman primates.

BoNT are unique as a biowarfare threat agent in that the mechanism of action is consistent across species regardless of the route of exposure; it is a blood-borne toxicosis. In addition, it is widely accepted that the presence of neutralizing antibodies indicates protection and thus a serological correlate of protection. Over the last several decades, the Centers for Disease Control and Prevention, The Salk Institute, and the US Army Medical Research Institute of Infectious Disease, have standardized neutralization bioassay to measure circulating neutralizing antibodies in volunteers vaccinated with Pentavalent Botulinum Toxoid. Standards are available from the World Health Organization (WHO). The uniformity of the disease across species and a correlation between neutralizing antibody titer and protection from disease has led the Food and Drug Administration to consider neutralizing antibody levels in humans as a surrogate endpoint for clinical efficacy (Federal Register/Vol. 62, No. 147/Thursday, July 31, 1997). This is further supported by demonstration of protection against aerosol challenge of guinea pigs through passive transfer of human antibodies.

5.4. Staphylococcal Enterotoxin B

SEB belong to a family of microbial products known as bacterial superantigens because they have drastic effects on the immune system. SEB binds to class II major histocompatibility complex proteins and the T-lymphocyte antigen-binding receptor β-chain. This binding to cells associated with immune responses activates antigen-presenting cells, overstimulating the immune response. This is marked by excessive T-cell proliferation, release of various mediators such as histamine and leukotriene from mast cells, and induction of proinflammatory cytokine gene expression for various of cytokines (interferon-γ, interleukin-6, and tumor necrosis factor-α). The pathological basis of SEB lethality is the physiological impact of the cytokines and other mediators on the body.

Exposing human volunteers to known amounts of SEB by inhalation showed how exquisitely sensitive they are. SEB is considered both a lethal and incapacitating biowarfare agent. Rodents are resistant to the toxic effects of SEB, whereas nonhuman primates succumb to the toxin with similar clinical signs as humans. As a febrile toxicosis, elevated body temperature was the most consistent surrogate endpoint correlating with human incapacitation.

The nonhuman primate rhesus macaque model is used as both an incapacitating and a lethal model after aerosol exposure of SEB. Because rhesus macaques display similar disease found in SEB-exposed humans, the dose range for incapacitation and lethality is very different. Rhesus macaques are not nearly as sensitive to the toxin as humans, with the incapacitation to lethality being very tight in the microgram/kilogram dose range *(64)*. In humans, however, the dose range from incapacitant to lethality is more than 3 logs, from picogram/kilogram to nanogram/kilogram. In addition, definitions of incapacitation that would be clinically relevant in humans make meaningful extrapolation of toxicity data even more complicated. Suppression of a febrile response in the rhesus macaque has been used in determining vaccine SEB dose schedule *(65)*. Although a mouse model has been developed, an additional agent has to be coadministered to increase the sensitivity of mice to SEB. Several agents have been reported to do this; lipopolysaccharide (LPS) was the agent of choice in these studies *(66)*. The mechanism of action for this increase in sensitivity is not totally understood. It is likely that the induction and release of cytokines in response to LPS sublethally prime a mouse for superantigen-induced release of cytokines. This leads to additive effects and subsequent lethal toxic shock. The native or inbred mouse is an inadequate model for aerosol challenge, as it is relatively insensitive to SEB. Transgenic strains of mice bearing human leukocyte antigen loci (HLA)-DR and -DQ and human CD4 receptors are being developed. These are a lethal model, although logs are less sensitive than rhesus macaques and do not involve clinical signs *(67)*.

6. SUMMARY

Aerosol delivery of biological agents by terrorists is a real threat. However, our knowledge of the resulting disease or intoxication in humans caused by this route of exposure is extremely limited. We have to rely on data collected from animal experiments. It is very important to develop relevant animal models but still recognize their limitations. The fate of inhaled biological agents are likely to differ when comparing humans to animals based on both anatomical and susceptibility factors. Despite the shortcomings of using imperfect animal models and extrapolation from a laboratory setting, the data generated are extremely important.

In the analysis of the potential biological threat agents and the development of medical countermeasures to these threats, care must be taken in the extrapolation of this data from nonhuman animal models. Misinterpretation of such information may lead to nonefficacious countermeasures or the oversight of potential, valuable pre- and posttherapies.

REFERENCES

1. Schlesinger, R. B. (1985) Comparative deposition of inhaled aerosols in experimental animals and humans: a review. *J. Toxicol. Environ. Health* **15**, 197–214.
2. Asgharian, B., Wood, R., and Schlesinger, R. B. (1995) Empirical modeling of particle deposition in the alveolar region of the lungs: a basis for interspecies extrapolation. *Fundam. Appl. Toxicol.* **27**, 232–238.
3. Lippmann, M. and Schlesinger, R. B. (1984) Interspecies comparisons of particle deposition and mucociliary clearance in tracheobronchial airways. *J. Toxicol. Environ. Health* **13**, 441–469.
4. Schlesinger, R. B., Gurman, J. L., and Lippmann, M. (1982) Particle deposition within bronchial airways: comparisons using constant and cyclic inspiratory flows. *Ann. Occup. Hyg.* **26**, 47–64.
5. Yeates, D. B., Gerrity, T. R., and Garrard, C. S. (1981) Particle deposition and clearance in the bronchial tree. *Ann. Biomed. Eng.* **9**, 577–592.
6. Lippmann, M., Yeates, D. B., and Albert, R. E. (1980) Deposition, retention, and clearance of inhaled particles. *Br. J. Ind. Med.* **37**, 337–362.
7. Oberdorster, G., Ferin, J., and Lehnert, B. E. (1994) Correlation between particle size, in vivo particle persistence, and lung injury. *Environ. Health Perspect.* **102(Suppl 5)**, 173–179.
8. Schlesinger, R. B. (1985) Clearance from the respiratory tract. *Fundam. Appl. Toxicol.* **5**, 435–450.
9. Stuart, B. O. (1976) Deposition and clearance of inhaled particles. *Environ. Health Perspect.* **16**, 41–53.
10. Stuart, B. O. (1984) Deposition and clearance of inhaled particles. *Environ. Health Perspect.* **55**, 369–390.
11. Swift, D. L. (1981) Aerosol deposition and clearance in the human upper airways. *Ann. Biomed. Eng.* **9**, 593–604.
12. Wilkey, D. D., Lee, P. S., Hass, F. J., et al. (1980) Mucociliary clearance of deposited particles from the human lung: intra- and inter-subject reproductivity, total and regional lung clearance, and model comparisons. *Arch. Environ. Health* **35**, 294–303.
13. (1966) Task Group on Lung Dynamics for Committee II of the International Commision on Radiological Protection, Deposition and Retention Models. *Health Physics* **12**, 173–208.
14. Hounam, R. F. and Morgan, A. (1977) Particle deposition, in: *Lung Biology in Health and Disease*. Vol. 5 Respiratory Defense Mechanisms, Part I. (Lenfant, C., ed.), Marcal Dekker, Bethesda, Maryland, pp. 125–156.

15. Proctor, D. F. (1977) The upper airways. I. Nasal physiology and defense of the lungs. *Am. Rev. Respir. Dis.* **115,** 97–129.
16. Proctor, D. F., Adams, G. K., Andersen, I., and Man, S. F. (1978) Nasal mucociliary clearance in man. *Ciba Found. Symp.* **54,** 219–234.
17. Schlesinger, R. B. and Lippmann, M. (1972) Particle deposition in casts of the human upper tracheobronchial tree. *Am. Ind. Hyg. Assoc. J.* **33,** 237–251.
18. Svartengren, K., Philipson, K., Svartengren, M., Anderson, M., and Camner, P. (1996) Tracheobronchial deposition and clearance in small airways in asthmatic subjects. *Eur. Respir. J.* **9,** 1123–1129.
19. Oldham, M. J. and Phalen, R. F. (2002) Dosimetry implications of upper tracheobronchial airway anatomy in two mouse varieties. *Anat. Rec.* **268,** 59–65.
20. Spritzer, A. A., Watson, J. A., Auld, J. A. (1967) Mucociliary clearance rates. Deposition and clearance in the tracheobronchial tree of rats. *Arch. Environ. Health.* **15,** 39–47.
21. Ilowite, J. S., Smaldone, G. C., Perry, R. J., Bennett, W. D., and Foster, W. M. (1989) Relationship between tracheobronchial particle clearance rates and sites of initial deposition in man. *Arch. Environ. Health* **44,** 267–273.
22. Bachofen, H. and Schurch, S. (2001) Alveolar surface forces and lung architecture. *Comp. Biochem. Physiol. A Mol. Integr. Physiol.* **129,** 183–193.
23. Oberdorster, G. (1992) Pulmonary deposition, clearance and effects of inhaled soluble and insoluble cadmium compounds. *IARC Sci. Publ.* **118,** 189–204.
24. Gehr, P., Green, F. H., Geiser, M., Im Hof, V., Lee, M. M., and Schurch, S. (1996) Airway surfactant, a primary defense barrier: mechanical and immunological aspects. *J. Aerosol Med.* **9,** 163–181.
25. Schlesinger, R. B., Vollmuth, T. A., Naumann, B. D., and Driscoll, K. E. (1986) Measurement of particle clearance from the alveolar region of the rabbit respiratory tract. *Fundam. Appl. Toxicol.* **7,** 256–263.
26. Pavia, D. (1991) Bronchoalveolar clearance. *Respiration* **58(Suppl 1),** 13–17.
27. Lehnert, B. E. (1992) Pulmonary and thoracic macrophage subpopulations and clearance of particles from the lung. *Environ. Health Perspect.* **97,** 17–46.
28. Gradon, L. and Podgorski, A. (1995) Displacement of alveolar macrophages in air space of human lung. *Med. Biol. Eng. Comput.* **33,** 575–581.
29. Kaltreider, H. B. (1976) Expression of immune mechanisms in the lung. *Am. Rev. Respir. Dis.* **113,** 347–379.
30. Bienenstock, J., Johnston, N., and Perey, D. Y. (1973) Bronchial lymphoid tissue. I. Morphologic characteristics. *Lab. Invest.* **28,** 686–692.
31. Bienenstock, J., Johnston, N., and Perey, D. Y. (1973) Bronchial lymphoid tissue. II. Functional characterisitics. *Lab. Invest.* **28,** 693–698.
32. Bienenstock, J., McDermott, M. R., and Befus, A. D. (1982) The significance of bronchus-associated lymphoid tissue. *Bull. Eur. Physiopathol. Respir.* **18,** 153–177.
33. Murray, M. J. and Driscoll, K. E. (1992) Immunology of the respiratory system, in: *Comparative Biology of the Normal Lung.* Vol. 1. (Parent, R. A., ed.), CRC, Baton Rouge, LA, pp. 725–746.
34. Holt, P. G. (2000) Antigen presentation in the lung. *Am. J. Respir. Crit. Care Med.* **162,** S151–S156.
35. Geiser, M. (2002) Morphological aspects of particle uptake by lung phagocytes. *Microsc. Res. Tech.* **57,** 512–522.
36. Holt, P. G. and Stumbles, P. A. (2000) Characterization of dendritic cell populations in the respiratory tract. *J. Aerosol Med.* **13,** 361–367.
37. Kradin, R., MacLean, J., Duckett, S., Schneeberger, E. E., Waeber, C., and Pinto, C. (1997) Pulmonary response to inhaled antigen: neuroimmune interactions promote the recruitment of dendritic cells to the lung and the cellular immune response to inhaled antigen. *Am. J. Pathol.* **150,** 1735–1743.

38. Reynolds, H. Y. (2000) Advances in understanding pulmonary host defense mechanisms: dendritic cell function and immunomodulation. *Curr. Opin. Pulm. Med.* **6,** 209–216.
39. Wilkes, D. S. and Twigg, H. L. B-lymphocytes in the lung: a topic to be revisited. *Sarcoidosis Vasc. Diffuse. Lung Dis.* **18,** 34–49.
40. Palliser, D., Lowrey, J. A., Lamb, J. R., and Hoyne, G. F. (1998) T-cell response to inhaled antigen. *Chem. Immunol.* **71,** 161–177.
41. Lowell, G. H., Colleton, C., Frost, D., et al. (1996) Immunogenicity and efficacy against lethal aerosol staphylococcal enterotoxin B challenge in monkeys by intramuscular and respiratory delivery of proteosome-toxoid vaccines. *Infect. Immun.* **64,** 4686–4693.
42. Boles, J. W., Pitt, M. L., LeClaire, R. D., et al. (2003) Generation of protective immunity by inactivated recombinant staphylococcal enterotoxin B vaccine in nonhuman primates and identification of correlates of immunity. *Clin. Immunol.* **108,** 51–59.
43. Stiles, B. G., Garza, A. R., Ulrich, R. G., and Boles, J. W. (2001) Mucosal vaccination with recombinantly attenuated staphylococcal enterotoxin B and protection in a murine model. *Infect. Immun.* **69,** 2031–2036.
44. Vogel, P., Abplanalp, D., Kell, W., et al. (1996) Venezuelan equine encephalitis in BALB/c mice: kinetic analysis of central nervous system infection following aerosol or subcutaneous inoculation. *Arch. Pathol. Lab. Med.* **120,** 164–172.
45. Hart, M. K., Pratt, W., Panelo, F., Tammariello, R., and Dertzbaugh, M. (1997) Venezuelan equine encephalitis virus vaccine induce mucosal IgA responses and protection from airborne infection in BALB/c, but not C3H/HeN mice. *Vaccine* **15,** 363–369.
46. Hart, M. K., Caswell-Stephan, K., Bakken, R., et al. (2000) Improved mucosal protection against Venezuelan equine encephalitis virus is induced by the molecularly defined, live-attenuated V3526 vaccine candidate. *Vaccine* **18,** 3067–3075.
47. Druett, H. A., Henderson, D. W., and Peacock, S. (1956) Studies on respiratory infection. III. Experiments with *Brucella suis. J. Hyg. Camb. 54,* 49–57.
48. Druett, H. A., Henderson, D. W., Packman, L., and Peacock, S. (1953) Studies on respiratory infection. I. The influence of particle size on respiratory infection with anthrax spores. *J. Hyg. Camb.* **54,** 359–371.
49. Druett, H. A., Henderson, D. W., Packman, L., and Peacock, S. (1956) Studies on respiratory infection. I. The influence of aerosol particle size on infection of guinea-pig with *Pasturella Pestis. J. Hyg.* **54,** 37–48.
50. Roy, C. J., Hale, M., Hartings, J. M., Pitt, L., and Duniho, S. (2003) Impact of inhalation exposure modality and particle size on the respiratory deposition of ricin in BALB/c mice. *Inhal. Toxicol.* **15,** 619–638.
51. Fritz, D. L., Jaax, N. K., Lawrence, W. B., et al. (1995) Pathology of experimental inhalation anthrax in the rhesus monkey. *Lab. Invest.* **73,** 691–702.
52. Ivins, B. E., Fellows, P. F., Pitt, M. L. M., et al. (1996) Efficacy of a standard human anthrax vaccine against Bacillus anthracis aerosol spore challenge in rhesus monkeys. *Salisbury Med. Bull.* **Special Suppl 87,** 125,126.
53. Welkos, S. L., Keener, T. J., and Gibbs, P. H. (1986) Differences in susceptibility of inbred mice to Bacillus anthracis. *Infect. Immun.* **51,** 795–800.
54. Welkos, S. L. anf Friedlander, A. M. (1988) Comparative safety and efficacy against *Bacillus anthracis* of protective antigen and live vaccines in mice. *Microb. Pathog.* **5,** 127–139.
55. Haines, B. W., Kleain, F., and Lincoln, R. E. (1965) Quantitiative assay for crude anthrax toxins. *J. Bacteriol.* **89,** 74–83.
56. Lincoln, R. E., Walker, J. S., Klein, F., Rosenwald, A. J., and Jones, W. I., Jr. (1967) Value of field data for extrapolation in anthrax. *Fed. Proc. 26,* 1558–1562.
57. Ivins, B. E., Fellows, P. F., and Nelson, G. O. (1994) Efficacy of a standard human anthrax vaccine against *Bacillus anthracis* spore challenge in guinea-pigs. *Vaccine* **12,** 872–874.

58. Fellows, P. F., Linscott, M. K., Ivins, B. E., et al. (2001) Efficacy of a human anthrax vaccine in guinea pigs, rabbits, and rhesus macaques against challenge by *Bacillus anthracis* isolates of diverse geographical origin. *Vaccine* **19,** 3241–3247.

59. Zaucha, G. M., Pitt, L. M., Estep, J., Ivins, B. E., and Friedlander, A. M. (1998) The pathology of experimental anthrax in rabbits exposed by inhalation and subcutaneous inoculation. *Arch. Pathol. Lab. Med.* **122,** 982–992.

60. Pitt, M. L., Little, S. F., Ivins, B. E., et al. (2001) In vitro correlate of immunity in a rabbit model of inhalational anthrax. *Vaccine* **19,** 4768–4773.

61. Yersin, N. B. and Carre, M. (1904) Sur la vaccination contre la peste au moyen du virus attenue, Congress International de Medecine. Section de Medecine et Chirurgie Militaires. 17 Soussection coloniale, Paris.

62. Davis, K. J., Fritz, D. L., Pitt, M. L., Welkos, S. L., Worsham, P. L., and Friedlander, A. M. (1996) Pathology of experimental pneumonic plague produced by fraction 1-positive and fraction 1-negative *Yersinia pestis* in African green monkeys (Cercopithecus aethiops). *Arch. Pathol. Lab. Med.* **120,** 156–163.

63. Middlebrook, J. L. and Franz, D. R. (1997) Botulinum toxins, in: *Textbook of Military Medicine: Medical Aspects of Chemical and Biological Warfare.* (Zatjchuk, R., ed.), Borden Institute, Washington, D.C., pp. 645.

64. Bavari, S., Hunt, R. E., and Ulrich, R. G. (1995) Divergence of human and nonhuman primate lymphocyte responses to bacterial superantigens. *Clin. Immunol. Immunopathol.* **76,** 248–254.

65. Boles, J. W., Pitt, M. L., LeClaire, R. D., Gibbs, P. H., Ulrich, R. G., and Bavari, S. (2003) Correlation of body temperature with protection against staphylococcal enterotoxin B exposure and use in determining vaccine dose-schedule. *Vaccine* **21,** 2791–2796.

66. Stiles, B. G., Bavari, S., Krakauer, T., and Ulrich, R. G. (1993) Toxicity of staphylococcal enterotoxins potentiated by lipopolysaccharide: major histocompatibility complex class II molecule dependency and cytokine release. *Infect. Immun.* **61,** 5333–5338.

67. DaSilva, L., Welcher, B. C., Ulrich, R. G., Aman, M. J., David, C. S., and Bavari, S. (2002) Humanlike immune response of human leukocyte antigen-DR3 transgenic mice to staphylococcal enterotoxins: a novel model for superantigen vaccines. *J. Infect. Dis.* **185,** 1754–1760.

5

Bacillus anthracis and the Pathogenesis of Anthrax

Dominique M. Missiakas and Olaf Schneewind

1. INTRODUCTION

Bacillus anthracis is the causative agent of anthrax, a disease of animals that is transmissible to humans. Because *B. anthracis* forms spores that can be aerosolized and sprayed with the intent to kill, this pathogen can also be viewed as an agent of biological warfare and bioterrorism *(1)*. The accidental release of spores into the air in Sverdlosk, Russia, and the recent mail attacks in the United States in the Fall of 2001 led to human casualties that sadly document the pathogenic potential and bioterrorism threat of *B. anthracis (2,3)*. Furthermore, it appears that *B. anthracis* has been a research focus of biological warfare industries and subject to genetic manipulation with the intent of generating pathogen variants with increased virulence or with resistance to medical therapies and vaccine prevention strategies *(1,4,5)*. *B. anthracis* can be obtained from infected animals or soil and anthrax spores are easily prepared. Furthermore, *B. anthracis* spores display very low visibility when delivered as an aerosol spray or powder. Inhalational anthrax is the primary target disease of biological warfare schemes *(6)*. The LD_{50} for human inhalation of anthrax is not known, but has been estimated from animal studies to be of the order of 10,000 spores, corresponding to approx 0.01 μg *(2,7)*, and a kilogram amount of spores, if sprayed intentionally on an urban area, is capable of killing hundreds of thousands of people. Biological warfare is an evolving research enterprise, and *B. anthracis* strains resistant to the commonly used antibiotic therapies may be available to several countries and terrorist organizations *(6)*. American defense strategies against bioterrorist or biological warfare attacks must focus on the development of novel therapies that circumvent drug and vaccine-resistant *B. anthracis* strains *(8)*. Much attention is directed toward finding inhibitors that disrupt the function of anthrax toxin. Anthrax toxin is the major virulence factor of *B. anthracis (9)* and consists of three proteins: lethal factor (LF), edema factor (EF), and protective antigen (PA). PA combines with either LF or EF enzymes to mediate their translocation across the plasma membrane *(10)*. The combination of PA and LF forms lethal toxin (LeTx) and that of PA and EF forms edema toxin (EdTx). Once bacteria have secreted a large amount of anthrax toxin, antibiotic treatment becomes far less effective. At this later stage of anthrax pathogenesis, it might be useful to disrupt the biological activity of the toxin. This chapter reviews current knowledge of the factors that contribute to the pathogenesis of *B. anthracis* and highlights recent reports of possible strategies for blocking toxin action *(11–13)*. Additionally, based on the known mechanisms of list-

From: *Infectious Diseases: Biological Weapons Defense: Infectious Diseases and Counterterrorism*
Edited by: L. E. Lindler, F. J. Lebeda, and G. W. Korch © Humana Press Inc., Totowa, NJ

eria-mediated invasion and virulence, the currently available genome sequences of *B. anthracis* were searched in an attempt to identify *B. anthracis* genes that may act early during pathogenesis by contributing to bacterial attachment to host tissues or to toxin secretion.

2. HISTORY AND BACTERIOLOGY

B. anthracis was shown to be the etiologic agent of anthrax disease by Robert Koch *(14)*. The zoonotic disease anthrax offered several advantages for studying the causative agent. First, anthrax is caused by a very large microorganism, which facilitated detection by light microscopy. Second, although anthrax is found primarily in cattle and sheep, the disease can be transmitted to smaller and less expensive animals. Third, *B. anthracis* is a hardy organism that can grow on many different media in the laboratory. Finally, *B. anthracis* multiplies to great density in the terminal stages of the disease, which again facilitated detection by microscopy. In 1850, Davaine observed rod-shaped bodies in the blood of sheep that died from anthrax, and he later transmitted the disease by inoculating as little as 10^{-6} mL of blood. Nonetheless, skeptics argued that the microscopic bodies were a result rather than the cause of the disease. Koch provided unequivocal proof that the rod-shaped bodies were the cause of the disease *(14)*. He was able to isolate these microorganisms in pure culture and used them to infect animals. This approach became the key to establishing various bacteria as pathogens. After identifying the bacterium *B. anthracis* as the etiologic agent of anthrax, Koch formulated four postulates for identifying microbes as the causative agents of infectious diseases. The powerful methodology that arose from this work laid the foundation for many future successes of medical microbiology and is still applied in today's experimental strategies.

B. anthracis derives from the Greek word for coal, anthrakis, because of the black skin lesions that arise during the course of cutaneous infections. *B. anthracis* is a Gram-positive, aerobic, spore-forming bacillus *(14)*. The vegetative cell is rather large (1–8 μm long, 1–1.5 μm wide) whereas the spore size is approx 1 μm (*see* Fig. 1). Herbivores are the natural host of *B. anthracis (15)*. Unlike *B. subtilis* and *B. cereus*, *B. anthracis* is nonmotile, nonhemolytic on sheepblood agar, and grows on all ordinary laboratory media at 37°C. *B. anthracis* forms large colonies with irregularly tapered outgrowths. The bacteria grow as long chains in vitro and form mucoid colonies. This is because of the production of a prominent capsule. Capsule formation can be observed by growing bacteria on nutrient agar containing 0.7% sodium bicarbonate in the presence of 5–20% carbon dioxide. When nutrients are exhausted, resistant spores are formed that can survive in the soil for decades *(16)*. *B. anthracis* spores ingested by herbivores germinate within the host as they enter an environment rich in amino acids, nucleosides, and glucose. *B. anthracis* cells appear as single organisms or as extended chains of several incompletely separated bacilli in the host. Vegetative bacilli multiply rapidly in the host and express virulence factors that kill the host. The bacilli sporulate in the cadaver once in contact with air and then contaminate the soil, anticipating another host. Vegetative bacteria have poor survival outside of an animal or human host. For example, when inoculated into water, colony counts decline rapidly within 24 h *(17)*.

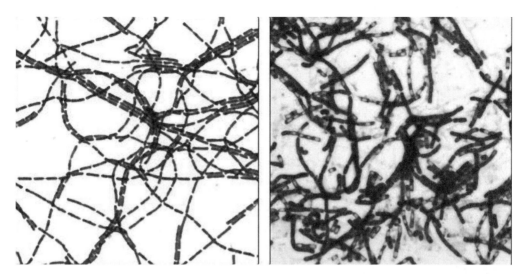

Fig. 1. Photomicrograph of Gram-stained bacilli. *Left panel*: vegetative cells of *B. anthracis*; *right panel*: sporulating cells of *B. anthracis*.

3. ANTHRAX OUTBREAKS

Anthrax is primarily a disease of herbivores, and, prior to the advent of an effective vaccine, it caused substantial losses in cattle, sheep, goats, horses, and donkeys worldwide *(18,19)*. Humans are accidental hosts of *B. anthracis*. Infection is initiated with the introduction of spores into skin lesions or entry, through the intestinal or respiratory mucosa. Depending on the route of entry either cutaneaous, gastrointestinal, or inhalational anthrax disease can be distinguished *(20)*. Humans acquire anthrax infections from contact with infected animals or contaminated animal products, such as hides, wool, hair, and ivory tusks. Ingestion of poorly cooked infected meat may lead to gastrointestinal anthrax. Cases of inhalational anthrax have been observed in individuals that process animal products such as hides and wool (woolsorters' disease) in enclosed factory spaces, where aerosolized anthrax spores may be inhaled.

From 1979 until 1985, a large outbreak of anthrax (about 10,000 cases) occurred in Zimbabwe *(21)*. At this time, a civil war caused the interruption of veterinary and public health services in Zimbabwe, which contributed significantly to the magnitude of this outbreak. Noticeably, most of the human-reported cases represented cutaneous infections and this epidemic was directly related to a major epizootic in cattle. These events underscore the importance of livestock vaccination in endemic areas as an effort to prevent anthrax in humans. It was also observed that treatment with penicillin could prevent complications of human disease such as bacteremia, meningitis, and lethality.

In 1979, 66 people died in Sverdlovsk in the former Soviet Union from inhalational anthrax. These deaths were attributed to the accidental release of anthrax spores into the atmosphere by a research facility involved in "weaponizing" anthrax. The spores had been finely milled, and rendered electrostatically neutral for optimal dissemination. The accident demonstrated that inhalation of anthrax spores can cause human

disease even without the conventional exposure to infected animals or animal products, and provided clear evidence for the notion that anthrax is a weapon for biological
warfare and bioterrorism *(2)*.

In October 2001, the United States experienced a series of attacks with anthrax
(7,22). A publishing company in Boca Raton, FL, the NBC news desk in New York
City, and the office of Senator Tom Daschle in Washington, DC, received letters or
packages laden with anthrax spores. At the onset of these attacks, five people died of
inhalational anthrax *(23)*. Two of the five victims that succumbed to anthrax were sent
home because the disease had been mistaken for a stomach virus or bad cold. As the
anthrax threat became obvious, six additional patients with inhalational anthrax were
saved following proper antibiotic treatment. This represents an impressive success rate.

With the deliberate dissemination of spores through the US mail, public health officials were presented with two challenges: how to rapidly detect spores and how to treat
surfaces, buildings, and individuals contaminated with spores. Preventive antibiotic
treatment (ciprofloxacin) was prescribed to the thousands of people who might have
been exposed to anthrax. It appears that the effectiveness of this intervention relied on
the fact that the same strain had been used in all these attacks: a strain sensitive to
antibiotic treatment. Indeed, comparative sequence analysis of highly variable genomic
regions (a strain-typing tool developed by Keim and coworkers; ref. *24*) has recently
revealed that the Florida, New York, and Washington, DC, isolates originated from the
same strain isolated from a dead cow in Texas in 1981 *(25)*. This strain of *B. anthracis*,
designated Ames strain, contains two extrachromosomal elements (plasmids) required
for virulence (*see* Subheading 6.2.) and has been used by the US Army Medical Research Institute for Infectious Diseases in Fort Detrick, MD, as well as several research
laboratories in the United States and Europe *(25)*.

4. HUMAN DISEASE

4.1. Inhalational Anthrax

Human inhalation of spores leads to bacterial germination in the hilar and mediastinal lymph nodes *(20)*. The classic clinical description of inhalational anthrax is that of
a biphasic illness. Following an incubation period of 1–6 d, mild fever, malaise, myalgia, nonproductive cough, and some chest or abdominal pain can be observed. As the
illness progresses further, fever, acute dyspnea, diaphoresis, and cyanosis occur. Some
patients present a dry cough and stridor because of extrinsic obstruction of the trachea
by enlarged lymph nodes, mediastinal widening, and subcutaneous edema of the chest
and neck. *B. anthracis* entry into the bloodstream results in systemic spread of the
disease to the intestines and meninges. Obtundation and nuchal rigidity is observed in
half of the infected individuals as a result of anthrax meningitis. During the meningitis,
the cerebrospinal fluid is hemorrhagic with polymorphonuclear pleocytosis. This disease invariably results in an excitus lethalis within 1–2 d. Very rarely, the primary
lesion of inhalational anthrax has occurred in the nasal mucosa or a nasal accessory
sinus. Marked facial edema and a thick, gelatinous nasal discharge have been prominent findings for such cases. When used as a biological warfare agent, *B. anthracis*
spores are dispersed into respiratory droplets and disseminated within target populations to cause respiratory infections. As aforementioned, spore preparations of *B.
anthracis* also have been used during the recent terrorist attacks in the United States

and either mailed to targeted institutions or placed in areas that lead to the infection of targeted individuals *(23)*.

4.2. Cutaneous Anthrax

B. anthracis spores enter through a small abrasion or wound in the human skin, typically in the face, hands, or neck and cause cutaneous anthrax *(20)*. Cutaneous anthrax represents 95% of all naturally occurring anthrax. The primary lesion, a pruritic papule, appears within a few days (1–7 d). It develops into an ulcer with surrounding vesicles *(20)*. Sometimes a single larger vesicle forms (1–2 cm in diameter). It is filled with clear or serosanguineous fluid containing occasional leukocytes and numerous large, Gram-positive bacilli. In about 20% of all cases, regional lymphadenitis and lymphadenopathy can be observed, which are followed by systemic symptoms such as fever, malaise, and headache. After 2 d, the vesicle ruptures and undergoes necrosis and a painless characteristic black eschar with a surrounding edema can be seen. The edema may become massive, particularly when the lesions are on the face or neck, and occasionally, multiple bullae develop along with marked toxic effects. Incision of such lesions should be avoided to prevent possible bacteremia. After 1 or 2 wk, the lesion dries and the eschar separates, revealing an underlying scar. Systemic infections are almost always lethal if left untreated. Antibiotic therapy does not prevent the progression of the skin lesion but abbreviates or prevents systemic infection.

4.3. Gastrointestinal Anthrax

Human consumption of food that is contaminated with *B. anthracis* spores results in gastrointestinal anthrax *(20)*. The characteristic skin lesion is not present and the establishment of a definitive diagnosis outside of an epidemic is difficult. The incubation period of gastrointestinal anthrax is only 3–7 d. Abdominal symptoms with nausea, vomiting, anorexia, and fever may develop. The manifestations progress rapidly and patients present with severe, bloody diarrhea. The primary intestinal lesions are ulcerative and occur mainly in the terminal ileum or caecum. Hemorrhagic mesenteric lymphadenitis is also a feature of gastrointestinal anthrax, and marked ascites may occur. The associated mortality is greater than 50%, and death can occur within 2–5 d after the onset of symptoms.

5. ANTHRAX PROPHYLAXIS

Prior to the availability of antibiotics, anthrax was treated with the chemotherapeutic agents neoarsphenamine and sulphonamides in large repeated doses. Additionally, small doses of antianthrax horse serum were injected around the malignant pustule, as well as intravenously *(26)*. With the availability of antibiotics, penicillin became the preferred agent for anthrax treatment *(27)*. Successful chemotherapy relies on the prompt uptake of antibiotics. As noted earlier, antibiotic treatment does not prevent the formation of the eschar in cutaneous anthrax. Chemotherapy is rarely effective in the case of inhalational anthrax, simply because exposure to spores might go unrecognized for some time. The first stages of infection are often mistaken for bronchitis, and the second stages for cardiac failure or cerebrovascular accidents. Spores engulfed by alveolar macrophages are carried to local lymph nodes, germinate, and rapidly multiply in the bloodstream. Dense bacterial growth is associated with the accumulation of anthrax toxin, and toxin activity is unaffected by antibiotic treatments. Animal studies have shown that prolonged antibiotic treatment is necessary for therapeutic success, because the spores can persist in the lungs for prolonged periods of time. Immediate vaccination of infected individuals tackles this problem as protective immunity develops during antibiotic treatment *(28)*. Most importantly, during the anthrax outbreak in the United States in 2001 we learned that when diagnosed early, anthrax can be efficiently treated with antibiotics. The antimicrobial susceptibility patterns of 11 *B. anthracis* isolates associated with intentional exposures in Florida, New York City, and Washington, DC, have been determined. All isolates displayed susceptibility to ciprofloxacin, doxycycline, chloramphenicol, clindamycin, tetracycline, rifampin, vancomycin, penicillin, and amoxicillin *(29)*. This susceptibility spectrum is in agreement with the recent genetic analysis suggesting that all isolates originated from the same source *(25)*. Because of the mortality associated with inhalational anthrax, the Centers for Disease Control and Prevention (CDC) recommends that two or more antimicrobial agents be used for effective treatment, and that ciprofloxacin or doxycycline be used for initial intravenous therapy. Duration of therapy should be prolonged over 60 d *(29)*. Treatment of systemic *B. anthracis* infection using penicillin alone is no longer recommended because *B. anthracis* genome encodes for at least two β-lactamases: a penicillinase and a cephalosporinase *(29)*.

Sterne isolated *B. anthracis* variants lacking the characteristic capsule and used these attenuated strains as live vaccine in cattle or other animals, which effectively prevented anthrax disease in animals *(19,30)*. The vaccine strains had been cured of pXO2, one of the two virulence plasmids that is required for capsule expression but not for production of anthrax toxins *(see* Subheading 6.2.). Anthrax vaccine adsorbed (AVA) is an adjuvant absorbed preparation of the culture supernatant of vaccine strains and has been licensed by the Food and Drug Administration (FDA) for the prevention of anthrax disease in humans *(31)*. The AVA vaccine has been successfully employed to prevent laboratory infections in the United States and its effectiveness in preventing anthrax following a respiratory challenge has been demonstrated in rodents and nonhuman primates *(8,28)*. The active vaccine component, anti-PA IgG, is believed to exert some sporicidal effect; however, the use of the AVA vaccine in preventing human anthrax following bioterrorist or biological warfare use of *B. anthracis* spores is hitherto unknown *(32,33)*.

6. PATHOGENESIS

6.1. Bacillus Anthracis *Lifestyle*

Despite the early identification of *B. anthracis* as the etiologic agent of anthrax, the pathogenic mechanisms of human or animal disease remain poorly understood. Experiments with laboratory animals have shown that bacterial invasion of intestinal epithelia is followed by macrophage engulfment of the spores *(14,34)*. It is not clear whether a specific property of the spores, for example, a surface ligand, targets spores into endocytic or phagocytic pathways. Alternatively, macrophage phagocytosis of anthrax spores may occur by a universal mechanism that targets all nonpathogenic microbes for killing by the innate immune response.

During inhalation anthrax, the spores are engulfed by alveolar macrophages *(20,35)*. Engulfment of ingested spores may be achieved by *M* cells in the intestines. These lymphoid cells deliver intestinal contents to macrophages and adjacent lymph follicles (Peyer's patches). The spores survive the harsh environment of the macrophage and phagocytosis and instead germinate within phagosomes. Vegetative bacilli escape from the infected cell and bacteria spread to regional lymph nodes and eventually the bloodstream.

The vegetative form of *B. anthracis* elaborates a capsule that confers an antiphagocytic property on the bacilli *(36,37)* and secretes the three-component protein toxin, PA (*pagA* encoded), LF (*lef* encoded), and EF (*cya* encoded) *(38)*. The combined action of the protein toxins is believed to kill infected animals by triggering the release of interleukin (IL)-1 and tumor necrosis factor-α from intoxicated macrophages *(39)*. Vegetative bacilli secrete the PA toxin as a precursor, PA83 *(40,41)*. PA83 binds to the anthrax toxin receptor (ATR), a membrane protein on the surface of macrophage *(11)*. Cellular proteases, furin or furin-like, cleave PA83 to the mature, active PA63 form, a mechanism that promotes PA63 assembly into a heptameric form *(42)*. This species interacts with either EF or LF and promotes transport of EF and LF across the endocytic vesicle into the cytosol of intoxicated cells. The two binary exotoxins are referred to as LeTx when comprising PA and LF, and EdTx when encompassing PA and EF.

LeTx is implicated in both macrophage and host death *(43–45)*. LeTx acts as a zinc protease and cleaves mitogen-activated protease kinase kinase (MAPKK), presumably interfering with signal transduction events of the p38 pathway and causing apoptosis of activated macrophage and release of IL-1 cytokine *(44,46)*. In addition to ATR and MAPKK, the proteasome *(47)* and Kif1C, a kinesin motor protein *(48)*, may also be required for LeTx intoxication; the molecular events that cause macrophage-mediated host killing by the LeTx pathway are not yet understood *(39)*.

EdTx is thought to be responsible for phagocyte inhibition and the massive edema observed upon anthrax infection *(49)*. EF is an adenylate cyclase *(50)*. After binding to calmodulin, EdTx cleaves adenosine triphosphate (ATP) to generate the second messenger cyclic adenosine monophosphate (cAMP), thereby presumably interfering with the normal immune function of macrophage *(50)*. At this stage, the bacilli multiply in the lymph system and in the blood but not within macrophages *(14)*.

6.2. Virulence Plasmids

Virulence of all *B. anthracis* strains requires two large plasmids, pXO1 and pXO2, respectively *(51,52)*. pXO1 carries the genetic determinants that are responsible for the synthesis of the anthrax exotoxin complexes (PA, LF, and EF) *(53)*, whereas pXO2 is responsible for capsule production *(54)*. Plasmid pXO1 has been sequenced *(55)*. It is a circular DNA sequence of 181,654 bp of which only 61% can be translated into 143 open reading frames (ORFs). More than two-thirds of pXO1 ORFs do not have significant similarity to sequences available in databases. The three-toxin genes *cya*, *lef*, and *pagA* are encoded within a pathogenicity island defined by a 44.8-kb region that is bordered by inverted IS*1627* elements at each end of pXO1. This island also contains regulatory elements controlling the toxin genes such as *atxA*, *pagA*, and *pagR*, a three-gene germination operon (*gerX*), and 19 additional ORFs. Plasmid pXO2 has been sequenced from strain A2012 (accession no. AE011191). It is a 94,829-bp long circular DNA molecule that encodes 113 ORFs. The *capB*, *capC*, *capA*, and *dep* genes are involved in capsule synthesis and degradation *(56,57)* and are located on plasmid pXO2 along with a regulatory gene *acpA (58)*.

B. anthracis lacking plasmid pXO2 can be isolated easily under laboratory growth conditions. Epidemiological investigations during an anthrax outbreak show that bacilli resembling *B. anthracis* are often dismissed in clinical and veterinary laboratories as *B. cereus* or unidentified *Bacillus spp. (59)*. Such bacilli fail to produce a capsule and do not induce anthrax in test animals. Loss of pXO2 can be scored on agar plates by observing colony morphology. The Sterne strain 34F2 *(30)*, which is used as an animal vaccine, represents one of those avirulent nonencapsulated strains lacking pXO2 plasmid.

On the other hand, the spontaneous loss of pXO1 is a rare event. Bacterial growth at 43°C or incubation in the presence of antibiotics favors curing of pXO1 under laboratory conditions. The curing of pXO1 obviously leads to the loss of toxin production and, when combined with the loss of the *gerX* locus, results in attenuated virulence. Spores of mutants lacking only the *gerX* operon do not germinate efficiently in macrophages *(60)*. The *gerX* operon is organized as a tricistronic operon (*gerXB*, *gerXA* and *gerXC*), located between the *pag* and *atxA* genes. The three predicted proteins (40, 55, and 37 kDa in size) have significant sequence similarities to *B. subtilis*, *B. cereus*, and *B. megaterium* germination proteins. As for the other bacilli species, *B. anthracis* encodes more paralogs of the *gerX*-like operon on its chromosome. Blast searches suggest that it may, in fact, encode six additional such operons on the chromosome. The *gerX* operon is expressed exclusively in the forespore 2.5–3 h after the initiation of sporulation *(60)*. Strains lacking pXO1 are also less capsulated, because capsule expression is partly controlled by *pXO1* genes (*see* Subheading 6.4.).

6.3. Surface Structures

The surface structures of spores have been characterized for *B. subtilis*. The spore coat is assembled by the surrounding mother cell, as the spore resides within its cytoplasm. The spore is surrounded by spore peptidoglycan, a heteropolymer that is similar to the peptidoglycan of vegetative cells, with the exception of some spore-specific aminosugar modifications. The surrounding mother cell synthesizes the coat proteins that are layered onto the spore surface. Spore release occurs on lysis of the mother cell. Coat assembly in *B. subtilis* is coupled to the well-described developmental program driving spore formation *(61,62)*. Comparison of *B. subtilis* and *B. anthracis* genomes suggests that coat assembly follows a similar program in the pathogen and that anthrax also possesses an inner and outer coat, although the morphological distinction between these two layers by electron microscopy is not as obvious *(63)*. In addition, spores of *B. anthracis*, *B. cereus*, and *B. thuringiensis* are surrounded by an additional structure, the exosporium *(64)*. The mother cell is also responsible for the synthesis and assembly of the exosporium. This structure truly represents the outermost integument of the mature spore. It is composed of proteins, lipids, and carbohydrates *(65,66)*, and its surface is decorated with filamentous appendages *(67)*. Several of the protein components of the exosporium have been described for *B. thurengiensis* and *B. cereus*, some of which are in fact glycoproteins *(66,68,69)*. Glycosylation of protein is rarely observed in the microbial world. The exosporium of *B. anthracis* spores also contains an abundant glycoprotein designated BclA *(70)*. BclA presents striking similarities with collagen at the amino acid level, and it is the major constituent of the filamentous appendages protruding from the exosporium *(70)*. Although structurally reminiscent of the pili of Gram-negative bacteria, it is not clear whether these appendages play a role during spore invasion across mucosal surfaces or macrophage engulfment. Thus, the precise function of individual exosporium components is not yet known but can be established by comparing pairs of isogenic mutant and wildtype strains in an animal experiment.

Two structures surround the vegetative cell of *B. anthracis*: an *S*-layer and a capsule. The *S*-layer can be observed clearly when *B. anthracis* does not produce its capsule. *S*-layers are proteinaceous paracrystalline sheaths that completely cover the cell surface in a highly organized two-dimensional array *(71)*. The *S*-layer of *B. anthracis* is composed of two proteins, surface array protein (Sap) and extractable antigen (EA1) *(72)*. The expression and assembly of Sap and EA1 arrays seem regulated. As cells enter stationary phase, EA1 progressively replaces Sap, which is shed into the surrounding medium, suggesting developmental regulation of *S*-layer assembly *(73)*. The *S*-layer proteins interact noncovalently with the underlying peptidoglycan and the pyruvyl of a peptidoglycan-associated polysaccharide, without which the *S*-layer proteins EA1 and Sap cannot assemble *(74)*. Various functions have been attributed to *S*-layers, including bacterial shape, barrier for molecular diffusion, and virulence; however, much of the thought in this area has not been tested experimentally yet *(75)*. It should be noted that deletion of *S*-layer genes does not impair the ability of *B. anthracis* variants to cause animal disease.

The encapsulation of *B. anthracis* bacilli does not require a functional *S*-layer *(76)*. Anthrax variants lacking the genes required for capsule assembly (*capABC*) are avirulent. Preisz was the first to correlate the presence of a capsule with the virulence of *B. anthracis* strains *(37)*. By virtue of its negative charge, the capsule is presumed to inhibit the phagocytic host defense *(36,53,77)*. The capsule is a linear polymer of poly-γ-D-glutamic acid peptide which is weakly immunogenic *(36,78)*. Capsular synthesis occurs via the expression of three gene products, CapA, CapB, and CapC *(56)*. The nonpathogenic organism *B. licheniformis* appears to synthesize a similar capsule as *B. anthracis*. It follows that the capsule of *B. anthracis* may be necessary for bacterial pathogenesis, but it clearly cannot be sufficient to promote the establishment of anthrax disease. No specific enzymatic activity has thus far been attributed to the CapABC factors, which are shared with the nonpathogenic *B. licheniformis*. *B. anthracis* synthesizes an additional factor Dep (the *dep* gene is located downstream of the *cap* region and is absent in *B. licheniformis*), which presumably acts as a depolymerase and hydrolyzes poly-γ-D-glutamic acid polymers to generate lower molecular weight glutamates. These compounds are thought to interfere with host defense mechanisms *(79)*.

6.4. Regulation of B. anthracis *Virulence*

During infection, vegetative bacilli synthesize and secrete both the capsule and the toxins. In vitro, their synthesis can be induced by the addition of bicarbonate and changes in temperature. This induction has been shown to be regulated at the level of

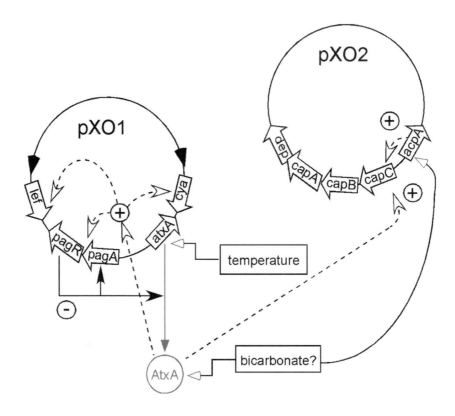

Fig. 2. Schematic representation of plasmids pXO1 and pXO2 and of AtxA-mediated regulation of the toxin genes. Plasmid pXO1 encodes for 143 open reading ORFs. The two IS1627 inverted elements at each end of the pXO1 pathogenicity island are shown as black arrows. The three toxin genes *cya*, *lef*, and *pagA* and the regulatory elements *atxA* and *pagR* controlling the toxin genes are indicated. Plasmid pXO2 encodes 113 ORFs. The *capB*, *capC*, *capA*, and *dep* genes involved in capsule synthesis and degradation as well as the regulatory gene *acpA* are shown. Question marks indicate putative or uncharacterized regulation. (Adapted from ref. *76*.)

transcription by the AtxA factor *(80,81)*. AtxA is a transcriptional activator encoded by the pXO1 plasmid *(see* Fig. 2). It is required to induce the expression of both the toxin genes on the pXO1 plasmid and the capsule operon on pXO2 *(82,83)*. AtxA synthesis is not affected by bicarbonate. However, in the absence of AtxA, induction of *pagA* transcription is not observed in the presence of bicarbonate *(82)*. Most importantly, *atxA* mutant bacilli are avirulent in the mouse model of anthrax *(84)*. *pagR*, the second gene of the *pag* operon, represses the expression of the *pag* operon *(85)* and appears to influence the expression of other pXO1-encoded genes *(86)*. A chromosomally encoded *abrB* gene negatively regulates the expression of the three anthrax toxin genes and of the *pagA* gene *(87)*. The *B. anthracis abrB* gene is an ortholog of the well-studied *abrB* gene of *B. subtilis*. AbrB is referred to as "transition state regulator," a term used to describe regulatory proteins that repress or activate genes during the transition from active growth into stationary phase *(88)*. Capsule synthesis is also regulated by a pXO2-encoded transcriptional activator, AcpA *(58)*. Environmental stimuli during infection are likely to be sensed by chromosomally encoded factors as well. For example, *B.*

anthracis encodes the stress-transcription factor σ^B (*sigB* gene) along with two regulatory proteins RsbV and RsbW *(89)*. The finding that a *B. anthracis-* σ^B mutant is less virulent than the parental strain *(89)* suggests that σ^B, along with additional factors, must be involved in the adaptation of *B. anthracis* to its varying and extreme lifestyles, either in the host or during prolonged survival outside of the host.

6.5. Potential Virulence Factors

Although the toxins play a major role in *B. anthracis* pathogenesis, much remains to be understood. Because of its complex life cycle, it seems reasonable to assume that other genes will contribute to *B. anthracis* pathogenesis. For example, how do spores travel through epithelia and become engulfed by macrophages? Do they display surface receptors? What are the factors that are sensed by the engulfed spores and trigger germination? How do vegetative bacilli escape the phagolysosome and survive in the macrophage?

It seems worthwhile comparing anthrax to other Gram-positive pathogens and their invasive strategies. One may distinguish extracellular from intracellular pathogens such as staphylococci and *Listeria monocytogenes*, respectively. In fact, because of its complex life cycle, *B. anthracis* may employ strategies from both organisms, as spores may be considered to be intracellular pathogens whereas vegetative bacilli are equivalents of extracellular pathogens. Bearing this in mind, we have searched the unfinished genome of *B. anthracis* (available from the TIGR website; http://www.ncbi. nlm.nih.gov./entrez/viewer.fcgi?db=nucleotide&val=30407125), for possible virulence factors by comparing sequences with the genome data of *S. aureus* and *L. monocytogenes* (these genomes are also available from the TIGR website; http:// www.ncbi.nlm.nih.gov/entrez/viewer.fcgi?db=nucleotide&val=15922990 and http:// www.ncbi.nlm.nih.gov/entrez/viewer.fcgi?db=nucleotide&val=21397375, respectively).

First, *B. anthracis* genome sequence was searched for the presence of sortase-like genes. Sortases are transpeptidase enzymes that are required for the covalent attachment of proteins in the cell wall of Gram-positive bacteria. Gram-positive bacteria use cell surface displayed proteins to mediate specific receptor–ligand interactions *(90)*. For example, one could envision that engulfment of spores require receptor proteins that are anchored in the spore wall. *S. aureus* encodes two sortases, sortase A and B. Sortase A cleaves the LPXTG motif in the C-terminal sorting signal of surface proteins and is responsible for the covalent attachment of polypeptides to the cell wall envelope *(91,92)*. Although most surface proteins of *S. aureus* are attached to the cell wall in a sortase A-dependent manner, the cell surface display of three proteins IsdA, IsdB, and IsdC specifically requires the second enzyme, sortase B *(93)*. In this manner, Sortase B and the Isd proteins contribute to a mechanism of heme-iron transport across the bacterial envelope (94). Iron is essential for bacteria and limiting in host cells.

The genome of *L. monocytogenes* (GenBank/EMBL accession no. AL591824), a close relative of *B. anthracis*, encodes two transpeptidases, sortase A and B, which seem to function similar to those reported for staphylococci *(95,96)*. Searching the genome sequence of *B. anthracis* (GenBank accession no. NC_003995) revealed 10 genes that may encode possible surface proteins. Of these 10 surface protein genes, we believe that two represent homologs of the *L. monocytogenes* internalin gene family (*see* Table 1). Internalin A, a sortase A anchored surface protein, mediates the invasion

Table 1
Suface Proteins Encoded in the Genome of *B. anthracis:* Potential Virulence Factors

Protein	Homolog	Sortase	Sorting signal		AA
BasA*	Internalin E	SrtA	LPKTG	TNVASTIGAGLAFIGAGFLLLFRRKKANR	304
BasB	Protein A	SrtA	LPATG	HDMNYLPFIGFALVLLGIRLRFMTKNN	898
BasC	Lmo0159	SrtA	LPATG	GVSNQFTSLFVLGISFIIAGAYVLRMKNRKEM	632
BasD	Lmo0159	SrtA	LPNTG	HKNDSTQTVGIILLLAGLLSVLATKRKKY	880
BasE	None	SrtA	LPKTG	AASPWMVSVGAGISFLVGGVLFVLGRRRKQ	1448
BasR	None	SrtA	LPKTG	ASSHSAATEVGMGVLCIASAYVLWRRK	358
BasG/IsdC	IsdC	SrtB	NPKTG	DEARIGLFAALILISGVFLIRKVKLSK	237
BasH	None	SrtB	NSKTA	DTAQLGLTMVLLLGSLALLVRKTRAGRL	875
BasI	Internalin A	SrtC	LGATG	GQENTSTLLSGLALVLSALSMFVFRKRLFKK	1066
BasJ	None	SrtC	LPTQS	WETSSNSDYSNASYYYQCQHGNNKPYKIR	1354

*Bas, *Bacillus anthracis* surface protein.

of *L. monocytogenes* into epithelial cells by binding to its E-cadherin receptor during host infection *(97–99)*. In contrast to staphylococci and listeria, *B. anthracis* harbors at least three sortase genes *(100)*. Whereas the sortase A and B homologs of *B. anthracis* likely exert functions similar to those reported for *S. aureus*, elucidating the role of the third sortase gene requires some innovative experimental work (*see* Table 1). Is it possible that anchored surface proteins of *B. anthracis* are involved in targeting spores or bacilli to distinct locations within the infected host? Is it possible that *B. anthracis* sortases are active even during spore development and serve to anchor proteins to the spore wall? Although these hypotheses are somewhat iconoclastic, a definitive answer can only be obtained with experimental work.

Surface proteins of *L. monocytogenes* provide not only for invasion mechanisms during host entry but also aid listerial evasion of the immune response by facilitating bacterial spread within the cytoplasm of infected host cells *(101)*. The latter pathway requires, in addition to internalins, several other gene products that provide for listerial escape from the phagosome (*hlyA* or *llo*) *(102)*, actin-polymerization and spread between cells (*actA*) *(103)*, and lysis of host cell double-membrane vacuoles after bacterial transmission into neighboring cells (*plcB*) *(104,105)*. Could similar strategies be employed by *B. anthracis*? Ingested spores of *B. anthracis* are transported via lymphatic to mediastinal lymph nodes and resist phagocytic killing. Instead, they begin to germinate within macrophages *(106,107)*. Similar to listeria, newly germinated bacilli escape from the phagocytic vacuole and replicate within the cytoplasm of macrophages. Experiments performed with cultured macrophages show that bacilli replicate and escape from the cells within 6 h following endospore phagocytosis. The kinetics of these events correlate with the timing of disease symptoms during infection of laboratory animals *(108)*.

We have searched the available genome of *B. anthracis* and found that it carries homologs of both listeriolysin O (*llo*) and C-type phospholipase (*plcB*), but the *actA* gene could not be identified. Although host cell invasion may be a common strategy between *listeria* and *B. anthracis*, bacterial spread through cytoplasmic compartments presumably is not. But how are the vegetative bacilli released from the macrophages?

It is interesting that the listeriolysin homolog of *B. anthracis* does not contain a PEST-like sequence (P, Pro; E, Glu; S, Ser; T, Thr) as is observed for listerial LLO (W. Williams, personal communication), a secreted pore-forming polypeptide. LLO variants lacking the PEST-like sequence accumulate in the host-cell cytosol, suggesting that the PEST motif targets LLO for degradation. The aberrantly stabilized LLO mutants cause the subsequent permeabilization of the host-cell membrane and bacterial exposure to the environment *(109)*. One wonders whether this strategy is the means by which *B. anthracis* perforates both phagolysosome and host-cell membranes. Other reports have proposed that macrophage lysis may be a consequence of early LeTx and EdTx production *(46,110)*. However, this view is challenged by a third report claiming that the toxin genes are not required for release from the macrophage *(108)*. These dissensions likely result from differences in the model systems that were used. So far, most data were obtained using cultured macrophages and the Sterne strain. Better comprehension of the system is likely to be achieved with experiments using the fully virulent strain and appropriate animal systems.

7. OUTLOOK

B. anthracis has captured the attention and imagination of microbiologists around the globe. Its elaborate cell cycle allows it to multiply undetected by the host and to produce large quantities of anthrax toxin. Currently available antibiotic treatments aim to kill multiplying bacteria but are unable to interfere with toxin-mediated killing of the host. Microbiologists are exploring the possibility of combining passive immunization of infected patients with aggressive antibiotic treatments. Most attempts described so far aim at interfering with the correct functioning of the PA subunit. For example, an antibody library generated by phage display has been screened by panning with the PA subunit of anthrax toxin. The antibody with the highest affinity for PA prevented anthrax toxin from binding to its receptor on cultured alveolar macrophages as well as protected rats against anthrax toxin *(111)*. However, no matter how effective a vaccine may be, multiple immunizations are required for protection to build up. The recent discovery of the ATR has uncovered new exciting avenues *(11)*. The demonstration that the soluble region of ATR blocks killing by PA suggests that the design of a receptor decoy may represent a new therapeutic strategy. However, because the physiological function of ATR (TEM8) is not known, it is unclear whether such therapeutic agents will also affect the host. Another means for blocking PA's function takes advantage of mutant PA exhibiting a dominant negative phenotype. Such mutants coassemble with the wildtype protein in a test tube, and prevent pore formation and translocation of EF and LF into cultured cells. Injection of the mutant PA in rats challenged with anthrax conferred protection from disease *(112)*. It is conceivable that administration of mutant PA into individuals infected with anthrax may block the progression of the disease even at more advanced stages of disease.

Finally, one must mention the elegant strategy recently explored by Fischetti et al. *(113)*. These authors took advantage of the inherent binding specificity and lytic action of bacteriophage enzymes called lysins. As a normal part of their life cycle, bacteriophages multiply in host cells and their progeny is released upon lysis of the cell wall. Purified PlyG, an enzyme synthesized by bacteriophage-γ, was found to destroy the cell wall of both vegetative cells and germinating spores of *B. anthracis (113)*. PlyG is a virus specific lysin for *B. anthracis* and other members of the *B. anthracis* "cluster" of bacilli. The lytic specificity of PlyG could be exploited as a tool for the treatment and detection of *B. anthracis*.

In summary, *B. anthracis* is the causative agent of anthrax, a terrifying disease that can be inflicted by man. Anthrax can be viewed as a series of astonishingly complex interactions between a microbial pathogen and its hosts. By gaining new insights in the biology of this microbe, bioterrorism or biological warfare may be prevented and one may appreciate intricate molecular mechanisms that presumably govern the interplay between microbe and host. Thus, *B. anthracis* could once again serve as model microbe to further our understanding of human and animal infectious diseases.

REFERENCES

1. Meselson, M. (1999) The challenge of biological and chemical weapons. *Bull. World Health Organ.* **77,** 102,103.
2. Meselson, M., Guillemin, J., Hugh-Jones, M., et al. (1994) The Sverdlovsk anthrax outbreak of 1979. *Science* **266,** 1202–1208.
3. Brown, K. (2001) Anthrax. A 'sure killer' yields to medicine. *Science* **294,** 1813,1814.
4. Edsall, J. T. and Meselson, M. (1967) Proliferation of CB warfare. *Science* **156,** 1029,1030.
5. Harris, S. H. (1994) *Factories of death: Japanese secret biological warfare, 1932–1945, and the American cover-up.* Routledge, London.
6. Inglesby, T. V., Henderson, D. A., Bartlett, J. G., et al. (1999) Anthrax as a biological weapon: medical and public health management. Working group on civilian defense. *JAMA* **281,** 2127–2137.
7. Enserink, M. (2001) This time it was real: knowledge of anthrax put to the test. *Science* **294,** 490,491.
8. Friedlander, A. M. (2001) Tackling anthrax. *Nature* **414,** 160,161.
9. Leppla, S. H. (2000) Anthrax toxin, in: *Bacterial Protein Toxins.* (Aktories, K. and Just, I., eds.), Springer, p. 445–472.
10. Chaudry, G. J., Moayeri, M., Liu, S., and Leppla, S. H. (2001) Quickening the pace of anthrax research: three advances point towars possible therapies. *Trends Microbiol.* **10,** 58–62.
11. Bradley, K. A., Mogridge, J., Mourez, M., Collier, R. J., and Young, J. A. (2001) Identification of the cellular receptor for anthrax toxin. *Nature* **414,** 225–229.
12. Pannifer, A. D., Wong, T. Y., Schwarzenbacher, R., et al. (2001) Crystal structure of the anthrax lethal factor. *Nature* **414,** 229–233.
13. Watters, J. W., Dewar, K., Lehoczky, J., Boyartchuk, V., and Dietrich, W. F. (2001) Kif1C, a kinesin-like motor protein, mediates mouse macrophage resistance to anthrax lethal factor. *Curr. Biol.* **11,** 1503–1511.
14. Koch, R. (1876) Die Aetiologie der Milzbrand-Krankheit, begruendet auf die Entwicklungsgeschichte des *Bacillus Anthracis. Beitraege zur Biologie der Pflanzen* **2,** 277–310.
15. Pasteur, L. (1881) De l'attenuation des virus et de leur retour a la virulence. *C.R. Acad. Sci. III* **92,** 429–435.
16. Williams, R. *(1986) Bacillus anthracis* and other spore forming bacilli, in: *Infectious Disease and Medical Microbiology.* (Braude, A., Davis, L., and Fierer, J., eds.), WB Saunders, Philadelphia, PA, pp. 270–278.
17. Titball, R. W., Turnbull, P. C., and Hutson, R. A. (1991) The monitoring and detection of Bacillus anthracis in the environment. *Soc. Appl. Bacteriol. Symp. Ser.* **20,** 9S–18S.

18. Turnbull, P. C. B. (1996) Anthrax is alive and well. *PHLS Microbiol. Dig.* **9,** 103–106.
19. Sterne, M. (1967) Distribution and economic importance of anthrax. *Fed. Proceed.* **26,** 1493–1495.
20. Dixon, T. C., Meselson, M., Guillemin, J., and Hanna, P. C. (1999) Anthrax. *N. Engl. J. Med.* **341,** 815–826.
21. Swartz, M. N. (2001) Recognition and management of anthrax—an update. *N. Engl. J. Med.* **345,** 1621–1626.
22. Dewan, P. K., Fry, A. M., Laserson, K., et al. (2002) Inhalational anthrax outbreak among postal workers, Washington, D.C., 2001. *Emerg. Infect. Dis.* **8,** 1066–1072.
23. Borio, L., Frank, D., Mani, V., et al. (2001) Death due to bioterrorism-related inhalational anthrax: report of two patients. *JAMA* **285,** 2763–2773.
24. Keim, P., Price, L. B., Klevytska, A. M., et al. (2000) Multiple-locus variable-number tandem repeat analysis reveals genetic relationships within *Bacillus anthracis. J. Bacteriol.* **182,** 2928–2936.
25. Read, T. D., Salzberg, S. L., Pop, M., et al. Comparative genome sequencing for discovery of novel polymorphisms in Bacillus anthracis. *Science* **296,** 2028–2033.
26. Gold, H. (1967) Treatment of anthrax. *Fed. Proc.* **26,** 1563–1568.
27. Lightfoot, N. F., Scott, R. J. D., and Turnbull, P. C. B. (1989) Antimicrobial susceptibility of Bacillus anthracis, in: *Proceedings of the International Workshop on Anthrax.* Salisbury Medical Bulletin, Winchester, UK, pp. 95–98.
28. Friedlander, A. M., Welkos, S. L., Pitt, M. L. M., et al. (1993) Postexposure prophylaxis against experimental inhalation anthrax. *J. Infect. Dis.* **167,** 1239–1242.
29. Centers for Disease Control. (2001) Update: Investigation of Bioterrorism-Related Anthrax and Interim Guidelines for Exposure Management and Antimicrobial Therapy, October 2001. *Morb. Mortal. Wkly Rep.* **50,** 909–919.
30. Sterne, M. (1937) Avirulent anthrax vaccine. *Onderstepoort J. Vet. Sci Animal Ind.* **21,** 41–43.
31. Pittman, P. R., Kim-Ahn, G., Pifat, D. Y., et al. (2002) Anthrax vaccine: immunogenicity and safety of a dose-reduction, route-change comparison study in humans. *Vaccine* **20,** 1412–1420.
32. Welkos, S., Little, S., Friedlander, A., Fritz, D., and Fellows, P. (2001) The role of antibodies to *Bacillus anthracis* and anthrax toxin components in inhibiting the early stages of infection by anthrax spores. *Microbiology* **147,** 1677–1685.
33. Welkos, S., Friedlander, A. M., Weeks, S., Little, S., and Mendelson, I. (2002) In-vitro characterization of the phagocytosis and fate of anthrax spores in macrophages and the effects of anti-PA antibody. *J. Med. Microbiol.* **51,** 821–831.
34. Metchnikoff, E. (1905) *Immunity in Infectious Diseases.* Cambridge University Press, Cambridge.
35. Guidi-Rontani, C. (2002) The alveolar macrophage: the Trojan horse of *Bacillus anthracis. Trends Microbiol.* **10,** 405–409.
36. Zwartouw, H. T. and Smith, H. (1956) Polyglutamic acid from *Bacillus anthracis* grown *in vivo*: structure and aggressin activity. *Biochem. J.* **63,** 437–454.
37. Preisz, H. (1909) Experimentelle studien ueber virulenz, empfaenglichkeit und immunitaet beim milzbrand. *Zeitschr. Immunitaet.-Forsch.* **5,** 341–452.
38. Leppla, S. H. (1991) The anthrax toxin complex, in: *Scourcebook of Bacterial Protein Toxins.* (Alouf, J. and Freer, J. H., eds.), Academic Press, London, pp. 277–302.
39. Hanna, P. C., Acosta, D., and Collier, R. J. (1993) On the role of macrophages in anthrax. *Proc. Natl. Acad. Sci. USA* **90,** 10,198–10,201.
40. Vodkin, M. H. and Leppla, S. H. (1983) Cloning of the protective antigen gene of *Bacillus anthracis. Cell* **34,** 693–697.
41. Welkos, S. L., Lowe, J. R., Eden-McCutchan, F., Vodkin, M., Leppla, S. H., and Schmidt, J. J. (1988) Sequence and analysis of the DNA encoding the protective antigen of *Bacillus anthracis. Gene* **69,** 287–300.

42. Milne, J., Furlong, D., Hanna, P. C., Wall, J. S., and Collier, R. J. (1994) Anthrax protective antigen forms oligomers during intoxication of mammalian cells. *J. Biol. Chem.* **269,** 20,607–20,612.

43. Klimpel, K. R., Arora, N., and Leppla, S. H. (1994) Anthrax toxin lethal factor contains a zinc metalloprotease consensus sequence which is required for lethal toxin activity. *Mol. Microbiol.* **13,** 1093–1100.

44. Duesbery, N. S., Webb, C. P., Leppla, S. H., et al. (1998) Proteolytic inactivation of Map-kinase-kinase by anthrax lethal factor. *Science* **280,** 734–737.

45. Vitale, G., Pellizzari, R., Recchi, C., Napolitani, G., Mock, M., and Montecucco, C. (1998) Anthrax lethal factor cleaves the N-terminus of MAPKKs and induces tyrosine/threonine phosphorylation of MAPKs in cultured macrophages. *Biochem. Biophys. Res. Commun.* **248,** 706–711.

46. Park, J. M., Greten, F. R., Li, Z. W., and Karin, M. (2002) Macrophage apoptosis by anthrax lethal factor through p38 MAP kinase inhibition. *Science* **297,** 2048–2051.

47. Tang, G. and Leppla, S. H. (1999) Proteasome activity is required for anthrax toxin to kill macrophages. *Infect. Immun.* **67,** 3055–3060.

48. Watters, J. W., Dewar, K., Lehoczky, J., Boyartchuk, V., and Dietrich, W. F. (2001) Kif1C, a kinesin-like motor protein, mediates mouse macrophage resistance to anthrax lethal factor. *Curr. Biol.* **11,** 1503–1511.

49. Leppla, S. H. *(1984) Bacillus anthracis* calmodulin-dependent adenylate cyclase: chemical and enzymatic properties and interactions with eucaryotic cells. Adv. *Cyclic Nucleotide Protein Phosphorylation Res.* **17,** 189–198.

50. Leppla, S. H. (1982) Anthrax toxin edema factor: a bacterial adenylate cyclase that increases cyclin AMP concentrations in eukaryotic cells. *Proc. Natl. Acad. Sci. USA* **79,** 3162–3166.

51. Green, B. D., Battisti, L., Koehler, T. M., Thorne, C. B., and Ivins, B. E. (1985) Demonstration of a capsule plasmid in *Bacillus anthracis. Infect. Immun.* **49,** 291–297.

52. Mikesell, P., Ivins, B. E., Ristroph, J. D., and Dreier, T. M. (1983) Evidence for plasmid-mediated toxin production in *Bacillus anthracis. Infect. Immun.* **39,** 371–376.

53. Smith, H., Keppie, H. S., and Stanley, J. I. (1953) The chemical basis of the virulence of *Bacillus anthracis.* I. Properties of bacteria grown in vivo and preparation of extracts. *Br. J. Exp. Pathol.* **34,** 477–485.

54. Keppie, J., Smith, H., and Harris-Smith, P. W. (1963) The chemical basis of the virulence of *Bacillus anthracis.* II. Some biological properties of bacterial products. *Br. J. Exp. Pathol.* **34,** 486–496.

55. Okinaka, R. T., Cloud, K., Hampton, O., et al. (1999) Sequence and organization of pXO1, the large *Bacillus anthracis* plasmid harboring the anthrax toxin genes. *J. Bacteriol.* **181,** 6509–6515.

56. Makino, S., Uchida, I., Terakado, N., Sasakawa, C., and Yoshikawa, M. (1989) Molecular characterization and protein analysis of the *cap* region, which is essential for encapsulation in *Bacillus anthracis. J. Bacteriol.* **171,** 722–730.

57. Uchida, I., Makino, S., Sasakawa, C., Yoshikawa, M., Sugimoto, C., and Terakado, N. (1993) Identification of a novel gene, *dep,* associated with depolymerization of the capsular polymer in *Bacillus anthracis. Mol. Microbiol.* **9,** 487–496.

58. Vietri, N. J., Marrero, R., Hoover, T. A., and Welkos, S. L. (1995) Identification and characterization of a trans-activator involved in the regulation of encapsulation by *Bacillus anthracis. Gene* **152,** 1–9.

59. Turnbull, P. C., Hutson, R. A., Ward, M. J., et al. (1992) Bacillus anthracis but not always anthrax. *J. Appl. Bacteriol.* **72,** 21–28.

60. Guidi-Rontani, C., Pereira, Y., Ruffie, S., Sirard, J. C., Weber-Levy, M., and Mock, M. (1999) Identification and characterization of a germination operon on the virulence plasmid pXO1 of *Bacillus anthracis. Mol. Microbiol.* **33,** 407–414.

61. Driks, A. *(1999) Bacillus subtilis* spore coat. *Microbiol. Mol. Biol. Rev.* **63,** 1–20.
62. Piggot, P. and Losick, R. (2002) Sporulation genes and intercompartmental regulation, in: *Bacillus subtilis and its Closest Relatives: From Genes to Cells.* (Sonenshein, A. L., Hoch, J. A., and Losick, R., eds.), ASM, Washington, DC, pp. 483–517.
63. Driks, A. (2002) Maximum shields: the assembly and function of the bacterial spore coat. *Trends Microbiol.* **10,** 251–254.
64. Hachisuka, Y., Kozuka, S., and Tsujikawa, M. (1984) Exosporia and appendages of spores of Bacillus species. *Microbiol. Immunol.* **28,** 619–624.
65. Matz, L. L., Beaman, T. C., and Gerhardt, P. (1970) Chemical composition of exosporium from spores of *Bacillus cereus. J. Bacteriol.* **101,** 196–201.
66. Beaman, T. C., Pankratz, H. S., and Gerhardt, P. (1971) Paracrystalline sheets reaggregated from solubilized exosporium of *Bacillus cereus. J. Bacteriol.* **107,** 320–324.
67. Hachisuka, Y., Kojima, K., and Sato, T. (1966) Fine filaments on the outside of the exosporium of *Bacillus anthracis* spores. *J. Bacteriol.* **91,** 2382–2384.
68. Charlton, S., Moir, A. J., Baillie, L., and Moir, A. Characterization of the exosporium of Bacillus cereus. *J. Appl. Microbiol.* **87,** 241–245.
69. Garcia-Patrone, M. and Tandecarz, J. S. (1995) A glycoprotein multimer from *Bacillus thuringiensis* sporangia: dissociation into subunits and sugar composition. *Mol. Cell. Biochem.* **145,** 29–37.
70. Sylvestre, P., Couture-Tosi, E., and Mock, M. (2002) A collagen-like surface glycoprotein is a structural component of the *Bacillus anthracis* exosporium. *Mol. Microbiol.* **45,** 169–178.
71. Gerhardt, P. (1967) Cytology of *Bacillus anthracis. Fed. Proc.* **26,** 1504–1517.
72. Ezzell, J. W. and Abshire, T. G. J. (1988) Immunological analysis of cell-associated antigens of *Bacillus anthracis. Infect. Immun.* **56,** 349–356.
73. Mignot, T., Mesnage, S., Couture-Tosi, E., Mock, M., and Fouet, A. (2002) Developmental switch of S-layer protein synthesis in *Bacillus anthracis. Mol. Microbiol.* **43,** 1615–1627.
74. Mesnage, S., Fontaine, T., Mignot, T., Delepierre, M., Mock, M., and Fouet, A. (2000) Bacterial SLH domain proteins are non-covalently anchored to the cell surface via a conserved mechanism involving wall polysaccharide pyruvylation. *EMBO J.* **19,** 4473–4484.
75. Sára, M. and Sleytr, U. B. (2000) S-layer proteins. *J. Bacteriol.* **182,** 859–868.
76. Mock, M. and Fouet, A. (2001) Anthrax. *Annu. Rev. Microbiol.* **55,** 647–671.
77. Hanby, W. E. and Rydon, HNTcsoBaBJ-. (1946) The capsular substance of *Bacillus anthracis. Biochem. J.* **40,** 297–309.
78. Goodman, J. W. and Nitecki, D. E. (1967) Studies on the relation of a prior immune response to immunogenicity. *Immunology* **13,** 577–583.
79. Ezzel, J. W. and Welkos, S. L. (1999) The capsule of bacillus anthracis, a review. *J. Appl. Microbiol.* **87,** 250.
80. Bartkus, J. M. and Leppla, S. H. (1989) Transcriptional regulation of the protective antigen gene of *Bacillus anthracis. Infect. Immun.* **57,** 2295–2300.
81. Cataldi, A., Labruyère, E., and Mock, M. (1990) Construction and characterization of a protective antigen-deficient *Bacillus anthracis* strain. *Mol. Microbiol.* **4,** 1111–1117.
82. Koehler, T. M., Dai, Z., and Kaufman-Yarbray, M. (1994) Regulation of the *Bacillus anthracis* protective antigen gene: CO2 and a trans-acting element activate transcription from one of two promoters. *J. Bacteriol.* **176,** 586–595.
83. Uchida, I., Makino, S., Sekizaki, T., and Terakado, N. (1997) Cross-talk to the genes for *Bacillus anthracis* capsule synthesis by *atxA*, the gene encoding the trans-activator of anthrax toxin synthesis. *Mol. Microbiol.* **23,** 1229–1240.
84. Dai, Z., Sirard, J.-C., Mock, M., and Koehler, T. M. (1995) The *atxA* gene product activates transcription of the anthrax toxin genes and is essential for virulence. *Mol. Microbiol.* **16,** 1171–1181.

85. Hoffmaster, A. R. and Koehler, T. M. (1999) Autogenous regulation of the *Bacillus anthracis pag* operon. *J. Bacteriol.* **181,** 4485–4492.

86. Hoffmaster, A. R. and Koehler, T. M. (1999) Control of virulence gene expression in *Bacillus anthracis. J. Appl. Microbiol.* **87,** 279–281.

87. Saile, E. and Koehler, T. M. (2002) Control of anthrax gene expression by the transition state regulator *abrB. J. Bacteriol.* **184,** 370–380.

88. Strauch, M. A. and Hoch, J. A. (1993) Transition-state regulators: sentinels of *Bacillus subtilis* post-exponential gene expression. *Mol. Microbiol.* **7,** 337–342.

89. Fouet, A., Namy, O., and Lambert, G. (2000) Characterization of the operon encoding the alternative σ^B factor from *Bacillus anthracis* and its role in virulence. *J. Bacteriol.* **182,** 5036–5045.

90. Navarre, W. W. and Schneewind, O. (1999) Surface proteins of Gram-positive bacteria and the mechanisms of their targeting to the cell wall envelope. *Microbiol. Mol. Biol. Rev.* **63,** 174–229.

91. Mazmanian, S. K., Liu, G., Ton-That, H., and Schneewind, O. *(1999) Staphylococcus aureus* sortase, an enzyme that anchors surface proteins to the cell wall. *Science* **285,** 760–763.

92. Mazmanian, S. K., Liu, G., Jensen, E. R., Lenoy, E., and Schneewind, O. *(2000) Staphylococcus aureus* mutants defective in the display of surface proteins and in the pathogenesis of animal infections. *Proc. Natl. Acad. Sci. USA* **97,** 5510–5515.

93. Mazmanian, S. K., Ton-That, H., Su, K., and Schneewind, O. (2002) An iron-regulated sortase enzyme anchors a class of surface protein during *Staphylococcus aureus* pathogenesis. *Proc. Natl. Acad. Sci. USA* **99,** 2293–2298.

94. Mazmanian, S. K., Skaar, E. P., Gasper, A. H., et al. (2003) Passage of heme-iron across the envelope of *Staphylococcus aureus. Science* **299,** 906–909.

95. Glaser, P., Frangeul, L., Buchrieser, C., et al. (2001) Comparative genomics of *Listeria* species. *Science* **294,** 849–852.

96. Bierne, H., Mazmanian, S. K., Trost, M., et al. (2002) Inactivation of the *srtA* gene in *Listeria monocytogenes* inhibits anchoring of surface proteins and affects virulence. *Mol. Microbiol.* **43,** 869–881.

97. Gaillard, J.-L., Berche, P., Frehel, C., Gouin, E., and Cossart, P. (1991) Entry of *L. monocytogenes* into cells is mediated by internalin, a repeat protein reminiscent of surface antigens from gram-positive cocci. *Cell* **65,** 1127–1141.

98. Mengaud, J., Ohayon, H., Gounon, P., Mege, M., and Cossart, P. (1996) E-cadherin is the receptor for internalin, a surface protein required for entry of Listeria monocytogenes into epithelial cells. *Cell* **84,** 923–932.

99. Lecuit, M., Vandormael-Pournin, S., Lefort, J., et al. (2001) A transgenic model for listeriosis: role of internalin in crossing the intestinal barrier. *Science* **292,** 1722–1725.

100. Pallen, M. J., Lam, A. C., Antonio, M., and Dunbar, K. (2001) An embarrassment of sortases - a richness of substrates. *Trends Microbiol.* **9,** 97–101.

101. Dramsi, S. and Cossart, P. (1998) Intracellular pathogens and the actin cytoskeleton. *Annu. Rev. Cell Dev. Biol.* **14,** 137–166.

102. Portnoy, D. A., Jacks, P. A., and Hinrichs, D. J. (1988) Role of hemolysin for the intracellular growth of *Listeria monocytogenes. J. Exp. Med.* **167,** 1459–1471.

103. Kocks, C., Gouin, E., Tabouret, M., Berche, P., Ohayon, H., and Cossart, P. *(1992) L. monocytogenes*-induced actin assembly requires the *actA* gene product, a surface protein. *Cell* **68,** 521–531.

104. Camilli, A., Tilney, L. G., and Portnoy, D. A. (1993) Dual roles of *plcA* in *Listeria monocytogenes* pathogenesis. *Mol. Microbiol.* **8,** 143–157.

105. Cossart, P. and Lecuit, M. (1998) Interactions of Listeria monocytogenes with mammalian cells during the entry and actin-based movement: bacterial factors, cellular ligands and signaling. *EMBO J.* **17,** 3797–3806.

106. Hanna, P. C.(1997) Anthrax pathogenesis and host response. *Curr. Top. Microbiol. Immunol.* **225,** 13–35.
107. Guidi-Rontani, C., Weber-Levy, M., Labruyere, E., and Mock, M. (1999) Germination of *Bacillus anthracis* spores within alveolar macrophages. *Mol. Microbiol.* **31,** 9–17.
108. Dixon, T. C., Fadl, A. A., Koehler, T. M., Swanson, J. A., and Hanna, P. C. (2000) Early Bacillus anthracis-macrophage interactions: intracellular survival survival and escape. *Cell. Microbiol.* **2,** 453–463.
109. Decatur, A. L. and Portnoy, D. A. (2000) A PEST-like sequence in listeriolysin O essential for *Listeria monocytogenes* pathogenicity. *Science* **290,** 992–995.
110. Guidi-Rontani, C., Levy, M., Ohayon, H., and Mock, M. (2001) Fate of germinated Bacillus anthracis spores in primary murine macrophages. *Mol. Microbiol.* **42,** 931–938.
111. Maynard, J., Maassen, C., Leppla, S., et al. (2002) Protection against anthrax toxin by recombinant antibody fragments correlates with antigen affinity. *Nat. Biotechnol.* **20,** 597–601.
112. Sellman, B. R., Mourez, M., and Collier, R. J. (2001) Dominant-negative mutants of a toxin subunit: an approach to therapy of anthrax. *Science* **292,** 695–697.
113. Schuch, R., Nelson, D., and Fischetti, V. A. (2002) A bacteriolytic agent that detects and kills Bacillus anthracis. *Nature* **418,** 884–889.

6

Virologic and Pathogenic Aspects of the *Variola* Virus (Smallpox) as a Bioweapon

Robert G. Darling, Timothy H. Burgess, James V. Lawler, and Timothy P. Endy

1. INTRODUCTION

"The end of smallpox—but for the World Health Organization (WHO), it is only the end of the beginning. It has been said that if we had known beforehand "the heart-aches and the thousand natural shocks" that awaited us, we would never have undertaken the smallpox eradication programme….Victory over smallpox has implications that go far beyond the individuals directly concerned, however. It reasserts our ability to change the world around us for the better, through mutual collaboration and mobilization of resources, allied to human energies and the will to succeed. It comes like a freshening wind for a vessel to long becalmed, creating hopeful new impetus as we set our course towards Health for All by the Year 2000," as written by then Director-General of The WHO, Dr. Halfdan Mahler, in celebration of the global eradication of smallpox *(1)*.

October 1977 was a seminal time in the 3000-yr history of smallpox, because that was the year when the world's last naturally acquired case of smallpox occurred in Somalia, Africa *(2)*. The last case of smallpox (a laboratory-associated infection), occurred in England in September 1978. After a worldwide program to verify the eradication of smallpox in May 1980, the 33rd World Health Assembly accepted the report of the Global Commission for the Certification of Smallpox Eradication that smallpox had been eradicated. The elimination of smallpox was a landmark event in the history of public health and a culmination of intensive planning, geopolitical cooperation, and an effective vaccine to eradicate a disease responsible for human pain, suffering, and death *(3)*. By all rights, this celebration of humanity should have been a bookmark for students of history, yet smallpox remains a public health concern. Now the threat comes not as a naturally occurring disease, but as a bioweapon to introduce smallpox in a now immunologically naïve population. This concern, catalyzed by the intentional introduction of anthrax into the US postal system in September 2001, resulted in the rejuvenation of the smallpox vaccine, Dryvax, and the vaccination of more than 628,000 US serviceman and health care providers *(4–6)*. This chapter reviews the history and the current knowledge on the virology and pathogenesis of smallpox, highlighting its unique characteristics that makes it an ideal biological weapon.

From: *Infectious Diseases: Biological Weapons Defense: Infectious Diseases and Counterterrorism*
Edited by: L. E. Lindler, F. J. Lebeda, and G. W. Korch © Humana Press Inc., Totowa, NJ

2. HISTORY OF SMALLPOX

Until its eradication in 1980, smallpox was one of the most universally feared of all diseases. *Variola major*, the causative virus of smallpox, was probably responsible for more deaths and disability than any other pathogen *(2)*. Those fortunate enough to survive the infection often faced lifelong complications and sequelae, including blindness, arthritis, encephalitis, permanent osteoarticular anomalies, and a severely scarred complexion *(7)*.

The unique clinical manifestations of smallpox and its dramatic spread and mortality have made this disease easily identifiable in history. It is thought that *Variola* virus evolved as a human pathogen from an orthopoxvirus of animals in the Central African rain forests and established itself in the valley of the Nile and Fertile Crescent of Egypt thousands of years ago *(2)*. Examination of Egyptian mummified remains demonstrated the typical pustular eruptions of smallpox *(8)*. Historical descriptions of smallpox place it in China during the 4th century, in India and the Mediterranean during the 7th century and in southwestern Asia during the 10th century. Smallpox became established in Europe during the times of the crusades, and explorations from Europe aided its spread to the Americas *(2)*.

Before the development of the cowpox vaccine by Dr. Edward Jenner in 1796, there was no safe and consistently effective prevention method for this dreaded disease *(9)*. Variolation, the process of inoculating a subject with live *Variola* virus, probably originated in China around the 10th century but was frequently either ineffective or lethal *(10)*. Traditional therapies included "cupping," bloodletting, and a "sweating" regimen in which the heavily clothed patient was swaddled in blankets and placed in an overheated room and administered "heating medicines and cordials"*(11)*.

Between 1966 and 1980, Donald ("D. A") Henderson led the WHO effort to eradicate smallpox from the face of the Earth *(12)*. In 1976, the last naturally occurring case of *Variola major* was isolated in India, and in 1977, the last naturally occurring case of *Variola minor* was isolated in Somalia *(2)*. In 1980, the WHO declared the disease eradicated worldwide, and routine vaccination was discontinued shortly thereafter *(13)*. The United States ceased routine childhood smallpox vaccination in 1972, although the US military continued to vaccinate recruits until 1990. According to US Census Bureau data, approx 40% of the US population age 29 yr old or younger and, having never received a smallpox vaccination, would be susceptible to infection.

Global terrorism, the continued research and development of biological weapons, and other geopolitical events have generated a concern that smallpox could be directed against a susceptible population. Dr. Ken Alibek, the former deputy director of Biopreparat, the biological weapons program in the former Soviet Union, reported at the time of his defection to the United States in 1992 that the Soviet Union had produced massive amounts of smallpox since the WHO declaration and that Russia was continuing to attempt to genetically engineer the organism *(14)*. Evaluations of North Korean soldiers raised other concerns. Some showed signs of recent smallpox vaccination, suggesting that country's involvement in smallpox weapons research *(15)*. These and other findings led federal officials to conclude that the threat of a smallpox biological warfare attack is significant enough to warrant the reinstitution of a vaccination program for selected members of the US population, including members of the military, healthcare workers, and certain emergency responders, with the possibility of making the vaccine available to the general population on a volunteer basis in the near future *(16)*.

3. SMALLPOX AS A BIOLOGICAL WEAPON

The first documented attempt to use smallpox as a biological weapon occurred during the French and Indian Wars (1754–1767) in North America *(17)*. British colonial commanders serving under Sir Jeffrey Amherst allegedly gave blankets from smallpox victims as gifts to susceptible North American Indians. Although the actual cause is suspect, epidemics raged among the indigenous population, and in some areas, 50% mortality was not uncommon. During World War II, the Japanese Military Unit 731 experimented with the use of smallpox as a bioweapon *(18)*. The former Soviet Union had a massive biological weapons program *(14)*. At one point, as many as 50,000 scientists and technicians performed research on various bacteria, viruses, and toxins in as many as 40 facilities scattered throughout the country. Allegedly, the Soviets perfected large-scale industrial production of smallpox and considered it so important that they maintained an annual stockpile of 20 tons. They produced a weapon that was stable in an aerosol and could be delivered in warheads on intercontinental ballistic missiles *(14)*. There is some evidence that the release of aerosolized smallpox in the Aral Sea may have caused an accidental epidemic *(19)*.

In 1992, President Boris Yeltsin admitted that the Soviet Union had been pursuing development of biological weapons, prohibited by the Biological Weapons and Toxin Convention of 1972 *(20)*. Ironically, the Biopreparat program was established the same year that the Biological and Toxin Weapons Convention was ratified. President Yeltsin further stated at that time that the program would be promptly terminated.

Subsequent to the WHO declaration of smallpox eradication in 1980, signatory nations agreed to destroy all laboratory stores of the virus or surrender them to one of two officially sanctioned WHO reference laboratories: The Centers for Disease Control and prevention in Atlanta, GA, or the Institute of Virus Preparations in Moscow, Russia. Although remaining stocks at these laboratories were scheduled for destruction in 1996, controversy continued concerning this issue, and both Presidents Clinton and Bush placed destruction in abeyance (http://www.newsmax.com/archives/articles/2001/11/16/193250.shtml; http://www.fas.org/spp/starwars/program/news99/990429-smallpox-usia.htm; http://www.cbsnews.com/stories/1999/04/22/health/main42900.shtml).

In 2002, the World Health Assembly, the WHO decision-making body, accepted a recommendation that the remaining stocks be retained and that the issue be reviewed not later than 2005. Those arguing against destruction have put forth numerous compelling arguments: (a) destruction would hinder investigation into the mechanisms of viral pathogenesis and impede the development of medical countermeasures; (b) detailed molecular epidemiological studies to establish precise phylogenetic relationships of an isolate to known strains would be impossible, thus impairing forensic analysis and potentially assignment of attribution; (c) extinction of the smallpox virus would disallow study of its unique proteins that interfere with host immune and regulatory functions; and (d) mankind has never intentionally destroyed a species of life *(21)*.

Even if legally sanctioned repositories were destroyed, other potential sources of smallpox could exist, including clandestine stockpiles, cadavers in permafrost, and strains reverse engineered by scientists using data obtained from genetically sequenced strains. In short, most authorities agree that the likelihood of smallpox virus existing outside the WHO-sanctioned laboratories is high.

4. VIROLOGY

4.1. Classification of Variola Virus

Variola virus is a member of the family *Poxviridae*, subfamily *Chordopoxvirinae*, genera *Orthopoxvirus*. The genus *Orthopoxvirus* is composed of many related viruses and includes *Vaccinia* virus (virus used in the smallpox vaccine), cowpox, monkeypox, ectromelia, camelpox, taterapox, Uasin Gishu disease, and racoonpox (22). *Variola* virus is exclusively a human disease with no known animal reservoir. Other members within this genus produce disease primarily in their respective animal host. However, because of the close interrelationship of the viruses, species jumping can occur, as evidenced by cowpox and monkeypox, with the latter virus capable of producing large outbreaks of human disease with clinical manifestations very similar to *V. major* and a mortality of 10–15% *(23)*. Monkeypox has recently been implicated in an extensive outbreak of human disease in the United States with the source of the virus being imported, infected Gambian rats *(24)*.

4.2. Morphology

Poxviruses are the largest of all viruses with a genome consisting of a single molecule of double-stranded DNA crosslinked with a hairpin loop at the ends. Their genomes vary in size from 130 to 300 kbp *(25)*. The physical properties of the poxviruses are quite similar. They are described as "brick-shaped" or ovoid and are 200–400 nm long. The external surface of the virus contains an envelope consisting of host cell membrane lipoprotein plus virus-specific polypeptides such as hemagglutinin. Based on knowledge gained from the study of *Vaccinia* virus, the presence or absence of an outer envelope defines two major infectious forms of the virus: the intracellular mature virion (IMV), and the extracellular enveloped virion (EEV) *(26)*. The IMV form is stable in the environment and plays a predominant role in host-to-host transmission. The EEV form plays an important role in dissemination within the host. Below the envelope is the outer membrane consisting of a complex of surface tubules and globular proteins and encloses large lateral bodies. The nucleosome of the virus is contained within a core membrane and the core itself consists of double-stranded DNA. The DNA is unique to each virus by restriction fragment length polymorphism analysis; genomes of these viruses have a very well-preserved central region, allowing classification within the genus, whereas heterology in the terminal regions can be used to differentiate species *(27–29)*. The morphology of the orthopoxviruses is unique. Electron micrographs demonstrating a brick-shaped virus with a biconcave core with two lateral bodies are diagnostic for this genus of viruses but not specifically for *Variola*.

4.3. Antigenic Structure

The *Orthopoxviruses* contain a large number of polypeptides that define cellular receptors and antigenic sites for protective immunity. Some antigens are highly crossreactive across the viruses within this genus and others are virus-specific *(27)*. The close relation of these viruses and serologic crossreactivity helps to explain why species, as is the case with *Vaccinia* virus and *Variola* virus. Studies of *Vaccinia* demonstrate the importance of the type of antigen required for protective immunogencity. Mice vaccinated with VACV L1R (IMV immunogen) and A33R (EEV immunogen) were protected from a lethal poxvirus challenge *(26)*. Both antigens induced greater protection than either antigen alone, suggesting that for complete protective immunity, both IMV and EEV antigens are required.

4.4. Replication

Orthopoxviruses, like all viruses are dependent on host cellular mechanisms for DNA replication, protein synthesis, and viral assembly and release. The first event is the attachment of the virus to the host cell through specific cellular receptors on the outer surface of the virus. IMV and EEV forms are both infectious but differ in their attachment and entry into cells *(22)*. The EEV form has a more rapid cellular entry and requires uncoating of the virus in the cellular cytoplasm. The IMV form can enter either through the host-cell outer membrane or within a vacuole formed by invagination of the plasma membrane releasing its core directly into the cytoplasm. Once the core enters the host cytoplasm, there is an immediate transcription of viral enzymes that results in the uncoating of the virus and the release of the DNA into the cytoplasm. DNA replication occurs followed by translation of both structural and nonstructural polyproteins leading to viral assembly first as IMV, which are then wrapped in modified Golgi membranes and transported to the periphery of the cell with release of the EEV form of the mature virion *(25)*.

4.5. Virulence

Variola virus is a collection of numerous distinct strains. Although difficult to differentiate antigenically or serologically, the existence of distinct strains is suggested by clinical evidence, notably the wide variation in mortality from epidemics in different areas *(30)*. These differences did not appear to be related to host factors and persisted when the particular strain was transported to a different region *(22)*. The clearest distinction was between strains of the virus that caused outbreaks with mortality between 5 and 40% and strains associated with a mortality of 0.1–2%. This led to the classifications of *V. major* and *V. minor* *(22)*. Virulence among the strains of *Variola* virus was first noted in vitro with chick embryo cultures. Viral titers were higher for Asian variants of *V. major* as compared to *V. minor* isolates *(31)*. The genetic differences between strains have been analyzed by restricted fragment length polymorphism (RFLP) mapping *(28,29)*. These studies found that strains of *V. minor* were similar but differed from strains of *V. major*. Genetic differences among the strains presumably reflect differences in viral replication and host-cell assembly, leading to greater or lesser virulence. A variant of *Variola* virus has been described that produces a unique late polypeptide of different size and endonuclease cleavage site *(32)*. This marker was demonstrated to be genetically independent, expressed by 14 of the 48 *Variola* strains examined and correlated to *V. major* strains and not *V. minor*.

4.6. Immune Evasion Strategies

The poxviruses are notable for their ability to manipulate the immune response mechanisms of the vertebrate hosts in which they replicate. These adaptations likely play an important role in the pathogenesis of poxvirus diseases and the virulence observed among the strains. Most notable is the ability of the poxviruses to produce many proteins that interact with the host at both the cellular and systemic levels *(33,34)*. *Vaccinia* virus produces a viral homolog of epidermal growth factor, several serine protease inhibitors thought to block a host pathway for generating a chemotactic response, and proteins, which interfere with the activation of the classical complement pathway *(34,35)*. Direct inhibition of the host cellular immune response has been demonstrated by the orthopoxviruses through the production of soluble receptors for gamma interferon (IFN)-γ which prevents host-produced IFN-γ from binding to its receptor *(36)*.

The potential for genetic manipulation of the orthopoxviruses leading to expression of novel proteins and evasion of the host immune system introduces the potential that an engineered *Variola* virus may be used as a bioweapon. Recombinant *Vaccinia* viruses that were engineered to express genes encoding cytokines and chemokines have been studied extensively to understand the pathogenesis of the orthopoxviruses *(37)*. For example, the introduction of the interleukin (IL)-4 gene, a human interleukin involved in the type-2 immune response, greatly increased viral virulence by downregulating the cellular, type-1, immune responses. Similarly, IL-4 expressing engineered ectromelia virus was found to overcome genetic resistance to this virus in mice and produced an infection characterized by a high mortality similar to the disease seen when genetically sensitive mice are infected with wildtype virus *(38)*.

5. EPIDEMIOLOGY

5.1. Incidence

Before the 1959 WHO resolution on global eradication, smallpox went from an endemic disease in most countries of the world to a disease primarily of Asia, Africa, and the Indian subcontinent with an estimated 50 million cases per year *(22)*. By 1967, smallpox was eliminated in 125 of 156 countries, with 31 countries in South America, Africa, and the Indian subcontinent reporting incidence rates of greater than five cases per 100,000 and an estimated 10–15 million cases of smallpox per year.

The incidence of smallpox varies by year and season. In endemic countries, epidemic years of higher incidence of disease were observed with periodic fluctuations of 4–8 yr *(22,39)*. Smallpox in temperate countries was primarily a disease of the winter and spring and varied in tropical countries. Peak incidence in Bangladesh, for example, occurred from January through April, in Brazil from August through October, and in Indonesia during January.

5.2. Morbidity and Mortality

The morbidity and mortality of smallpox is dependent on numerous factors to include the type of smallpox virus (*V. minor* or *major*), clinical manifestation, previous smallpox vaccination, age, geography, urban or rural setting, underlying immune status, and, for women, pregnancy. A retrospective analysis was performed in 243 smallpox patients admitted to the Southampton Street smallpox hospital in Boston, MA during the 1901–1903 epidemic *(7)*. Mortality data were available in 206 patients for an overall mortality of 17.5%. Significant factors associated with survival were vaccination status, disease severity, and age. Recovery from smallpox took weeks, with most deaths occurring 7–14 d after the onset of symptoms.

V. minor, a milder form of smallpox, is associated with less severe disease and a mortality of 1% as compared to *V. major*, which has an average associated mortality of 35% in the unvaccinated population *(22)*. Within *V. major*, ordinary smallpox in the unvaccinated population is associated with an overall mortality of 30%, (confluent smallpox 62%, semiconfluent 37%, and discrete 42%), modified-type smallpox 0%, flat type 96%, and hemorrhagic type 96% *(22)*. In the smallpox-vaccinated population, disease severity is lower, with an overall average mortality of 6%. Ordinary smallpox in the smallpox-vaccinated population has an overall mortality of 3% (confluent smallpox 26%, semiconfluent 8%, and discrete 1%), modified-type smallpox 0%, flat type 67%, and hemorrhagic type 94% *(22)*.

Age is an important determinant of morbidity and mortality. More severe disease and higher mortality were observed in the very young and in older age groups. Mortality in Western and Central African patients ages less than 1 yr, 1–4 yr, 5–14 yr, 15–44 yr, and older than 44 yr, were 29, 12, 8, 15, and 32%, respectively.

Variation in the morbidity and mortality of smallpox was observed for different geographic areas and between urban or rural settings *(22)*. In general, urban areas had higher mortality rates than rural areas and Asian *V. major* was associated with a mortality of 20% in the smallpox-unvaccinated population. Asia, Bangladesh, India, Afghanistan, Pakistan, and Indonesia reported mortality rates of 19, 17, 16, 9–24, and 8–20%, respectively. In comparison, African countries reported mortalities of 5–10%, and South America reported less than 1%.

Smallpox in the pregnant patient is associated with more severe disease and a higher rate of mortality, abortions, and stillbirths *(22)*. For ordinary smallpox in the pregnant patient, mortality was 65%, for flat smallpox it was 95%, hemorrhagic and modified smallpox mortality was 99% *(40,41)*. The high mortality observed during pregnancy is presumably the result of defects in cell-mediated immunity. Similar mortality from smallpox could be anticipated in patients with defects in cell-mediated immunity from cancer, chemotherapy, organ transplants, and in those infected with the human immunodeficiency virus.

5.3. Infection and Infectivity

Variola virus gains entry to its human host through the oropharynx or respiratory tract. Direct inoculation in the skin can occur as demonstrated by the practice of variolation. *Variola* virus can be readily aerosolized from infected patients by coughing or sneezing. Viral particles are then deposited in the nasal cavity, oropharynx, and the lower respiratory tract. Direct inoculation can occur from contaminated fingers into the nasal cavity, mouth, or conjunctiva. The infectious dose 50% of *Variola* virus is not known. In studies performed with *Vaccinia* virus delivered by scarification, it was demonstrated that the infectious dose 50% was 3×10^5 pock-forming units per milliliter *(42)*.

The period and degree of infectivity of a patient with smallpox is determined by the quantity of virus shed in secretions, pustules, and scabs, which is dependent on the clinical manifestation of smallpox (*V. minor* or *major*) and day of clinical illness. From the time of inoculation with *Variola* virus, there follows an incubation period of 10–14 d *(43)*. During this time period, the virus replicates in the respiratory tract and disseminates throughout the body during viremia. Transmission of *Variola* virus from infected patients rarely occurs during the incubation period. With the onset of rash a period of maximum infectivity begins and gradually wanes until the rash evolves to the point where all scabs have separated *(22)*. Patients with a severe rash and enanthem were more infectious than patients with mild disease such as modified-type smallpox or *V. minor*. Patients with ordinary and flat-type smallpox are highly infectious during the rash and scabbing of lesions. As noted, the onset of the enanthem and exanthem of smallpox marks the period of maximum infectivity and viral shedding. Smallpox lesions within the mouth and pharynx release a large amount of virus into the oral and pharyngeal secretions. Virus can be recovered from patients from the 3rd to the 14th day of rash with maximum shedding on the 3rd and 4th day *(44)*. Virus shedding from the skin occurs during the pustular and scabbing stages of the rash with high titers of virus present in the pustular fluid and in the scabs that form during the convalescent period. *Variola* virus is present within scabs throughout the convalescent period, leading to the practice of patient isolation until the last scab has become separated *(22)*.

5.4. Transmission

Direct transmission of *Variola* virus occurs by inhalation of aerosolized virus or by direct transfer from contaminated fingers from infected material or surfaces. Individuals at high risk for secondary infections are those with close contact to the infected patient such as family contacts and hospital personnel *(22)*. Indirect transmission is defined as transmission of viral particles, which have traveled considerable distances by air or contaminated material (fomites). Indirect transmission of *Variola* virus by the aerosol route can occur over short distances as evidenced by the airborne spread of smallpox in the Meschede Hospital, Federal Republic of Germany, in 1970 *(45)*. During the Meschede outbreak, a patient with smallpox was admitted to the isolation ward. Secondary indirect transmission occurred in 17 health care personnel or visitors to the hospital who were removed from the index patient by several floors. Smoke analysis of the ventilation system demonstrated air ventilation from the index patient room to the upper level rooms. Factors that favored indirect transmission were the severity of disease by the index patient who had a confluent rash, severe bronchitis with cough, low humidity in the hospital (which favored survival of the virus) and the design of the hospital heating system that created strong air currents *(45)*. Indirect transmission of *Variola* virus can occur through fomites such as clothing and bed linen as evidenced by documented transmission of virus to laundry personnel *(22)*.

5.5. Factors Determining Population Spread

Numerous factors determine the spread of smallpox, including individual susceptibility within the population, social, demographic, political, and economic factors. Genetic predisposition to smallpox is suggested by observation of severe epidemics among certain groups, such as American Indians and Polynesians. Age is an important determinant of individual susceptibility, with more severe disease observed at the extremes of age *(22)*. Physiological factors that increase susceptibility include immunodeficiency and nutritional deficiency. Social factors include the time of year when close contact is maximal, such as during winter or rainy seasons, and societies where large families live in proximity. For densely concentrated populations, even vaccination rates of 80% do not mitigate the risk of epidemics *(46)*. Political and economic factors are important in determining the population spread of smallpox. Developed nations with a higher economic status have better access to healthcare and a developed infrastructure to more effectively identify cases of smallpox and more quickly institute containment of cases and vaccination of immune susceptible individuals.

5.6. Summary of Epidemiology

The epidemiological characteristics of smallpox suggest that this virus is a potential bioweapon. Based on naturally occurring smallpox before its global eradication and the low rate of smallpox vaccination in the current population, the intentional introduction of *V. major* can be expected to result in epidemic disease and produce a high degree of morbidity and mortality in the very young and elderly as well as in those with an underlying immunodeficiency or pregnancy. The presumed high severity of disease will result in a high degree of infectivity of cases and thus high rates of secondary transmission. The density of the population and the time of year will determine its spread, and because of the mobility of today's population, it is expected that spread will be rapid and difficult to contain once identified.

6. CLINICAL MANIFESTATION

6.1. Clinical Smallpox

For the past century, two distinct types of smallpox were recognized: major and minor (*see* Table 1). The prototypical disease, *Variola major*/ordinary smallpox resulted in a mortality of approx 30% in unvaccinated victims. Other clinical forms associated with *V. major*, such as flat-type and hemorrhagic-type smallpox, were notable for severe mortality. The incubation period of ordinary smallpox averaged 12 d, although it could range from 7 to 19 d after exposure. Clinical manifestations begin acutely with malaise, fever, rigors, vomiting, headache, backache, and as many as 15% of patients develop delirium. Approximately 10% of light-skinned patients exhibited an erythematous rash during this phase. Two to three days later, an enanthem (rash in the oropharynx) appeared concomitantly with a cutaneous rash (exanthem) about the face, hands, and forearms. The exanthem then spreads to the lower extremities, and subsequently to the trunk. Lesions quickly progress from macules to papules to vesicles and eventually to pustular vesicles. Lesions are more abundant on the extremities (including palms and soles) and face, and this centrifugal distribution is an important diagnostic feature. In distinct contrast to *Varicella* (chickenpox), lesions on various segments of the body remain generally synchronous in their stages of development. From 8 to 14 d after onset of exanthem, the pustules scab to leave depressed depigmented scars upon healing. Although *Variola* virus shedding from the throat, conjunctiva, and urine diminishes with time, it can be readily recovered from scabs throughout convalescence. The major sequelae of smallpox are permanent pockmarks, ranging from barely discernable scarring to an extremely disfiguring complexion. This results from fibrosis within the dermis and is seen in 65–80% of survivors. Corneal scarring leading to blindness occurs in 1–4% of patients. The second form, *V. minor*, was distinguished by milder systemic toxicity and more diminutive pox lesions and caused only 1% mortality in unvaccinated victims. Although the viral exanthem is the most prominent feature of both diseases, when patients with *V. major* and *V. minor* were matched for the same extent of exanthem, mortality rates differed substantially.

Table 1
Clinical Distinction Between *V. major* and *V. minor*

Characteristic	*V. major*	*V. minor*
Symptoms	Severe	Mild
Mortality	10–30%	1–2%
Use as a possible BW/BT weapon	Weaponized by former Soviet Union and produced in multiton quantities	Not suitable as a weapon because of low mortality
Consequence of release	Public health emergency with national security consequences	Public health emergency
Variants	Purpura variolosa (hemorrhagic smallpox) 3% of *V. major* Flat type 5% of *V. major*	Rare

Modified from ref. *22*.

6.2. Ordinary or Classic Smallpox

This was the most common form of smallpox caused by *V. major*. In the pre-eradication era, it accounted for 90% of cases with an overall case fatality rate of 30% among the unvaccinated. Some have noted differences in disease severity and prognosis that correlated with the density of the rash *(47)*. Ordinary smallpox can be stratified into three distinct clinical presentations or types: discrete, in which individual lesions are separated by normal appearing skin; confluent, in which lesions on any part of the body coalesce; and semiconfluent, in which lesions on the face are confluent but are discrete on the rest of the body. Those victims with discrete lesions tended to have a significantly lower case fatality rate than those with confluent lesions (9 vs 62% in unvaccinated cases in Rao's clinical series).

6.3. Hemorrhagic Smallpox

This form accounted for about 2–3% of all cases, although the percentage was higher in some outbreaks *(47)*. Hemorrhagic smallpox could be subdivided into early and late hemorrhagic smallpox. Early hemorrhagic smallpox had a different clinical presentation than ordinary smallpox and would often kill patients before they exhibited the focal rash *(47)*. In late hemorrhagic smallpox, the typical focal rash appeared, but hemorrhages would occur between the pustules. Illness was more common in adults, and pregnant women appeared to be at greater risk *(47)*. In early hemorrhagic smallpox, patients developed a toxic clinical picture resembling disseminated intravascular coagulation and in most cases rapidly succumbed to their disease. Death occurred in excess of 95% in unvaccinated persons with hemorrhagic smallpox. Host factors, such as some form of immune system deficiency, rather than a unique pathogenic strain of virus, are thought to be responsible for the development of this form of smallpox illness; however, immunological data generally are lacking *(48)*.

6.4. Flat-Type or Malignant Smallpox

Flat-type smallpox accounted for about 6% of cases in the pre-eradication era and occurred most commonly in children *(47)*. The illness was more than 95% fatal in unvaccinated persons. The rash characteristically involved flattened, confluent lesions rather than the characteristic firm pustules seen with ordinary smallpox. As in the hemorrhagic form, flat-type smallpox is thought to have been associated with a deficient cellular immune response to the virus *(48)*.

6.5. Modified Smallpox

Modified smallpox was most likely to be seen in patients who had been vaccinated previously but whose immunity had waned with time. According to the WHO definition of modified smallpox, the modification is related to the character and development of the focal eruption, with crusting being complete within 10 d. The prodrome may or may not be shortened or lessened in severity, but the secondary fever is typically absent *(27)*. There are typically fewer skin lesions and the lesions tend to be more superficial, evolve more rapidly, and not show the typical uniformity seen in ordinary smallpox. Modified smallpox presented diagnostic difficulties, and patients were still contagious, although often ambulatory.

6.6. Variola *sine eruptione*

This occurred in vaccinated contacts of cases and was characterized by sudden onset of fever, headache, and backache, but no rash followed the prodrome. Illness was short-lived and resolved in 1–2 d, but patients could transmit virus to others for a short period of time.

6.7. Smallpox in Children

Smallpox in children was clinically similar to that seen in adults, with several notable exceptions. In infants, the overall mortality was often greater than 40% *(27)* and in one series reached 85% *(49)*. Children had a higher incidence of vomiting, conjunctivitis, seizures, and cough *(50)*. Infections during pregnancy were associated with uterine hemorrhage, premature labor, and fetal demise, although no distinct congenital syndrome has been associated with smallpox infection *in utero (27)*.

6.8. V. minor

V. minor represents a strain of the *Variola* virus that is distinct from *V. major*. It causes a milder form of smallpox, and these patients can be confused with patients presenting with modified smallpox.

7. CLINICAL PATHOGENESIS

The brick-shaped smallpox virion is readily transmitted from person to person via respiratory particles. The virus initially replicates in respiratory tract epithelial cells, and then migrates to regional lymph nodes. From there, a massive asymptomatic viremia ensues 3–4 d later and may result in focal infections involving lymphoid tissues, skin, intestines, lungs, kidneys, and/or brain. After an incubation period of approx 12 d (range: 7–17 d), a second viremia, lasting 2–5 d, results in prodromal symptoms of high fever, malaise, headache, severe backache, rigors, vomiting, and prostration. Some patients (approx 15%) will become delirious. The virus localizes in the small blood vessels of the oropharyngeal mucosa and dermis, leading to the initial onset of an enanthem and exanthem. At the tissue level, dilatation of the capillaries in the papillary layer of the dermis occurs initially, followed by swelling of the endothelial cells in the vessel walls. Perivascular cuffing with lymphocytes, plasma cells, and macrophages can be seen. Lesions then develop in the epidermis and cells become swollen and vacuolated. Cell membranes soon rupture, leading to the characteristic vesicular stage of the rash. Pustulation results from the migration of polymorphonuclear cells into the vesicle. Patients often develop a secondary fever as the lesions evolve from vesicles to pustules. The contents of the pustule gradually desiccate, resulting in crusting and scabbing of the lesions with loss of pigment and scar formation within the dermis. Death most commonly results from overwhelming toxemia probably associated with circulating immune complexes *(51)*. Other causes of death include secondary bacterial infections, sepsis, and dehydration.

8. DIAGNOSIS

Research and development of easy-to-use rapid diagnostic tests for smallpox is ongoing, but no such tests were commercially available at the time of this writing. The initial diagnosis of smallpox remains a clinical one, and physicians or other healthcare providers should not await laboratory confirmation before instituting appropriate infection-control and public-health measures. However, confirmation of alternative diagnoses, particularly chickenpox or monkeypox, can be rapidly accomplished by means of techniques such as direct fluorescent antibody staining. Such alternative diagnoses should be expeditiously pursued in the appropriate settings, because confirmation would avert unnecessary public health measures. Laboratory diagnosis of *Variola* requires the handling of potentially infectious samples and should be done only in reference laboratories under biosafety level (BSL)-4 safety containment *(48)*.

The most rapid diagnostic tools available are light and electron microscopy. Scrapings of the vesicular or pustular lesions or scabs can be examined for characteristic findings. An experienced microscopist may be able to discern Guanieri bodies using Giemsa or Gispen's modified silver stains under light microscopy *(30,52)*. Guanieri bodies are aggregates of virions within the cytoplasm of infected cells. Electron microscopy using a negative staining technique is a much more sensitive test. The recognition of the large, brick-shaped virions is diagnostic of a poxvirus, although the particular species may not be identified. This technique can easily differentiate poxviruses from other viruses (such as herpesviruses) and was used extensively in the Intensified Smallpox Eradication Program *(27)*.

Antigen-detection methods and serologic tests for antibodies to *Variola* can also be used for diagnosis. The most widely used method for antigen detection was gel precipitation, which detected the presence of viral antigen in vesicular or pustular fluid by using *Vaccinia* hyperimmune serum *(27)*. This test was rapid and did not require a microscope. However, it required a supply of *Vaccinia* hyperimmune serum, a laboratory, and technicians capable of performing the test. It was unable to differentiate species of orthopoxviruses (smallpox, *Vaccinia*, cowpox, monkeypox). Serologic testing can be accomplished by various of means, such as ELISA, Western blot, or virus neutralization assay, but these are most useful in retrospective diagnosis *(53)*. Neutralization assays, requiring viable virus, can only be performed under BSL-4 conditions.

Historically, the definitive identification of *Variola* virus was made by viral culture. Poxviruses replicate on various of cell lines, but the most useful substrate has been the chick chorioallantoic membrane. All orthopoxviruses that infect humans produce unique pockmarks on the chick chorioallantoic membrane, permitting identification by experienced personnel *(27)*.

Nucleic acid techniques have been used for specific virus identification. Endonuclease digestion and RFLP are established techniques that can provide unequivocal identification *(28,29)*. Modern nucleic acid amplification tests such as polymerase chain reaction are available in specialized laboratories and may be able to give a very rapid diagnosis *(48,54)*.

9. DIFFERENTIAL DIAGNOSIS

In the majority of cases, initial diagnosis of smallpox can be made on clinical grounds. During the eruptive phase, the distribution and evolution of the skin lesions are extremely valuable clues to the diagnosis of smallpox. After the onset of the rash in the buccal and pharyngeal mucosa, the first maculopapular skin lesions appear on the face and/or hands and forearms. Lesions spread to the trunk and lower limbs in a centrifugal distribution. Skin lesions evolve from macules, to papules, to vesicles, followed by pustules, which ultimately desiccate and fall off. The lesions in any one area are all at the same stage of development. The history of a severe febrile pre-eruptive illness lasting 2–4 d is usual, and contact with a previous case should be sought. Diseases with similar skin manifestations must be considered in the differential diagnosis. The rash of smallpox is most likely to be mistaken for chickenpox (*Varicella*) during the vesicular stage. However, there are two important distinctions. First, the rash of smallpox develops synchronously, in contrast to the asynchronous development observed with *Varicella*. Second, the rash of smallpox is concentrated on the face and extremities (centrifugal distribution, as opposed to the trunk (centripetal distribution), as occurs in chickenpox. The pustules of smallpox are also notable for a characteristic central umbilication, which is sometimes—but not always—present.

Monkeypox produces a disease in humans very similar to smallpox. The emergence of monkeypox in equatorial Africa as a human disease resulted in large epidemic outbreaks with a mortality that ranged between 10 and 15% *(23)*. In part, the emergence of monkeypox is thought to be caused by the population loss of cross-protective immunity from the *Vaccinia* virus vaccine during the smallpox eradication campaign *(55)*. Monkeypox causes a lymphadenopathy not ordinarily seen in smallpox but is otherwise clinically indistinguishable from smallpox *(55)*. A travel history could aid in distinguishing a monkeypox patient just returning from equatorial Africa versus an intentional introduction of *Variola* virus; however, recently a monkeypox outbreak caused by the importation of infected Gambian rats as household pets was described *(24)*.

10. SPECIMEN COLLECTION AND HANDLING

If a patient presents with a condition suggesting smallpox and is considered to be at high risk, healthcare providers should immediately contact their hospital infection control officer and either their state or local health department for instructions before attempting to collect specimens. Only recently vaccinated persons (positive take within 3 yr) should collect specimens, and only if directed to do so by public health personnel. If only unvaccinated personnel are available, the collector should wear a fit-tested, high-efficiency particulate air (HEPA)-filtered mask at the N95 level or higher and should be vaccinated within 24 hr if at all possible. Regardless of vaccination status, barrier precautions (gloves, gowns, shoe covers) should be worn while collecting specimens. The Centers for Disease Control and Prevention (CDC) has established guidelines for specimen collection, handling, and shipping, which have been included in its Smallpox Response Plan and Guidelines. Specimens collected depend on at what stage of development the patient presents. At all skin stages, punch biopsies should be taken. At maculopapular stages, skin scrapings should be obtained; in the vesicular/pustular stages, fluid or pus should be collected; and during the crusting stage, a minimum of 3–10 crusts should be collected.

Initial evaluation of clinical specimens obtained from patients at risk for smallpox must be performed at a level D laboratory within the Laboratory Response Network (LRN). The LRN represents a network of laboratories organized into four levels (A–D) of increasing sophistication and biosafety. Level D labs operate under the highest BSL (BSL-4). There are only two such laboratories in the United States—one at the CDC in Atlanta, GA; and the other at the US Army Medical Research Institute of Infectious Diseases (USAMRIID) in Fort Detrick, MD. These labs may be accessed via local or state health department laboratories. Once smallpox is confirmed in a geographic area, additional cases can be diagnosed clinically.

11. INFECTION CONTROL

During a small-scale attack, infected patients should be admitted to the hospital in negative-pressure isolation rooms with HEPA filtration. In larger outbreaks, home care and patient isolation may have to be considered. Although modeling and simulation matrices developed at the CDC indicate a more rapid control of outbreaks with restriction of movement campaigns in conjunction with vaccination programs, the institution of quarantine of potentially infected individuals in today's society would pose numerous problems and raise a myriad of legal issues. In an attempt to address these issues, the CDC has recently published a model quarantine law, developed after a comprehensive review of existing state laws (http://www.phppo.cdc.gov/od/phlp/resources.asp).

Airborne and contact precautions are important infection-control adjuncts to standard precautions. Healthcare workers at risk of exposure should also be vaccinated (*see* Section 13). All contaminated material (i.e., laundry and waste) should be placed in biohazard bags and should be autoclaved before incineration or washing. Standard hospital tuberculocidal solutions can be used to clean surfaces and reusable medical equipment.

12. TREATMENT

12.1. General Measures

In the pre-eradication era, only general supportive measures were available to care for the smallpox victim. Attention to hydration status, fever and pain control, and meticulous care of the skin to prevent bacterial superinfection were performed when possible. Intravenous lines should be established early during the course of disease, as placement of lines in the presence of confluent vesicles is both difficult and painful. Patients are extremely sensitive to light, so a darkened environment is important. The skin lesions are extremely pruritic, so pain relief is important to help prevent scratching. In confluent cases especially, the throat may be very sore, making it difficult for the patient to swallow.

12.2. Antiviral Therapy

Through the last human case of smallpox infection in 1978, standard treatment for smallpox patients remained primarily supportive. Almost all data regarding clinical outcome were garnered from patients in underdeveloped countries before the advent of modern medical practice. The effect of modern supportive care upon outcome in small-pox cases is unknown. Some studies of the efficacy of early antiviral drugs were performed, and a few showed some evidence of benefit *(27)*. These studies set the stage for modern efforts to find effective therapy for smallpox and related poxviruses. These efforts have now found new momentum as the threat of biological weapons attack has been more fully appreciated.

Orthopoxviruses were the first targets of antiviral chemotherapy research *(56,57)*. Few drugs actually advanced to the stage of human trials, and the results of these trials were disappointing *(27)*. Among the more potentially toxic drugs used without success were cytosine arabinoside and adenine arabinoside. The most promising agents tested against human smallpox were the thiosemicarbazones, in particular methisazone (Marboran) and its relative M & B 7714. These had excellent activity in mouse models of *Vaccinia* and *Variola (56,57)*. However, randomized, placebo-controlled human trials for treating smallpox infection yielded disappointing results *(57a,b)*. A statistically insignificant decrease in mortality was seen in vaccinated individuals, but no difference was detected in unvaccinated subjects. In addition, side effects of nausea and vomiting were sometimes severe. Trials of these agents for chemoprophylaxis were problematic. Some early trials showed dramatic reductions in smallpox infection and death, but later randomized trials showed only a small benefit *(57c–h)*. In addition, the severe gastrointestinal side effects and the expense of the thiosemicarbazones were prohibitive *(56,57)*. Vaccination was clearly superior in its effectiveness and ease of administration, and these agents never experienced significant use for prophylaxis or treatment *(27)*.

Since the eradication of smallpox, a wide variety of antiviral compounds with activity against many different viruses have become available. Antiviral classes that have shown in vitro activity against orthopoxviruses include inosine monophosphate (IMP) dehydrogenase inhibitors, *s*-adenosylhomocysteine hydrolase inhibitors, orotidine monophosphate decarboxylase inhibitors, cytosine triphosphate synthetase inhibitors, thymidylate synthetase inhibitors, nucleoside analogs, thiosemicarbazones, and acyclic nucleoside phosphonates *(56–58)*. Most of this work has been performed with orthopoxviruses other than *Variola*, but several available antiviral drugs have demonstrated in vitro activity specifically against *Variola* virus in addition to other orthopoxviruses. Of the current commercially available drugs, HPMPC (cidofovir), *bis*-POM PMEA (adefovir dipivoxil), and ribavirin have been shown to have an IC_{50} in cell culture assays well below levels associated with cytotoxicity *(58)*. Ribavirin and to a greater extent cidofovir have demonstrated in vivo efficacy against orthopoxvirus infection in animal models *(56,57)*. The potency of these drugs against *Variola* virus in vitro is many times that of methisazone, one of the only drugs used with minimal success in human smallpox infection *(58)*.

Adefovir dipivoxil is the orally bioavailable form of adefovir, a cytidine analog originally developed as an antiretroviral drug for use against HIV. Trials of adefovir dipivoxil for HIV were stopped because of nephrotoxicity and other side effects encountered with doses (usually 60 mg/d or greater) required for reverse-transcriptase inhibition. However, adefovir has been used at lower doses (10–30 mg/d) against hepatitis B infection without significant adverse effects. It has recently been approved by the FDA for use against hepatitis B. Adefovir dipivoxil has shown in vitro activity against cowpox, monkeypox, camelpox, and *Variola* viruses at concentrations many times below cytotoxic levels but failed to show efficacy against *Vaccinia (58)*. To date, no published study has looked at adefovir's efficacy in a live animal model.

Cidofovir is a nucleotide analogue with significant activity against DNA viruses, including members of the adenovirus, papillomavirus, and herpesvirus families *(59)* It has been approved for use in cytomegalovirus retinitis in AIDS patients. It has the advantage of a very long intracellular half-life, requiring dosing only every other week. It has been associated with severe nephrotoxicity in some instances, but this may be ameliorated with aggressive hydration and concomitant administration of probenicid. Iritis and uveitis has been seen with relative frequency in postmarketing studies *(60,61)*. Cidofovir has been tested in various in vitro and in vivo models. In cell culture assays, cidofovir has been effective against a spectrum of poxvirus infections, including *Vaccinia* and *Variola (56–58)*. It has been shown to be effective in preventing tail lesion formation in mice after *Vaccinia* infection and was effective in preventing end-organ replication of *Vaccinia* and mouse death in *Vaccinia*-infected severe combined immunodeficient (SCID) mice *(62)*.

The most important and most promising studies of cidofovir treatment of poxvirus infections have been done with respiratory inoculation cowpox infections in mice. In one study, mice were exposed to aerosolized cowpox virus and were treated with cidofovir or placebo *(63)*. All of the control mice died, whereas in mice given a subcutaneous (sc) injection of 100 mg/kg of cidofovir anywhere from 4 d before to 3 d after infection, survival was 80–100%. In another study, intranasal cidofovir from 2.5–40 mg/kg given in a single dose was shown to be effective in reducing mortality in mice given an intranasal inoculation of cowpox virus *(64)*. The protection was dose- and time-dependent. Of mice treated 1 d after infection with 10–40 mg/kg of cidofovir, survival was 29 of 30 compared to 0 of 10 in controls. Even when treated 3 d after infection, mice given 40 mg/kg of cidofovir had a 60% survival rate, a statistically significant difference compared to the 100% mortality in controls. Finally, Bray et al. looked at the administration of aerosolized cidofovir for mice infected with aerosolized cowpox *(65)*. They found that aerosolized cidofovir was as efficacious as subcutaneous cidofovir at much lower doses (0.5–5.0 mg/kg) if given early in the course of infection, on d 0 or 1. However, later administration of aerosolized cidofovir appeared to have a less protective effect compared to sc administration.

Obviously, no human data exist for cidofovir for treating smallpox; however, case reports have documented several successes in its use in other poxvirus infections. Topical and parenteral cidofovir has effectively treated patients with severe immunodeficiency disorders (AIDS and Wiskott–Aldrich Syndrome) and disfiguring molluscum contagiosum *(66,67)*. Topical cidofovir has also been associated with complete resolution of human orf (ecthyma contagiosum,) another poxvirus infection *(68)*.

Ribavirin is an IMP dehydrogenase inhibitor that has been studied for several decades. It has clinical utility against respiratory syncytial virus and hepatitis C, influenza A and B, Lassa fever, measles, Hantaan virus, Junin virus, and other viral infections. Ribavirin is associated with bone marrow suppression that can be dose limiting. It is also potentially teratogenic and cannot be used in pregnancy. In orthopoxvirus infections, animal data for ribavirin therapy are less convincing than data for cidofovir. Studies found varying activity against orthopoxviruses in vitro *(56,57,69)*. In live animal models, topical ribavirin was effective in treating *Vaccinia* keratitis in rabbits and in preventing tail lesions in *Vaccinia*-infected mice *(57,70)*. Ribavirin alone can delay or prevent death in studies of intranasal, cowpox infection in mice, depending upon inoculation dose of virus and dose of drug *(64,69)*. Subcutaneous injections of ribavirin, 100 mg/kg/d for 5 d, followed by one dose of cidofovir (75 mg/kg on d 6) did significantly improve survival over placebo or either of the drugs used individually on the same schedule *(64)*. There are no published data regarding the use of ribavirin in human orthopoxvirus infections.

13. VACCINATION

Several different *Vaccinia* strains have been used in vaccine production. Currently in the United States, Dryvax vaccine (Wyeth) is the only licensed *Vaccinia* vaccine. The vaccine consists of a lyophilized (freeze-dried) preparation of live *Vaccinia* virus obtained from New York City calf lymph, which is derived from a seed virus of the New York City Board of Health (NYCBH) strain. During the smallpox eradication campaign of the 1960s and 1970s, other strains were used including the New York City chorioallantoic membrane, which is also derived from the NYCBH strain. Other strains used throughout the world included EM-63 (USSR), the Temple of Heaven strain (China) and the Lister or Elestree strain (United Kingdom). All strains were probably equally effective in preventing smallpox; differences seemed to be related to rates of adverse reactions.

Detailed information on the efficacy of Dryvax vaccine can be obtained from the Advisory Committee on Immunization Practices. The current supplies of Dryvax were produced in the 1970s and have been in lyophilized storage since that time. Approximately 15.4 million doses are currently available and largely under the control of the Department of Health and Human Services. When it was recognized that this supply would not be adequate to effectively manage a smallpox bioterrorism event, studies were initiated to see if the supply could be diluted without losing potency. In 2002, Frey reported that the vaccine could be diluted both 1:5 and 1:10 and still elicit an adequate immune response in the vast majority of patients *(71)*. However, as the 1:10 dilution left only a small margin for error in the administration of an effective dose to individual patients, it was felt that if necessary, the 1:5 dilution would be employed in an emergency situation requiring mass vaccination. A 1:5 dilution would effectively increase the supply to 77 million doses, but under current FDA guidelines, diluted vaccine would have to be administered under an Investigational New Drug (IND) protocol. The diluent originally used for reconstituting the vaccine also expired from FDA license and was replaced for current usage. In 2002, the drug company Aventis located 85 million doses of frozen vaccine that was produced from the same NYCBH strain as Dryvax. These stores were donated to the federal government. This vaccine is not licensed and there are no plans at this time to initiate the FDA licensure process. However, it could be administered under an IND Protocol. It is likely that the Aventis vaccine could also be diluted fivefold, effectively increasing this supply to 425 million doses.

New *Vaccinia* vaccines include a cell-culture-derived *Vaccinia* vaccine in production by Acambis. It uses the same NYCBH *Vaccinia* strain as was used in the older Wyeth Dryvax product in the 1970s and is expected to have similar immunogenicity and a similar side effect profile *(72)*. The production contract calls for a delivery of 209 million doses sometime in 2003. Until FDA licensing is complete, this vaccine will have to be administered under an IND protocol. A strain of *Vaccinia* referred to as Modified *Vaccinia* Ankara (MVA) was used with apparent success in Europe, particularly in Germany, through the 1970s. This attenuated virus appeared to demonstrate less virulence than other vaccine strains of vaccinia, in particular with regard to post-vaccinal encephalitis. Subsequent to the eradication of smallpox, the virus has been investigated extensively as a platform for inducing heterologous immune responses, especially against tumor antigens but also in other infectious disease systems. Efforts are now underway to examine the potency of the MVA-induced immune response against vaccinia challenge, thought to be a surrogate for *Variola* protection.

14. SUMMARY

Who could have predicted in 1980 when Halfdan Mahler wrote, "Victory over smallpox has implications that go far beyond the individuals directly concerned...." It reasserts our ability to change the world around us for the better, through mutual collaboration and mobilization of resources, allied to human energies and the will to succeed" that 23 yr later smallpox would still be a major public health concern not as a natural occurring disease but as a potential bioweapon *(1)*? Little did we know that the forces of humanity that "reassert our ability to change the world around us for the better" are equally likely to reassert our ability to change the world for the worse. This chapter presented the unique virologic, epidemiologic and clinical characteristics of *Variola* virus that make it an ideal bioweapon. Hopefully, understanding these basic concepts, will increase our awareness of *Variola* virus the bioweapon, leading to early recognition, appropriate isolation and treatment, and, thus, minimizing the population impact of smallpox.

REFERENCES

1. Mahler, H. (1980) *Towards the Year 2000.* World Health: Magazine of the World Health Organization **May,** 19.
2. Fenner, F. (1993) Smallpox: emergence, global spread, and eradication. *Hist. Philos. Life. Sci.* **15,** 397–420.
3. Hopkins, J. (1988) The eradication of smallpox: organizational learning and innovation in international health administration. *J. Dev. Areas* **22,** 321–332.
4. Winkenwerder, W. (2003) First Department of Defense Smallpox Vaccination Program Report. *Miss RN* **65,** 8.
5. Wharton, M., Strikas, R., Harpaz, R., et al. Recommendations for using smallpox vaccine in a pre-event vaccination program. Supplemental recommendations of the Advisory Committee on Immunization Practices (ACIP) and the Healthcare Infection Control Practices Advisory Committee (HICPAC). *MMWR Recomm. Rep.* **52,** 1–16.
6. Grabenstein, J. and Winkenwerder, W. (2003) US military smallpox vaccination program experience. *JAMA* **289,** 3278–3282.
7. Albert, M., Ostheimer, K., Liewehr, D., Steinberg, S., and Breman, J. (2002) Smallpox manifestations and survival during the Boston epidemic of 1901 to 1903. *Ann. Intern. Med.* **137,** 993–1000.

8. (1988) Smallpox and its eradication, in *The History of Smallpox and its Spread Around the World*. World Health Organization, Geneva.

9. Baxby, D. (1996) The Jenner bicentenary: the introduction and early distribution of small-pox vaccine. *FEMS Immunol. Med. Microbiol.* **16**, 1–10.

10. Horton, R. (1995) Myths in medicine. Jenner did not discover vaccination. *BMJ* **310**, 62.

11. Radetsky, M. (1999) Smallpox: a history of its rise and fall. *Pediatr. Infect. Dis. J.* **18**, 85–93.

12. Henderson, D. (1998) Smallpox eradication—a cold war victory. *World Health Forum* **19**, 113–119.

13. (2002) 25th Anniversary of the last case of naturally acquired smallpox. *MMWR Morb. Mortal. Wkly. Rep.* **51**, 952.

14. Alibek, K., S H. (1999) *Biohazard*. Random House, New York.

15. Gellmam, B. (2002) *Four nations thought to possess smallpox: Irac, North Korea named two officials say*. Washington Post, Washington, DC, 1.

16. Bicknell, W. J. (2002) The case for voluntary smallpox vaccination. *N. Engl. J. Med.* **346**, 1323–1325.

17. Parkman, F. (1969) *The Conspiracy of Pontiac*. Litle Brown, Boston, MA.

18. Williams, P. and Wallace, D. (1989) *Unit 731 the Japanese Army's Secret of Secrets*. Hodder and Stoughton, London.

19. Enserink, M. (2002) Biowarfare. Did bioweapons test cause a deadly smallpox outbreak? *Science* **296**, 2116, 2117.

20. Smith, R. J. (1992) *"Our military development was the cause", Yeltsin blames '79 anthrax on germ warfare efforts*. Washington Post, Washington, DC, p. 1.

21. Baxby, D. (1996) Should smallpox virus be destroyed? The relevance of the origins of vaccinia virus. *Soc. Hist. Med.* **9**, 117–119.

22. (1988) *Smallpox and its Eradication*. World Health Organization, Geneva.

23. (1997) Human monkeypox in Kasai Oriental, Zaire (1996–1997). *Wkly. Epidemiol. Rec.* **72**, 101–104.

24. (2003) Multistate outbreak of monkeypox—Illinois, Indiana, and Wisconsin, 2003. *MMWR Morb. Mortal. Wkly. Rep.* **52**, 537–540.

25. Moss, B. (2001) Poxviridae: the viruses and their replication, in *Fields Virology*. 4th ed. (Knipe, D. M. and Howley, P. M., eds.), Lippincot Williams & Wilkins, Philadelphia, pp. 2849–2883.

26. Hooper, J., Custer, D., and Thompson, E. (2003) Four-gene-combination DNA vaccine protects mice against a lethal vaccinia virus challenge and elicits appropriate antibody responses in nonhuman primates. *Virology* **306**, 181–195.

27. Fenner, F., Henderson, D. A., Arita, I., Jezek, Z., and Ladnyi, I. D. (1988) *Smallpox and its Eradication*. World Health Organization, Geneva.

28. Esposito, J., Obijeski, J., and Nakano, J. (1978) Orthopoxvirus DNA: strain differentiation by electrophoresis of restriction endonuclease fragmented virion DNA. *Virology* **89**, 53–66.

29. Esposito, J. and Knight, J. (1985) Orthopoxvirus DNA: a comparison of restriction profiles and maps. *Virology* **143**, 230–251.

30. Dixon, C. W. (1962) *Smallpox*. J & A Churchill, London.

31. Dumbell, D. R. and Huq, F. (1986) The virology of variola minor: correlation of laboratory tests with the geographic distribution and human virulence of variola isolates. *Am. J. Epidemiol.* **123**, 403–415.

32. Dumbell, K., Harper, L., Buchan, A., Douglass, N., and Bedson, H. (1999) A variant of variola virus, characterized by changes in polypeptide and endonuclease profiles. *Epidemiol. Infect.* **122**, 287–290.

33. Smith, V. and Alcami, A. (2000) Expression of secreted cytokine and chemokine inhibitors by ectromelia virus. *J. Virol.* **74**, 8460–8471.

34. Buller, R. and Palumbo, G. (1991) Poxvirus pathogenesis. *Microbiol. Rev.* **55**, 80–122.

35. Mahalingam, S. and Karupiah, G. Modulation of chemokines by poxvirus infections. *Curr. Opin. Immunol.* **12,** 409–12.

36. Alcami, A. and Smith, G. (1995) Vaccinia, cowpox, and camelpox viruses encode soluble gamma interferon receptors with novel broad species specificity. *J. Virol.* **69,** 4633–4639.

37. Ramshaw, I., Ramsay, A., Karupiah, G., Rolph, M., Mahalingam, S., and Ruby, J. (1997) Cytokines and immunity to viral infections. *Immunol. Rev.* **159,** 119–135.

38. Jackson, R., Ramsay, A., Christensen, C., Beaton, S., Hall, D., and Ramshaw, I. Expression of mouse interleukin-4 by a recombinant ectromelia virus suppresses cytolytic lymphocyte responses and overcomes genetic resistance to mousepox. *J. Virol.* **75,** 1205–1210.

39. Mielke, J., Jorde, L., Trapp, G., Anderton, D., Pitkanene, K., and Erikson, A. (1984) Historical epidemiology of smallpox in Aland, Finland: 1751-1890. *Demography* **21,** 271–295.

40. Rao, A. R., Prahlad, I., Swaminathan, M., and Lakshmi, A. (1963) Pregnancy and smallpox. *J. Indian Med. Assoc.* **40,** 353–363.

41. Suarez, V. and Hankins, G. Smallpox and pregnancy: from eradicated disease to bioterrorist threat. *Obstet. Gynecol.* **100,** 87–93.

42. Cockburn, W. C., Cross, R. M., Downie, A. W., et al. (1957) Laboratory and vaccination studies with dried smallpox vaccines. *Bull. World Health Org.* **16,** 63–77.

43. Mack, T. M. (1972) Smallpox in Europe, 1950-1971. *J. Infect. Dis.* **125,** 161–169.

44. Sarkar, J. K., Mitra, A. C., Mukherjee, M. K., De, S. K., and Guha Mazumdar, D. (1973) Virus excretion in smallpox. 1. Excretion in the throat, urine and conjunctiva of patients. *Bull. World Health Org.* **48,** 517–522.

45. Wehrle, P. F., Posch, J., Richter, K. H., and Henderson, D. A. (1970) An airborne outbreak of smallpox in a German hospital and its significance with respect to other recent outbreaks in Europe. *Bull. World Health Org.* **43,** 669–679.

46. Arita, I., Wickett, J., and Fenner, F. (1986) Impact of population density on immunization programmes. *J. Hyg.* **96,** 459–466.

47. Rao, A. R.(1972) *Smallpox.* Kothari Book Depot, Bombay.

48. Henderson, D., Inglesby, T., Bartlett, J., et al. (1999) Smallpox as a biological weapon: medical and public health management. Working Group on Civilian Biodefense. *JAMA* **281,** 2127–2137.

49. Mazumder, D. N., Mitra, A. C., and Mukherjee, M. K. (1975) Clinical observations on smallpox: a study of 1233 patients admitted to the Infectious Diseases Hospital, Calcutta, during 1973. *Bull. World Health Org.* **52,** 301–306.

50. Sheth, S. C., Maruthi, V., Tibrewala, N. S., and Pai, P. M. (1971) Smallpox in children. A clinical study of 100 cases. *Indian J. Pediatr.* **38,** 128–131.

51. Martin, D. (2002) The cause of death in smallpox: an examination of the pathology record. *Mil. Med.* **167,** 546–551.

52. Henderson, D. (2002) Smallpox: clinical and epidemiologic features. *Med. Health R. I.* **85,** 107, 108.

53. Esposito, J. J. and Fenner, F. (2001) Poxviruses, in *Fields Virology.* 4th ed. (Knipe, D. M. and Howley, P. M., eds.), Lippincott Williams & Wilkins, Philadelphia, pp. 2885–2921.

54. Ibrahim, M., Lofts, R., Jahrling, P., et al. (1998) Real-time microchip PCR for detecting single-base differences in viral and human DNA. *Anal. Chem.* **70,** 2013–2017.

55. Arita, I., Jezek, Z., Khodakevich, L., and Ruti, K. (1985) Human monkeypox: a newly emerged orthopoxvirus zoonosis in the tropical rain forests of Africa. *Am. J. Trop. Med. Hyg.* **34,** 781–789.

56. De Clercq, E. (2002) Cidofovir in the therapy and short-term prophylaxis of poxvirus infections. *Trends Pharmacol. Sci.* **23,** 456.

57. De Clercq, E., Luczak, M., Shugar, D., Torrence, P. F., Waters, J. A., and Witkop, B. (1976) Effect of cytosine, arabinoside, iododeoxyuridine, ethyldeoxyuridine, thiocyanatodeoxyuridine, and ribavirin on tail lesion formation in mice infected with vaccinia virus. *Proc. Soc. Exp. Biol. Med.* **151,** 487–490.

57a. Rao, A. R., McFadzean, J. A., and Kamalakshi, K. (1966) An isothiazole thiosemi-carbazone in the treatment of *variola major* in man. A controlled clinical trial and laboratory investigations. *Lancet* **1,** 1068–1072.

57b. Rao, A. R., Jacobs, E. S., Kamalakshi, S., Bradbury, and Swamy, A. (1969) Chemoprophylaxis and chemotherapy in *variola major*. II. Therapeutic assessment of CG662 and Marboran in treatment of *variola major* in man. *Indian J. Med. Res.* **57,** 484–494.

57c. Bauer, D. J., St. Vincent, L., Kempe, C. H., and Downie, A. W., (1963) Prophylactic treatment of smallpox contacts with *N*-methylisatin β-thiosemicarbazone (compound 33T57, Marboran). *Lancet* **2,** 494–496

57d. doValle, L. A., DeMelo, P. R., deGomes, L. F., and Proenca, L. M. (1965) Methiszaone in prevention of *variola minor* among contacts. *Lancet* **2,** 976–978.

57e. Rao, A. R., McKendrick, G. D., Velayudhan, L., and Kamalakshi, K. (1966) Assessment of an isothiazole thiosemicarbazone in the prophylaxis of contacts of *variola major*. *Lancet* **1,** 1072–1074.

57f. Bauer, D. J., St. Vincent, L., Kempe, C. H., Young, P. A., and Downie, A. W. (1969) Prophylaxis of smallpox with methisazone. *Am. J. Epidemiol.* **90,** 130–145.

57g. Rao, A. R., Jacobs, E. S., Kamalakshi, S., Bradbury, and Swamy, A. (1969) Chemoprophylaxis and chemotherapy in *variola major*. I. An assessment of CG662 and Marboran in prophylaxis of contacts of *variola major*. *Indian J. Med. Res.* **57,** 477–483.

57h. Heiner, G. G., Fatima, N., Russell, P. K., et al. (1971) Field trials of methisazone as a prophylactic agent against smallpox. *Am. J. Epidemiol.* **94,** 435–449.

58. Jahrling, P. B., Zaucha, G. M., and Huggins, J. W. (2000) Contermeasures to the reemergence of smallpox virus as an agent of bioterrorism, in *Emerging Infections 4.* (Scheld, W. M., Craig, W. A., and Hughes, J. M., eds.), ASM, Washington, DC.

59. Naesens, L. (1997) HPMPC (cidofovir), PMEA (adefovir) and related acyclic nucleoside phosphonate analogues: a review of their pharmacology and clinical potential in the treatment of viral infections. *Antivir. Chem. Chemotherap.* **8,** 1–23.

60. Wachsman, M., Petty, B. G., Cundy, K. C., et al. (1996) Pharmacokinetics, safety and bioavailability of HPMPC (cidofovir) in human immunodeficiency virus-infected subjects. *Antivir. Res.* **29,** 153–161.

61. Plosker, G. L. and Noble, S. (1999) Cidofovir: a review of its use in cytomegalovirus retinitis in patients with AIDS. *Drugs* **58,** 325–345.

62. Neyts, J. and De Clercq, E. (1993) Efficacy of (S)-1-(3-hydroxy-2-phosphonylmethoxypropyl)cytosine for the treatment of lethal vaccinia virus infections in severe combined immune deficiency (SCID) mice. *J. Med. Virol.* **41,** 242–246.

63. Bray, M., Martinez, M., Smee, D., Kefauver, D., Thompson, E., and Huggins, J. (2000) Cidofovir protects mice against lethal aerosol or intranasal cowpox virus challenge. *J. Infect. Dis.* **181,** 10–19.

64. Smee, D., Bailey, K., Wong, M., and Sidwell, R. (2000) Intranasal treatment of cowpox virus respiratory infections in mice with cidofovir. *Antivir. Res.* **47,** 171–177.

65. Bray, M., Martinez, M., Kefauver, D., West, M., and Roy, C. (2002) Treatment of aerosolized cowpox virus infection in mice with aerosolized cidofovir. *Antivir. Res.* **54,** 129–142.

66. Meadows, K. P., Tyring, S. K., Pavia, A. T., and Rallis, T. M. (1997) Resolution of recalcitrant molluscum contagiosum virus lesions in human immunodeficiency virus-infected patients treated with cidofovir. *Arch. Dermatol.* **133,** 987–990.

67. Davies, E. G., Thrasher, A., Lacey, K., and Harper, J. (1999) Topical cidofovir for severe molluscum contagiosum. *Lancet* **353,** 2042.

68. Geerinck, K., Lukito, G., Snoeck, R., et al. A case of human orf in an immunocompromised patient treated successfully with cidofovir cream. *J. Med. Virol.* **64,** 543–549.

69. Smee, D. F. and Huggins, J.W. (1998) Potential of the IMP dehydrogenase inhibitors for intiviral therapies of poxvirus infections ABSTRACT. Eleventh International Conference on Antiviral Research. International Society for Antiviral Research, San Diego, CA.

70. Huffman, J. H., Sidwell, R. W., Khare, G. P., Witkowski, J. T., Allen, L. B., and Robins, R. K. (1973) In vitro effect of 1-beta-D-ribofuranosyl-1,2,4-triazole-3-carboxamide (virazole, ICN 1229) on deoxyribonucleic acid and ribonucleic acid viruses. *Antimicrob. Agents Chemother.* **3,** 235–241.

71. Frey, S., Couch, R., Tacket, C., et al. (2002) Clinical responses to undiluted and diluted smallpox vaccine. *N. Engl. J. Med.* **346,** 1265–1274.

72. Bicknell, W. and James, K. (2003) The new cell culture smallpox vaccine should be offered to the general population. *Rev. Med. Virol.* **13,** 5–15.

7

Plague Vaccines

Retrospective Analysis and Future Developments

Jeffrey J. Adamovicz and Gerard P. Andrews

1. INTRODUCTION

Plague has had a long and remarkable association with humankind, causing incalculable pain and suffering, thus it should not be surprising that some of the first vaccine efforts were directed against this dreaded disease. The first effective plague vaccines were developed through the efforts of the Pasteur Institute in the late 1890s. Although the first products were whole-cell killed vaccines, live-attenuated plague vaccines soon followed. Both types of vaccines met with varying degrees of success. The true efficacy of these early vaccines remains difficult to determine as no large controlled efficacy trials were recorded. These early vaccine products were empirical attempts to prevent disease given at a time when the pathogenesis of the organism and the basis for immunity were not fully understood. Although more than 100 yr has passed since these initial attempts, we still do not have an effective licensed human plague vaccine with demonstrated efficacy against both bubonic and pneumonic plague, with acceptable reactogenicity, nor a full understanding of pathogenesis or the true nature of immunity to the disease. Our understanding of plague immunity in humans is hampered by the lack of established correlates between observations in animal models and humans. Furthermore, it is clear that vaccines that protect against bubonic plague may not protect against pneumonic plague. A significant effort was made to accurately describe older plague vaccines and establish a more fundamental understanding of how the next plague vaccine should/should not be designed. This chapter is a summary of plague vaccine development, a discussion of our current understanding of immunity to plague, and recent attempts to develop a safe and effective plague vaccine with an eye toward the future.

2. PATHOLOGY OF BUBONIC AND PNEUMONIC PLAGUE

Animal models for plague vaccine studies were chosen on the basis of similarities in pathology to the disease in humans. Whereas early studies used numerous animal models, those that exhibit the closest relationship to pathology in humans include the mouse and the nonhuman primate (NHP) models *(1–4)*. The pathology of plague infection in NHPs and humans is strikingly similar. What is not appreciated are the dissimilarities

From: *Infectious Diseases: Biological Weapons Defense: Infectious Diseases and Counterterrorism*
Edited by: L. E. Lindler, F. J. Lebeda, and G. W. Korch © Humana Press Inc., Totowa, NJ

in pathology between bubonic and pneumonic plague. The infection and pathology of plague from parenteral or aerosol exposure is illustrated in Fig. 1.

2.1. Bubonic Plague

Bubonic plague is a Gram-negative endotoxemia that in a certain sense presents as a generalized Swartzman reaction *(5,6)*, with detectable levels of endotoxin in the blood of patients *(7)*. Patients with bubonic plague typically exhibit defined enlarged painful lymph nodes. Detection of these "bubos" varies, reported to occur in 50% of American Indians and close to 100% of South Vietnamese in two small studies *(6,8,9)*. In both studies, patients with bubonic plague exhibited fever, tachycardia, hypotension, and depending on length of infection, symptoms of disseminated intravascular coagulation (DIC). Disease most often results from the bite of an infected flea. The current paradigm for disease after inoculation from an infected flea is either the development of "bubonic" or septicemic forms *(10)*. Although some of the cellular and molecular events that follow initial infection are still undefined, there is a generally accepted sequence of events.

After dermal inoculation, the bacterial virulence factors required for survival in a mammalian host are not expressed; the bacteria are unencapsulated and lack the virulence-associated effector proteins *Yersinia* outer proteins (Yops) *(11–14)*. The majority of inoculated bacteria are not initially resistant to phagocytosis by tissue macrophages or polymorphonuclear leukocytes (PMNs). In previous studies *(11,15)*, it was shown that phagocytosed organisms are either killed or transported to the regional lymph nodes. Plague bacilli injected into the peritoneal cavity of mice were rapidly

---

Fig. 1. *(opposite page)* Plague pathogenesis. Humans become incidental hosts for plague through the bite of an infected flea (middle). Plague bacilli replicate at the site of infection and/ or are transported by phagocytic cells to the draining lymph nodes. Organisms in the lymph nodes replicate and cause a destructive necrotic process marked by intense swelling and pain in the infected nodes. A histological representation of this necrotic process in the infected lymph node is compared to normal tissue. Numerous organisms can be seen in the lesion. Organisms may seed from the infected node to other nodes and possibly to multiple distal organs. Conversely, in septicemic plague, there is no apparent lymph node involvement and the organisms spread hematogenously to multiple organs. The organ spread usually progresses first to the liver and spleen and then to other organs inducing secondary pneumonia upon reaching the lungs or meningitis/encephalitis after infection of the meninges. Exposure to infected aerosols (top) may occur as a result of person-to-person spread or intentional aerosolization. This usually leads to a rapid and fatal pneumonia. The histological lesions are representative of the destruction of the alveolar spaces. As compared to normal tissue the infected tissue contains numerous neutrophils and plague bacilli and edematous fluid. However, as with bubonic plague, the bacilli can spread hematogenously from the lung to multiple organs. The concept of increasing symptomology with its relationship to death as an outcome for all disease manifestations is illustrated at the bottom of the figure. The most rapid time-course for disease progression occurs following exposure to an infected aerosol. Although many factors affect the time-course disease progression in an immunologically naïve person usually manifests within 2–4 d. The time-course for bubonic or septicemic plague is generally more protracted, taking from 3 to 10 d. Without medical intervention, death as an outcome occurs in almost 100% of aerosol exposures and about 50% of parenteral exposures.

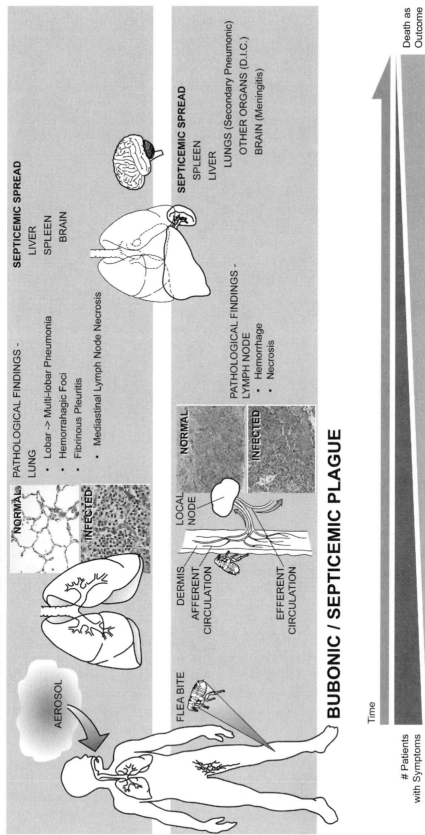

phagocytized and killed by PMNs; however, the rate of phagocytosis decreased to zero, 5 h after injection *(15)*. Intracellular bacteria are probably initially killed by some professional phagocytes (e.g., PMNs) *(11,16)* but not by others (e.g., macrophages) *(12,17,18)*. The surviving bacteria, like *Salmonella*, can grow within phagolysosomes *(19,20)*. Intracellular *Yersinia* survive by an undefined mechanism but most eventually escape their intracellular captivity within the lymph nodes. Within hours of infection, extracellular bacteria in the lymph nodes express a range of antihost proteins *(21,22)*, including the proteinacious Fraction One (F1) capsule *(13)*. Some bacteria may also remain at the site of inoculation and establish a local infection. This focus of infection grows and the resulting progeny, regardless of location, actively resist phagocytosis by PMNs *(1,23,24)*. The invading bacteria rapidly kill host phagocytes and lymphocytes, resulting in local necrosis and swelling of the infected node at the site of inoculation *(11)*. During the development of septicemic plague, it is not clear if the invading bacteria actually avoid the regional lymph nodes or, if infection of the nodes does occur, the invading bacteria fail to induce gross pathological or physiological changes *(25)*. Infection may directly proceed from the infection site to the peripheral circulation with or without subsequent seeding of the lymph nodes. As the duration of bubonic or septicemic infection increases, bacteria may disseminate to multiple organs. Distal sites of infection can include the lungs and/or the meninges *(26,27)*. Infection of the lungs by this route may induce a secondary pneumonia. Persons in close contact to a patient with secondary plague pneumonia can acquire primary plague pneumonia by exposure to small droplet nuclei during coughing or sneezing *(28)*.

2.2. Pnuemonic Plague

Clinical disease after exposure to "intentionally" aerosolized plague is markedly different. It has been known for some time that inhaling plague bacilli after exposure to a person with pneumonic plague induces primary plague pneumonia and death within 2–4 d *(29)*. Primary pneumonic plague occurs after inhaling plague bacilli dispersed in the size that can reach the deep lungs, (1–10 μm in diameter). Deposited bacilli may be unencapsulated and phenotypically negative for the virulence-associated Yop proteins or, if transmitted from an infected person, may be expressing both. The effect of expressing or not expressing capsule and/or Yops in the lungs at the time of infection is unclear. It is tempting to speculate that expression of virulence factors may lead to a more rapidly fatal pneumonia. Evidence for this hypothesis comes from a primary pneumonic plague outbreak in Mukden, China *(30)*. In this outbreak, most close contacts of primary cases died from pneumonic plague as early as 2–3 d after exposure. In our experience, NHPs exposed to aerosolized plague grown at 26°C do not die until day 4–5 postexposure. The relevance of these observations requires additional investigation.

In either form, the majority of inhaled bacteria may be cleared by host nonspecific defense mechanisms *(18)*. Some bacteria in the alveolar spaces are phagocytosed by alveolar macrophages and transported to the mediastinal lymph nodes. The remaining bacteria rapidly become resistant to phagocytosis and establish an infection in the lungs, which leads to frank pneumonia. Bacteria that are transported outside of the lungs must rapidly escape to induce the massive necrosis observed in the mediastinal lymph nodes. As time progresses, bacteria may escape the nodes via the blood and seed to other organs, principally the liver and spleen *(1)*.

The dissemination of bacteria from the lungs after aerosol exposure to plague bacilli has been modeled in the laboratory. A comparative study of intracutaneous and intratracheal infection of rhesus macaques revealed significant differences in hepatic function, an important temporal marker of dissemination/physiological stress. Monkeys infected intertracheally with virulent plague bacilli had diminished liver function by the second day of infection and associated hepatic infection. In contrast, monkeys with bubonic infections maintained normal hepatic function and were free from hepatic infection up to day 5 after infection, suggesting a more rapid septicemia in animals exposed via the lungs *(31)*. Exposure of rhesus macaques to true aerosolized plague revealed little difference in disease pathology compared to rhesus that were infected via intratracheal instillation or to humans with primary pneumonic plague *(32)*. The 50% lethal dose (LD_{50}) for rhesus monkeys was determined to be 20,000 colony-forming units (CFU) via aerosol but only 100 CFUs by intratracheal instillation *(31,32)*. It is tempting to speculate on the reasons for the difference in LD_{50}. The most likely reason is that an aerosol dose is not entirely retained by the animal. In fact, Speck proposes that the retained dose might be only 30% of the exposed dose *(32)*. Regardless of the route of infection, a confounding factor is the disruption of normal platelet function manifested as DIC. Evidence of DIC and fibrin thrombi in the liver and glomerular capillaries in NHPs and humans is notable *(33,34)* and probably contributes to mortality especially in late-course disease.

The histopathology can be compared between the monkey and the mouse models. In mice, aerosolized plague bacilli are rapidly cleared from the lungs. Only 5% of the challenge inoculum are detectable in the lungs from 30 min to 16 h postexposure. The bacteria were not trapped in the upper respiratory system, as the trachea and oropharynx contained only a small percentage of the inoculum *(35)*. Between 16 and 48 h after exposure, the number of plague bacilli increased exponentially in the lungs. Microorganisms outside the lungs were first seen in the liver (16 h), then the heart circulation (24 h) and peripheral blood and spleen. The rapid dissemination of bacilli from the lungs to the liver was likely caused by cells of the reticuloendothelial system or the deposition of fibrin-bacteria thrombi. PMNs appear to play an important role in preventing dissemination of plague bacilli from the lungs principally through an antibody-dependent mechanism *(1,36)*. Mice passively protected with antiserum to whole bacilli or to capsule, F1, had an intense neutrophilic response that was apparently not associated with increased phagocytosis *(36)*. The massive influx of neutrophils to the infected lungs of nonimmune individuals most likely induces detrimental pathology for the host, although the mechanism has not yet been clearly demonstrated. The histopathology of aerosolized or intratracheal plague in untreated mice is extremely similar to pneumonic plague in humans *(1)*. In both mice and humans, the infected lungs have extensive, consolidated, necrotic lesions containing massive numbers of neutrophils, bacteria, and fibrinous fluid. The plague pathology of rhesus *(24,33)* and African green monkeys *(4)* is similar to the observations in humans. These observations support the use of both the mouse and the NHP for plague studies.

An asymptomatic infection in some humans and NHP, presumably exposed to aerosolized plague, is the development of pharyngeal plague *(37,38)*. Pharyngeal carriage is thought to eventually resolve asymptomatically or progress after an extended time to fulminate plague pneumonia. In rhesus macaques, exposure to aerosolized plague resulted in subacute or chronic disease in some animals up to the termination of the experiment (at day 54), with no relationship between the severity of lesions and the challenge dose *(37)*. In Vietnam, 15% of patients with bubonic plague and some of their close contacts were noted to carry plague by pharyngeal swab. Resolution of this carriage state is difficult to interpret as most patients and contacts were treated with antibiotics; five that were not treated resolved their carriage without disease. The role of previous vaccination on disease resolution was not discussed, but residual vaccine immunity may be a factor that leads to resolution of pharyngeal infection *(38)* or aerosol exposure *(39,40)*. This human carriage state may play a role in spreading infection during human outbreaks and must be considered in future outbreaks.

The histopathological data and comments provided by Ransom and Krueger suggest that the lesions of chronic plague may be the result of a more appropriate host immune response that minimizes damage to host tissue *(37)*. The ability to minimize the necrotic host response to plague bacilli may be the unstated goal of an effective plague vaccine. However, the ultimate goal of any plague vaccine should be the prevention of replication and elimination of any invading bacteria regardless of route of exposure. Although natural immunity in patients that survive plague infection generally prevents reinfection, some individuals may become reinfected with bubonic plague *(9)*. Large portions of the world are still endemic for bubonic plague, emphasizing the need for an effective vaccine. Also, because of the short time-course for onset of clinical disease, the risk of person-to-person transmission and the potential for use as a weapon, the importance of developing an effective vaccine against aerosolized plague cannot be overemphasized.

3. KILLED WHOLE-CELL PLAGUE VACCINES

3.1. The Haffkine Vaccine

3.1.1. Description

The development and use of effective plague vaccines began in the late 19th century. The first widely used plague vaccine was developed in India by W.M.W. Haffkine *(41,42)*. The original Haffkine vaccine was a whole-cell killed vaccine made from stationary phase broth cultures of the virulent Indian strain of *Y. pestis* 195/P. An improved Haffkine vaccine was subsequently produced using log-phase broth cultures grown at 37°C. These organisms were formalin-killed and mixed with phenyl-nitrate as a preservative. The vaccine was given subcutaneously in a range of primary doses (2.5–12 mL) with 0.4-mL boosts. A retrospective comparison of the old and new Haffkine vaccines revealed that the latter contained four times the amount of F1 antigen as the former. The importance of the amount of F1 antigen in whole-cell vaccines has subsequently been directly linked to their efficacy *(43)*. The Haffkine vaccine was the first plague vaccine to address consistency among production lots. This was done with a direct mouse potency assay. The potency test used for Haffkine vaccine *(44,45)* was later adopted and modified for inclusion in the United States Pharmacopoeia (USP) for Plague Vaccine USP *(46)*.

3.1.2. Efficacy/Comparability

The Haffkine-type vaccines were tested in numerous animal models including mice, rats, guinea pigs, and cynomolgus macaques. It was also the first vaccine to be tested in a manner that approximates modern field trials. These field studies, although not conducted as rigorously as they would be today, represented a significant step forward in scientific method. During three partially controlled field tests, the Haffkine vaccine was shown to reduce the morbidity and mortality in vaccinates as compared to the nonvaccinated controls *(42)*. The reduction of the incidence of bubonic plague with Haffkine's vaccine was also associated with severe local and systemic vaccine reactions *(43)*. The local and systemic reactions were most likely a result of the route of administration, the preservative, and other impurities in the vaccine itself. The Haffkine vaccine was reported to be 62–65% effective in reducing bubonic plague during human trials conducted in Kenya after a single 2-mL inoculation of a locally prepared batch of vaccine *(47)*. In a field trial conducted from 1933–1934 in the East Indies, the Haffkine vaccinates experienced only 38 bubonic plague deaths while the unvaccinated population experienced 213 deaths, a degree of protection similar to that observed in the Kenyan trial *(48)*.

Vaccinates were able to establish a memory response to the vaccine preparation as boosts of Haffkine vaccine were noted to induce hemagglutination titers associated with protection. Also, serum from human vaccinates with as much as 20 yr between inoculations passively protected mice, indicating that antibody is important in immunity and that individuals that made an anamastic response to plague antigens may be protected from subsequent challenge. Although the Haffkine vaccine was reported to be relatively effective, it fell out of favor outside of India because of severe side effects, high numbers of vaccine failures, contamination of some vaccine preparations and, in the 1930s, the development of new, live-attenuated plague vaccines. There is no evidence that Haffkine-type vaccines were effective against aerosol challenge. The Haffkine vaccine was used extensively in and around the Indian cities of Surat and Bombay after the plague outbreak in 1994. A related vaccine is in use in Australia, manufactured by Commonwealth Serum Laboratories. It is recommended as a traveler's vaccine, but little efficacy data are available *(49)*.

3.1.3. Immunogenicity/Reactigenicity

Haffkine selected his vaccine's dosage based on the induction of a postvaccination fever of 102°F persisting for 24–48 h. Other noted side effects included localized pain, swelling, erythema, and lymphadenopathy. Local and systemic side effects including incapacitation were noted in vaccinated persons after subsequent boosts *(42)*. Because of the high levels of reactigenicity in some vaccinates, the health authorities in the Pacific Islands and Hawaii eventually banned the use of Haffkine vaccine imported from India *(43)*.

3.2. The "Army" Vaccine

3.2.1. Description

In the United States, whole-cell killed vaccines were favored over the live-attenuated vaccines, and in 1941, the US National Research Council recommended the use of a new "Army" whole-cell killed vaccine for deploying US troops. This decision was not based on a head-to-head comparison with live-attenuated vaccines but rather on the less-severe vaccine reactions in humans as compared to Haffkine vaccine. The Army vaccine was the first US plague vaccine manufactured for human use in 1942. Like the Haffkine vaccine, the vaccine was a whole-cell, formalin-killed preparation of agar-grown *Y. pestis,* although a different strain, Shasta, was used for the inoculum. It is not clear what was the basis for selection of Shasta. The vaccination regimen varied, although it was generally given as a 1.5-mL primary dose with 1-mL boosts 5–11 mo later. The vaccine contained 2 billion killed plague bacilli per milliliter that reportedly included approx 0.4 mg of F1 antigen *(50).*

3.2.2. Efficacy/Comparability

The Army vaccine, with minor modifications, became the Plague Vaccine USP. It is credited, retrospectively, with reduction in plague (bubonic) morbidity and mortality of US soldiers in the Mediterranean and the Far East during World War II, as no vaccinated US soldiers were diagnosed with plague. Nonimmune British forces in the Middle East experienced 26 clinical cases of bubonic plague with five deaths *(51).* Like the Haffkine vaccine, there is no evidence that this vaccine was effective against pneumonic plague.

3.2.3. Immunogenicity/Reactigenicity

The mouse potency index (MPI) was developed as an indirect potency assay by measuring the protective efficacy of human immune sera passively transferred to mice during early vaccine trials. As opposed to the direct potency test used for the Haffkine vaccine, this assay was used to predict potency of plague vaccine in humans and for comparison to other plague vaccines. The MPI value is calculated by dividing the percentage mortality by the average day of death of the mice during a 14-d observation period. Thus, MPI values less than 10 were associated with protection from bubonic plague *(52).* Eight human volunteers vaccinated with two or three doses of Army vaccine routinely developed protective antibodies. In these studies, the MPI decreased from a prevaccine average of 18.2 to 8.6 ($n = 6$) for two doses or 1.9 for three doses ($n = 2$) *(50).* A similar result was found for volunteers vaccinated with three doses of a F1 subunit vaccine (*see* Subheading 3.3.2.); their postinoculation MPI values decreased from 15.5 to 6.3 *(53).*

3.3. The Cutter/Greer Vaccine

3.3.1. Description

The first US licensed plague vaccine was manufactured by Cutter (Berkley, CA). This vaccine was an adaptation of the Army product. Cutter went through several modifications of its vaccine product from the original Army vaccine in 1942–1945 to a first-generation vaccine made from 1950 to 1967 with a final formulation used in 1967 and subsequent manufacture by Greer Laboratories (Lenoir, NC) from 1993 to 1999. The final version of Cutter/Greer vaccine was an aqueous, formalin-killed suspension of agar-grown *Y. pestis* 195/P. The organisms were grown at 37°C for 48 h on agar and mixed with formaldehyde at 0.5%, then mixed with physiological saline and adjusted to 2.0×10^9 organisms/mL in 20-mL vials. The Greer vaccine was prepared from fully virulent *Y. pestis* 195/P grown on E-broth agar overlay production medium, killed with 0.019% formaldehyde, and mixed with 0.5% phenol as a preservative. The final concentration was adjusted to 10^9 bacilli/mL with saline. The vaccine was packaged in 20-mL bottles and stored under refrigeration *(54,55).*

The recommended schedule for persons age 18–61 yr was 1.0 mL intramuscular primary dose with 0.2 mL boosters at 1–3 mo after the primary dose and a second boost

5–6 mo after the first. Annual booster shots were recommended for personnel with an occupational or travel-related risk of exposure *(52)*. The potency assay for Cutter and Greer was a direct potency assay for comparison of a test lot of vaccine with a reference standard lot of vaccine. The test lot effective dose 50% (ED_{50}) value must be greater than 0.5 of the ED_{50} of the reference lot *(46)*. As with the Army vaccine, an indirect potency test was also used as a surrogate measure of efficacy. Cutter and Greer vaccines routinely generated geometric mean MPI values less than 10 in approx 55% of human subjects after a primary and single boost *(52)*. Unfortunately, the Plague USP vaccine is no longer manufactured.

3.3.2. Efficacy/Comparability

The majority of direct efficacy data available for Cutter/Greer vaccines are from animal models. The vaccine, when given in two doses of 0.2 mL was efficacious against a modest subcutaneous (SC) challenge in mice but not in guinea pigs. Efficacy in guinea pigs was improved with increased dosages and the addition of adjuvants such as aluminum potassium sulfate (alum) or aluminum hydroxide but not calcium phosphate. A 1-mL dose and 0.2-mL boost of Plague USP manufactured by Cutter was able to protect six of nine langur monkeys from 131,000 CFU of 195/P by SC inoculation. The surviving subjects had an average MPI value of 3.4 at the time of challenge; those that did not survive had an average MPI of 13.7. The nonsurvivors had an extended time to death when compared to the unvaccinated controls and also different disease pathology, succumbing to metastatic pulmonary plague vs the controls which died on day 5 of bubonic-septicemic plague *(51)*. The delay in time to death is related to the altered disease pathology and is similar to observations in our laboratory with this vaccine in both the mouse and NHP models. The same lot of vaccine used in the above NHPs was used to vaccinate 25 human volunteers. Eleven weeks after a basic 1-mL dose, the vaccinates were given 0.2-mL booster, the boost increased the ability of human sera to passively vaccinate mice, increasing the percent with MPI values of less than 10 from 20% at day 28 to 91% 4 wk after the boost *(51)*. These data indicate that the Cutter vaccine may be effective in protecting humans from bubonic plague.

The majority of the human efficacy data was collected retrospectively from US service personnel deployed to Vietnam. Soldiers who received the Cutter vaccine had a much lower incidence of bubonic plague than their nonimmune South Vietnamese counterparts *(56)*. There were only seven cases of plague in US personnel or one case per one million human years of exposure compared to the 333 cases per one million human years in the South Vietnamese Army. The different rates of disease were most likely a result of the protection induced by vaccination and not because of other differences such as personnel cleanliness or site sanitation. When examined for rates of a second vectorborne disease, murine typhus, both the US and South Vietnamese forces experienced the same incidence of disease. It was not possible to determine if the vaccine protected against pneumonic plague because of the low incidence of pneumonic disease.

We tested the ability of Cutter/Greer vaccine to protect animals against pneumonic plague. Three doses of Cutter/Greer vaccine given on days 0, 28, and 90 did not protect vaccinated mice, guinea pigs, or African green monkeys from aerosolized plague (US Army Medical Researcg Institute of Infectios Disease [USAMRIID], unpublished data). The basis for the complete failure of the Cutter vaccine to protect three different animal species from aerosol challenge is unknown but could be related to the qualitative antibody response to F1 because rF1 alone has been shown to protect mice from a similarly modest aerosol challenge *(57)*.

3.3.3. Immunogenicity/Reactigenicity

Vaccine-associated sequelae have not been noted in mice or langur monkeys vaccinated with the recommended human dose. However, local and systemic reactions to this vaccine have been reported in humans vaccinated at or above the recommended dose *(51)*. The clinical symptoms of a local reaction include edema, tenderness, decreased motion, warmth, and/or induration at the site of inoculation, lasting for less than 48 h. Systemic reactions include three or more of the following: malaise, headache, dizziness, chills, generalized muscle or joint aches, feverishness, anorexia, nausea, and vomiting *(52)*.

A comprehensive study on adverse clinical reactions in 1219 persons to early preparations of killed plague vaccine made by Cutter from 1942 to 1974 noted local reactions in 29% and a systemic reaction in 20% of vaccinates. This study also indicated a close relationship between antigenic mass (of the vaccine) and local and systemic reactions as the early Army/Cutter lots induced more systemic and local reactions than more recently produced lots. Early lots of vaccine contained twice as many organisms per dose (4×10^9) than more recent lots. As a consequence, it was shown that reductions in both the primary and booster doses from 2 to 1 mL and from 1 to 0.5 mL, respectively, of early lots of Cutter vaccine resulted in a concomitant reduction in local and systemic reactions *(58)*. The induction of local and systemic reactions was not always viewed unfavorably. The induction of local reactogenicity was viewed as a measure of "vaccine take" after administration of both the Haffkine vaccine and live-attenuated vaccines. The higher reactivity of early Cutter vaccine lots may have been caused by the presence of A- and/or B-blood group antigens, contaminants of the production process. The blood group antigens were removed by an improved production process in 1967.

The principal protective antigen in plague vaccines produced by both Cutter and Greer is the capsular antigen F1. It was understood in the early days of plague vaccine development that the induction of antibodies to F1 was important for a protective immune response. Amazingly, the vaccine preparations are standardized for nitrogen content and colony counts but are not standardized for F1 content and, therefore, the amount of detectible F1 antigen may vary greatly from lot to lot. An indirect measure of the F1 content between lots is the mouse potency assay, as it is believed that protecting mice depends on the F1 in the vaccine preparation. Because Plague Vaccine USP was administered in a primary series of two to three injections, the relevance of F1 variation between lots is unclear. The geometric mean titer for anti-F1 passive hemagglutination (PHA) values of human immune sera increases with the number of doses over a course of three injections of the vaccine. This again indicates the importance of F1 in the vaccine preparation.

One aspect of using serological data to predict immunity in humans is the duration of positive correlative antibody values. The anti-F1 titer in humans may be relatively short-lived in that it rapidly decreases 3–6 mo after each boost. Also of concern was the observation that two of 29 (7%) human subjects failed to make a detectable PHA titer even after three doses of Cutter vaccine *(59)*. In a related, but larger, study the PHA titers and MPI values of 117 human subjects were followed over the course of repeated inoculations and potential exposures from 1952 to 1972. This study revealed a pattern of human sero-conversion to the Cutter vaccine based on the reciprocal of the PHA titer that included the definition of three levels of responsiveness: 72% high responders (reciprocal titer = 1024 – 16,382), 20% intermediate responders (64–512), and 8% nonresponders (<16) *(54)*. The anti-F1 response appeared to plateau after five doses of vaccine, but in contrast to the study with three doses, the antibody titers were maintained for the 6 mo between boosts. Even individuals with interrupted vaccine regimens maintained PHA titers up to 6 yr after their last boosts. This observation is similar to that reported earlier for Haffkine vaccinates. The US Public Health Service Immunization Practices Advisory Committee recognizes a PHA titer of 1:128 to F1 as a correlate of immunity in animals *(60)*, and by extension this titer is predictive of immunity in humans.

4. LIVE-ATTENUATED PLAGUE VACCINES

4.1. Description

The first live vaccines were used in the Philippines in 1908, but the first large-scale trials were conducted in the 1930s. These trials were conducted with the Tjiwidej strain developed by Otten and tested in Indonesia, and the EV strain developed by Girard and Robic and tested in Madagascar. The EV-type vaccine was more extensively used and reported to be more effective *(61)*. The new live-attenuated vaccines were reported to substantially reduce both rates of infection and death in vaccinees living in plague-endemic areas *(61–63)*. Initial reports on the effectiveness of the live-attenuated vaccines did not include lengthy descriptions of the associated side effects, although it is reasonable to assume that they were widely known. The molecular basis for the attenuation of the EV-type strains is unknown, but the parent strain was selected for reduced virulence by SC inoculation in Hartley guinea pigs. The Tjiwidej strain of Otten was reported to be negative for the production of V antigen (VW–) *(63)*, whereas the EV-type vaccine of Girard did produce V-antigen (VW+) *(64)*. The phenotypic criteria for EV strains are listed in Table 1. These include the ability to immunize guinea pigs, the possession of F1 and V (VW) antigens, and uracil independence for growth and pigmentation-negative reaction on agar with hemin *(51)*. The genetic relatedness of the numerous EV strains is still unclear.

The current dose regimen for the Russian EV-type vaccines in adults is dependent on the route of administration. A 0.5-mL injection (containing 300 million organisms) is given SC, 0.1 mL intracutaneously, or 0.15 mL (containing 3 billion organisms) supracutaneously with boosts to be given yearly *(65)*. Children and adults over age 60 yr receive reduced doses of the vaccine per the package insert instructions. The dose and schedule for EV-type attenuated plague vaccines by aerosol is variable. Several studies of aerosol vaccination with EV-type vaccines from the 1960s and 1970s are described *(66)*. The vaccines were manufactured by the Mechnikov Vaccine and Sera Scientific Research Institutes or the Sanitary Scientific Research Institute (NIIS). The effectiveness of these vaccines was determined from studies in baboons

Table 1
Characteristics of EV-Type Live-Attenuated Plague Vaccines

Strain	Pigmentation	Capsule	Calcium dependence	Uracil dependence	PD_{50} guinea pigs[a]	PD_{50} mice[a]	LD_{50} mice[b]
EV76 WR (Saigon)	–	+	+	+	–	2500	–
EV76 (Paris)	–	+	+	–	33	2800	>100,000
EV76 (51f) (Madagascar)	–	+	+	–	5	3600	1300

[a]50% protective dose (CFU) by SC route.
[b]50% lethal dose (CFU) by iv route.
(Adapted from ref. *51*.)

and was related to the percent of organisms in the respirable range (1–10 μm) and the size of the inoculum *(66,67)*. The problems with vaccine-induced morbidity, questionable effectiveness in humans, duration of immunity, and anticipated problems with US licensure make additional testing of the EV-type live-attenuated vaccines inadvisable.

4.2. Efficacy/Comparability

Trials in NHPs indicate that the EV-type attenuated vaccines may significantly protect them from bubonic plague *(see* Table 2). The data in this table were adapted from summarized data *(51,68)*. These data reflect the efficacy of EV-type plague vaccines in different NHP species after parenteral challenge. These experiments are difficult to compare to one another because of variations in the challenge strain, route, vaccination regimen, or other variables; however, collectively they indicate efficacy of EV-type vaccines against bubonic plague *(51,68)*. Of particular relevance is the ability of serum from different vaccinated NHP species to passively protect mice. As with the whole-cell killed vaccines, MPI values are below 10 and or anti-F1 hemagglutination titers are greater than 1:128 (experiments 1–7, Table 2).

The data in Table 2 also reveal a pattern of vaccine and species-dependent mortality. Although it may not be possible to directly compare the experiments to each other, the authors cite a pattern of vaccine-related sequelae in the NHPs that are linked to vaccine-dependent mortality. The most severe vaccine reactions occur in the langurs and the least severe in the macaques. As noted in experiments 1 and 3, the vaccination itself induced a significant mortality in the grivet and langur monkeys. Conversely, the survivors of the vaccination process were relatively (although not completely) protected from subsequent challenge. This poses an interesting question: are humans more like langurs, macaques, or something in between?

What is also apparent, in retrospect, is that many of the strains used to prepare EV-type vaccines, although fulfilling "EV-phenotype" requirements; either consisted of mixed cultures, were not sufficiently attenuated, or were inherently unstable. The strain designated as 51f was derived from passage of the "parent" EV 76 strain through guinea pigs treated with iron salts. This treatment served to decrease the attenuation of the vaccine by lowering the protective dose 50% (PD_{50}) for guinea pigs and the intrave-

Table 2
Efficacy of Live Attenuated Plague Vaccines in NHPs

Exp #	Species	Vaccine	Dose	Route	Challenge strain	Challenge dose (#CFU)	Challenge route	Time of challenge (days)	Survival/ total	MTD (day)	Ref.
1	Grivets (South Africa)	EV76 51f	10^2–10^8	sc	NA	NA	NA	NA	37/50	10	
	Vaccine survivors	–	–	–	F357	8770	sc	170	7/10	10	72
2	Langurs	Plague USP+EV Saigon boost D+60	2×10^9 4×10^8	im im	195/P	6.4×10^4	sc	94	2/7	11*	
	"	EV Saigon	1.8×10^4–10^6	id	195/P	2.3×10^5	sc	69	5/11	10*	73
3	Langurs	195P	10^2–10^5	sc	NA	NA	NA	NA	7/13	9	
	Vaccine survivors	–	–	–	195/P	10^2–10^4	id	105	4/5	8	74
4	Presbytis	–	–	–	195/P	81–810,00	sc	–	2/28	N/S	
	Grivets (Kenya)	–	–	–	195/P	209–2,090,000	sc	–	3/14	N/S	73
5	Grivets	EV76 F	1–10^6 2–10^9	Oral	195/P	8646	id	159	1/6	N/S	
6	"	EV76 F	3×10^9	Oral	195/P	12,875	id	166	3/3	–	75
7	Grivets	EV76 F	1.2×10^9	Oral	195/P	3.2×10^6	Aerosol	42	3/6	4	77
	Langurs	EV 76	2.7×10^7	id	195/P	3.4×10^5	sc	42	4/4 0/2(?)	– 4.0	
	Grivets (Kenya)	EV 76	2.7×10^7	id	195/P	1.6×10^5	sc	77	6/6 0/2 controls	– 3.5	

(continued)

Table 2 (continued)

Exp #	Species	Vaccine	Dose	Route	Challenge strain	Challenge dose (#CFU)	Challenge route	Time of challenge (days)	Survival/ total	MTD (day)	Ref.
7	Macaques	EV76	2.7×10^7	id	195/P	7.2×10^6	ip	119	2/2 2/5 controls	–	68
8	Langurs	M$_{23}$	4×10^7	i.d.	–	–	–	–	0/4	12	
	Grivets (Kenya)	M$_{23}$	4×10^7	4-id (2/4 died) 2-sc	195/P	1.6×10^5	sc	161	1/4 0/2 controls	6	
	Macaques	M$_{23}$	3.8×10^7	4-id 2-sc	195/P	7.2×10^6	ip	210	6/6 2/5 controls		68

*denotes statistical significance

nous LD$_{50}$ for mice (experiment 1, Table 2). The classical EV 76 vaccine and its many homologs are invasive and have produced many local and systemic side effects in NHPs. The presence of local and systemic reactions in NHPs often mimics clinical observations in vaccinated humans.

There is evidence in the literature that the live-attenuated plague vaccine is effective for reducing the incidence of bubonic plague in humans *(50,63,69,70)*. A field trial of the Tjiwidej strain of vaccine in South Africa in the 1930s reported an 82% decrease in disease in vaccinates *(69)*. A second field trial of Tjiwidej vaccine in 37,000 people in Java reported 50–75% reduction in plague mortality *(63)*. Note that neither of these field trials were properly controlled. There were no exclusion criteria nor were adverse events properly reported. A potential problem with EV-type vaccines is the maintenance of seed cultures because it is clear that the EV 76 strain has undergone several changes since its original isolation. These cultures are known to change phenotypes. For example, when passaged through animals, many of the attenuated vaccine strains will revert to the virulence of the parent strain *(71)*. On average, only about 30% of a delivered dose of EV-type vaccines is viable. There is currently no methodology to control for this fluctuation in viability. This aspect of the EV-type vaccine has significant implications for vaccinating populations of the old, young, and inmunocompromised.

Few data have been published concerning protection from pneumonic plague with live-attenuated plague vaccines. There is one published report of EV-76-dependent protection in rhesus monkeys intratracheally challenged *(76)*. Resistance in vaccinated monkeys was related to circulating levels of anti-F1 antibody. In another study, partial protection (3 of 6; 50%) from aerosolized plague was noted in orally exposed African green monkeys (experiment 6, Table 2) *(77)*. This experiment is interesting in that attempts to vaccinate this species of monkey by other routes with the same type of vaccine produced significant vaccine-dependent mortality *(51)*. Otten *(63)* observed that the live Tjiwidej vaccine strain did not reduce the incidence of pneumonic plague in humans. Alternatively, investigators recently attempted to genetically construct a better live-attenuated plague vaccine. A vaccine consisting of *Y. pestis* with defined deletion of the 102-kb pigmentation *(pgm)* locus was used to subcutaneously vaccinate mice; this vaccine protected the animals against aerosolized wildtype challenge. As with the EV-type vaccines, the *pgm* vaccine strain was lethal in 50% of the 16 African green monkeys exposed by the aerosol route *(78)*. The lethality of this vaccine strain was abolished by adding a second defined point mutation in *pla;* however, systemic sequelae were still noted. The double mutant vaccine strain was immunogenic and protective for all four NHP vaccinates in that all made potent antibodies to F1 *(78)*. Whereas the construction of a defined, live, nonreverting attenuated vaccine is theoretically possible, it has not been accomplished. A recent review summarizes the attempts to construct defined plague auxotrophic mutants or mutants in two component sensor systems *(79)*. These efforts have met with little success.

4.3. Immunogenicity/Reactigenicity

The first report to describe the serious side effects caused by live-attenuated plague vaccines was published in French Senegal *(80)*. The investigators described fever, lymphadenopathy, malaise, headaches, and sloughing of skin at the inoculation site, in addition to other severe local and systemic reactions for European recipients. The significance of this report is that the authors noted a significant difference in vaccine-related side effects between the native and European vaccinees. Whether the difference in vaccine side effects between Africans and Europeans was real or artificial is unclear. It was noted that in general, prior vaccination with a killed plague vaccine had an ameliorating effect on subjects given live vaccine. The vaccine status of the native population was not often known. The reports of serious side effects may have had an adverse effect on the acceptability of live plague vaccines in the United States and pushed the development of the killed Army vaccine. In 1939, the Soviet Union adopted the live-attenuated EV-type plague vaccine. However, there were serious side effects from EV-76 vaccinations. These effects, similar to those described in Senegal, included painful erythema up to 225 cm^2, fever, lymphadenopathy, headache, weakness, and malaise, which required hospitalization for some vaccinates. Because of the severe local and systemic reactions, the Russians attempted to ameliorate the side effects by changing the route of administration. These experiments tested SC, intracutaneous, scarification, oral, conjunctival, and aerosol vaccination. The outcome of aerosol vaccination studies is provocative in that it was reported that aerosol route was safer than cutaneous vaccination. In the first study, there were no adverse events reported for 534 test subjects. A second study reported only pyrexia in five of 68 test subjects *(81,82)*. It is difficult to determine if the aerosol route of exposure provided significant mucosal or systemic immunity to plague. The oral route of administration was tested in approx 4600 subjects in a field trial with a live EV-type plague vaccine. The study concluded that reactigenicity was low (5.2%) and efficacy was estimated to be 79% by extrapolation of PHA titers to F1 *(83)*.

The results of experiments to alter the route of EV-76 administration, summarized by Meyer *(71)*, indicate the preferred method of vaccination was intracutaneous or cutaneous (by abrasion) and that although the side effects are downplayed, it is clear that there were still significant vaccine-induced side effects with SC or cutaneous vaccination. The results of the Soviet studies led the United States to conduct its own small trial in the 1960s. Twelve volunteers were vaccinated with a single SC dose of Russian-type live-attenuated plague vaccine. Six vaccinates were unable to work for 72 h with two requiring hospitalization. These results, among others, led the physicians who supervised the clinical trial to conclude that mass vaccinations with EV-type live-attenuated plague vaccine would not be prudent *(51)*. The duration of immunity in EV-vaccinated NHPs is associated with maintenance of a PHA titer to F1 *(51)* and, as in humans, is believed to be short-lived. Two to three months after vaccination, antibody titers to F1 decline, as does the predicted protection. However, frequent boosters with live-attenuated, whole-cell killed or F1 antigen can maintain protective levels of antibody. This indicates that the induction of long-term immunity may be a problem with EV-type vaccines. An indirect method to measure duration of immunity in humans to live plague vaccines is to test the recall response to bacterial fractions after vaccination. The recall response to Russian EV-type vaccination, as determined by intradermal inoculation of pestin, indicates that immunity may wane in 60% of vaccinees between 6 mo and 1 yr *(84)*. Efforts to improve the efficacy and reduce the side effects of the EV-type vaccine continue *(85)*.

5. SUBUNIT VACCINES

Although much work has been done over the decades on developing an efficacious vaccine against bubonic and pneumonic plague, efforts on designing a well-defined subunit vaccine have only recently moved to the forefront. Consequently, there are far fewer data in this area of plague vaccine development; however, it is quite rapidly gaining momentum and will most likely dominate in the years to come.

Subunit vaccines, as the name implies, are essentially acellular preparations that contain one or a number of bacterial antigens, proteins, and/or carbohydrates, formulated with a characterized adjuvant. These preparations may be well-defined by combining highly purified components in specific amounts, or they may simply be crude preparations of ill-defined composition. Because a subunit vaccine by today's standards should most certainly be the former, the focus of this section will be on the application of purified plague antigens, alone or in combination, as potential subunit vaccines candidates. The basis for selecting these candidates is obviously immunogenicity in the host during infection, although as discussed in Subheadings 5.1.–5.7., not all plague immunogens by any means induce a protective response in the host.

5.1. Capsular Antigen

Y. pestis has long been known to produce a highly immunogenic, proteinacious capsule that is actively synthesized in vitro as well as in vivo *(53,86,87)*. Evidence for the latter comes from numerous serological surveys of convalescent human and animal sera, as well as anti-F1 reactivity in infected tissues *(88,89)*. Antibody to at least one epitope of the capsular protein is also protective *(90)*. The capsule can be readily visualized by phase-contrast microscopy of India ink-stained live bacteria *(91)*. Baker et al. *(92)* have reported the use of crude preparations of the capsular antigen to induce protective immunity against infection by virulent organisms in a mouse plague model. For these studies (and others), capsule was easily isolated from cultures of the bacteria by acetone drying, extracting the dried organisms with a toluene-saturated buffer, and centrifugation of the sample. Differential ammonium sulfate precipitation of the resulting "supernatant" then yielded a precipitate, designated "F1," rich with capsular protein, but also containing significant levels of carbohydrate (from lipopolysaccharide [LPS]). Further processing of F1 yielded a subfraction (#1B) composed almost entirely of protein, highly enriched for the capsular antigen but also containing other contaminating proteins. Biochemically, the capsule is a macromolecular aggregate of a single protein subunit of 17 kilodaltons *(93–95)*.

Capsular antigen, or F1 antigen, has also been observed to be spontaneously sloughed from the bacteria in vitro *(96)*. This cell-free F1 represents between 30 and 50% the total F1 synthesized by the organism when the protein is harvested from stationary-phase cultures *(93)*. There appear to be no differences between the cell-free and cell-associated material in terms of immunogenicity and protection. Table 3 shows the results of such an experiment in an outbred mouse model, using highly pure, LPS-free preparations of F1, derived from either a recombinant F1-producing *Escherichia coli* strain or avirulent *Y. pestis*. As shown, F1, regardless of the source and whether cell-associated or cell-free, affords a high degree of protection against either lethal parenteral (SC) or aerosolized plague infection. These results are consistent with an

Table 3
Efficacy of Purified (F1) From *Y. pestis* or *E. coli*
Against Parenteral or Aerosol Lethal Plague Challenge
in the Outbred Mouse Model

Treatment	Challenge[a]	Survivors	MDT ± SD[b] (d)
E. coli F1cell	sc	7/10	15.3 ± 3.5
E. coli F1sup		10/10	
Y pestis F1cell		10/10	
Y. pestis F1sup		10/10	
Plague USP		5/10	20.6 ± 4.6
Adjuvant only[a]		0/10	4.9 ± 0.7
E. coli F1cell	Aerosol	8/10	14.0 ± 12.2
E. coli F1sup		9/10	10.0 ± 0.0
Y. pestis F1cell		7/10	13.3 ± 11.9
Y. pestis F1sup		7/10	12.0 ± 11.4
Plague USP		1/9	11.8 ± 7.0
Adjuvant only[a]		0/10	3.3 ± 0.7

[a]Dose = 100 LD_{50}.
[b]Mean-time-to-death ± standard deviation.
[c]Alhydrogel.
(Adapted from ref. *93*.)

earlier study that reported protection in BALB/c mice against an intraperitoneal plague challenge with a recombinant F1 preparation *(97)*.

The role of the F1 capsule in virulence is a conundrum, as some virulent natural isolates are nonencapsulated, and laboratory-generated, nonencapsulated isogenic mutants still retain virulence *(4,98,99)*. Despite these observations, expression of F1 is temperature-regulated, with synthesis and secretion actively occurring at 37°C, thus, favoring the mammalian host environment. In fact, F1 can evoke antiphagocytic properties on the microorganism *(100,101)*. Therefore, it appears that F1 is useful to the microorganism, at least at one point in its evolution as a mammalian pathogen. It is provocative to speculate that the capsule has a more relevant role in the nonprimate host, such as facilitating persistence of the microorganism in a chronic or asymptomatic (cryptic) infection, such as that observed in laboratory rats *(102)*.

Not surprisingly, immunity to F1 fails to protect laboratory animals against nonencapsulated virulent *Y. pestis (103)*. In this regard, inoculating with an F1-only vaccine does not represent a prudent strategy for protecting against a biological weapons threat in light of the possibility of alteration of the organism to a nonencapsulated virulent variant. An analysis of Plague USP in our laboratory suggests that the bulk of the protein antigen in the preparation consists of F1 (unpublished data) and also that it fails to protect mice against an F1⁻ strain. Additionally, analytical gel filtration chromatography showed that F1 in Plague USP appears to be in a different aggregation state than freshly prepared protein (Andrews, unpublished data). Furthermore, Miller et al. *(104)*, reported significantly less efficacy elicited by the monomeric form of the protein compared to the aggregate, which is consistent with a loss of immunogenicity upon disaggregation as observed by others *(95)*. Taken together, these observations may have some bearing on why Plague USP also fails to protect against lethal aerosol challenges with F1⁺ strains (unpublished data).

Early studies suggested that F1 is not the only virulence determinant that induces protective immunity in the host *(100)*. Thus, although the basis for an acellular vaccine against plague may be F1, additional protective components could certainly be included, which may give an added advantage to the protected host.

5.2. Lipopolysaccharide

In addition to large amounts of the F1 capsule, Plague USP also possesses very high levels of LPS, which may have been a contributing factor to the reactogenicity of this product observed in many recipients of the vaccine *(58,59)*. Like most Gram-negative bacteria, the *Y. pestis* LPS contains 2-keto-3-deoxy-octulosonic acid; however, it may more appropriately be referred to a lipooligosaccharide as it lacks a true *O*-side chain antigen *(105,106)*. In fact, the complete lack of *O*-antigen ("rough" LPS phenotype) in some strains of *Y. pestis* is a result of mutations in existing genes required for the biosynthesis of the *O*-antigen *(107)*. Although the immunomodulatory effects of the molecule are unquestionable, the contribution of *Y. pestis* LPS in the development of a protective immune response in the host is tenuous, particularly in light of recent evidence that purified material failed to protect mice *(108)*.

5.3. pH 6.0 Antigen

Another macromolecular surface structure unique to *Y. pestis* that has intrigued vaccinologists over the years is a fibrillar-like protein polymer, known as pH 6.0 antigen. Like the F1 capsule, this protein appears across the surface of the organism as "wiry," filamentous strands only at 37°C *(109)*. However, in contrast with F1 another environmental cue is required, that of low pH. This phenomenon is highly suggestive of selective expression of the antigen in acidified host cell compartments, such as the phagolysosome of a macrophage, which was subsequently demonstrated to be the case by Lindler et al. *(110)*. A mutation in the pH 6.0 antigen structural gene *psaA* confers an attenuated phenotype on *Y. pestis (111)*. Despite this observation, purified preparations of recombinant pH 6.0 antigen failed to protect inoculated mice against a parenteral plague challenge, although the protein induced very high levels of circulating antibody (Andrews, unpublished data). However, it is quite possible that immunity to this virulence factor is more important in the lungs, although antibody responses to pH 6.0 antigen, during experimental aerosol infection of laboratory mice, were inconsistent at best *(112)*. Further examination of this intriguing protein is warranted, as studies involving aerosol challenges of pH 6.0 antigen-vaccinated laboratory animals have yet to be completed.

5.4. Plasminogen Activator

The small virulence plasmid, unique to *Y. pestis,* encodes a protein known as plasminogen activator, or Pla. As the name implies, it possesses an enzymatic activity that leads to clot lysis by converting plasminogen to the plasmin protease *(113)*. Bacterial plasminogen activator activity is not unique to *Y. pestis* and is associated with the virulence of many bacterial species *(114,115)*. A coagulase activity is also associated with the *Y. pestis* Pla but at temperatures below that of the mammalian host. In light of these findings, it was hypothesized that Pla has a dual enzymatic function: that of dissemination factor in the mammal and that of a clotting factor in the flea. Recently, *Y. pestis* Pla was shown to mediate invasion of the microorganism into host endothelial cells (114). The proteolytic activity of Pla also has been shown to affect degradation of certain immunogenic outer-membrane proteins of *Y. pestis*, associated with virulence *(116)*. More intriguingly, *Y. pestis* membrane preparations containing biologically active Pla cleaved certain cytokines *(117)*. Although the implications of these phenomena in the mammalian host may lead one to speculate on an immune avoidance strategy, they have only been observed in vitro. A mutation in *pla* confers an attenuated phenotype to *Y. pestis* (by the intradermal route of infection), with significantly reduced pathology, despite the fact that the mutant survived well in sera of mice *(116)*. However, as with pH 6.0 antigen, a preliminary study in our laboratory evaluating the efficacy of recombinant Pla in mice yielded inconclusive results, although a delay in time-to-death was observed (unpublished data). This finding in itself warrants further evaluation of the antigen as a potential protective component of the next-generation plague vaccine.

5.5. V Antigen

The virulence determinant known as V antigen, present in *Y. pestis* (as well as other *Yersinia* species), is required for full virulence of the bacterium, and its existence has been reported as far back as 1956 *(86,118–120)*. This polypeptide was later shown to be encoded by the medium molecular weight virulence plasmid pLCR and is temperature-regulated (expressed only at 37°C), as well as induced in vitro only in the absence of calcium cations, hence the term "low calcium response." The function of V antigen has been the subject of intense study for decades. Although many believe that the protein is involved in regulatory functions associated with secretion of other virulence proteins *(121,122)*, others have presented experimental evidence suggesting host immunomodulatory effects *(123–126)*. Recently, V antigen from *Y. enterocolitica* was shown to bind a host–cell pattern recognition receptor, toll-like receptor (TLR)2. Binding of TLR2 by V antigen was shown to induce the expression of interleukin-10 and may be responsible for other TLR2-dependent immunomodulatory effects *(127)*.

The use of V antigen as a protective immunogen was documented nearly 40 yr ago *(53)*. Later studies, demonstrating passive protection in mice with monoclonal antibody to V antigen, supported these earlier findings *(128)*. A more recent study with purified recombinant V antigen demonstrated excellent efficacy against high-level parenteral, as well as aerosol challenges *(129)*. Table 4 shows survival ranging from 80 to 100% in V-inoculated outbred mice against an F1+ subcutaneous challenge from 60 to more than 10^6 LD$_{50}$. There was 87–100% survival against F1+ aerosol challenges ranging from 59 to roughly 1000 LD$_{50}$. In contrast to F1 alone, this protection was equally as effective against an F1− virulent *Y. pestis* variant, C12 (*see* Table 4). This impressive protection lends support to the rationale of using V antigen as at least one of the components in a new acellular plague vaccine.

5.6. Other pLCR-Encoded Proteins

Additional antigenic proteins have also been identified on pLCR that may make promising subunit vaccine candidates. A group of effector proteins that are translo-

Table 4
**Protection by Recombinant V Antigen Against Parenteral
and Aerosol Lethal Challenge by F1$^+$ (CO92) and F1$^-$ (C12)
Y. pestis in a Mouse Model**

Treatment	Challenge	LD$_{50}$	Survival	MTD ± SD (d)
V antigen	F1$^+$, sc	61	10/10	
		6.1×10^3	10/10	
		1.2×10^6	8/10	5.0 ± 1.4
Adjuvant only		61	1/10	6.1 ± 0.9
V antigen	F1$^+$, aero.	59	9/10	4.0
		9.7×10^2	10/10	
Adjuvant only		59	0/9	3.3 ± 0.5
V antigen	F1$^-$, sc	37	10/10	
		3.7×10^3	10/10	
		7.4×10^5	9/10	7.0
Adjuvant only		37	1/10	11.4 ± 7.0
V antigen	F1$^-$, aero.	84	7/8	11.0
		1.9×10^2	9/10	5.0
Adjuvant only		84	0/10	3.7 ± 0.7

(Adapted from ref. *129*.)

cated extracellularly by a type-III secretion apparatus are known as the *Yersinia* outer proteins, or Yops. Alleles of the *yop* loci are found on pLCR in all three species of pathogenic *Yersinia (14)*. Various of biochemical functions have been associated with these proteins to include apoptosis (YopJ; *130,131*), cytolysis (YopB/D; *132,133*), dephosphorylation of host cell proteins (YopH; *134–136*), serine/threonine kinase activity (YpkA; *137–139*), actin microfilament disruption (YopE; *140,141*), and inhibition of platelet aggregation (YopM; *142,143*). Studies have shown that at least some of the Yops are immunogenic, as antibodies to these proteins have been detected in human convalescent sera *(144,145)*. Furthermore, culture supernatants containing a mixture of secreted Yops protected mice from lethal challenge with *Y. pestis (146)*. In a series of experiments designed to identify *Y. pestis* immunogens in a mouse model for aerosol infection, followed by antibiotic rescue, Benner et al. *(112)* examined the immune response to six secreted pLCR proteins. Whereas all infected animals consistently responded to V antigen, the humoral response to other pLCR proteins was variable. Despite these data, a systematic evaluation of the ability of individual recombinant Yops to induce a protective immune response shows promise. Our laboratory has examined seven purified *Y. pestis* recombinant pLCR proteins and has thus far found at least one interesting candidate, YopD. Although only partial protection and a delay in time-to-death were seen in YopD-vaccinated mice parenterally challenged with an F1$^+$ strain, there was significant protection (survival) against the nonencapsulated virulent isogenic strain, C12 (*see* Table 5). Despite these results, in the previous study *(112)* naïve mice were poorly responsive to this antigen compared to their responses to V antigen, F1, and Pla. In the above scenarios, differences in the immune response to the

Table 5
Efficacy of Vaccination With *Yersinia* Outer Proteins Against
Lethal Parenteral Plague Challenge With Nonencapsulated
***Y. pestis* (C12)**

Exp. #	Treatment group	Survivors total (%)[a]	MST ± S.E. (d)[b]
1	YopD	7/9(78)	22.4 ± 3.1
	YopH	2/9(22)	12.9 ± 3.5
	F1 (recombinant)	0/9(0)	7.7 ± 1.4
	Plague USP	2/9(22)	11.2 ± 3.3
	Adjuvant only	2/9(22)	10.8 ± 3.4
2	YopD	9/10(90)	26.2 ± 1.7
	Adjuvant only	1/10(10)	10.4 ± 2.2
3	YpkA	3/10(30)	14.1 ± 3.4
	YopE	4/14(29)	11.8 ± 2.9
	Adjuvant only	0/10(0)	5.4 ± 0.5
4	YopK	1/10(10)	10.0 ± 2.3
	Adjuvant only	1/10(0)	7.9 ± 0.4
5	YopM	2/10(20)	10.4 ± 3.0
	Adjuvant only	0/10(0)	6.9 ± 1.4
6	YopN	0/9(0)	8.0 ± 1.7
	Adjuvant only	0/10(0)	5.4 ± 0.4

[a]Challenge = 55–195 LD_{50}, SC.
[b]Mean Survival Time ± Standard Error. Day 28, the last day of observation
was used in the calculation for the mice that survived.
(Adapted from ref. *150*.)

various antigens and their ability to protect may possibly be due to differences in route of infection between the two studies.

In contrast to YopD, other recombinant Yops, although immunogenic, so far have failed to provide good protection in vaccinated animals. This observation is not surprising in light of the fact that the molecular mechanism of delivery of these effector proteins may prevent an antibody-dependent immune response *(147,148)*. Given this most recent model, a somewhat more selective approach may be taken in a continuing search for protective pLCR gene products. Therefore, the second component, YopB, of a cytolytic complex may also afford protection as does the first, YopD, although like this antigen, the consistency of the humoral response in the aerosol challenge mouse model is poor for YopB *(112)*. Additionally, a crude preparation of recombinant YopB failed to protect mice *(149)*. A poor immune response to the recombinant product was likely a contributing factor in these experiments, which may have been caused by the difficulty in obtaining stable expression (proteolysis of the product during processing was almost invariably observed). Therefore, a Yop B/D complex *(133)* may represent a better vaccine candidate compared to the individual antigens. An examination of some of the additional "translocator" gene products of the actual type III secretion apparatus would also be prudent. One such protein, YscC, is believed to be a surface-expressed molecule that spans the bacterial outer membrane *(14)* and may represent a target for antibody that can potentially disrupt secretion of multiple effectors.

5.7. Multiple Subunit Vaccines

The preponderance of data collected throughout the decades strongly suggests that a rational platform for a new cell-free plague vaccine would consist of both the F1 capsule and V antigens *(13,88,151)*. In light of this strategy, Heath et al. *(152)* developed a unique recombinant hybrid protein, consisting of a gene fusion between the F1 structural gene *caf1* and *lcrV* encoding V antigen. The gene product was expressed in *E. coli* to reasonably high levels and purified by standard chromatographic techniques. In a single-dose vaccination study, the fusion protein was subsequently compared to a F1 + V cocktail, F1, or V alone in an outbred mouse model for immunogenicity and protective efficacy *(103)*. As shown in Table 6, F1 and V alone provided some protection to vaccinated mice against moderate parenteral challenges, and it is interesting that protection afforded by F1 alone breaks down with parenteral challenge doses above 100 LD_{50} (*see* Tables 3 and 6). However, a synergistic effect was observed with the F1-V fusion protein and to a lesser extent with the two-antigen cocktail, as demonstrated by their ability to protect against very high doses of virulent organisms (*see* Table 6). In another study, vaccination with a single dose of F1-V protected outbred mice to 1 yr postvaccination *(57)*.

The greatest advantage of the fusion protein over separate components is the relative ease of manufacturing, the components of an F1 + V mixture would be considered as separate products. In this regard, the fusion protein will likely represent the licensed, next-generation plague vaccine in the United States.

Although the direct efficacy of the F1-V in NHP models has been variable, the fusion vaccine candidate, given in a three-dose regimen combined with Alhydrogel™, adjuvant, offers significant protection over Plague USP, which has historically performed very poorly against pneumonic plague infection. In two studies conducted at USAMRIID in the African green monkey (vervet) model, F1-V provided statistically significant protection against a high aerosol challenge dose with *Y. pestis* strain C12, a fully virulent F1$^-$ variant. In a different experiment using cynomolgus macaques, 80% (8 of 10) of the vaccinated animals were protected against a moderate aerosol challenge (70 LD_{50}) using a F1$^+$ virulent strain. The results in the African green monkey aerosol protection studies suggest that at challenge doses (below 100 LD_{50}), F1-V may be equally effective at protecting the African green monkey as the macaque.

A further refinement of the F1-V fusion protein vaccine is the addition of another allele of lcrV (from *Y. enterocolitica*) to the C-terminal end of the *Y. pestis* V antigen coding sequence. This new fusion protein, designated F1-Vp-Ve, would thus induce immune responses not only to epitopes of *Y. pestis* F1 and V antigens but also to those of *Y. enterocolitica* V antigen. The rationale for this "extension" is that any attempt to evade immunity to *Y. pestis* V antigen by genetically altering the V-phenotype and maintaining full virulence would be thwarted. Although in theory, a fusion protein of this nature seems the next likely step to improve the vaccine candidate, in practice, there are size limitations to what recombinant proteins *E. coli* is capable of synthesizing. Therefore, a more practical approach to improving the vaccine would be to add additional individual purified proteins to F1-V, such as other V antigens, YopD, YscC, or others.

Efforts by Williamson et al. *(153)* have also demonstrated excellent performance of a UK version of the F1 + V cocktail in mice and have even successfully vaccinated

Table 6
Comparative Efficacy of F1-V, F1 + V, V, or
F1 Alone, Against Lethal Parenteral or
Aerosol Challenge With *Y. pestis* **CO92 in**
the Mouse Model

Treatment	Challenge	LD_{50}	Survival (%)
F1-V	$F1^+$, SC	10^7	14/14 (100)
F1-V	$F1^+$, SC	10^8	9/15 (60)
F1 + V	$F1^+$, SC	10^7	12/15 (80)
F1 + V	$F1^+$, SC	10^8	3/14 (21)
V alone	$F1^+$, SC	10^7	10/15 (67)
V alone	$F1^+$, SC	10^8	5/15 (33)
F1 alone	$F1^+$, SC	10^4	3/15 (20)
Adjuvant only	$F1^+$, SC	10^2	0/15 (0)

(Adapted from ref. 57.)

mice with the mixture of antigens in biodegradable microspheres *(154,155)*. Consequently, this product is ultimately destined for European licensure. Both the UK and US products will ultimately make reasonable platforms for multicomponent, improved variations of a recombinant plague vaccine.

Another approach to a multiple subunit vaccine is the use of a "complex" of antigens. In the case of the *Yersinia*, the most likely candidate would be the YopB/D cytolytic porin. This bipartite complex attaches to the target host cell and forms a "portal of entry" for the pathogen's effector proteins *(133)*. Although limited success has been obtained by vaccinating with the individual proteins, it is provocative to hypothesize that an improved/synergistic immune response may be developed if the YopB/D complex is used (with the caveat of potential toxicity to the host). Our laboratory is currently pursuing this idea using tandomly expressed recombinant genes. Expression of these recombinant proteins together (and subsequent *in situ* complex formation) may facilitate stable recovery of both proteins, particularly the more proteolytically labile YopB. Regardless of what combinations of protective antigens are selected, the use of state-of-the-art molecular techniques combined with recent genomic sequencing data *(156,157)* should facilitate development of a well-defined and -characterized subunit vaccine candidate.

6. CONCLUSIONS

Historically, whole-cell plague vaccines are effective in preventing bubonic plague in humans. The basis for their inability to protect against pneumonic plague is unclear but may be caused by alterations in the quality or quantity of F1 and the limited presence of other important antigens. It is also probable that the type of immune response to the killed organism is not optimal because of the route of administration and/or the choice of adjuvants. A major criticism of whole-cell plague vaccines is the predicted duration of "immunity" and the inability to induce a mucosal immune response. Whereas live-attenuated plague vaccines are believed to induce a more potent immune response of longer duration, they have not significantly reduced plague morbidity and mortality. Current live plague vaccines are associated with severe local and systemic reactions in humans and NHPs and significant mortality in some species of NHPs. The efficacy of live-attenuated plague vaccines against bubonic plague is significant, but is not adequately demonstrated against pneumonic plague. The Russian EV-type live-attenuated plague vaccine was evaluated and not recommended for use in the United States because of significant local and systemic reactigenicity. Additional testing of EV-type live-attenuated plague vaccines is not recommended; however, the development and testing of other live-attenuated plague vaccines remains an exciting possibility.

Of more immediate interest are vaccines composed of recombinant subunits. Immunity to plague clearly requires antibody to V antigen and for typical plague isolates to F1 antigen. Although it is clear that a vaccine containing F1 and V antigen is a powerful platform for inducing a protective response in animal models of plague, future identification and addition of other protective antigens are paramount to ensuring maximal protection, particularly in light of technical capabilities to artificially alter the virulence of microorganisms.

The basis for comparison of vaccine efficacy results in animals to humans is unclear. Some animals appear to more suitable for pathological studies (NHPs), others for immunogenicity/potency assays (mice/rats), and still others may be needed for efficacy studies or the development of surrogate markers of immunity. Criteria for the comparison of vaccine efficacy in animals to humans should be established. A molecular comparison of characteristics of the immune response (i.e., MHC, antibody, T-cell proliferation, pathology, plus others singularly or in combination) are likely to be more effective predictors of immunity in humans. The differential response of animals of different species and even within the same species to plague vaccines is unclear. The antibody response to plague antigen(s) formed the basis of predictive protection to all previous plague vaccines. However, it is clear that protection (at least in rodents) is not dependent on the presence of large amounts of circulating antibody. It has been shown that vaccinated animals that have little to no detectable circulating antibody to plague antigens are still protected. Absolute correlation of antibody response in animals to those in humans remains difficult. The interpretation of data from passive transfer of human immune sera to animals provides information about protective levels of antibody for the animal. A dangerous corollary is the assumption that these levels would also be protective to humans. Although using the correlation between protective antibody levels in animals and predicting immunity in humans may be dangerous, there is no readily available alternative short of challenging vaccinated human volunteers; a study that would have little chance for approval within any clinical protocol. There remain large areas endemic for plague throughout the world; this coupled with the very real threat of intentional use of aerosolized plague makes the development of an effective plague vaccine a top medical priority.

REFERENCES

1. Smith, P. N. (1959) Pneumonic plague in mice: gross and histopathology in untreated and passively immunized animals. *J. Infect Dis.* **104,** 78–84.
2. Chen, T. H. and Meyer, K. F. (1965) Susceptibility of the Langur monkey (*Semnopithecus entellus*) to experimental plague: pathology and immunity. *J. Infect Dis.* **115,** 456–464.
3. Smith, J. H. (1976) Plague, in *Pathology of Tropical and Extraordinary Diseases. An Atlas.* Vol. 1. (Binford, C. H. and Connor, D. H., eds.), Armed Forces Institute of Pathology, Washington D.C., pp. 130–134.

4. Davis, K. J., Fritz, D. L., Pitt, M. L., Welkos, S. L., Worsham, P. L., and Friedlander, A. M. (1996) Pathology of experimental pneumonic plague produced by fraction 1-positive and fraction 1-negative *Yersinia pestis* in African green monkeys (*Cercopithecus aethiops*). *Arch. Pathol. Lab. Med.* **120,** 156–163.

5. Walker, R. V. (1968) Comparative physiopathology of plague endotoxin in mice, guinea pigs and monkeys. *J. Infect. Dis.* **118,** 188–196.

6. Butler ,T. (1972) A clinical study of bubonic plague observations of the 1970 Vietnam epidemic with emphasis on coagulation studies, skin histology and electrocardiograms. *Am. J. Med.* **53,** 268–276.

7. Butler, T., Levin, J., and Cu, D. Q. (1973) Bubonic plague: detection of endotoxemia with the Limulus test. *Ann. Int. Med.* **79,** 642–646.

8. Crook, L. D. and Tempest, B. (1992) Plague. A clinical review of 27 cases. *Arch. Intern. Med.* **152,** 1253–1256.

9. Butler, T., Bell, W. R., Linh, N. N., Tiep, N. D., and Arnold, K. (1974) *Yersinia pestis* infection in Vietnam. I. Clinical and hematologic aspects. *J. Infect. Dis.* **129(Suppl.),** S78–S84.

10. McGovern, T. W. and Friedlander, A. M. (1997) Plague, in *Textbook of Military Medicine. Part 1. Weaponry, Warfare and the Casualty; Medical Aspects of Chemical and Biological Warfare.* (Sidell, F. R., Takafuji, E. T., and Franz, D. R., eds.), Office of the Surgeon General at TMM Publications, Borden Institute, pp. 479–502.

11. Burrows, T. W. and Bacon, G. A. (1956) The basis of virulence in *Pasteurella pestis*: the development of resistance to phagocytosis *in vitro. Br. J. Exp. Pathol.* **37,** 286–299.

12. Cavanaugh, D. C. and Randall, R. (1959) The role of multiplication of *Pasteurella pestis* in mononuclear phagocytes in the pathogenesis of flea-borne plague. *J. Immunol.* **83,** 348–363.

13. Perry, R. D. and Featherston, J. D. (1997) *Yersinia pestis*-etiologic agent of plague. *Clin. Micro. Rev.* **10,** 35–66.

14. Cornelis, G. R., Boland, A., Boyd, A. P., et al. (1998) The virulence plasmid of *Yersinia*, an anti-host genome. *Microbiol. Mol. Biol. Rev.* **62,** 1315–1352.

15. Burrows, T. W. and Bacon, G. A. (1954) The basis of virulence in *Pasteurella pestis*: comparative behavior of virulent and avirulent strains in vitro. *Br. J. Exp. Pathol.* **35,** 134–143.

16. Janssen, W. A., Lawton, W. D., Fuku, G. M., and Surgalla, M. J. (1963) The pathogenesis of plague, 1. A study of the correlation between virulence and relative phagocytosis resistance of some strains of *Pasteurella pestis. J. Infect. Dis.* **113,** 139–143.

17. Janssen, W. A. and Surgalla, M. J. (1969) Plague bacillus: survival within host phagocytes. *Science* **163,** 950–952.

18. Green, G. M. and Kass, E. H. (1964) The role of the alveolar macrophage in the clearance of bacteria from the lung. *J. Exp. Med.* **119,** 167–175.

19. Straley, S. C. and Harmon, P. A. (1984) *Yersinia pestis* grows within phagolysosomes in mouse peritoneal macrophages. *Infect. Immun.* **45,** 655–659.

20. Charnetzky, W. T. and Shuford, W. W. (1985) Survival and growth of *Yersinia pestis* within macrophages and an effect of the loss of the 47-megadalton plasmid on growth in macrophages. *Infect. Immun.* **47,** 234–241.

21. Pollack, C., Straley, S. C., and Klempner, M. S. (1986) Probing the phagolysosomal environment of human macrophages with a Ca^{2+}-responsive operon fusion in *Yersinia pestis. Nature* **322,** 834–836.

22. Straley, S. C. and Perry, R. D. (1995) Environmental modulation of gene expression and pathogenesis in *Yersinia. Trends Microbiol.* **3,** 310–317.

23. Jawetz, E. and Meyer, K. F. (1944) Studies on plague immunity in experimental animals II. Some factors of the immunity mechanism in bubonic plague. *J. Immunol.* **39,** 15–30.

24. Finegold, M. J. (1969) Pneumonic plague in monkeys an electron microscopic study. *Am. J. Pathol.* **54,** 167–185.

25. Butler ,T. (1983) Plague and other *Yersinia* infections, in: *Current Topics in Infectious Disease.* (Greenough, W. B. and Marigan, T. C., eds.), Plenum Press, New York, pp. 73–108.

26. Feeley, E. J. and Kriz, J. J. (1965) Plague meningitis in an American serviceman. *JAMA* **191,** 140, 141.

27. Cleri, D. J., Vernaleo, J. R., Lombardi, L. J., Rabbat, M. S., Mathew, A., Marton, R., and Reyelt, M. C. (1997) Plague pneumonia disease caused by *Yersinia pestis. Sem. Res. Infect.* **12,** 12–23.

28. Inglesby, T. V., Dennis, D. T., Henderson, D. A., et al. (2000) Plague as a biological weapon. Medical and public health management. *JAMA* **283,** 2281–2290.

29. Strong, R. P. and Teague, O. (1912) Studies on pneumonic plague and plague immunization. IV. Portal of entry of infection and method of development of the lesions in pneumonic and primary septic plague: experimental pathology. *Phillip. J. Sci.* **7,** 173–180.

30. Tieh, T. H., Landauer, E., Miyagawa, F., Kobayashi, G., and Okayasu, G. (1948) Primary pneumonic plague in Mukden, 1946, and report of 39 cases with 3 recoveries. *J. Infect. Dis.* **82,** 52–58.

31. Ehrenkranz, N. J. and White, L. P. (1954) Hepatic function and other physiologic studies in monkeys with experimental pneumonic plague. *J. Infect. Dis.* **95,** 226–231.

32. Speak, R. S. and Wolochow, H. (1957) Studies on the experimental epidemiology of respiratory infections. VIII. Experimental pneumonic plague in *Macacus Rhesus. J. Infect. Dis.* **100,** 58–69.

33. Finegold, M. J. (1968) Studies on the pathogenesis of plague. Blood coagulation and tissue responses of *Macaca mulatta* following exposure to aerosols of *Pasteurella pestis. Am. J. Med.* **53,** 99–114.

34. Finegold, M. J. (1968) Pathogenesis of plague. A review of plague deaths in the United States during the last decade. *Am. J. Med.* **45,** 549–554.

35. Smith, P. N., McCamish, J., Seely, J., and Cooke, G. M. (1957) The development of pneumonic plague in mice and the effect of paralysis of respiratory cilia upon the course of infection. *J. Infect. Dis.* **100,** 215–222.

36. Smith, P. N. (1959) Pneumonic plague in mice: modification of the infection by antibody against specific components of *Pasteurella pestis. J. Infect. Dis.* **104,** 85–91.

37. Ransom, J. P. and Krueger, A. P. (1954) Chronic Pneumonic plague in *Macaca mulatta. Am. J. Trop. Med. Hyg.* **3,** 1040–1054.

38. Marshall, J. D., Quy, D. V., and Gibson, F. L. (1967) Asymptomatic pharyngeal plague in Vietnamese. *Am. J. Trop. Med.* **16,** 175–177.

39. Burmeister, R. W., Tigertt, W. D., and Overholt, E. L. (1962) Laboratory-acquired pneumonic plague report of a case and review of previous cases. *Ann. Int. Med.* **56,** 789–800.

40. Cohen, R. J. and Stockard, J. L. (1967) Pneumonic plague in an untreated plague-vaccinated individual. *JAMA* **202,** 217, 218.

41. Haffkine, W. M. (1897) Remarks on the plague prophylactic fluid. *Br. Med. J.* **1,** 1461.

42. Taylor, J. (1933) Haffkine's plague vaccine. *Indian Med. Res. Memoirs* **27,** 3–125.

43. Meyer, K. F., Smith, G., Foster, L. E., Marshall, J. D. Jr., and Cavanaugh, D. C. Plague immunization IV. Clinical reactions and serological response to inoculations of Haffkine and freeze-dried plague. *J. Infect. Dis.* **129(Suppl.),** S30–35.

44. Sokey, S. S. and Maurice, H. (1935) Biological method used to standardize anti-plague vaccination and discussion on the relative protection offered by various anti-plague vaccines, measured according to this method. *Bull. Off. Inst. Hyg. Publ.* **27,** 1534–1545.

45. Hubbu, M. K., Nimbkar, Y. S., and Jhala, H. I. (1968) Selection of a suitable batch of plague vaccine for use as a standard. *Indian J. Path. Bacteriol.* **11,** 152–159.

46. Plague vaccine. *United States Pharmacopoeia* **23,** 1235.
47. Smidt, F. P. G. de. (1929) Laboratory notes on plague in Kenya. *J. Hyg. (Lond).* **29,** 201–218.
48. Otten, L. (1936) Immunization against plague with live vaccine. *Ind. J. Med. Res.* **24,** 73–101.
49. Product Insert. Plague Vaccine. Commonwealth Serum Laboratories, Limited, Victoria Australia.
50. Meyer, K. F. and Foster, L. E. (1948) Measurement of protective serum antibodies in human volunteers inoculated with plague prophylactics. *Stan. Med. Bull.* **6,** 75–79.
51. Meyer, K. F. (1970) Effectiveness of live or killed plague vaccines in man. *Bull. Wld. Hlth. Org.* **42,** 653–666.
52. Gage, K. L., Dennis, D. T., and Tsai, T. F. (1996) Prevention of Plague. Recommendations of the advisory committee on immunization practices (ACIP). *MMWR* **45,** RR14.
53. Lawton, W. D., Fukui, G. M., and Surgalla, M. J. (1960) Studies on antigens of *Pasteurella pestis* and *Pasteurella pseudotuberculosis. J. Immunol.* **84,** 475–479.
54. Marshall, J. D. Jr., Cavanaugh, D. C., Bartelloni, P. J., and Meyer, K. F. (1974) Plague Immunization III. Serological response to multiple inoculations of vaccine. *J. Inf. Dis.* **129(Suppl.),** S26–S29.
55. Product Insert. Plague Vaccine USP. Greer Laboratories, Lenoir, NC.
56. Cavanaugh, D. C., Elisberg, B. L., Llewellyn, C. H., et al. (1974) Plague immunization V. Indirect evidence for the efficacy of plague vaccine. *J. Inf. Dis.* **129(Suppl.),** S37–40.
57. Anderson, G. W. Jr., Heath, D. G., Bolt, C. R., Welkos, S. L., and Friedlander, A. M. (1998) Short- and long-term efficacy of single-dose subunit vaccines against *Yersinia pestis* in mice. *Am. J. Trop. Med. Hyg.* **58,** 793–799.
58. Marshall, J. D. Jr., Bartelloni, P. J., Cavanaugh, D. C., Kadull, P. J., and Meyer, K. F. (1974) Plague immunization II. Relation of adverse clinical reactions to multiple immunizations with killed vaccine. *J. Inf. Dis.* **129(Suppl.),** S19–S25.
59. Bartelloni, P. J., Marshall, J. D., and Cavanaugh, D. C. (1973) Clinical and serological responses to plague vaccine U.S.P. *Military Med.* **138,** 720–722.
60. Product Insert. Plague Vaccine USP. Miles Inc. Cutter Biologicals, Elkhart, IN.
61. Grasset, E. (1942) Plague immunization with live vaccine in South Africa. *Trans. R. Soc. Trop. Med. Hyg.* **35,** 203–211.
62. Girard, G. and Robic, J. (1938) La vaccination antipesteuse avec le vaccin vivant EV a Madagascar (The plague; Madagascar's contribution to current knowledge). *Proc. Third Int. Cong. Trop. Med. Malar.* **1,** 335–353.
63. Otten, L. (1941) A live plague vaccine and the results. Mededeel. *Dienst Volksgezondheidt Nederland Indie* **30,** 961–110.
64. Girard, G. and Robic, J. (1936) La vaccination de l'homme contre la peste au moyen de bacilles vivants (virus vaccin E.V.): son application a Madagascar. *Bull. Off. Int. Hyg. Publ.* **28,** 1078.
65. Translation, E. V. Plague vaccine product insert. 2001 Ministry of Education, Culture and Health, R.K. Kazakh Anti-plague Scientific Research Institute, Almaty, Kapalskaya.
66. Stepanov, A. V., Marinin, L. I., and Vorob'ev, A. A. (1999) Aerosol vaccination against dangerous infectious diseases. *Vestn. Ross. Akad. Med. Nauk.* **8,** 47–54.
67. Byvalov, A. A., Plutov, V. N., and Chicherin, Y. V. (1984) Effectiveness of the revaccination of Hamadryas baboons with dried live plague vaccine NIIS and *Yersinia pestis* fraction 1. *Z. Mikrobiol. Epidem. Immunobiol.* **4,** 74–76.
68. Meyer, K. F., Smith, G., Foster, L., Brookman, M., and Sung, M. (1974) Live, attenuated *Yersinia pestis* vaccine: virulent in nonhuman primates, harmless to guinea pigs. *J. Inf. Dis.* **129(Suppl.),** S85–S120.
69. Grasset, E. (1942) Plague immunization with live vaccine in South Africa. *Trans. R. Soc. Trop. Med. Hyg.* **35,** 203–211.
70. Grasset, E. (1946) Control of plague by means of live avirulent plague vaccine in southern Africa (1941–44). *Trans. R. Soc. Trop. Med. Hyg.* **40,** 275–294.

71. Meyer, K. F., Cavanaugh, D. C., Bartelloni, P. J., and Marshall, J. D. Jr. (1974) Plague immunization I. Past and present trends. *J. Inf. Dis.* **129(Suppl.),** S13–S17.

72. Hallett, A. F., Isaacson, M., and Meyer, K. F. (1973) Pathogenicity and immunogenic efficacy of a live attenuated plague vaccine in vervet monkeys. *Inf. Imm.* **8,** 876–881.

73. Chen, T. H. and Meyer, K. F. (1974) Susceptibility and immune response to experimental plague in two species of langurs and in African green (Grivet) monkeys. *J. Inf. Dis.* **129(Suppl.),** S46–S51.

74. Chen, T. H., Elberg, S. S., and Eisler, D. M. (1976) Immunity in plague: protection induced in *Cercopithecus aethiops* by oral administration of live, attenuated *Yersinia pestis. J. Inf. Dis.* **133,** 302–309.

75. Ehrenkranz, N. J. and Meyer, K. F. (1955) Studies on immunization against plague. VIII. Study of three immunizing preparations in protecting primates against pneumonic plague. *J. Inf. Dis.* **96,** 138–144.

76. Chen, T. H., Elberg, S. S., and Eisler, D. M. (1977) Immunity in plague: protection of the Vervet (*Cercopithecus aethiops*) against pneumonic plague by the oral administration of live attenuated *Yersinia pestis. J. Inf. Dis.* **135,** 289–293.

77. Welkos, S., Pitt, M. L. M., Martinez, M., Friedlander, A., Vogel, P., and Tammariello, R. (2002) Determination of the virulence of the pigmentation-deficient and pigmentation-/ plasminogen activator-deficient strains of *Yersinia pestis* in non-human primate and mouse models of pneumonic plague. *Vaccine* **20,** 2206–2214.

78. Titball, R. W. and Williams, E. D. (2001) Vaccination against bubonic and pneumonic plague. *Vaccine* **19,** 4175–4184.

79. Rotman, C. M. H. (1945) Bubonic plague in Dakar. *Royal. Nav. Med. Ser.* **31,** 155.

80. Aleksandrov, N. I., Gefen, N. E., Gapochko, K. G., Grain, N. S., Sergeyev, V. M., and Lasareva, E. S. (1961) Aerosol immunization with dry living vaccines and toxoids. Report VI. A study of postvaccinal reaction and immunological efficacy of aerosol immunization with pulverized vaccines (Brucellosis, Tularemia, Anthrax and Plague) in man. *J. Mikrobiol. Epidemiol. Immunobiol.* **32,** 1245–1252.

81. Aleksandrov, N. I., Gefen, N. E., Gapochko, K. G., et al. (1962) Aerosol immunization with dry dust vaccines and toxoids. Communication VIII. A study of the method of aerosol immunization with dust anti-plague vaccine during mass immunization. *J. Mikrobiol. Epidemiol. Immunobiol.* **33,** 46–50.

82. Vorob'ev, A. A., Zemskov, E. M., Kutyrev, P. A., et al. (1973) New data on oral immunization with live Plague vaccine EB. *J. Mikrobiol. Epidemiol. Immunobiol.* **50,** 77–82.

83. Kozlov, M. P., Lemekhova, A. E., and Norovd, D. (1960) The relationship between the vaccine reaction and allergic reactions in persons inoculated with plague vaccine. *Zh. Mikrobiol. Epidemiol. Immunobiol.* **31,** 102–105.

84. Anisimov, A. P., Nikiforov, A. K., Yeremin, S. A., and Drozdov, I. G. (1995) Design of the strain *Yersinia pestis* with improved level of protection. *Bull. Exp. Biol. Med.* **120,** 532–534.

85. Burrows, T. W. and Bacon, G. A. (1956) The basis of virulence in *Pasteurella pestis*: an antigen determining virulence. *Br. J. Exp. Path.* **37,** 481–493.

86. Sheremet, O. V., Terent'ev, A. N., Shatova, I. N., and Morozova, L. N. (1987) Levels of fraction 1 and VW antigens in cultures of the plague microbe grown on Yeats-casein, yeast-Hottinger broth and yeast-sunflower oil cake media. *Zh. Mikrobiol. Epidemiol. Immunobiol.* **6,** 18–22.

87. Meyer, K. F., Hightower, J. A., and McCrumb, F. R. (1974) Plague immunization. VI. Vaccination with the fraction 1 antigen of *Yersinia pestis. J. Infect. Dis.* **129(Suppl.),** S41–S45.

88. Guarner, J., Shieh, W. J., Greer, P. W., et al. (2002) *Am. J. Clin. Pathol.* **117,** 205–209.

89. Anderson, G. W., Worsham, P. L., Bolt, C. R., Andrews, G. P., Welkos, S. L., Friedlander, A. M., and Burans, J. P. (1997) Protection of mice from fatal bubonic and pneu-

monic plague by passive administration with monoclonal antibodies against the F1 protein of *Yersinia pestis. Am. J. Trop. Med. Hyg.* **56,** 471–473.

90. Atlas, R. M,, Brown, A. E., and Dobra, K. W. (1984) In *Experimental Microbiology: Fundamentals and Applications.* (Miller, L., ed.), Macmillan, New York, p. 54.

91. Baker, E. E., Sommer, H., Foster, L. E., Meyer, E., and Meyer, K. F. (1952) Studies on immunization against plague. I. The isolation and characterization of the soluble antigen of *Pasteurella pestis. J. Immunol.* **68,** 131–145.

92. Andrews, G. P., Heath, D. G., Anderson, G. W. Jr., Welkos, S. L., and Friedlander A. M. (1996) Fraction 1 capsular antigen (F1) purification from *Yersinia pestis* and from an *Escherichia coli* recombinant strain and efficacy against lethal plague challenge. *Infect. Immun.* **64,** 2180–2187.

93. Bennett, L. G. and Tornabene, T. G. (1974) Characterization of the antigenic subunits of the envelope protein of *Yersinia pestis. J. Bacteriol.* **117,** 48–55.

94. Voronstov, E. D., Dubichev, A. G., Serdobinstev, L. N., and Naumov, A. V. (1990) Association-dissociation processes and supramolecular organization of the capsule antigen (protein F1) of *Yersinia pestis. Biomed. Sci.* **1,** 391–396.

95. Englesberg, E. and Levy, J. B. (1954) Studies on the immunization against plague. VI. Growth of *Pasteurella pestis* and the production of the envelope and other soluble antigens in a casein hydrolysate mineral glucose medium. *J. Bacteriol.* **67,** 438–449.

96. Simpson, W. J., Thomas, R. E., and Schwan, T. G. (1990) Recombinant capsular antigen (fraction 1) from *Yersinia pestis* induces a protective antibody response in BALB/C mice. *Am. J. Trop. Med. Hyg.* **43,** 389–396.

97. Friedlander, A. M., Welkos, S. L., Worsham, P. L., et al. (1995) Relationship between virulence and immunity as revealed in recent studies of the F1 capsule of *Yersinia pestis. Clin. Inf. Dis.* **21(Suppl. 2),** S178–S181.

98. Drozdov, I. G., Anisimov, A. P., Samoilova, S. V., et al. (1995) Virulent non-capsulate *Yersinia pestis* variants constructed by insertion mutagenesis. *J. Med. Microbiol.* **42,** 264–268.

99. Smith, H., Keppie, J., Cocking, E. C., and Witt, K. (1960) The chemical basis of the virulence of *Pasteurella pestis.* I. The isolation and the aggressive properties of *Pasteurella pestis* and its products from infected Guinea pigs. *Br. J. Exp. Path.* **41,** 452–458.

100. Du, Y., Rosqvist, R., and Forsberg, A. (2002) Role of fraction 1 antigen of *Yersinia pestis* in inhibition of phagocytosis. *Infect. Immun.* **70,** 1453–1460.

101. Williams, J. E., Harrison, D. N., and Cavanaugh, D. C. (1975) Cryptic infection of rats with non-encapsulated variants of *Yersinia pestis. Trans. R. Soc. Trop. Med. Hyg.* **43,** 389–396.

102. Heath, D. G., Anderson, G. W. Jr., Mauro, J. M., et al. (1998) Protection against experimental bubonic and pneumonic plague by a recombinant capsular F1-V antigen fusion protein vaccine. *Vaccine* **11/12,** 1131–1137.

103. Miller, J., Williamson, E. D., Lakey, J. H., Pearce, M. J., Jones, S. M., and Titball, R. W. (1998) Macromolecular organization of recombinant *Yersinia pestis* F1 antigen and the effect of structure on immunogenecity. *FEMS Immunol. Med. Microbiol.* **21,** 213–221.

104. Hartley, J. L., Adams, G. A., and Tornabene, T. G. (1974) Chemical and physical properties of lipopolysaccharide of *Yersinia pestis. J. Bacteriol.* **118,** 848–854.

105. Hitchen, P. G., Prior, J. L., Oyston, P. C., et al. (2002) Structural characterization of lipoologosaccharide (LOS) from *Yersinia pestis*: regulation of LOS structure by the PhoPQ system. *Mol. Microbiol.* **44,** 1637–1650.

106. Prior, J. L., Hitchen, P. G., Willliamson, D. E., et al. (2001) Characterization of the lipopolysaccharide of *Yersinia pestis. Microb. Pathog.* **30,** 49–57.

107. Prior, J. L., Parkhill, J., Hitchen, P. G., et al. (2001) The failure of different strains of *Yersinia pestis* to produce lipopolysaccharide O-antigen under different growth conditions is due to mutations in the O-antigen gene cluster. *FEMS Microbiol. Lett.* **197,** 229–233.

108. Ben-Efraim, S., Aronson, M., and Bichowsky-Slomnicki, L. (1961) New antigenic component of *Pasteurella pestis* formed under specific conditions of pH and temperature. *J. Bacteriol.* **81**, 704–714.

109. Lindler, L. E. and Tall, B. D. (1993) *Yersinia pestis* pH 6 antigen forms fimbriae and is induced by intracellular association with macrophages. *Mol. Microbiol.* **8**, 311–324.

110. Lindler, L. E., Klempner, M. S., and Straley, S. C. (1990) *Yersinia pestis* pH 6 antigen: Genetic, biochemical, and virulence characterization of a protein involved in the pathogenesis of bubonic plague. *Infect. Immun.* **58**, 2569–2577.

111. Benner, G. E., Andrews, G. P., Byrne, W. R., Strachan, S. D., Sample, A. K., Heath, D. G., and Friedlander, A. M. (1999) Immune response to *Yersinia* outer proteins and other *Yersinia pestis* antigens after experimental plague infection in mice. *Infect. Immun.* **67**, 1922–1928.

112. Francis, C. W. and Marder, V. J. (1996) Concepts of clot lysis. *Ann. Rev. Med.* **37**, 187–204.

113. Lahteenmaki, K., Kukkonen, M., and Korhonen, T. K. (2001) The Pla surface protease/adhesin of *Yersinia pestis* mediates bacterial invasion into human endothelial cells. *FEBS Lett.* **504**, 69–72.

114. Lahteenmaki, K., Kuusela, P., and Kornhonen, T. K. (2001) Bacterial plasminogen activators and receptors. *FEMS Microbiol. Rev.* **25**, 531–552.

115. Sodeinde, O. A., Sample, A. K., Brubaker, R. R., and Goguen, J. D. (1988) Plasminogen activator/coagulase gene of *Yersinia pestis* is responsible for degradation of plasmid-encoded outer membrane proteins. *Science.* **258**, 1004–1007.

116. Sample, A. K. and Friedlander, A. M. (1996) Degradation of proinflammatory cytokines by the plasminogen activator protease of *Yersinia pestis*. Abstracts of the 96th General Meeting of the American Society for Microbiology. New Orleans, LA. (Poster Session).

117. Burrows, T. W. (1956) An antigen determining virulence in *Pasteurella pestis*. *Nature* **177**, 426, 427.

118. Burrows, T. W. (1957) Virulence in *Pasteurella pestis*. *Nature* **179**, 1246, 1247.

119. Burrows, T. W. and Bacon, G. A. (1958) The effects of loss of different virulence determinants on the virulence and immunogenicity of strains of *Pasteurella pestis*. *Br. J. Exp. Path.* **39**, 278–291.

120. Bergmen, T., Hakansson, S., Forsberg, A., et al. (1991) Analysis of the V antigen lcrGVH-yopBD operon of *Yersinia pseudotuberculosis*: evidence for a regulatory role of LcrH and LcrV. *J. Bacteriol.* **173**, 1607–1616.

121. Price, S. B., Cowan, C., Perry, R. D., and Straley, S. C. (1991) The *Yersinia pestis* V antigen is a regulatory protein necessary for Ca^{2+}-dependent growth and maximal expression of low-Ca^{2+} response virulence genes. *J. Bacteriol.* **173**, 2649–2657.

122. Nakajima, R. and Brubaker, R. R. (1993) Association between virulence of *Yersinia pestis* and suppression of gamma interferon and tumor necrosis factor alpha. *Infect. Immun.* **61**, 23–31.

123. Nedialkov, Y. A., Motin, V. L., and Brubaker, R. R. (1997) Resistance to lipopolysaccharide mediated by the *Yersinia pestis* V antigen-polyhistidine fusion peptide: amplification of Interleukin-10. *Infect. Immun.* **65**, 1196–1203.

124. Schmidt, A., Rollinghoff, M., Beuscher, H. U. (1999) Suppression of TNF by V antigen of *Yersinia spp.* involves activated T cells. *Eur. J. Immunol.* **29**, 1149–1157.

125. Sing, A., Roggenkamp, A., Geiger, A. M., and Heesemann, J. (2002) Yersinia enterocolitica evasion of the host innate immune response by V antigen-induced IL-10 production of macrophages is abrogated in IL-10-deficient mice. *J. Immunol.* **168**, 1315–1321.

126. Sing, A., Rost, D., Tvardovskaia, N., et al. (2002) *Yersinia* V-antigen exploits toll-like receptor 2 and CD14 for Interleukin 10-mediated immunosuppression. *J. Exp. Med.* **196**, 1017–1024.

127. Motin, V. L., Nakajima, R., Smirnov, G. B., and Brubaker, R. R. (1994) Passive immunity to *Yersiniae* mediated by anti-recombinant V antigen and protein A-V antigen fusion peptide. *Infect. Immun.* **62**, 4192–4201.

128. Anderson, G. W. Jr, Leary, S. E., Williamson, E. D., et al. (1996) Recombinant V antigen protects mice against pneumonic and bubonic plague caused by F1-capsule-positive and -negative strains of *Yersinia pestis*. *Infect. Immun.* **64,** 4580–4585.

129. Orth, K. (2002) Function of the *Yersinia* effector YopJ. Curr. Opin. Microbiol. 5(1), 38–43.

130. Orth, K., Xu, Z., Mudgett, M. B., et al. (2000) Disruption of signaling by *Yersinia* effector YopJ, a ubiquitin-like protein protease. *Science.* **290,** 1594–1597.

131. Hakansson, S., Bergman, T., Vanooteghem, J. C., Cornelis, G., and Wolf-Watz, H. (1993) YopB and YopD constitute a novel class of *Yersinia* Yop proteins. *Infect. Immun.* **61,** 71–80.

132. Hakansson, S., Persson, C., Schesser, K., Galyov, E. E., Rosqvist, R., and Wolf-Watz, H. (1996) The YopB protein of *Yersinia pseudotuberculosis* is essential for translocation of Yop effector proteins across the target cell plasma membrane and displays contact-dependent membrane-disrupting activity. *EMBO J.* **15,** 5812–5823.

133. Persson, C., Nordfelth, R., Holmstrom, A., Hakansson, S., Rosqvist, R., and Wolf-Watz, H. (1995) Cell-surface-bound *Yersinia* translocate the protein tyrosine phosphatase YopH by a polarized mechanism into the target cell. *Mol. Microbiol.* **18,** 135–150.

134. Andersson, K., Carballeira, N., Magnusson, K. E., Persson, C., Stendhal, O., Wolf-Watz, H., and Fallman, M. (1996) YopH of *Yersinia pseudotuberculosis* interrupts early phosphotyrosine signaling associated with phagocytosis. *Mol. Microbiol.* **20,** 1057–1069.

135. Black, D. S. and Bliska, J. B. (1997) Identification of p130^{Cas4} as a substrate of *Yersinia* YopH (Yop51), a bacterial protein tyrosine phosphatase that translocates into mammalian cells and targets focal adhesions. *EMBO J.* **16,** 2730–2744.

136. Galyov, E. E., Hakansson, S., Forsberg, A., and Wolf-Watz, H. (1993) A secreted protein kinase of *Yersinia pseudotuberculosis* is an indispensable virulence determinant. *Nature* **361,** 730–732.

137. Galyov, E. E., Hakansson, S., and Wolf-Watz, H. (1994) Characterization of the operon encoding the YpkA Ser/Thr protein kinase and the YopJ protein of *Yersinia pseudotuberculosis*. *J. Bacteriol.* **176,** 4543–4548.

138. Hakansson, S., Galyov, E. E., Rosqvist, R., and Wolf-Watz, H. (1996) The *Yersinia* YpkA Ser/Thr kinase is translocated and subsequently targeted to the inner surface of the HeLa cell plasma membrane. *Mol. Microbiol.* **20,** 593–603.

139. Rosqvist, R., Forsberg, A., and Wolf-Watz, H. (1991) Intracellular targeting of the *Yersinia* YopE cytotoxin in mammalian cells induces actin microfilament disruption. *Infect. Immun.* **59,** 4562–4569.

140. Rosqvist, R., Magnusson, K. E., and Wolf-Watz, H. (1994) Target cell contact triggers expression and polarized transfer of *Yersinia* YopE cytotoxin into mammalian cells. *EMBO J.* **13,** 964–972.

141. Boland, A., Sory, M. P., Iriate, M., Kerbourch, C., Wattiau, P., and Cornelis, G. R. (1996) Status of YopM and YopN in the *Yersinia* Yop virulon: YopM of *Y. enterocolitica* is internalized inside the cytosol of PU5-1.8 macrophages by the YopB, D, N delivery apparatus. *EMBO J.* **15,** 5191–5201.

142. Reisner, B. S. and Straley, S. C. (1992) *Yersinia pestis* YopM: thrombin binding and over expression. *Infect. Immun.* **60,** 5242–5252.

143. Drobkov, V. I., Marakulin, I. V., Pogorelsky, I. P., Darmov, I. V., and Smirnov, E. V. (1996) Antibody spectrum after the inoculation of *Yersinia pestis* and *Yersinia pseudotuberculosis* to susceptible animals. *Zh. Mikrobiol. (Moscow)* **2,** 81–85.

144. Mazza, G., Karu, A. E., and Kingsbury, D. T. (1985) Immune response to plasmid- and chromosome-encoded *Yersinia* antigens. *Infect. Immun.* **48,** 676–685.

145. Michel, P., Rasoamanana, B., Rasolofonorina, N., and Roux, J. (1992) Plague disease and vaccine. *Dakar Med.* **37,** 2–18.

146. Forsberg, A., Viitanen, A. M., Skurnik, M., and Wolf-Watz, H. (1991) The surface-located YopN protein is involved in calcium signal transduction in *Yersinia pseudotuberculosis*. *Mol. Microbiol.* **5,** 977–986.

147. Holmstrom, A., Pettersson, J., Rosqvist, R., Hakansson, S., Tafazoli, F., Magnusson, K. E., Wolf-Watz, H., and Forsberg, A. (1997) YopK of *Yersinia pseudotuberculosis* controls translocation of Yop effectors across the eukaryotic cell membrane. *Mol. Microbiol.* **24,** 73–91.

148. Strachan, S. D., Andrews, G. P., and Friedlander, A. M. (1996) Cloning, expression, and characterization of the *Yersinia* outer membrane protein B (YopB) from *Yersinia pestis.* Abstracts of the 96th annual meeting of the American Society for Microbiology. New Orleans, LA. (Poster Session).

149. Andrews, G. P., Strachan, S. D., Benner, G. E., et al. (1999) Protective efficacy of recombinant *Yersinia* outer proteins against bubonic plague caused by encapsulated and nonencapsulated *Yersinia pestis. Infect. Immun.* **67,** 1533–1537.

150. Burrows, T. W. (1963) Virulence of *Pasteurella pestis* and immunity to plague, In *Ergebnisse Der Mikrobiologie Immunitatsforschung und Experimentellen Therapie.* (Henle, W., Kikuth, W., Meyer, K. F., Nauck, E. G., and Tomscik, J., eds.), Springer-Verlag, Berlin, pp. 59–113.

151. Heath, D. G., Anderson, G. W. Jr., Welkos, S. L., Andrews, G. P., Friedlander, A. M., and Mauro, J. M. (1997) A recombinant capsular F1-V antigen fusion protein vaccine protects against experimental bubonic and pneumonic plague, in *Vaccines 97.* (Brown, F., Burton, D., Doherty, .P, Mekalanos, J., and Norrby, E.. eds.), Cold Spring Harbor Laboratory Press, NY, 197–200.

152. Williamson, E. D., Eley, S. M., and Griffin, K. F. (1995) A new improved sub-unit vaccine for plague: the basis of protection. *FEMS Immun. Med. Microbiol.* **12,** 223–230.

153. Eyles, J. E., Williamson, E. D., Spiers, I. D., and Alpar, H. O. (2000) Protection studies following bronchopulmonary and intramuscular immunization with *Yersinia pestis* F1 and V subunit vaccines coencapsulated in biodegradable microspheres: a comparison of efficacy. *Vaccine* **18,** 3266–3271.

154. Alpar, H. O., Eyles, J. E., Williamson, E. D., and Somavarapu, S. (2001) Intranasal vaccination against plague, tetanus and diphtheria. *Adv. Drug. Rev.* **51,** 173–201.

155. Deng, W., Burland, V., Plunkett, G. 3rd, et al. (2002) Genome sequence of *Yersinia pestis* KIM. *J. Bacteriol.* **184,** 4601–4611.

156. Parkhill, J., Wren, B. W., Thomson, N. R., et al. (2001) Genome sequence of *Yersinia pestis*, the causative agent of plague. *Nature* **413,** 467, 469, 470.

8

Medical Protection Against Brucellosis*

David L. Hoover and Richard H. Borschel

1. INTRODUCTION

Human brucellosis is a systemic, febrile illness caused by at least five different species of *Brucella*, a Gram-negative, aerobic, nonmotile, nonspore-forming coccobacillus. It has long been considered a prime biowarfare threat agent. As an intracellular parasite of mononuclear phagocytes, it successfully evades many host immune responses and resists easy eradication by antimicrobial agents. These characteristics both increase the need for effective strategies to protect against infection and create challenges to development of vaccines and other antimicrobial countermeasures against the organism.

2. HISTORY OF *BRUCELLA* AS A BIOWEAPON

The potential use of *Brucella* as a bioweapon derives from its great infectivity, ability to incapacitate infected individuals, and the stubborn persistent nature of human disease. Both the United States and the former Soviet Union weaponized *Brucella* in the 1940s.

2.1. US Army Biowarfare Research During World War II

The US Army's research on biowarfare defense began as part of the biowarfare program. This program was instituted during World War II after intelligence reports indicated that the Japanese were intensively researching biological weapons *(1)*. The National Academy of Sciences (NAS), at the request of the War Department, appointed a committee known as the War Bureau of Consultants Committee to prepare a report regarding the potential threat and what appropriate steps should be taken to protect US soldiers against biological agents. This report stated: "The value of biological warfare will be a deliberate question until it has been clearly proven or disproven by experience. The wide assumption is that any method which appears to offer advantages to a

---

*The views of the authors do not purport to reflect the position of the Department of the Army or the Department of Defense (para 4-3, AR 360-5). Data discussed from unpublished manuscripts was conducted in compliance with the Animal Welfare Act and other federal statutes and regulations relating to animals and experiments involving animals and adheres to principles stated in the *Guide for the Care and Use of Laboratory Animals*, NRC Publication, 1996 edition.

From: *Infectious Diseases: Biological Weapons Defense: Infectious Diseases and Counterterrorism*
Edited by: L. E. Lindler, F. J. Lebeda, and G. W. Korch © Humana Press Inc., Totowa, NJ

nation at war will be vigorously employed by that nation. There is only one logical course to pursue, namely, to study the possibilities of such warfare from every angle, make every preparation for reducing its effectiveness, and thereby reduce the likelihood of its use." President Roosevelt subsequently ordered the creation of a civilian agency to take full charge of all aspects of biowarfare including research for offensive use and defensive countermeasures. This agency, known as the War Research Service, was created in 1942 and attached to the Federal Security Agency operating under the authority of the War Department. In January 1943, the NAS formed a second committee on biowarfare, the ABC Committee, to advise the War Research Service on its work in locating and developing agents suitable for use in biowarfare. With the disbanding of the War Research Service in June 1944, the ABC Committee was discontinued. The ABC Committee was followed by the third NAS biowarfare committee, the DEF Committee, which was organized in September 1944, and finally disbanded in 1948. (Because their work was so secretive, the second and third NAS committees on biowarfare were given names that would be unrevealing. Thus, "ABC and "DEF" are not acronyms; they are simply arbitrarily chosen letters that deliberately stood for nothing *[2]*.)

In November 1942, Secretary of War Stimson requested the Chemical Warfare Services (CWS) to prepare to assume responsibility for biowarfare research and development under the supervision of the War Research Service. Subsequently, the Army chose Camp Detrick in Frederick, MD, as the site for the biowarfare research program, and construction began in April 1943. The emphasis of the program was protection of soldiers. To achieve this goal, CWS created the Special Projects Division (SPD). The SPD built and operated numerous of facilities, including Camp Detrick in April 1943 with the parent research and pilot plant; Field Testing Facility in Horn Island Mississippi in June 1943; Vigo Ordinance Plant in Terre Haute, IN in May 1944; Granite Peak Test Site at Dugway Proving Grounds for field testing in June 1944; and Fort Terry in Plum Island, NY for Veterinary Testing in 1944. Work with brucellosis performed at Camp Detrick and Dugway Proving Ground during the war was focused on aerosol dispersion patterns, infective dosages, and development of vaccine products in an attempt to develop countermeasures and offensive weapons.

2.2. US Army Biowarfare Research From the End of World War II to 1969

During the period after World War II and particularly after the Korean War, there was a major expansion of the offensive biowarfare research effort, with an expansion of the bioweapons production facility in Pine Bluff, AR. The Mississippi facility and Vigo Ordinance Plant were closed in 1946 and the facility at Plum Island was turned over to the US Department of Agriculture. Later, in November 1953, a biowarfare Ordinance Plant was built at Pine Bluff under the Directorate of Biological Operations.

A series of studies for aerosol dispersion was carried out at Dugway Proving Grounds from 1952 to 1954, and offensive weapons using *Brucella suis* were produced in quantity at Pine Bluff Arsenal beginning in 1954. The US Army discontinued all offensive work in 1969 and all weapons were destroyed, after which work was limited to defensive projects. The first production of weaponized *B. suis* was begun in 1953 *(1)* in the newly constructed facility at Pine Bluff. Defensive work continued at Fort Detrick, including human volunteer testing begun in 1955 as the CD-22 program. Participants in program CD-22 were assigned to the Walter Reed Army Medical Center (WRAMC). The work under CD-22 was terminated in 1956, but important human data were acquired during this program. This research included the establishment of minimum infective doses, effectiveness of prophylactic and therapeutic measures, serological response to infection, as well as the effectiveness of various doses of inoculum. Following the completion of program CD-22, the human volunteer program was developed further to incorporate additional legal requirements for human subject research and the subsequent implementation of Operation WHITECOAT. A new unit, the United States Army Medical Unit (USAMU) was created and activated on June 20, 1956 at Camp Detrick to conduct human research on defense against bioweapons under the control of WRAMC. Part of the involvement of WRAMC included the creation of Ward 200 at USAMU to provide a medical treatment facility, including an inpatient hospital for military personnel assigned to Camp Detrick. By 1957, there were 110 research volunteers participating in the research program *(1)*. In 1958, USAMU was assigned to the United States Army Medical Research and Development Command. In 1963, it was internally reorganized and in 1969 was renamed the United States Army Medical Research Institute of Infectious Diseases (USAMRIID). Operation WHITECOAT ended in 1969 as well. Other than classified research data developed during CD-22, no further work was conducted on brucellosis until 1992, when the US Army tasked the Walter Reed Army Institute of Research (WRAIR) to develop a vaccine to protect soldiers from aerosol exposure to *Brucella*.

3. PATHOGENESIS

Many features of the disease may be understood by examining pathogenetic aspects of the relationship between mammalian hosts and the bacterium. Brucellae produce no exotoxins and do not naturally harbor plasmids or phages. The bacterium's most remarkable virulence factor is its outer membrane lipopolysaccharide (LPS). At least two features of LPS contribute to its ability to enhance bacterial survival in the host. First, its endotoxic activity (ability to trigger a systemic inflammatory response) is much less than that of typical enteric Gram-negative organisms, so innate immune responses are poorly activated by encounter with the bacterium. Second, smooth strains of *Brucella*, which have long chains of *O*-polysaccharide (OPS) on their LPS, fix small amounts of serum complement to their surface, but are resistant to complement-mediated lysis *(3)*. Furthermore, smooth strains have reduced ability to induce cytokine responses from monocytes, perhaps because of steric interference by their surface OPS with binding of the lipid A, endotoxic component, of LPS to mononuclear phagocyte surface receptors (C. Fernandez-Prada, personal communication). Smooth, virulent brucellae that have been coated with complement are readily phagocytosed by mononuclear phagocytes *(4)*. Inside these cells, bacteria foster phagosomal acidification *(5)*, inhibit the fusion of phagosomes with lysosomes *(6–8)*, remain in the phagosomes, and replicate to enormous numbers inside their host cells.

Following lysis of infected cells, the bacteria are ingested by other mononuclear phagocytes and the cycle of bacterial proliferation continues. With the development of an effective host response, presumably triggered by a sufficient bacterial load to provide a "danger" signal *(9)*, bacterial proliferation is controlled and brucellae are gradually eliminated. However, the bacteria may persist in their host cells for months or years, and recommence replication if the activity of immunological control mechanisms declines. In addition to mononuclear phagocytes, placental trophoblasts are highly susceptible to infection with *Brucella* and support rampant intracellular proliferation of the organism. In this location, bacteria associate with the rough endoplasmic reticulum *(10)*, where they may have access to more nutrients than are available in the macrophage phagosome. Recent studies have demonstrated that phagosomal maturation in both HeLa cells and J774 murine macrophage-like cells and establishment of the endoplasmic reticulum replicative niche in HeLa cells are controlled by the VirB type IV secretion apparatus *(11,12)*.

Numerous of host cell activities, including production of reactive oxygen intermediates or nitric oxide (NO), cell-mediated cytotoxicity for infected macrophages, and T-cell or T-cell subset responsiveness have been shown to have antimicrobial consequences; however, an absolute requirement for any one of these activities has not been described. Whether antibodies play a significant role in recovery from primary infection is also unknown. The single factor that is clearly required for an effective host response against primary infection is interferon (IFN)-γ. Treatment of mice with anti-IFN-γ antibody exacerbates infection *(13)*, and mice lacking the gene encoding IFN-γ succumb to uncontrolled infection *(14)*. Delineation of the mechanisms by which IFN-γ mediates its antibrucella effects is a topic of ongoing research.

4. DISEASE

These interactions of *Brucella* and its host largely explain the clinical manifestations and course of brucellosis. Although members of the genus infect a wide range of mammalian hosts, each *Brucella* species has a predilection for certain animals and tends to be more or less virulent for humans (*see* Table 1). In humans, *B. melitensis* is the most virulent species, followed by *B. suis* and *B. abortus*. *Brucella canis* and an organism (proposed name *Brucella maris*) isolated from marine mammals appear to be approximately as virulent as *B. abortus*. Despite these generalizations, in any given patient, the causative species cannot be predicted by clinical criteria alone. *Brucella ovis* and *Brucella neotomae* are not known to cause human disease.

4.1. Clinical Manifestations

When susceptible hosts encounter *Brucella*, the bacterium enters across mucus membranes, is ingested by mononuclear phagocytes, travels to local lymph nodes, and then disseminates via the thoracic duct and blood throughout the mononuclear phagocyte system *(15)*. At the time of dissemination, humans typically develop fever, chills, and malaise. In addition, neuropsychiatric abnormalities, including depression and inability to concentrate on task performance are common *(16)*. Rarely, overt psychosis may occur. Focal disease may occur in almost any organ, because resident mononuclear phagocytes are widely distributed, but tend to develop in sites where blood supply is particularly rich. Approximately one-third of human patients have disease in vertebrae or one or more joints, especially the sacroiliacs. *Brucella* vertebral osteomyelitis, which may be indistinguishable clinically from tuberculous disease, tends to occur in older patients *(17–19)*. Epididymitis or epididymoorchitis occurs in about 2–10% of males *(20)*. Endocarditis and central nervous disease, including meningitis, occur in less than 2% of patients; endocarditis is the major cause of death. Minor hematological abnor-

Table 1
Host Specificity of *Brucella*

Species	Animal host	Virulence for humans
B. suis	Swine	High
B. melitensis	Sheep, goats	High
B. abortus	Cattle, bison, camels	Intermediate
B. canis	Dogs	Intermediate
B. maris[a]	Marine mammals	Intermediate
B. ovis	Sheep	None
B. neotomae	Rodents	None

[a]Proposed name, probably more than one species,

malities, especially leukopenia or lymphopenia, are common. Thrombocytopenia is also common and may be severe. Brucellae have been recovered from human fetuses and products of conception, and brucellosis in pregnancy is associated with early- to midterm abortion, which may be prevented by antimicrobial therapy *(21)*.

In contrast to humans, livestock do not show systemic signs of illness during the dissemination phase. Involvement of the male genitoruinary tract can cause clinical epididymoorchitis and infertility, especially in boars and rams. However, the major economic consequence of infection derives from infection of the placental trophoblasts, leading to abortion, stillbirth, runting, and early death of offspring. Brucellae are also found in milk macrophages, leading to infection of young animals and providing a source of human infection. Some measure of immunity against placental infection develops, because the incidence of abortion declines in subsequent pregnancies.

4.2. Diagnosis

Diagnosis of human infection is usually made serologically, based on detection of antibodies directed against the OPS. The gold standard, tube agglutination, is time-consuming and requires experience for accurate interpretation. A number of variants of this test, including indirect Coombs, rose bengal, and slide agglutination, have been developed. In addition, enzyme-linked immunosorbent assays have recently been produced and commercialized. A novel fluorescence polarization assay has also been described and tested for veterinary applications *(22)*. A major difficulty in interpretation of nonagglutination tests is the lack of antigen standardization and/or inadequate clinical data to determine their accuracy. Polymerase chain reaction has also found adherents (reviewed in Chapter 26) but is presently an experimental test. Culture of blood or sites of suspected infection provides the most firm diagnosis. The sensitivity of blood culture varies, ranging from 10 to 90%. Automated blood culture detection systems are highly efficient in detecting brucellae in blood cultures. In contrast to older methods using solid or biphasic media, cultures with automated systems become positive within 7 d *(23)*.

4.3. Treatment

The essential requirement for successful treatment of brucellosis is the use of at least two effective antimicrobial agents for a sufficient length of time. The most effective regimens include oral administration of doxycycline or tetracycline for 45 d and an aminoglycoside antibiotic (traditionally streptomycin, but more recently, gentamicin or netilmicin) intramuscularly for the first 7–14 d *(24)*. Oral treatment with a combination of rifampin and doxycycline is also effective but is less satisfactory for localized infection and may be associated with a higher frequency of relapse *(24)*. Other combinations, including trimethoprim-sulfamethoxazole plus rifampin and rifampin plus gentamicin, may also be used. In complicated infections, surgical debridement and prolonged antimicrobial therapy may be necessary. Treatment of endocarditis usually requires both antimicrobial therapy and valve replacement *(25)*. Brucellosis treatment is covered more extensively in Chapter 13.

4.4. Epidemiology and Prevention of Naturally Occurring Disease

In nature, human disease is acquired either by occupational exposure to infected animals (e.g., slaughterhouse workers, herdsmen, veterinarians) or by ingestion of infected food, especially nonpasteurized dairy products. In addition, brucellosis is a common cause of infection in laboratory workers, a testament to its high infectivity by the aerosol or conjunctival route. Not counting a biological attack, the most effective means to prevent human brucellosis is to eliminate brucellosis in animals used for food. Indeed, an aggressive strategy of vaccination, testing of herds and individual animals for *Brucella* infection, and slaughter of infected herds has been highly successful in minimizing or eliminating brucellosis in industrialized nations. In the United States, for example, fewer than 150 cases per year have been reported since 1985 *(26)*. Moreover, most of the cases seen in the United States are acquired by travelers outside the country or derive from ingestion of imported, nonpasteurized dairy products *(27)*. Laboratory workers can be protected by handling the organism under appropriate biosafety level (BSL) conditions (BSL-2 for clinical samples, BSL-3 for most other activities).

4.5. Estimates of Consequences of a Biological Attack With Brucella

A recent review *(28)* estimated 413 deaths, 82,500 casualties and a cost of $478 million per 100,000 persons exposed based on an ID_{50} of 10^3 and assuming that the organisms used were sensitive to antibiotics. Using an ID_{50} estimate of 10^4 colony forming units (CFU), the World Health Organization estimated that an attack with *Brucella* on a city with a population of 1 million in a developed country would result in 200 deaths and 50,000 ill patients *(29)*. These scenarios may be optimistic. First, it is likely that the WHO estimate on the number of cases is too low, because the ID_{50} is probably substantially lower than assumed. The $ID_{50}0$ for guinea pigs after aerosol exposure is approx 36 CFU *(30)* and that for nonhuman primates (NHPs) is about 1.3 ¥ 10^3 CFUs *(31)*, consistent with our own studies as described later. Second, although nearly all naturally occurring strains of *Brucella* are sensitive to commonly used antibiotics, preparation of strains with multiple drug resistance is not difficult. Indeed, a vaccine strain resistant to tetracycline, doxycycline, rifampin, streptomycin, and ampicillin was developed in the former Soviet Union *(32)*. Use of a multiple drug-resistant strain for a bioterror attack would vastly complicate treatment and raise the cost substantially above that estimated by Kauffmann et al. *(28)*. Moreover, even standard treatment using a combination of oral antibiotics might be met with great public resistance and poor compliance with a prolonged antibiotic regimen, resulting in increased frequency of relapse and development of focal complications. One should also note that introduction of *B. melitensis* or *B. suis* might also cause infection of livestock and additional economic damage.

5. DEVELOPMENT OF MEDICAL COUNTERMEASURES AGAINST BRUCELLOSIS

Numerous of countermeasures may be taken to prevent or mitigate illness after biological attack with *Brucella*. None of these is entirely satisfactory. Early warning and use of physical protective measures may be effective, if available. Prophylactic treatment after the first index cases appeared could also be used; this strategy could be expensive and incur significant morbidity from side effects if an antibiotic-resistant organism were used. Vaccination has the advantage of protecting individuals prior to infection, albeit at high cost and with some adverse side effects. It is a particularly attractive strategy for use in military personnel, especially if the vaccine platform can be used to immunize against other threat agents. The remainder of this chapter examines immune phenomena that are relevant to vaccine development and focuses on recent *Brucella* vaccine strategies at the WRAIR.

5.1. Secondary (Acquired) Immunity to Brucella Infection

Vaccine development requires an understanding of the immune processes that prevent infection in hosts previously exposed to the organism or its components. These processes may be distinct from those described in the pathogenesis section earlier, which are involved in recovery from established infection. Recovery from infection may require elimination of infected host cells and destruction of intracellular parasites but may or may not require active prevention of spread of bacteria to uninfected host cells. In addition, recovery probably requires little interaction of host defense mechanisms with the mucosa and submucosa once bacteria have established themselves in deep tissues. In contrast, mechanisms that prevent infection of an immune host may involve natural barriers and mucosal, submucosal, and lymph node immune cells and soluble factors. Modulation of host response in these areas when bacteria first arrive may play a profound role in determining the subsequent course of infection and development of disease. Models to explore these processes are limited and applicability to interactions of humans and *Brucella* is incompletely understood.

5.1.1. Models of Infection and Protection

Defense against reinfection or vaccine-induced immunity can be partially mediated by both antibody and cellular immune components. Development of models to dissect the interactions of these components is complicated by several issues. First, there is great subtlety in the manifestations and pathogenesis of brucellosis among *Brucella* species and their mammalian hosts. Certain species preferentially infect certain hosts, but are capable of infecting a wide range of hosts. Moreover, the manifestations of disease may be quite different when the same strain of *Brucella* infects different hosts. For example, mice infected with *B. melitensis* strain 16M, a strain highly virulent for humans, do not show signs of distress, although they harbor virulent organisms at high numbers in their spleens for long periods after challenge *(33)*. Goats infected with the same strain also show no systemic symptoms but have a high frequency of abortion *(34)*. Genetically defined mutant strains may also behave differently in different hosts. PHE1, a *htrAcycL* mutant of *B. abortus* 2308, is slightly attenuated in mice *(35)*. It is cleared more readily than the parent strain from goats, but causes abortion in these animals *(36)*. In contrast, PHE1 has markedly increased clearance and does not cause abortion in cattle *(37)*. WR201, a *purEK* mutant of 16M, is attenuated in mice *(33)* and NPHs, as described below. In goats, its degree of attenuation is less clear. After subcutaneous (SC) injection, it colonizes the local draining lymph nodes like 16M and is cleared from them at the same rate but induces less intense inflammatory response and may have less propensity to cause disseminated infection *(38)*.

A second difficulty in model development is the choice of challenge route. Ideally, one should use a mucosal challenge route to model the entry point of *Brucella* in naturally acquired or deliberately delivered infection. Unfortunately, a large body of work examining pathogenesis and vaccine efficacy in laboratory animals has used direct injection of organisms intravenously, intraperitoneally and subcutaneously. Bacteria injected by these routes bypass mucosal dendritic cells or macrophages, which are probably the first cellular targets of natural bacterial infection. The response of these phagocytic cells to bacterial invasion is likely to influence the pattern of tissue localization and tempo of infection, as well as the protective efficacy of vaccines. For this reason, the applicability of numerous studies of mechanisms of vaccine efficacy to defense against natural infection is highly conjectural. The historical failure to use mucosal challenge routes in laboratory animals is surprising, because these approaches have been used effectively in studies on livestock. In large food animals, conjunctival inoculation of brucellae leads to disseminated infection of mammary glands and lymph nodes in nonpregnant animals; in addition to these sites, the uterus and placenta of pregnant animals are infected *(39,40)*. Both conjunctival and oral challenge routes have proven useful to determine vaccine efficacy *(41–44)*. In other laboratory animal studies, conjunctival challenge of badgers *(45)* and beagles *(46)* leads to disseminated infection.

5.1.2. Immune Mechanisms

Despite these two drawbacks, animal models, mostly focused on *B. abortus*, have provided insight into antibacterial immune mechanisms that may play a role in protection against natural challenge infection. Perhaps surprisingly for an intracellular pathogen, *Brucella* appears to be susceptible to antibacterial antibody. Immunization of mice with killed, smooth strains of *B. abortus* or *B. melitensis* reduces the number of *B. abortus* CFU in spleen or liver when mice are challenged intravenously or intraperitoneally *(47–49)*. Cell lysate fractions that induce anti-LPS antibodies also reduce intensity of spleen and liver infection in animals challenged with smooth strains of *B. abortus* or *B. melitensis* intravenously or intraperitoneally *(50–55)*. These effects on the intensity of hepatic and splenic infection are most prominent 1–2 wk after challenge. Studies using monoclonal antibodies confirmed that anti-OPS antibodies mediate these antibacterial effects *(56,57)*. In contrast, monoclonal antibodies directed against outer membrane proteins have little effect on spleen infection by smooth strains *(58)*, but are highly effective against infection by *B. ovis (59)*, a naturally rough organism that lacks surface OPS. The mechanism of the effect of anti-OPS antibody on transiently reducing infection of liver and spleen may reflect redistribution of organisms to lymph nodes and killing of bacteria in the nodes. Sulitzeanu demonstrated that active immunization with live or dead brucellae, passive transfer of immune serum, or precoating of bacteria with immune serum leads to redirection of intraperitoneally administered ^{131}I-labeled brucellae away from liver and spleen and into mesenteric lymph nodes *(60)*. However, when live bacteria are injected intraperitoneally in passively immunized mice the number of live bacteria in mesenteric lymph nodes is greatly reduced in immune mice compared to nonimmune animals *(61)*.

In other studies, treatment with immune serum or immunization with live or dead brucellae restricted bacteria to the draining popliteal lymph node when low numbers of bacteria were injected subcutaneously into the footpads of mice *(62)* or guinea pigs *(63)* and inhibited the growth of bacteria in the node. These data do not clarify whether antibody works solely by redirecting bacteria to a site that may have enhanced "natural" antibrucella activity compared to other organs of the mononuclear phagocyte system, or if it sensitizes the bacteria to the antibrucella activity of the nodes or enhances lymph node antimicrobial capability. In vitro studies have not resolved this issue. Opsonization of brucellae by antibody or antibody plus complement enhances ingestion but does not inhibit the intracellular growth of bacteria in resting macrophages. On the other hand, opsonization enhances the antibrucella activity of macrophages activated by IFN-γ *(4,64,65)*. It is possible that, in a lymph node, natural killer cells or T cells that respond to relatively nonpolymorphic antigens might provide sufficient IFN-γ to activate macrophages to inhibit the replication of opsonized brucellae, but this issue has not been addressed experimentally. However, it is likely that an optimal protective response to *Brucella* challenge requires both anti-OPS antibody and specifically sensitized T cells that produce large amounts of IFN-γ Indeed, administration of *Brucella*-immune serum to recombination-activating gene (RAG)-1 knockout mice, which lack mature B and T cells, fails to modify the course of infection following intranasal challenge with 16M (Izadjoo et al., unpublished). These studies indicate that cellular, as well as humoral immune components are crucial for protective immunity.

Numerous studies using passive transfer of immune cells or serum have demonstrated a role for cellular immune effectors as mediators of antibrucella activity. Pavlov *(66)* demonstrated that adoptively transferred Ly1[+]2[+] (i.e., CD8) cells reduce the number of splenic bacteria following intravenous challenge with *B. abortus* strain 19. Araya found that both CD4 and CD8 immune T cells and serum obtained during the course of infection with strain 19 mediate approximately equivalent levels of protection against challenge with strain 19 in mice *(67)*. Plommet and Plommet *(68)* demonstrated that spleen cells obtained from mice immunized with a peptidoglycan fraction of *Brucella* protect against challenge with virulent *B. abortus* 544. Furthermore, they showed that immune serum is at least as efficacious as immune cells, and serum and cells do not have additive or synergistic protective effects. Immune serum is less effective against *B. abortus* strain 2308 than against strain 19, whereas immune T cells preferentially protect recipients against challenge with the same strain used to infect donor mice *(69)*. These studies suggest that immunization strategies that induce either antibody responses or sensitization of T lymphocytes will have anti-*Brucella* effects. Data from our laboratory (*see* Subheading 5.5.1.) suggest that induction of both T-cell and antibody responses may be better than antibody alone.

5.2. Vaccines in Livestock and Animal Models

The success of several of different vaccination strategies in livestock supports this concept. Early adjuvanted, whole, killed cell vaccines induced good antibody responses and provided effective protection. However, they also caused severe local reactions and had a limited duration of immunity. Although the ability of these vaccines to induce protein antigen-specific T-cell responses is unknown, it is likely that the primary basis of protection lay in induction of anti-OPS antibody. Live-attenuated vaccines based on smooth bacteria (*B. abortus* strain 19 and *B. melitensis* Rev1) supplanted killed vaccines because of reduced side effects and longer-lasting immunity *(70)*. Like killed vaccines, these live vaccines elicit antibody that renders vaccinated animals positive in the serological tests used to screen herds for brucellosis. They also induce lymphoproliferative responses to *Brucella* antigens that may contribute to vaccine efficacy *(71)*. Recently, a highly attenuated rough organism, *B. abortus* strain RB51, has replaced strain 19 for cattle vaccination in the United States. RB51 is a highly attenuated organism deficient in *wboA*, which encodes a glycosyl transferase, an enzyme required for synthesis of OPS. RB51 also lacks *wzt*, which encodes a transporter protein. This vaccine elicits lymphoproliferative responses to *Brucella* protein antigens *(72)* but does not usually induce sufficient antibody to interfere with veterinary diagnostic tests for brucellosis. However, because RB51 may express small amounts of OPS *(73)* and may induce low levels of antibody it is difficult to exclude the possibility that anti-*Brucella* antibody plays a role in protection of livestock immunized with it. Indeed, complementation of the *wboA* defect of RB51 leads to creation of a rough strain (RB51WboA) with unchanged survival, but which elicits antibody and enhanced antibrucella activity in mice *(74)*.

In mice, live-attenuated vaccines derived from smooth or rough *Brucella* reduce spleen infection after intravenous challenge with smooth, virulent homologous or heterologous strains *(75)*. Smooth strains (Rev1 or 19) are more effective vaccines, although persistence of rough and smooth strains in the mice is similar *(75)*. In these same studies, RB51 was less effective, probably because it persisted for a shorter period of time; killed vaccines were only marginally effective. These data further support the notion that anti-LPS antibody and T-cell-mediated immunity cooperate for maximal vaccine efficacy.

5.3. Experience With Human Vaccines

It is likely that a successful human vaccine will elicit both humoral and cellular immunity. Although several human vaccines have been tested to date, none is completely satisfactory. In an early experiment, immunization with killed *B. melitensis* led to transient protection against illness in two volunteers challenged with 450 million CFU of the homologous organisms, but one of the two volunteers developed brucellosis as a consequence of a laboratory accident 5 mo after immunization *(76)*. A nonliving vaccine comprising a delipidated, phenol-insoluble (PI) fraction of strain 19 was tested in volunteers *(77,78)* who had been previously screened and found nonreactive in intradermal skin tests. This vaccine was highly reactogenic, causing both local and systemic reactions (fever, chills, malaise). It induced little or no delayed type skin hypersensitivity response to melitin, but 18–25% developed a response to intradermally administered diluted vaccine. Blood mononuclear cells obtained from immunized subjects had weak lymphoproliferative responses to PI antigen unless donors had been occupationally exposed to *Brucella* for extended periods of time after vaccination *(79)*. The PI vaccine induced anti-*Brucella* antibodies, presumably directed against the OPS. Antibody titers peaked at 2 mo after immunization and gradually declined over the next 18 mo. There are no controlled trials indicating efficacy. The vaccine is no longer commercially available.

Live-attenuated vaccines for humans are theoretically attractive because, as indicated by experience in livestock, they are likely to elicit the most solid immunity against infection. However, a major hurdle to overcome is finding a strain that is both suitably attenuated and sufficiently immunogenic. At least three live-attenuated vaccines have been tested or fielded in humans. A streptomycin-dependent variant of *B. abortus* strain 19 induced agglutinating antibodies in volunteers. Serum passively transferred from these vaccinees to mice reduced spleen colonization in animals challenged with strain 2308 *(80)*. A derivative of strain 19, called 19-BA, was developed and used extensively in the former Soviet Union. This vaccine had both local and systemic side effects, but was credited with reducing the 5-yr incidence of brucellosis from 12.3% in nonvaccinated persons to 0.5% in vaccinated individuals *(81)*. However, when Spink et al. *(82)* tested it in US volunteers they found it to be insufficiently attenuated.

The Soviets studied use of the BA vaccine as an aerosolized dry powder. Aerogenic vaccination of guinea pigs led to protection of 80–90% of animals challenged subcutaneously with 5–10 infectious doses *(83)*. A similar level of protection was seen in animals immunized with the same vaccine subcutaneously. In contrast, only half of aerogenically immunized animals challenged with 100 infectious doses of *B. melitensis* by aerosol were protected. Of 153 volunteers immunized aerogenically, only one had a febrile, systemic reaction, compared to 9 of 25 volunteers immunized subcutaneously. Antibody titers were comparable after immunization by either route. Agglutination titers of 1:20 to 1:40 appeared in 20% of aerogenically immunized subjects as early as 7 d after vaccination *(83)*. At 30 d postimmunization, 96% were seropositive, with a median titer of 1:160. In other studies, of 1201 individuals vaccinated with the dry powder vaccine, systemic or respiratory reactions (laryngitis, tracheitis, bronchitis) occurred in 92 (7.6%). The systemic reactions, characterized by fever, slight lymphadenopathy, mucus membrane, and facial hyperemia and minor defects in ventilation and blood oxygenation, occurred more commonly in previously sensitized individuals *(84)* but were noted to be "harmless, of short duration" and "readily reversible."

In China, *B. abortus* strain 104M was used both subcutaneously and epicutaneously. This vaccine appears to be less attenuated than 19-BA. Both 19-BA and 104M may have increased side effects in individuals who have been previously sensitized to *Brucella* by previous infection *(85)*. Attempts to use the goat vaccine *B. melitensis* Rev1 for human vaccination were abandoned after studies in volunteers showed that the range between toxic and effective doses was too narrow *(82,86)*. These data suggest that vaccination of humans with live brucellae leads to protective immunity but that the vaccines used to date are not sufficiently attenuated. In addition, subcutaneous or cutaneous vaccination may have side effects that can be more severe in previously infected persons.

5.4. NHP Models and Studies With Live-Attenuated Strains of B. melitensis

Although Rev1 was eventually found to be too virulent for use in humans, a large number of vaccine development studies were done with it using mice, guinea pigs and

NHPs. These data, reviewed in detail below, provide important and fascinating benchmarks for current and future vaccine development efforts.

5.4.1. Early NHP Models

The earliest published work with NHP brucellosis was reported by Shaw, of the Mediterranean Fever Commission *(87)*, who observed that monkeys were susceptible to intranasal infection with *B. melitensis* only after repeated exposures. However, other than the ability of *Brucella* to infect nonhuman primates, no dose or pathogenicity data were provided in the report. Unfortunately, these studies led to the incorrect conclusion that monkeys had reduced sensitivity to infection.

In 1921, Fleischner and Meyer *(88)* conducted a series of experiments to study whether *Brucellae* from cattle (*B. abortus*) and swine (*B. suis*) could infect monkeys. They demonstrated that monkeys were susceptible to these organisms and that the disease was identical to that seen with *B. melitensis* as described by Shaw. However, their monkeys still required multiple applications of bacteria to establish an infection. In fact, many animals were never infected regardless of the number of brucellae given. This was the first report that the disease in monkeys caused by *B. abortus* was the same as that caused by *B. melitensis*.

The reported inability to establish infection in monkeys with a single exposure led Huddleson and Hallman in 1929 *(89)* to conduct a series of experiments on rhesus macaques using freshly isolated organisms, instead of multipassage laboratory isolates, as had been used in previous studies. By using freshly acquired organisms from infected animals (both milk and tissue samples), agar slants of freshly isolated organisms, and material from dead humans and animals, these investigators were able to establish acute brucellosis in monkeys. However, several animals still required additional exposure to become infected. Huddleson and Hallman observed that the various *Brucella* species differed in their ability to establish infection and disease. *B. abortus* was the least infective, with only two of eight animals developing brucellosis; however, all animals receiving *B. suis* and *B. melitensis* became infected. Animals developed positive serology and organisms were isolated from blood collected from the heart. Following euthanasia, cultures of the lung, liver, spleen, kidneys, and heart blood also yielded bacteria. In this model, fever was frequently observed but difficult to evaluate because only morning and afternoon measurements were taken. The amount of temperature change caused by diurnal variation prevented the use of these spot temperature measurements unless they were in excess of 2°F of elevation. This difficulty was also exacerbated by room temperature variations in the animal housing facility, with afternoon temperatures often exceeding 86°F. The authors concluded that all three *Brucella* species that cause brucellosis in humans can also establish brucellosis in rhesus macaques. *B. abortus* was the least virulent, followed by *B. melitensis,* then by *B. suis,* which was the most virulent.

5.4.2. NHP and Guinea Pig Aerosol Challenge Models

While at Camp Detrick, Henderson *(90)* developed an apparatus that produces aerosol suspensions of organisms in a cloud that is breathed by the subject animals. This work is the basis for the aerosol spray system currently in use at USAMRIID. It has the advantage of producing consistent cloud concentrations that can be varied as needed to achieve the desired delivery dose and is safe and simple as long as it is performed in a class III biosafety cabinet. However, the method has several disadvantages. Fragile organisms can be damaged, only clouds containing single organisms can be produced, and small numbers of organisms may escape even when a class III biosafety cabinet is used *(90)*. Using this apparatus, rhesus macaques were challenged with *B. melitensis* strain 6015 at doses from 6×10^3 to 1.22×10^5 CFU. The ID_{50} was determined to be 1.3×10^3 organisms (95% confidence interval = $1.2–1.5 \times 10^3$ organisms) *(31)*. This ID_{50} is consistent with earlier published data in the cavine model with *B. melitensis* and *B. suis (30)*. In the cavine model, the aerosol ID_{50} was determined to be 36 organisms for *B. suis*, only slightly more than the subcutaneous ID_{50} of six organisms. For *B. melitensis*, the aerosol ID_{50} is nearly identical to that of *B. suis*. To determine the potential for crossinfection, guinea pigs were subjected to an air wash for 48 h after aerosol exposure, then housed in open cages located adjacent to one another. There was no evidence of crossinfection in any animals including controls *(30)*. However, later studies by other investigators documented cross-contamination of monkeys resulting from presence of aerosolized inoculum on the fur. In the absence of vigorous air washing, brucellae could be recovered from the cage air for up to 30 h *(91)*. Additional studies in the late 1940s examined the effect of different suspension media on survival of aerosolized Gram-negative bacteria, including *B. suis*. *Brucella*e are more stable than any other Gram-negative bacteria tested; remarkably, their recovery from sprays in distilled water is similar to that of spore-forming bacteria. These data suggest that *Brucellae* are not destroyed by drying when aerosolized *(92)*.

5.4.3. Development of Rev1

B. melitensis Rev1, which is now the vaccine of choice to prevent caprine brucellosis, was originally developed circuitously as a candidate vaccine for humans.

5.4.3.1 STREPTOMYCIN-DEPENDENT *B. MELITENSIS*

An avirulent, naturally occurring mutant of *B. melitensis* that was dependent on streptomycin for growth *(93)* was suggested as an ideal vaccine candidate, because it should be require processing that would destroy its immunogenicity and should be avirulent in vaccinees, who would lack the antibiotic. The streptomycin-dependent mutant strain was developed from a single colony of *B. melitensis* strain 6056 and selected for growth in the presence of high concentrations of streptomycin. Only two per 1×10^8 streptomycin-dependent organisms reverted to streptomycin susceptibility in vitro. Guinea pigs inoculated with 1×10^{11} dependent organisms did not develop brucellosis up to 4 wk after injection. Mice remained infected for 2 wk but had mostly eliminated the organism from their spleens by 4 wk. Administration of 1×10^6 bacteria intravenously or 1×10^{10} cells subcutaneously to rhesus monkeys led to bacteremia 10 d later but no bacteremia at 14 and 25 d *(93)*.

To determine more accurately the ability of the streptomycin-dependent mutant to survive in monkeys, 13 rhesus macques were inoculated subcutaneously with 1×10^{10} CFU of the streptomycin-dependent mutant and sacrificed at 14, 28, 35, and 45 d for culture of tissues *(31)*. Bacteria were cleared from most, but not all, sites by 21 d. At 14 d, but not thereafter, organisms were recovered from the inguinal lymph node draining the injection site and from spleen, liver and right axillary lymph node in all animals. No organisms were recovered from blood cultures obtained weekly for 45 d. None of the mutant organisms recovered from the tissues had reverted to streptomycin independence. A 3–4 d febrile response that began within 72 h postinjection was seen in animals that received live mutant organisms but not in those that received killed organisms. Two animals were reinoculated with 1×10^{10} CFU of the mutant strain 21 d after the initial injection and organisms were recovered only from the inguinal lymph nodes at 11 d and only from the spleen at 21 d. This experiment indicated that primary infection limits the proliferation and dissemination on rechallenge with a homologous strain.

Initial enthusiasm for the streptomycin-dependent mutant vaccine was supported by avirulence, antibody production, and protection in mice, although there was little protection in guinea pigs *(94)*. However, this enthusiasm was soon tempered when mice *(95)* and rhesus monkeys *(31)* inoculated with steam-killed organisms also demonstrated appreciable serological titers to *Brucella* and were protected equally well by live and killed bacteria. This finding led the investigators to conclude that the vaccine mutant must replicate in the host to confer complete immunity.

5.4.3.2. STREPTOMYCIN-INDEPENDENT REVERTANT OF *B. MELITENSIS* (REV1)

Herzberg and Elberg also noted that some of the streptomycin-dependent *B. melitensis* strains that had reverted to streptomycin independence and senstitivity to killing by streptomycin were attenuated for growth in guinea pigs *(93)*. One of the mutants, named Rev1, multiplied in mice and guinea pigs during the first 5 wk but was cleared from guinea pigs and the Webster BRVS strain—but not the NAMRU strain—of mice by 8 wk. The virulent parent, strain 6015, caused splenomegaly and persisted in the spleen for at least 11 wk. Mice and guinea pigs immunized with Rev1 were protected against challenge with strain 6015 *(95)*. The nature of the mutation(s) in Rev1 is unknown. The strain grows more slowly in broth and on Albimi agar *(95)* and is sensitive to penicillin. Because of its significant attenuation in rodents, Rev1 was tested and found to be attenuated and immunogenic in goats *(96)*.

5.4.4. Studies With Rev1 in Monkeys

Elberg and Faunce *(97)* subsequently examined the attenuation and protective efficacy of Rev1 in *Cynomolgus phillippinensis* monkeys. Rev1 administered subcutaneously to monkeys at 1.8×10^9 CFU led to bacteremia that persisted for up to 4 wk, infection of spleen and liver for up to 4 wk, and infection with less than 10 CFU/lymph node for up to 8 wk. In a second series of experiments, animals were given 10^4, 10^6, or 10^8 CFU. Frequency of bacteremia was greatest (5 of 5 and 4 of 5 animals) in the two higher dose groups, compared to 2 of 5 animals in the lowest dose group. Interestingly, the duration of bacteremia was longer in the lowest-dose group (60 and 62 d) compared to the highest-dose group (8 of 9 animals with bacteremia from 20 to 34 d, 1 with bacteremia for 44 d). Spleen, liver, and deep cervical, inguinal, and axillary nodes were consistently positive for up to 44 d in the second series of experiments, with some animals positive in the nodes for up to 117 d. Monkeys in the first series and the high dose vaccinees in the second series also developed fever.

Monkeys from the first series of experiments were challenged with strain 6015 administered subcutaneously at graded doses ranging from 1×10^3 to 1×10^6 CFU. Unvaccinated controls received challenge doses of either 10^2 or 10^3 CFU. When examined 43–52 d after challenge, all nine control monkeys had heavy infection in liver, kidney, spleen, and nodes. In contrast, only one of 20 immunized animals had bacteria in liver, kidney, or spleen. No bacteria were recovered from 11 of 20 immunized animals, and these were present in low numbers in one or two lymph nodes. One animal had persistent infection of multiple nodes with the vaccine strain *(97)*.

Monkeys from the second series were exposed to the challenge strain via the respiratory route. The aerosol challenge dose consisted of either 1×10^8 strain 6015 for the vaccinates or 1×10^4 for the controls. Even using a large challenge dose, significant reduction in the challenge organisms was observed. More importantly, even when the vaccine dose was reduced 10,000-fold, there was only a slight reduction in the clearance capacity *(97)*. These important studies demonstrated that immunization with a live-attenuated vaccine could protect primates against both subcutaneous and aerosol challenge with virulent organisms, but also reflected the potential of Rev1 to persist in the lymph nodes. In that same report, strains from Spink's volunteer studies *(82)* were tested in guinea pigs. In these animals, the virulence of Rev1 was greater than that of BA-19, corresponding to results of the volunteer study,

Chen and Elberg *(98)* further characterized immune response and protection with orally administered Rev1 in Cynomolgus monkeys. Monkeys given 3.3×10^7 CFU by force feeding oral capsules did not become bacteremic, although those given 3.3×10^9, and 3.3×10^{11} did. All except the lowest dose resulted in anti-*Brucella* antibody. After SC challenge with 1.6×10^3 CFU of 6015, challenge strain organisms were recovered from half the animals in the high- and low-dose groups and 0 of 2 in the middle-dose group. In another study, three monkeys were immunized subcutaneously with 4.86×10^9 CFU Rev I. Two of the three became bacteremic. Animals were challenged subcutaneously with 6015 12 wk after immunization. Six weeks after challenge, no challenge organisms were recovered at necropsy from tissues of any of the three monkeys. An additional three animals were given two doses of Fraction 1 (F1) of Rev1 emulsified 1:1 with adjuvant 65 (86% peanut oil, 10% mannide monooleate, and 4% aluminum monostearate). F1 is a soluble protein extract of heat-killed, dried Rev1 that had demonstrated a protective response in guinea pigs. Compared to live Rev1, F1 elicited lower antibody titers and showed no protective efficacy. These studies suggested that vaccination with live organisms was effective, but vaccination with a product that elicited antibody was not. Interpretation of these data is complicated by the virulence of the live vaccine and the low antibody titers elicited by injection of the bacterial fraction.

In a subsequent study *(99)*, the same authors examined preimmunization with F1 followed by live vaccination with lower doses of Rev1 administered intradermally or cutaneously. Only 1 of 20 animals immunized developed Rev1 bacteremia. In challenge studies on immunized animals, no organisms were recovered from four of five animals challenged with 925 CFU of strain 6015. In a second experiment, no organisms were recovered from seven of eight animals challenged with 6625 CFU and none were recovered from five of eight animals challenged with 20,600 CFU. The three animals with positive cultures in the latter group had lower intensity of infection compared to nonimmunized controls. The authors proposed that a two-stage immunization strategy such as that used in their studies might overcome the difficulties of vaccine virulence.

5.5. Recent US Army Research on Brucellosis

Following the report by Chen et al. *(99)*, no further work was done on human vaccines by the Army and no additional nonhuman primate studies were conducted in Western countries. In 1992, renewed concern about the biowarfare threat of brucellosis prompted additional studies at the WRAIR, USAMRIID, and the Armed Forces Institute of Pathology. This work has focused on developing a genetically defined, live-attenuated vaccine that would protect against aerosol infection with *Brucella*.

5.5.1. Development of a New Murine Model and a Genetically Defined, Live-Attenuated Vaccine Candidate

To avoid the interpretive difficulties raised by the use of nonmucosal challenge routes, we first developed a murine intranasal challenge model using *B. melitensis* strain 16M. Administration of 10^3 CFU of 16M intranasally to anesthetized BALB/c mice leads to disseminated infection of liver and spleen in 50% of animals by 2 wk. A dose of 10^4 CFU leads to 100% infection of lungs but no apparent illness and no pneumonia *(100)*. Bacteria are gradually eliminated from the lungs; approx 60% of animals still have pulmonary infection after 8 wk (M. Izadjoo, unpublished observations). 16M disseminates to cause 90–100% splenic infection, which persists without clinical evidence of disease for months. Splenomegaly and increased splenic white pulp and marginal zones occur, as well as a mononuclear cell hepatitis. This infection model approximates the mucosal routes of bacterial entry expected after attack using aerosolized *Brucella* and permits analysis of vaccine-induced immunity across mucosal barriers.

The confinement of brucellae to phagosomes, where amino acids and nucleotides are limited, suggested that creation of mutations in genes encoding biosynthetic pathways for nutrients might lead to reliably attenuated live vaccines. The first mutant developed with this rationale targeted the *de novo* purine biosynthesis pathway. *B. melitensis* WR201 was made from 16M by replacement of most of *purE*, an intergenic region, and the first seven basepairs of *purK* with a kanamycin resistance cassette *(101)*. WR201 shows the expected purine auxotrophy when cultured on minimal medium. Moreover, in contrast to its parent 16M, WR201 fails to grow in human monocyte-derived macrophages, whereas 16M increases approx 100-fold in 72 h *(101)*.

WR201 is also markedly attenuated for growth in BALB/c mice. After intraperitoneal injection, it initially replicates in the animals, with increasing numbers of CFUs in the spleen for up to 3 d. The number of organisms in the spleen then begins to decline and bacteria are nearly completely cleared from liver, lungs, and spleens by 8 wk *(33)*. Mice immunized intraperitoneally with WR201 develop anti-LPS antibody and antigen-specific production of interleukin (IL)-2 and IFN-γ, but not IL-4, by cultured spleen cells *(102)*. These data suggest that immunization with this mutant leads to a Th1 immune response. In accord with this observation, intraperitoneal immunization of mice with WR201 reduces dissemination of intranasally administered 16M and slightly enhances clearance of the virulent organism from the lungs *(102)*. At a challenge dose of 10^4 CFUs of 16M, protective efficacy against dissemination ranged from 50–70%. Recently, WR201 was found to be slightly more attenuated and protective when given orally to mice (M. Izadjoo, personal communication). Parallel studies examined the ability of vaccines that elicit antibody against LPS to protect in this model. LPS prepared from both *B. melitensis* and *B. abortus* was given intranasally to mice as a noncovalent complex with outer membrane protein from *Niesseria meningitidis* group B, an excellent adjuvant for polysaccharide antigens. This LPS-GBOMP vaccine elicits both systemic and mucosal antibody *(103)* against *Brucella* LPS. Anti-LPS IgG, primarily of IgG1 and IgG3 subclasses, persists for at least 7 mo in blood. Like animals immunized with WR201, mice immunized with LPS-GBOMP vaccine are protected from dissemination to liver and spleen after intranasal challenge with 16M *(104)*. In contrast to those immunized with the live vaccine, however, they do not clear the challenge organisms more rapidly from their lungs. These data and additional, passive transfer studies of immune serum (M. Izadjoo, personal communication) indicated that vaccines that elicit antibody alone may be sufficient for inhibition of dissemination, but may not enhance destruction of bacteria at the site of entry.

5.5.2. Development of an Aerosol Challenge Model in Rhesus Macaques

The encouraging findings with WR201 in the mouse model suggested that this live-attenuated vaccine should be tested in NHPs. Building on the previous experience with brucellosis in NHPs and the ready availability of immunological reagents for *Macaca mulatta*, we initiated studies aimed at developing aerosol and mucosal challenge models using *B. melitensis* 16M. The first experiment (Borschel et al., unpublished observations) was designed to test the ability of 16M to cause acute brucellosis in rhesus macaques. Ten animals were divided into pairs and exposed to zero (controls), 1.25×10^2, 2.55×10^2, 3.60×10^3, 3.04×10^3, 9.6×10^4, 1.02×10^5, 1.45×10^5, or 3.34×10^5 using a head only exposure with the animals eyes taped open. Actual delivered dosages were calculated using plethysmographic data, duration of exposure and air samples obtained from the aerosol chamber via a sample port. All animals exposed to at least 1×10^3 CFU developed bacteremia. One of two exposed to 10^2 CFU also developed bacteremia. These data are consistent with the ID_{50} of 1.3×10^3 CFU described by Elberg et al. *(31)*. The day of onset of bacteremia was inversely related to the aerosol dose. Interestingly, the two challenge controls, housed upwind of the other animals in a room insert with directional airflow, also had evidence of infection. One control animal had a single positive blood culture and the other developed significant antibody titers. It is likely that these infections represent contamination from the fur of monkeys exposed to aerosols *(91)*.

Following the initial studies, four additional animals were challenged via aerosol with 1×10^7 organisms. Animals were monitored telemetrically using temperature recording devices implanted subcutaneously (Borschel, et al., unpublished observations). All became bacteremic within 14 d; two animals were positive by 7 d. Fever developed in two animals beginning by 10 d. The other two animals became febrile by 35 d postexposure. Histopathologic studies on the animals from these first two experiments showed inflammation in liver, kidney, spleen testis and epididymis of animals exposed to 16M (M. Mense et al., unpublished observations). Spleens were enlarged, with increased ratio of white to red pulp. This ratio was proportional to the challenge dose. In addition to histologic evidence of hepatitis, serum γ glutamyl transferase and alkaline phosphatase levels rose during the course of infection in challenged animals.

5.5.3. Testing of WR201 for Attenuation in Monkeys

To determine whether WR201 was attenuated in monkeys as well as in mice, rhesus macaques were given 10^{12} CFU of 16M or WR201 orally by gavage, followed for 4 wk, then necropsied (Borschel et al., unpublished observations). Animals given 16M became ill, decreased their food intake, and lost weight. Animals given WR201 appeared clinically normal. Serial quantitative blood cultures disclosed more than 10-fold higher CFU of 16M than WR201. Blood cultures remained positive until necropsy in animals given 16M, but became negative after 3 wk in those given WR201. At necropsy, animals given 16M had extensive infection of spleen and lymph nodes, which had colony counts 30-fold higher than counts in nodes from animals given WR201.

In another study (Borschel et al., unpublished observations), monkeys were given WR201 at the same dose and route and challenged via aerosol with 10^7 CFU of 16M 9 wk later. Four monkeys were necropsied 1 wk before challenge and found to have a mean of 30 CFU of WR201 in lymph nodes. Four of four nonimmunized monkeys challenged with 16M became bacteremic and febrile; none of four immunized animals did so. At necropsy 8 wk after challenge, 16M was recovered from nodes and other tissues of nonimmunized animals, but no 16M were recovered from immunized monkeys. Surprisingly, one colony of WR201 was recovered from a testis in one animal and one colony recovered from a lymph node of another animal.

These data indicate that WR201, whereas highly attenuated and protective against aerosol challenge with 16M in monkeys, may not be sufficiently attenuated for administration to humans. It is also possible, however, that the prolonged tissue persistence we observed may be caused by the high oral vaccine dose. A lower dose may result in less vaccine persistence and permit use of WR201 in future trials.

5.5.4. Implications of Experience With WR201

Three encouraging conclusions emerged from the murine and NHP studies with WR201. First, purine auxotrophy of *Brucella* is associated with a substantial degree of attenuation in two different animal species. Second, administration of this live vaccine leads to a combined humoral and cellular immune response to *Brucella*. Third, the vaccine provides sterile immunity and protection from disease when monkeys are challenged by aerosol at approx 10^4 times the ID_{50}. These conclusions further suggest that purine auxotrophy may be an excellent foundation for development of live, attenuated *Brucella* vaccines. Deletion of purine synthesis genes may be a more effective basis for attenuation in *Brucella* than in other facultative intracellular bacteria because of differences in rate of bacterial replication and location in the host. For example, *Shigella*, which is a rapid-growing organism, is not confined to the phagosome, but replicates in the cytoplasm. *Shigella purE* mutants are fully virulent *(105)*. *Salmonella*, like *Brucella*, is confined to phagosomes once ingested by macrophages. In contrast to *Brucella*, however, *Salmonella*, like *Shigella*, are fast growers. Hypoxanthine auxotrophic mutants of *S. typhimurium* are avirulent when injected into mice at low numbers, but not at high numbers *(106)*. Presumably, at high numbers, salmonellae can grow fast enough extracellularly to overwhelm the immune system before the bacteria are ingested and trapped inside the barren phagosome. On the other hand, *Brucella*, has little chance of dividing before it is ingested and sequestered in a phagosome. These unique characteristics of *Brucella* may permit development of a vaccine based on purine or other metabolite auxotrophy.

5.6. Other Attenuating Mutations in Brucella

Numerous of other attenuating mutations have been described in *Brucella*, which could be useful either alone or in combination to create additional strains with satisfactory characteristics of attenuation and immunogenicity. The powerful technique of signature-tagged mutagenesis has been used to identify mutants of *B. suis*, *B. abortus*, and *B. melitensis* that are attenuated for survival in mononuclear phagocytes or mice. Foulongne et al. *(107)* detected mutants of *B. suis* with reduced survival in THP1 and HeLa cells. Mutations were found in 14 different genes, including the VirB type IV secretion system (three genes), LPS biosynthesis, nucleotide biosynthesis, and metabolism of nitrogen and glucose metabolism. Hong *(108)* found that 13 *B. abortus* mutants with defects in genes encoding aromatic amino acid biosynthesis, LPS biosynthesis and the VirB region were not recovered 2 wk after injection into mice, but a mutant with a defect in glycine dehydrogenase, an enzyme induced during stationary phase, survived for a period between 2 and 8 wk. Lestrate et al. *(109)* found 18 attenuated mutants of *B. melitensis*, including 1 with a mutation in *virB* and others with mutations in transporters, amino acid and DNA metabolism, a two-component regulatory system, and a stress protein. Interestingly, no mutants were described with defects in LPS synthesis. This approach has provided a wealth of genes to examine more fully both for studies of pathogenesis and for development of attenuated vaccine candidates.

Table 2 shows more extensively characterized single gene deletion mutants that have reduced survival of *Brucella* in macrophages or animals. Attenuating mutations represent genes encoding LPS biosynthesis, the VirB pathway, synthesis of purines and aromatic compounds, regulators, and others. The LPS mutants are highly attenuated, but the requirement for anti-OPS antibody as an important contributor of an effective immune response may limit their utility as human vaccines. VirB is an attractive target for vaccine use. Whether mutations in VirB could be combined with those in purine or aromatic compound synthesis pathways to enhance attenuation is unknown. It is possible that these mutations might be antagonistic, if the VirB mutants localize to compartments in which they have better access to nutrients. Similarly, the possibility of combining deletions in regulatory operons with deletions in other pathways may be limited by compensatory mutations. At present, there is no obvious method to determine which mutations will be additive, antagonistic, or indifferent for affecting survival of *Brucella*. It is likely that numerous empiric attempts will be required to develop optimally attenuated candidates. The recent description of the complete genomic sequences of *B. melitensis (110)* and *B. suis (111)* should hasten vaccine development and provide numerous targets for gene deletion.

5.6.1. Nonattenuating Mutations

In several cases, gene interruption does not lead to attenuation. Deletions of genes encoding stress protein HtrA *(112–114)* carbohydrates (*chvE* or *gguA*) *(115)*, periplasmic protein BP26 *(116)*, bacterioferritin *(117)*, response regulator protein FeuP *(118)*, erythritol *(119)*, immunodominant protein P39 *(120)*, the siderophore 2,3 dihydroxybenzoic acid *(121)*, the nitrogen response regulator NtrC *(122)*, UDP-galactose-4-epimerase (*galE*) *(123)*, cytochrome bc(1) complex *(124)*, and ATP binding cassette (ABC) transporters *(125)* have little or no attenuation when tested in vivo or in mononuclear phagocytes. Deletion of the Lon protease from *B. abortus* leads to transient attenuation, similar to that seen with *cycL htrA* mutants but no effect on long-term persistence *(126)*. Deletion of *clpA*, which encodes a molecular chaperone, from *B. suis*, leads to enhanced persistence in vivo *(127)*.

Table 2
Attenuated *Brucella* Mutants

Parent strain	Mutant strain	Mutation	Gene product, function	Attenuation	Host or model showing anti-*Brucella* effect, model	Refs.
LPS mutants						
BM, BS	VTRM1, VTRS1	*wboA*	Glycosyltransferase required for OPS synthesis	BALB/c mice	Intraperitoneal challenge of BALB/c mice with BA,BS, BO, BM	75
BM	VTRM1	*wboA*	Glycosyltransferase required for OPS synthesis	Goats	Abortion, goats	36
BA2308	RA1	*wboA*	Glycosyltransferase required for OPS synthesis	Mice		128
BM 16M	B3B2		Perosamine synthetase, OPS synthesis	Mice, not bovine macrophages		129
BA2308	CA180, CA353, CA533, CA613	Various *lps* operon	OPS synthesis	BALB/c mice		130
BA2308	B2211	*pgm*	Phophoglucomutase, LPS and other glucose polymer synthesis	Mice, HeLa cells		131
Auxotrophic mutants						
BM16M	WR201	*purEK*	Purine synthesis	Human monocyte-derived macrophages; cleared from mice 8 wk	Intranasal challenge of BALB/c mice with 16M	101,102
BS		*aroC*	Aromatic compounds	Murine macrophages, mice		132

VirB mutants						
BA		*virB4*	Type IV secretion system	Murine macrophages, mice		*133*
BS1330		*virB*	Type IV secretion system	THP1 cells, human monocytes, mice		*134*
BA2308		*virB*	Type IV secretion system	HeLa cells, mice		*135*
BA		*dnaK*	Stress protein	Murine macrophages, mice		*136,137*
Other mutants						
BA2308	KL7	*bacA*	Cytoplasmic membrane transport protein	Murine macrophages, mice		*138*
BA2308	BvI129	*cgs*	Cyclic β(1-2) glucan synthesis	HeLa cells, mice		*139*
BA19	BAI129	*cgs*	Cyclic β(1-2) glucan synthesis	HeLa cells, mice	Intraperitoneal challenge of BALB/c mice with BA	*140*
BA2308		*bvr*	2-component regulatory system	Macrophages, HeLa cells, mice		*141*
BA2308	Hfq3	*hfq*	HF-I, stationary phase stress resistance	Murine resident peritoneal macrophages; BALB/c mice		*142*
BA		*hemH*	Ferrochetalase	J774 cells, mice		*143*
BA2308	PHE1	*cycL, htrA*	Cytochrome C maturation (CycL), stress protein (HtrA)	Murine macrophages, bovine neutrophils and macrophages, cattle; minimally attenuated in mice, goats		*35,37, 144,145*
BM16M	RWP5	*cycL, htrA*	Cytochrome C maturation (CycL), stress protein (HtrA)	Goats, minimal in mice	Abortion (goats), not colonization	*34,146*
BA	BA25	*omp*25	Omp25	Bovine macrophages, trophoblasts, pregnant cows		*147*

Abbreviations: BM, *B. melitensis;* BS, *B. suis*; BA, *B. abortus*.

6. SUMMARY AND OUTLOOK

Brucellae are highly infectious, incapacitating, but rarely lethal bioterror and biowarfare threat agents that have the potential to cause severe economic loss and interfere with civilian or military activities. The requirement for prolonged antibiotic treatment of patients with brucellosis and the known availability of antibiotic-resistant strains suggests that development of prophylactic countermeasures, including vaccines, is appropriate, particularly for individuals at high risk of attack. Human vaccine development is hampered by the lack of animal models that use routes of vaccination and challenge applicable to biodefense. The explosion in knowledge that will occur as a result of complete genome sequencing should greatly enhance understanding of pathogenetic mechanisms in brucellosis. It will also provide targets for deletion of genes for construction of live-attenuated mutant vaccines and proteins for use in subunit vaccines. In addition, more complete understanding of the role of antibody and various facets of cellular immunity in protection against challenge infection should assist in vaccine development. Better understanding of the complex interactions between *Brucella* and host immune systems should also enable development of novel vaccine strategies, including DNA vaccines or adjuvanted subunit vaccines. It is likely that any successful vaccine strategy will elicit anti-OPS antibody as well as cellular immune responses against protein antigens. Development of improved animal models and reliable in vitro correlates of protective immunity and early use of volunteers to examine safety and immunogenicity of vaccine candidates will be crucial for creation of effective vaccines to counter this threat. Other countermeasures will also need to be prepared. Specifically, more antimicrobial agents should be tested for activity against the organism and verified in animal models and clinical trials. Immunomodulators should also be studied more fully for their ability to delay onset or reduce severity of disease in exposed people. With a multifaceted approach, the risk of loss from a biological attack with *Brucella* should be mitigated substantially.

REFERENCES

1. United States Department of the Army. *U.S. Army Activity in the United States Biological Warfare Programs,* Vols 1 and 2, 24 February 1977 (Unclassified). 1977.
2. National Academy of Sciences (2002) *Committees on Biological Warfare.* Washington, DC: National Academy of Sciences.
3. Fernandez-Prada, C. M. Nikolich, M., Vemulapalli, R., et al. (2001) Deletion of wboA enhances activation of the lectin pathway of complement in Brucella abortus and Brucella melitensis. *Infect Immun.* **69(7),** 4407–4416.
4. Eze, M. O., Yuan, L., Crawford, R. M., et al. (2000) Effects of opsonization and gamma interferon on growth of Brucella melitensis 16M in mouse peritoneal macrophages in vitro. *Infect Immun.* **68(1),** 257–263.
5. Porte, F., Liautard, J. P., and Kohler, S. (1999) Early acidification of phagosomes containing Brucella suis is essential for intracellular survival in murine macrophages. *Infect Immun.* **67(8),** 4041–4047.
6. Rittig, M. G., Alvarez-Martinez, M. T., Porte, F., Liautard, J. P., and Rouot, B. (2001) Intracellular survival of Brucella spp. in human monocytes involves conventional uptake but special phagosomes. *Infect Immun.* **69(6),** 3995–4006.
7. Naroeni, A., Jouy, N., Ouahrani-Bettache, S., Liautard, J. P., and Porte, F. (2001) Brucella suis-impaired specific recognition of phagosomes by lysosomes due to phagosomal membrane modifications. *Infect Immun.* **69(1),** 486-493.

8. Pizarro-Cerda, J., Moreno, E., Sanguedolce, V., Mege, J. L., and Gorvel, J. P. (1998) Virulent Brucella abortus prevents lysosome fusion and is distributed within autophagosome-like compartments. *Infect Immun.* **66(5)**, 2387–2392.

9. Matzinger, P. (2002) The danger model: a renewed sense of self. *Science* **296(5566)**, 301–305.

10. Anderson, T. D., Cheville, N. F., and Meador, V. P. (1986) Pathogenesis of placentitis in the goat inoculated with Brucella abortus. II. Ultrastructural studies. *Vet. Pathol.* **23(3)**, 227–239.

11. Comerci, D. J., Martinez-Lorenzo, M. J., Sieira, R., Gorvel, J. P., and Ugalde, R. A. (2001) Essential role of the VirB machinery in the maturation of the Brucella abortus-containing vacuole. *Cell. Microbiol.* **3(3)**, 159–168.

12. Delrue, R. M., Martinez-Lorenzo, M., Lestrate, P., et al. (2001) Identification of Brucella spp. genes involved in intracellular trafficking. *Cell. Microbiol.* **3(7)**, 487–497.

13. Zhan, Y. and Cheers, C. (1993) Endogenous gamma interferon mediates resistance to Brucella abortus infection. *Infect. Immun.* **61(11)**, 4899–4901.

14. Murphy, E. A., Sathiyaseelan, J., Parent, M. A., Zou, B., and Baldwin, C. L. (2001) Interferon-gamma is crucial for surviving a Brucella abortus infection in both resistant C57BL/6 and susceptible BALB/c mice. *Immunology* **103(4)**, 511–518.

15. Enright, F. M. (1990) The pathogenesis and pathobiology of *Brucella* infection in domestic animals, in *Animal Brucellosis.* (Nielsen, K. and Duncan, J. R., eds.), CRC, Boca Raton, FL, pp. 301–320.

16. Spink, W. W. (1950) Clinical aspects of human brucellosis, in *Brucellosis.* (Larson, C. H. and Soule, M. H., eds.), Waverly, Baltimore, MD, pp. 1–8.

17. Malik, G. M. (1997) A clinical study of brucellosis in adults in the Asir region of southern Saudi Arabia. *Am. J. Trop. Med. Hyg.* **56(4)**, 375–377.

18. Mousa, A. R., Muhtaseb, S. A., Almudallal, D. S., Khodeir, S. M., and Marafie, A. A. (1987) Osteoarticular complications of brucellosis: a study of 169 cases. *Rev. Infect. Dis.* **9(3)**, 531–543.

19. Gotuzzo, E., Alarcon, G. S., Bocanegra, T. S., et al. (1982) Articular involvement in human brucellosis: a retrospective analysis of 304 cases. *Semin. Arthritis Rheum.* **12(2)**, 245–255.

20. Colmenero, J. D., Reguera, J. M., Martos, F., et al. (1996) Complications associated with Brucella melitensis infection: a study of 530 cases. *Medicine (Baltimore).* **75(4)**, 195–211.

21. Khan, M. Y., Mah, M. W., and Memish, Z. A. (2001) Brucellosis in pregnant women. *Clin. Infect. Dis.* **32(8)**, 1172–1177.

22. Nielsen, K. and Gall, D. (2001) Fluorescence polarization assay for the diagnosis of brucellosis: a review. *J. Immunoassay Immunochem.* **22(3)**, 183–201.

23. Yagupsky, P., Peled, N., Press, J., Abramson, O., and Abu, R. M. (1997) Comparison of BACTEC 9240 Peds Plus medium and isolator 1.5 microbial tube for detection of Brucella melitensis from blood cultures. *J. Clin. Microbiol.* **35(6)**, 1382–1384.

24. Solera, J., Rodriguez, Z. M., Geijo, P., et al. (1995) Doxycycline-rifampin versus doxycycline-streptomycin in treatment of human brucellosis due to Brucella melitensis. The GECMEI Group. Grupo de Estudio de Castilla-la Mancha de Enfermedades Infecciosas. *Antimicrob. Agents Chemother.* **39(9)**, 2061–2067.

25. Madkour, M. M. (2001) *Madkour's Brucellosis.* Springer-Verlag. Berlin.

26. (2002) Summary of notifiable diseases—United States, 2000. *MMWR Morb Mortal Wkly Rep.* **49(53)**, i–xxii, 1–100.

27. Chomel, B. B., DeBess, E. E., Mangiamele, D. M., et al. (1994) Changing trends in the epidemiology of human brucellosis in California from 1973 to 1992: a shift toward foodborne transmission. *J. Infect. Dis.* **170(5)**, 1216–1223.

28. Kaufmann, A. F., Meltzer, M. I., and Schmid, G. P. (1997) The economic impact of a bioterrorist attack: are prevention and postattack intervention programs justifiable? *Emerg. Infect. Dis.* **3(2)**, 83–94.

29. Anonymous. (1970) *Health Aspects of Chemical and Biological Weapons.* World Health Organization, Geneva.

30. Elberg, S. S. and Henderson, D. W. (1948) Respiratory pathogenicity of Brucella. *J. Infect. Dis.* **82,** 302–306.

31. Elberg, S. S., Henderson, D. W., Herzberg, M., and Peacock, S. (1955) Immunization against Brucella infection. IV. Response of monkeys to injection of a streptomycin-dependent strain of *Brucella melitensis. J. Bacteriol.* **69,** 643–648.

32. Gorelov, V. N., Gubina, E. A., Grekova, N. A., and Skavronskaia, A. G. (1991) [The possibility of creating a vaccinal strain of Brucella abortus 19-BA with multiple antibiotic resistance]. *Zh. Mikrobiol. Epidemiol. Immunobiol.* **9,** 2–4.

33. Crawford, R. M., Van De Verg, L., Yuan, L., et al. (1996) Deletion of purE attenuates Brucella melitensis infection in mice. *Infect Immun.* **64(6),** 2188–2192.

34. Phillips, R. W., Elzer, P. H., Robertson, G. T., et al. (1997) A Brucella melitensis high-temperature-requirement A (htrA) deletion mutant is attenuated in goats and protects against abortion. *Res. Vet. Sci.* **63(2),** 165–167.

35. Elzer, P. H., Phillips, R. W., Kovach, M. E., Peterson, K. M., Roop, R. n. (1994) Characterization and genetic complementation of a Brucella abortus high-temperature-requirement A (htrA) deletion mutant. *Infect. Immun.* **62(10),** 4135–4139.

36. Elzer, P. H., Enright, F. M., McQuiston, J. R., Boyle, S. M., and Schurig, G. G. (1998) Evaluation of a rough mutant of Brucella melitensis in pregnant goats. *Res. Vet. Sci.* **64(3),** 259, 260.

37. Edmonds, M., Booth, N., Hagius, S., et al. (2000) Attenuation and immunogenicity of a Brucella abortus htrA cycL double mutant in cattle. *Vet. Microbiol.* **76(1),** 81–90.

38. Cheville, N. F., Olsen, S. C., Jensen, A. E., et al. (1996) Bacterial persistence and immunity in goats vaccinated with a purE deletion mutant or the parental 16M strain of Brucella melitensis. *Infect. Immun.* **64(7),** 2431–2439.

39. Meador, V. P. and Deyoe, B. L. (1986) Experimentally induced Brucella abortus infection in pregnant goats. *Am. J. Vet. Res.* **47(11),** 2337–2342.

40. Corner, L. A., Alton, G. G., Iyer, H. (1987) Distribution of Brucella abortus in infected cattle. *Aust. Vet. J.* **64(8),** 241–244.

41. Fensterbank, R., Pardon, P., and Marly, J. (1985) Vaccination of ewes by a single conjunctival administration of Brucella melitensis Rev. 1 vaccine. *Ann. Rech. Vet.* **16(4),** 351–356.

42. Nicoletti, P. and Milward, F. W. (1983) Protection by oral administration of brucella abortus strain 19 against an oral challenge exposure with a pathogenic strain of Brucella. *Am. J. Vet. Res.* **44(9),** 1641–1643.

43. Plommet, M. and Plommet, A. M. (1975) Vaccination against bovine brucellosis with a low dose of strain 19 administered by the conjunctival route. I.—Protection demonstrated in guinea pigs. *Ann. Rech. Vet.* **6(4),** 345–356.

44. Fensterbank, R., Pardon, P., and Marly, J. (1982) Efficacy of Brucella melitensis Rev. 1 vaccine against Brucella ovis infection in rams. *Ann. Rech. Vet.* **13(2),** 185–190.

45. Corbel, M. J., Morris, J. A., Thorns, C. J., and Redwood, D. W. (1983) Response of the badger (Meles meles) to infection with Brucella abortus. *Res. Vet. Sci.* **34(3),** 296–300.

46. Carmichael, L. E., Zoha, S. J., and Flores-Castro, R. (1984) Biological properties and dog response to a variant (M-) strain of Brucella canis. *Dev. Biol. Stand.* **56,** 649–656.

47. Pardon, P. and Marly, J. (1976) Resistance of Brucella abortus infected mice to intravenous or intraperitoneal Brucella reinfection. *Ann. Immunol. (Paris)* **127(1),** 57–70.

48. Pardon, P. and Marly, J. (1976) Killed vaccine in adjuvant and protection of mice against an intraperitoneal challenge of Brucella: kinetic studies. *Ann. Rech. Vet.* **7(4),** 297–305.

49. Montaraz, J. A. and Winter, A. J. (1986) Comparison of living and nonliving vaccines for Brucella abortus in BALB/c mice. *Infect. Immun.* **53(2),** 245–251.

50. Dubray, G. and Bezard, G. (1980) Isolation of three Brucella abortus cell-wall antigens protective in murine experimental brucellosis. *Ann. Rech. Vet.* **11(4),** 367–373.

51. Jacques, I., Olivier, B. V., and Dubray, G. (1991)Induction of antibody and protective responses in mice by Brucella O-polysaccharide-BSA conjugate. *Vaccine* **9(12),** 896–900.

52. Phillips, M., Deyoe, B. L., and Canning, P. C. (1989) Protection of mice against *Brucella abortus* infection by inoculation with monoclonal antibodies recognizing *Brucella* O-antigen. *Am. J. Vet. Res.* **50,** 2158–2161.

53. Plommet, M. and Plommet, A. M. (1989) Immunity to Brucella abortus induced in mice by popliteal lymph node restricted strain 19 vaccination. *Ann. Rech. Vet.* **20(1),** 73–81.

54. Tabatabai, L. B., Pugh, G. J., Stevens, M. G., Phillips, M., and McDonald, T. J. (1992) Monophosphoryl lipid A-induced immune enhancement of Brucella abortus salt-extractable protein and lipopolysaccharide vaccines in BALB/c mice. *Am. J. Vet. Res.* **53(10),** 1900–1907.

55. Pugh, G. J., Tabatabai, L. B., Bricker, B. J., et al. (1990) Immunogenicity of Brucella-extracted and recombinant protein vaccines in CD-1 and BALB/c mice. *Am. J. Vet. Res.* **51(9),** 1413–1420.

56. Limet, J., Plommet, A. M., Dubray, G., and Plommet, M. (1987) Immunity conferred upon mice by anti-LPS monoclonal antibodies in murine brucellosis. *Ann. Inst. Pasteur Immunol.* **138(3),** 417–424.

57. Montaraz, J. A., Winter, A. J., Hunter, D. M., Sowa, B. A., Wu, A. M., and Adams, L. G. (1986) Protection against Brucella abortus in mice with O-polysaccharide-specific monoclonal antibodies. *Infect. Immun.* **51(3),** 961–963.

58. Jacques, I., Cloeckaert, A., Limet, J. N., and Dubray, G. (1992) Protection conferred on mice by combinations of monoclonal antibodies directed against outer-membrane proteins or smooth lipopolysaccharide of Brucella. *J. Med. Microbiol.* **37(2),** 100–103.

59. Bowden, R. A., Cloeckaert, A., Zygmunt, M. S., and Dubray, G. (1995) Outer-membrane protein- and rough lipopolysaccharide-specific monoclonal antibodies protect mice against Brucella ovis. *J. Med. Microbiol.* **43(5),** 344–347.

60. Sulitzeanu, D. (1959) The fate of killed, radioiodinated *Brucella abortus* injected into mice. *J. Immunol.* **82,** 304–312.

61. Sulitzeanu, D. (1965) Mechanism of immunity against *Brucella. Nature* **205,** 1086–1088.

62. Pardon, P. (1977) Resistance against a subcutaneous Brucella challenge of mice immunized with living or dead Brucella or by transfer of immune serum. *Ann. Immunol. (Paris)* **128(6),** 1025–1037.

63. Pardon, P. and Marly, J. (1978) Resistance of normal or immunized guinea pigs against a subcutaneous challenge of Brucella abortus. *Ann. Rech. Vet.* **9(3),** 419–425.

64. Jones, S. M. and Winter, A. J. (1992) Survival of virulent and attenuated strains of Brucella abortus in normal and gamma interferon-activated murine peritoneal macrophages. *Infect. Immun.* **60(7),** 3011–3014.

65. Gross, A., Spiesser, S., Terraza, A., Rouot, B., Caron, E., and Dornand, J. (1998) Expression and bactericidal activity of nitric oxide synthase in Brucella suis-infected murine macrophages. *Infect. Immun.* **66(4),** 1309–1316.

66. Pavlov, H., Hogarth, M., McKenzie, I. F., and Cheers, C. (1982) In vivo and in vitro effects of monoclonal antibody to Ly antigens on immunity to infection. *Cell. Immunol.* **71(1),** 127–138.

67. Araya, L. N., Elzer, P. H., Rowe, G. E., Enright, F. M., and Winter, A. J. (1989) Temporal development of protective cell-mediated and humoral immunity in BALB/c mice infected with Brucella abortus. *J. Immunol.* **143(10),** 3330–3337.

68. Plommet, M., Hue, I., and Plommet, A. M. (1986) [Anti-Brucella immunity transferred by immune serum and that transferred by splenic lymphocytes cannot be added]. *Ann. Rech. Vet.* **16(2),** 169–175.

69. Araya, L. N. and Winter, A. J. (1990) Comparative protection of mice against virulent and attenuated strains of Brucella abortus by passive transfer of immune T cells or serum. *Infect. Immun.* **58(1),** 254–256.

70. Nicoletti, P. (1990) Vaccination, in *Animal Brucellosis.* (Nielsen, K. and Duncan, J. R., eds.), CRC, Boca Raton, FL, pp. 283–300.

71. Kaneene, J. M., Anderson, R. K., Johnson, D. W., et al. (1978) Whole-blood lymphocyte stimulation assay for measurement of cell-mediated immune responses in bovine brucellosis. *J. Clin. Microbiol.* **7(6),** 550–557.

72. Stevens, M. G., Olsen, S. C., and Cheville, N. F. (1996) Lymphocyte proliferation in response to Brucella abortus RB51 and 2308 proteins in RB51-vaccinated or 2308-infected cattle. *Infect. Immun.* **64(3),** 1007–1010.

73. Cloeckaert, A., Zygmunt, M. S., and Guilloteau, L. A. (2002) Brucella abortus vaccine strain RB51 produces low levels of M-like O-antigen. *Vaccine* **20(13),** 1820–1822.

74. Vemulapalli, R., He, Y., Buccolo, L. S., Boyle, S. M., Sriranganathan, N., and Schurig, G. G. (2000) Complementation of Brucella abortus RB51 with a functional wboA gene results in O-antigen synthesis and enhanced vaccine efficacy but no change in rough phenotype and attenuation. *Infect. Immun.* **68(7),** 3927–3932.

75. Winter, A. J., Schurig, G. G., Boyle, S. M., et al. (1996) Protection of BALB/c mice against homologous and heterologous species of Brucella by rough strain vaccines derived from Brucella melitensis and Brucella suis biovar 4. *Am. J. Vet. Res.* **57(5),** 677–683.

76. Elberg, S. S. and Silverman, S. J. Immunology of Brucellosis, in *Brucellosis.* (Larson, C. H. and Soule, M. H., eds.), Waverly, Baltimore, MD, pp. 62–84.

77. Hadjichristodoulou, C., Voulgaris, P., Toulieres, L., et al. (1994) Tolerance of the human brucellosis vaccine and the intradermal reaction test for brucellosis. *Eur. J. Clin. Microbiol. Infect. Dis.* **13(2),** 129–134.

78. Bentejac, M. C., Biron, G., Bertrand, A., and Bascoul, S. (1984) [Vaccination against human brucellosis. 2 years of experience]. *Dev. Biol. Stand.* **56,** 531–535.

79. Bascoul, S., Peraldi, M., Merino, A. L., Lacave, C., Cannat, A., and Serre, A. (1976) Stimulating activity of Brucella fractions in a human lymphocyte transformation test. Correlation with humoral and cellular immunity. *Immunology* **31(5),** 717–722.

80. Sulitzeanu, D. (1955) Passive protection experiments with Brucella antisera. *J. Hygiene.* **53,** 133–142.

81. Elberg, S. S. (1973)Immunity to brucella infection. *Medicine (Baltimore)* **52(4),** 339–356.

82. Spink, W. W., Hall, J. W. I., Finstad, J., and Mallet, E. (1962) Immunization with viable *Brucella* organisms. Results of a safety test in humans. *Bull. WHO* **26,** 409–419.

83. Aleksandrov, N. I., Gefen, N. Y., Garin, N. S., Gapochko, K. G., Daal-Berg, I. I., and Sergeyev, V. M. (1958) Reactogenicity and effectiveness of aerogenic vaccination against certain zoonoses. *Voenno-Meditsinskii (USSR)* **12,** 51–59.

84. Aleksandrov, N. I., Gefen, N. Y., Gapochko, K. G., Garin, N. S., Maslov, A. I., and Mishchenko, V. V. (1962) A clinical study of postvaccinal reactions to aerosol immunization with powdered brucellosis vaccines. *Zhurnal. Mikrobiologii.* **33,** 31–37.

85. Elberg, S. S., ed. (1981) *A Guide to the Diagnosis, Treatment and Prevention of Human Brucellosis.* World Health Organization, Geneva.

86. Pappagianis, D., Elberg, S. S., and Crouch, D. (1966) Immunization against Brucella infections. Effects of graded doses of viable attenuated *Brucella melitensis* in humans. *Am. J. Epidemiol.* **84,** 21–31.

87. Shaw, E. A. (1907) *Immunity, serum, toxin, and vaccine experiments on monkeys with regard to Mediterranean Fever.* Mediterranean Fever Commission of the Royal Society (Great Britain); Part V.

88. Fleischner, E. C. and Meyer, K. F. (1920) Preliminary observations on the pathogenicity for monkeys of the *Bacillus abortus bovinus. Trans. Am. Pediatr. Soc.* **32,** 141–145.

89. Huddleson, I. F. and Hallman, E. T. (1929) The pathogenicity of the species of the genus Brucella for monkeys. *J. Infect. Dis.* **45**, 293–303.

90. Henderson, D. W. (1952) An apparatus for the study of airborne infection. *J. Hygiene.* **50**, 53–68.

91. Kruse, R. H. and Wedum, A. G. (1970) Cross infection with eighteen pathogens among caged laboratory animals. *Lab. Anim. Care.* **20(3)**, 541–560.

92. Rosebury, T. (1947) *Experimental Air-Borne Infection.* Williams and Wilkins, Baltimore, MD.

93. Herzberg, M. aand Elberg, S. (1953) Immunization against Brucella infection. I. Isolation and characterization of a streptomycin-dependent mutant. *J. Bacteriol.* **66**, 585–599.

94. Herzberg, M., Elberg, S. S., and Meyer, K. F. (1953) Immunization against Brucella infection. II. Effectiveness of a streptomycin-dependent strain of Brucella melitensis. *J. Bacteriol.* **66**, 600–605.

95. Herzberg, M. and Elberg, S. S. (1955) Immunization against Brucella infection. III. Response of mice and guinea pigs to injection of viable and nonviable suspensions of a streptomycin-dependent mutant of *Brucella melitensis. J. Bacteriol.* **69**, 432–435.

96. Elberg, S. S. and Meyer, K. F. (1958) Caprine immunization against brucellosis. *Bull. WHO* **19**, 711–724.

97. Elberg, S. S. and Faunce, W. K. (1962) Immunization against *Brucella* infection. 8. The response of *Cynomolgus phillipinensis*, guinea-pigs and pregnant goats to infection by the Rev I strain of *Brucella melitensis. Bull. WHO* **26**, 421–436.

98. Chen, T. H. and Elberg, S. S. (1970) Immunization against Brucella infections: immune response of mice, guinea pigs, and Cynomolgus philipinensis to live and killed Brucella melitensis strain Rev. I administered by various methods. *J. Infect. Dis.* **122(6)**, 489–500.

99. Chen, T. H. and Elberg, S. S. (1973) Immunization against Brucella infections. Priming of Cynomolgus philipinensis with purified antigen of Brucella melitensis prior to injection of Rev. I vaccine. *J. Comp. Pathol.* **83(3)**, 357–367.

100. Mense, M. G., Van De Verg, L. L., Bhattacharjee, A. K., et al. (2001) Bacteriologic and histologic features in mice after intranasal inoculation of Brucella melitensis. *Am. J. Vet. Res.* **62(3)**, 398–405.

101. Drazek, E. S., Houng, H. S., Crawford, R. M., Hadfield, T. L., Hoover, D. L., and Warren, R. L. (1995) Deletion of purE attenuates Brucella melitensis 16M for growth in human monocyte-derived macrophages. *Infect. Immun.* **63(9)**, 3297–3301.

102. Hoover, D. L., Crawford, R. M., Van De Verg, L. L., et al. (1999) Protection of mice against brucellosis by vaccination with Brucella melitensis WR201(16MDeltapurEK). *Infect. Immun.* **67(11)**, 5877–5884.

103. Van De Verg, L. L., Hartman, A. B., Bhattacharjee, A. K., et al. (1996) Outer membrane protein of Neisseria meningitidis as a mucosal adjuvant for lipopolysaccharide of Brucella melitensis in mouse and guinea pig intranasal immunization models. *Infect. Immun.* **64(12)**, 5263–5268.

104. Bhattacharjee, A. K., Van de Verg, L., Izadjoo, M. J., et al. (2002) Protection of mice against brucellosis by intranasal immunization with Brucella melitensis lipopolysaccharide as a noncovalent complex with Neisseria meningitidis group B outer membrane protein. *Infect. Immun.* **70(7)**, 3324–3329.

105. Formal, S. B., Gemski, P., Baron, L. S., and LaBrec, E. H. (1971) A Chromosomal Locus Which Controls the Ability of *Shigella flexneri* to Evoke Keratoconjunctivitis. *Infect. Immun.* **3(1)**, 73–79.

106. McFarland, W. C. and Stocker, B. A. (1987) Effect of different purine auxotrophic mutations on mouse-virulence of a Vi-positive strain of Salmonella dublin and of two strains of Salmonella typhimurium. *Microb. Pathog.* **3(2)**, 129–141.

107. Foulongne, V., Bourg, G., Cazevieille, C., Michaux-Charachon, S., and O'Callaghan, D. (2000) Identification of Brucella suis genes affecting intracellular survival in an in vitro human macrophage infection model by signature-tagged transposon mutagenesis. *Infect. Immun.* **68(3)**, 1297–1303.

108. Hong, P. C., Tsolis, R. M., and Ficht, T. A. (2000) Identification of Genes Required for Chronic Persistence of Brucella abortus in Mice. *Infect. Immun.* **68(7)**, 4102–4107.

109. Lestrate, P., Delrue, R. M., Danese, I., et al. (2000) Identification and characterization of in vivo attenuated mutants of Brucella melitensis. *Mol. Microbiol.* **38(3)**, 543–551.

110. DelVecchio, V. G., Kapatral, V., Redkar, R. J., et al. (2002) The genome sequence of the facultative intracellular pathogen Brucella melitensis. *Proc. Natl. Acad. Sci. USA* **99(1)**, 443–448.

111. Paulsen, I. T., Seshadri, R., Nelson, K. E., et al. (2002) The Brucella suis genome reveals fundamental similarities between animal and plant pathogens and symbionts. *Proc. Natl. Acad. Sci. USA* **99(20)**, 13,148–13,153.

112. Tatum, F. M., Cheville, N. F., and Morfitt, D. (1994) Cloning, characterization and construction of htrA and htrA-like mutants of Brucella abortus and their survival in BALB/c mice. *Microb. Pathog.* **17(1)**, 23–36.

113. Roop, R. M., 2nd, Phillips, R. W., Hagius, S., et al. (2001) Re-examination of the role of the Brucella melitensis HtrA stress response protease in virulence in pregnant goats. *Vet. Microbiol.* **82(1)**, 91–95.

114. Phillips, R. W. and Roop, R. M., 2nd. (2001) Brucella abortus HtrA functions as an authentic stress response protease but is not required for wild-type virulence in BALB/c mice. *Infect. Immun.* **69(9)**, 5911–5913.

115. Alvarez-Martinez, M. T., Machold, J., Weise, C., Schmidt-Eisenlohr, H., Baron, C., and Rouot, B. (2001) The Brucella suis homologue of the Agrobacterium tumefaciens chromosomal virulence operon chvE is essential for sugar utilization but not for survival in macrophages. *J. Bacteriol.* **183(18)**, 5343–5351.

116. Boschiroli, M. L., Cravero, S. L., Arese, A. I., Campos, E., and Rossetti, O. L. (1997) Protection against infection in mice vaccinated with a Brucella abortus mutant. *Infect. Immun.* **65(2)**, 798–800.

117. Denoel, P. A., Crawford, R. M., Zygmunt, M. S., et al. (1997) Survival of a bacterioferritin deletion mutant of Brucella melitensis 16M in human monocyte-derived macrophages. *Infect. Immun.* **65(10)**, 4337–4340.

118. Dorrell, N., Spencer, S., Foulonge, V., Guigue, T. P., O'Callaghan, D., and Wren, B. W. (1998) Identification, cloning and initial characterisation of FeuPQ in Brucella suis: a new sub-family of two-component regulatory systems. *FEMS Microbiol. Lett.* **162(1)**, 143–150.

119. Sangari, F. J., Grillo, M. J., Jimenez De Bagues, M. P., et al. (1998) The defect in the metabolism of erythritol of the Brucella abortus B19 vaccine strain is unrelated with its attenuated virulence in mice. *Vaccine* **16(17)**, 1640–1645.

120. Tibor, A., Jacques, I., Guilloteau, L., et al. (1998) Effect of P39 gene deletion in live Brucella vaccine strains on residual virulence and protective activity in mice. *Infect. Immun.* **66(11)**, 5561–5564.

121. Bellaire, B. H., Elzer, P. H., Baldwin, C. L., Roop, R. M., 2nd. (1999) The siderophore 2,3-dihydroxybenzoic acid is not required for virulence of Brucella abortus in BALB/c mice. *Infect. Immun.* **67(5)**, 2615–2618.

122. Dorrell, N., Guigue-Talet, P., Spencer, S., Foulonge, V., O'Callaghan, D., and Wren, B. W. (1999) Investigation into the role of the response regulator NtrC in the metabolism and virulence of Brucella suis. *Microb. Pathog.* **27(1)**, 1–11.

123. Petrovska, L., Hewinson, R. G., Dougan, G., Maskell, D. J., and Woodward, M. J. (1999) Brucella melitensis 16M: characterisation of the galE gene and mouse immunisation studies with a galE deficient mutant. *Vet. Microbiol.* **65(1)**, 21–36.

124. Ko, J. and Splitter, G. A. (2000) Residual virulence of Brucella abortus in the absence of the cytochrome bc(1)complex in a murine model in vitro and in vivo. *Microb. Pathog.* **29(3)**, 191–200.

125. Ko, J. and Splitter, G. A. (2000) Brucella abortus tandem repeated ATP-binding proteins, BapA and BapB, homologs of haemophilus influenzae LktB, are not necessary for intracellular survival. *Microb. Pathog.* **29(4)**, 245–253.

126. Robertson, G. T., Kovach, M. E., Allen, C. A., Ficht, T. A., and Roop, R. M., 2nd. (2000) The Brucella abortus Lon functions as a generalized stress response protease and is required for wild-type virulence in BALB/c mice. *Mol. Microbiol.* **35(3)**, 577–588.

127. Ekaza, E., Guilloteau, L., Teyssier, J., Liautard, J. P., and Kohler, S. (2000) Functional analysis of the ClpATPase ClpA of Brucella suis, and persistence of a knockout mutant in BALB/c mice. *Microbiology* **146(Pt 7)**, 1605–1616.

128. McQuiston, J. R., Vemulapalli, R., Inzana, T. J., et al. (1999) Genetic characterization of a Tn5-disrupted glycosyltransferase gene homolog in Brucella abortus and its effect on lipopolysaccharide composition and virulence. *Infect. Immun.* **67(8)**, 3830–3835.

129. Godfroid, F., Taminiau, B., Danese, I., et al. (1998) Identification of the perosamine synthetase gene of Brucella melitensis 16M and involvement of lipopolysaccharide O side chain in Brucella survival in mice and in macrophages. *Infect. Immun.* **66(11)**, 5485–5493.

130. Allen, C. A., Adams, L. G., and Ficht, T. A. (1998) Transposon-derived Brucella abortus rough mutants are attenuated and exhibit reduced intracellular survival. *Infect. Immun.* **66(3)**, 1008–1016.

131. Ugalde, J. E., Czibener, C., Feldman, M. F., and Ugalde, R. A. (2000) Identification and characterization of the Brucella abortus phosphoglucomutase gene: role of lipopolysaccharide in virulence and intracellular multiplication. *Infect. Immun.* **68(10)**, 5716–5723.

132. Foulongne, V., Walravens, K., Bourg, G., et al. (2001) Aromatic compound-dependent Brucella suis is attenuated in both cultured cells and mouse models. *Infect. Immun.* **69(1)**, 547–550.

133. Watarai, M., Makino, S., and Shirahata, T. (2002) An essential virulence protein of Brucella abortus, VirB4, requires an intact nucleoside-triphosphate-binding domain. *Microbiology* **148(Pt 5)**, 1439–1446.

134. O'Callaghan, D., Cazevieille, C., Allardet-Servent, A., et al. (1999) A homologue of the Agrobacterium tumefaciens VirB and Bordetella pertussis Ptl type IV secretion systems is essential for intracellular survival of Brucella suis. *Mol. Microbiol.* **33(6)**, 1210–1220.

135. Sieira, R., Comerci, D. J., Sanchez, D. O., and Ugalde, R. A. (2000) A homologue of an operon required for DNA transfer in Agrobacterium is required in Brucella abortus for virulence and intracellular multiplication. *J. Bacteriol.* **182(17)**, 4849–4855.

136. Kohler, S., Teyssier, J., Cloeckaert, A., Rouot, B., and Liautard, J. P. (1996) Participation of the molecular chaperone DnaK in intracellular growth of Brucella suis within U937-derived phagocytes. *Mol. Microbiol.* **20(4)**, 701–712.

137. Kohler, S., Ekaza, E., Paquet, J. Y., et al. (2002) Induction of dnaK through its native heat shock promoter is necessary for intramacrophagic replication of Brucella suis. *Infect. Immun.* **70(3)**, 1631–1634.

138. LeVier, K., Phillips, R. W., Grippe, V. K., Roop, R. M., 2nd, and Walker, G. C. (2000) Similar requirements of a plant symbiont and a mammalian pathogen for prolonged intracellular survival. *Science* **287(5462)**, 2492–2493.

139. Inon de Iannino, N., Briones, G., Tolmasky, M., and Ugalde, R. A. (1998) Molecular cloning and characterization of cgs, the Brucella abortus cyclic beta(1-2) glucan synthetase gene: genetic complementation of Rhizobium meliloti ndvB and Agrobacterium tumefaciens chvB mutants. *J. Bacteriol.* **180(17)**, 4392–4400.

140. Briones, G., Inon de Iannino, N., Roset, M., Vigliocco, A., Paulo, P. S., and Ugalde, R. A. (2001) Brucella abortus cyclic beta-1,2-glucan mutants have reduced virulence in mice and are defective in intracellular replication in HeLa cells. *Infect. Immun.* **69(7)**, 4528–4535.

141. Sola-Landa, A., Pizarro-Cerda, J., Grillo, M. J., et al. (1998) A two-component regulatory system playing a critical role in plant pathogens and endosymbionts is present in Brucella abortus and controls cell invasion and virulence. *Mol. Microbiol.* **29(1),** 125–138.

142. Robertson, G. T. and Roop, R. (1999) The Brucella abortus host factor I (HF-I) protein contributes to stress resistance during stationary phase and is a major determinant of virulence in mice. *Mol. Microbiol.* **34(4),** 690–700.

143. Almiron, M., Martinez, M., Sanjuan, N., and Ugalde, R. A. (2001) Ferrochelatase is present in Brucella abortus and is critical for its intracellular survival and virulence. *Infect. Immun.* **69(10),** 6225–6230.

144. Elzer, P. H., Phillips, R. W., Robertson, G. T., and Roop, R. n. (1996) The HtrA stress response protease contributes to resistance of Brucella abortus to killing by murine phagocytes. *Infect. Immun.* **64(11),** 4838–4841.

145. Elzer, P. H., Hagius, S. D., Robertson, G. T., et al. (1996) Behaviour of a high-temperature-requirement A (HtrA) deletion mutant of Brucella abortus in goats. *Res. Vet. Sci.* **60(1),** 48–50.

146. Phillips, R. W., Elzer, P. H., and Roop, R. I. (1995) A Brucella melitensis high temperature requirement A (htrA) deletion mutant demonstrates a stress response defective phenotype in vitro and transient attenuation in the BALB/c mouse model. *Microb. Pathog.* **19(5),** 227–284.

147. Edmonds, M. D., Cloeckaert, A., Booth, N. J., et al. (2001) Attenuation of a Brucella abortus mutant lacking a major 25 kDa outer membrane protein in cattle. *Am. J. Vet. Res.* **62(9),** 1461–1466.

9

Pathogenesis of and Immunity to *Coxiella burnetii*

David M. Waag and Herbert A. Thompson

1. INTRODUCTION

Q fever was discovered in both Australia and in the United States prior to the outbreak of World War II. In Australia, the disease was common in abattoir workers and farm workers *(1)* and persists today as an occupational problem *(2)*. The first described case in the United States was a lab infection caused by the "Nine Mile" agent *(3)*. This zoonotic disease is nearly worldwide in distribution. The etiological agent *Coxiella burnetii* has a surprisingly broad host range. Humans usually contract the disease by the inhalation of barnyard dust contaminated by dried ruminant parturition products or urine. Transmission can also occur by the ingestion of unpasteurized milk or cheese. The medical and veterinary concern for Q fever emanates from two syndromes. First, acute disease often presents with signs that overlap those seen in atypical pneumonia and, therefore, must be considered in the differential diagnosis when a history of animal contact can concomitantly be established with those signs. Second, some forms of the chronic disease are among the most difficult to treat of all human infectious diseases and, therefore, become life-threatening.

Because of its high infectivity and great external stability, the Q fever organism must be considered high on the probability list of potential terrorist agents. Here, we discuss the disease and the etiological agent and try to present information that is necessary when considering defensive strategies to counter its use as a bioweapon.

2. BACKGROUND

2.1. Discovery

In 1933, a fever of unknown origin was first observed in abattoir workers in Queensland, Australia. The disease was observed periodically for the next 2 yr and Dr. Edward Derrick, the Director of Health and Medical Services for Queensland, was sent to investigate the outbreak and determine the cause. Patients presented with fever, headache, and malaise. Serological tests for a wide variety of possible etiologic agents were negative *(1)*. Because the disease was thought to be previously undescribed, it was given the name Q fever (for Query). Blood and urine from patients elicited a febrile response after injection into guinea pigs, and the infection could be passed to successive animals. However, despite repeated attempts, no isolate could be obtained after

From: *Infectious Diseases: Biological Weapons Defense: Infectious Diseases and Counterterrorism*
Edited by: L. E. Lindler, F. J. Lebeda, and G. W. Korch © Humana Press Inc., Totowa, NJ

culture on bacteriological media. Derrick, therefore, surmized that the etiological agent was a virus.

At that time, half a world away in Montana, ticks were being collected as part of an ongoing investigation into Rocky Mountain Spotted Fever at the Rocky Mountain Laboratory (RML). Dr. Gordon Davis placed ticks collected from the Nine Mile Creek area onto guinea pigs, one of which became febrile. The infection could be passed to successive guinea pigs through injection of blood *(4)*. However, the disease picture observed in guinea pigs with this fever entity differed from that seen with classical spotted fever. In 1936, Dr. Herald Cox joined Davis at RML and identified rickettsia-like microorganisms in inflammatory cells from infected guinea pigs *(5)*. In 1938, Cox was able to cultivate *C. burnetii* in large numbers in yolk sacs of fertilized hen eggs *(6)*. Although an infectious microorganism was isolated, the disease that it caused was unknown.

So, in the United States, an infectious microorganism was isolated that caused no known disease, whereas in Australia, a disease was described of unknown etiology. In 1936, Derrick sent infected guinea pig tissues to Dr. Frank Macfarlane Burnet for assistance in determining the cause of Q fever. Burnet, although not able to culture the microorganism, was able to describe rickettsia-like bodies in the spleens of infected mice *(7)*. In 1938, a researcher was infected at RML while working with the Nine Mile isolate, and guinea pigs could be infected by injection of a sample of the patient's blood. Also in 1938, Burnet sent samples from infected mouse spleens to Dr. Rolla Dyer, who was Director of the National Institutes of Health. Dyer was able to confirm that the agent causing Q fever and the Nine Mile isolate were the same by demonstrating that guinea pigs previously challenged with the Nine Mile isolate were resistant to challenge with the Q fever agent *(3)*. The conclusion could also be made that Q fever was transmitted by ticks. This new disease was caused by a rickettsial organism that passed through filters, similar to a virus particle. Although initially named *Rickettsia diaporica (8)* and *Rickettsia burnetii (9)*, the microorganism was given the name *Coxiella burnetii* in 1948 in a fitting tribute to Cox and Burnet *(10)*.

Subsequently, Q fever disease investigations soon established its aerosol spread, its prevalence in slaughterhouses, and the hazards of laboratory work with the organism *(11–13)*. The successful culturing of the Q fever organism in embryos proved to be a very fortuitous breakthrough for advances in Q fever research, as well as for other rickettsias *(14)*.

2.2. Growth and Culture

C. burnetii is obligately intracellular and replicates only within the phagolysosomal vacuoles of animal cells, primarily macrophages. It cannot be grown on axenic mediums of any kind. During natural infections, the organism grows to high quantities in placental tissues of goats, sheep, and possibly cows *(15,16)*. Routine culture of most of the strains is accomplished in chicken embryo yolk sacs and in cell cultures *(17)*. It is also recovered in large numbers from spleens of experimentally infected mice and guinea pigs *(17)*. Regardless of the choice of experimental host, the organism is a slow grower, rarely growing at a generation time shorter than 8 h *(18)*. Reliable culture from clinical and environmental specimens is difficult, even for experienced laboratories. The standard (and most trusted) method of culturing from either clinical or environmental samples is sequential mouse passages that require weeks of time to accomplish *(17)*. Although less reliable, a tissue-culture shell vial technique may be used in culturing the organism from clinical samples and can be accomplished in 7–10 d *(19)*. This shell vial method grew organisms from 17% of confirmed acute infections (specimens obtained before therapy) and from 53% of chronic infections *(20)*.

2.3. Bacteriology and the Developmental Cycle

The organism usually grows as a small coccobacillus, approx 0.8–1.0 µm in length by 0.3–0.5 µm in width, and may occur either singly or in short chains. Although their gram stain reaction is variable, they possess an envelope structure similar to Gram-negative bacteria, including the presence of a lipopolysaccharide (LPS; refs. *21* and *22*). The LPS has not been fully characterized but plays a definite role in virulence and appears to be physically responsible for the well-known antigenic phase variation seen in this organism *(23,24)*. Although of average complexity, the LPS does contain some rare (methylated and branched) sugars and amino sugars *(21,25,26)*. *Coxiella* also possesses a gene that complements regulation of capsule production in *Escherichia coli* *(27)*. This suggests that the organism may possess the ability to form capsules under some circumstances.

The most important biological feature of the organism is the existence of small, compacted cell types within mature populations growing in animal hosts *(28)*. These forms, called small-cell variants (SCVs) are absolutely distinct from the large-cell variants (LCVs) in the population. The latter are probably the metabolizing stage in what is obviously a developmental life cycle in this organism. The SCVs possess an apparently condensed nucleoid that gives them a distinct "bull's eye" appearance when viewed in thin-section electron microscopy *(29)*. It is now generally agreed that this small form is a stage of a developmental cycle and *not* a stage within a standard microbial growth curve *(29,30)*. However, it appears to *not* be a classical spore. The SCV stage has been shown to contain a histone 1 protein homolog called Hq1 *(31)* that is very much like that discovered in Chlamydia elementary bodies *(32)*. Hq1 from *C. burnetii* has an isoelectric point of 13.1, contains 29% lysine, and is not found in LCVs. The *C. burnetii* SCV also contains a small basic protein, SCV protein A (ScvA), which is also unique to that stage. ScvA is only 30 amino acids long and contains 23% arginine, 23% glutamine, and 13% proline *(33)*. Other proteins presently under study are predominant or unique to the LCV stage of the organism *(29)*. These include the protein synthesis factors EF-Tu and EF-Ts and the surface protein OMP P1 *(34,35)*. Thus, it is important to stress that the SCV and LCV forms are antigenically distinct in addition to being metabolically and structurally distinct. It is suspected that the SCV accounts for the organism's high infectivity as well as its capability to survive relatively extreme environmental conditions. Moreover, the SCV structure, which in appearance resembles a Chlamydial elementary body, is likely responsible for *C. burnetii's* rather unique chemical resistance spectrum as well as its resistance to dessication, heat, sonication, and pressure *(29)*. We do not yet understand the full developmental cycle and the signals (if any) necessary to bring about small cell formation. There are some other stages or structural forms that may participate, such as the "small dense cell" *(28,29)* and the "spore-like particle" *(28,36)*; however, these are not yet defined, and until the spore-like particle can be isolated in pure form and then shown to germinate into a reproductive vegetative form, its role remains speculative. Nevertheless, the presence of significant numbers of SCVs within the late stages of infection is of importance to considerations of vaccine development and of organism detection by non-DNA methods (e.g., via surface antigens and structures). Certainly, the SCV surface differs considerably from that of the large metabolizing "vegetative" (LCV) form. Antibodies have been used to distinguish the two forms *(34,35)*.

2.4. Physical and Chemical Resistance

The SCV (and perhaps other stages) of the developmental cycle (above) is also believed to explain the unusual resistance characteristics of the Q fever organism, as well as its long-term durability within a number of different environments. In a study designed to determine *Coxiella's* chemical resistance properties, it was found that 10% household bleach (equivalent to a 0.5% concentration of the active ingredient hypochlorous acid) did not result in complete eradication all of 10^8 organisms during a 30-min exposure time *(37)*. Likewise, exposure of organisms for 30 min to 5% Lysol, 2% Roccal, or 5% formalin did not result in complete eradication *(37)*. Another early report found that 1.0% formalin for 24 h would not kill all *Coxiellae (38)*. *Coxiella* organisms are also more thermoduric than most mesophiles *(39)*. The stability of *C. burnetii* when in milk is remarkable because there is no decay of infectivity noted after weeks of storage at refrigerated temperature. The resistance of *Coxiella* to pressure and to osmotic lysis is also well-known. When breaking purified cells to obtain cytoplasmic extracts, we found that 10,000–12,000 psi was necessary, and even at this level, numerous unbroken particles remained *(40)*. It is now known that the resistant forms are represented by the SCV *(29,30)*. The use of osmotic lysis is a practical means of obtaining the SCV portion of the population, as the LCVs lyse on abrupt decreases in ionic strength *(29,30)*.

2.5. Metabolism

Coxiella's metabolism is acidophilic, presumably because most of its transport mechanisms required for import of required nutrient substrates from the vacuole environment will function in a pH range from 3.0 to 5.0. Purified organisms incubated without any host fractions or cells, at neutral or near neutral pH, will not transport or metabolize either glucose or glutamate, but it will readily do so at pH 4.5. This pH-dependent activity, termed "acid activation"of metabolism, was discovered by Hackstadt and Williams *(41)*. Transport or incorporation of several other substrates has been documented, including amino acids and nucleosides *(see* ref. *18)*, almost all of which required mild acid conditions. However, acid activation under numerous substrate conditions has not resulted in axenic growth, although considerable protein synthesis does occur during incubation in the presence of all 20 amino acids. This host-free accumulation of biomass by *Coxiella* organisms during acid activation is accompanied by DNA synthesis *(42)*.

3. DISEASE

3.1. Transmission and Occurrence

Q fever, caused by the intracellular bacterium, *C. burnetii*, is generally an acute and self-limited febrile illness that rarely causes a chronic debilitating disease. The case–fatality ratio is estimated to be less than 1% *(1)*. Q fever is a zoonotic disease that occurs worldwide. Although domestic ungulates, including cattle, sheep, and goats, usually acquire and transmit *C. burnetii*, domestic pets can also be a source of human infection *(43–47)*. Heavy concentrations of this organism are secreted in milk, urine, feces, and especially in parturient products of infected pregnant animals *(48)*. Infection is most commonly acquired by breathing infectious aerosols *(49–51)*. Less-frequent portals of entry include ingestion of infected milk *(52)* and parenteral acquisition caused by the bite of an infected tick *(4,51)*. The infectious dose for humans is estimated to be 10 microorganisms or less *(53)*. The route of infection may influence clinical presentation of the disease *(53a)*. In Europe, in regions where ingestion of raw milk is the more common transmission mode, acute Q fever is found mostly as a granulomatous hepatitis *(54)*. However, in Nova Scotia, where infection is predominantly by the aerosol route, Q fever pneumonia is more common *(55)*. Although *C. burnetii* strains display genetic heterogeneity by restriction fragment polymorphism analysis *(56)*, there may not be a strong association between genetic structure or plasmid type, and the disease type (chronic or acute) as was previously suggested *(57)*. Therefore, host-specific factors are thought to be more important in influencing the clinical form of Q fever *(58)*.

3.2. Disease Manifestations, Signs, and Symptoms

Human *C. burnetii* infections without overt clinical signs are common, especially among high-risk groups such as veterinary and abattoir workers, other livestock handlers, and laboratory workers *(59–62)*. Although clinical disease is infrequent, the vast majority of human cases are acute Q fever. The incubation period lasts from a few days to several weeks and the severity of infection varies in proportion to the dose *(63,64)*. Although no clinical feature is pathognomonic for Q fever, certain signs and symptoms tend to be prevalent in acute Q fever cases. Fever, headache (frontal or retroorbital), and chills are most commonly seen. The temperature generally peaks at 40°C and, in the majority of patients, the usual duration of fever is approx 13 d *(65)*. Fatigue and sweats are also frequently found *(66)*. Other symptoms reported in cases of acute Q fever include cough, nausea, vomiting, myalgia, arthralgia, chest pain, hepatitis, and occasionally, splenomegaly and meningoencephalitis *(66,67)*. The white blood cell count in acute Q fever is usually normal, but thrombocytopenia or mild anemia may be present *(68)*. The erythrocyte sedimentation rate is frequently elevated *(69)*.

A common clinical manifestation of Q fever is pneumonia *(70)*. Atypical pneumonia is most frequent, and asymptomatic patients can also exhibit radiologic changes *(71)*. These changes are usually nonspecific and, in Canadian studies, included rounded opacities and hilar adenopathy *(44)*. Although predominantly homogenous infiltrates were observed in a reported outbreak in England *(71)*, lobar consolidation was observed in cases in Crete *(72)*. Q fever may also manifest a syndrome resembling acute granulomatous hepatitis with elevations of the asparate transaminase and/or alanine transaminase *(66)*. Elevations in levels of alkaline phosphatase and total bilirubin are seen less commonly.

Chronic infection is rare but, unlike the acute disease, is often fatal. Chronic Q fever occurs almost exclusively in patients with prior coronary disease or in patients immunocompromised because of disease, such as AIDS, or therapy, such as immunosuppressive cancer therapy or antirejection therapy after organ transplant *(73,74)*.

Endocarditis is the main clinical manifestation of chronic Q fever, although other syndromes, such as chronic hepatitis *(75)* and infection of surgical lesions *(76)*, have been observed. Endocarditis usually affects the aortic and mitral valves *(77)*. In some individuals, the host immune system might not be sufficient to eradicate the microorganism and persistent infection results. Granulomas are not observed in cases of chronic Q fever hepatitis *(78)*. This finding is likely the result of the lack of a T-cell response in chronic Q fever patients *(79)*. Immunosuppression of host cellular immune responses is caused by a cell associated immunosuppressive complex (ISC) *(80)*. Although the chemical nature of this cellular component is not defined, it can be dissociated by extraction using chloroform:methanol. The resultant chloroform methanol residue (CMR) is not immunosuppressive after injection into the host, unlike *C. burnetii* phase I whole cells *(81)*. The mechanism of action of the ISC may involve stimulation of the production of prostaglandin E2 *(82)*. The stimulation of high levels of tumor necrosis factor, although possibly upregulating adhesion receptors on monocytes and macrophages may also have deleterious effects on the host *(83,84)*. In addition, an increase in interleukin-10 secretion is found in patients with chronic Q fever *(85)*. Suppression of host immunity may allow persistence of the microorganism in host cells during the development of chronic Q fever. Other pathological effects of chronic Q fever include the presence of circulating immune complexes, resulting in glomerulonephritis *(86)*.

Growth in the harsh phagolysosomal environment necessitates that this microorganism has coping strategies. This mechanism, although undefined, may involve the production of oxygen scavengers *(87)*. Stimulation of macrophage antimicrobial mechanisms by T-cell interferon (IFN)-γ production leads to control of infection *(88,89)*. Passive transfer of antibodies did not control infection *(90)*. Therefore, control of infection is dependent on cell-mediated immunity *(91)*.

4. DEFENSIVE STRATEGIES

4.1. Vaccines

An efficacious Q fever vaccine was developed in 1948, 12 yr after discovery of the etiologic agent. This preparation, consisting of formalin-killed and ether-extracted *C. burnetii* containing 10% yolk sac, was effective in protecting human volunteers from aerosol challenge *(92)*. In the early studies, the antigenic nature of the vaccine was not known. Stoker and Fiset discovered that *C. burnetii* displays LPS variations similar to the smooth-rough LPS variation in *E. coli (23)*. As bacterial isolates were passed in yolk sacs or other nonimmunocompetent hosts, the phase I (smooth) LPS character of the bacterial population gradually changed to the phase II (rough) form. Vaccines prepared from phase I microorganisms were found to be 100–300 times more potent than phase II vaccines *(93)* and form the basis for most current Q fever vaccines. Purification methods were improved over the years to separate bacterial cells from egg proteins and lipids. Vaccine efficacy of these more highly purified preparations was shown in human volunteers *(94)*. However, the use of this and other early phase I cellular vaccines was frequently accompanied by adverse reactions, including induration at the vaccination site or the formation of sterile abscesses or granulomas *(95,96)*. In addition, administration of cellular vaccine to persons previously infected could result in severe local reactions *(96)*. Approximately 3.6% of persons vaccinated for the 9th and 10th time developed severe persistent reactions *(97)*. In 1962, Lackman published a study that correlated a positive skin test with preexisting immunity to Q fever *(98)*. When skin-test-positive individuals were excluded from vaccination, the incidence of adverse reactions after vaccination decreased dramatically. Currently, potential for adverse vaccination reactions is usually assessed by skin testing, although some laboratories also measure the level of specific antibodies against *C. burnetii (99)*. Only individuals testing negative by either method are vaccinated. Evidence suggests that cellular *C. burnetii* vaccines are safe and efficacious if the recipients are not immune because of prior *C. burnetii* infection.

Attempts to maintain vaccine efficacy while decreasing potential for adverse reactions led to testing of cell extracts as vaccines. Phase I *C. burnetii* whole cells were extracted with dimethyl sulfoxide *(100)*, dimethylacetamide *(100)*, and trichloroacetic acid *(101)*. Although these extracted cellular antigens were less reactive than intact microorganisms after injection, they were also less efficacious as vaccines. For the most part, attenuated Q fever vaccines are not used. However, a phase II attenuated strain, designated M-44, was developed in the former Soviet Union *(102)*. This vaccine, used since 1960, was shown to cause myocarditis, hepatitis, liver necrosis, granuloma formation, and splenitis in guinea pigs *(103)*. In addition, in human vaccinees, no antiphase I antibodies were generated and antiphase II levels were variable and at low titer.

Prescreening of potential vaccinees by serology may not eliminate the risk of adverse vaccination reactions, as specific antibody titers wane after acute infection *(104)* and may not accurately reflect the immune status of the individual. In addition, skin tests are time consuming, costly, and may be incorrectly applied or misinterpreted. Therefore, efforts are underway to develop safer Q fever vaccines that will pose a lesser risk if given to someone with preexisting immunity. Such a vaccine could eliminate the requirement for prevaccination screening of potential vaccinees, yet retain vaccine efficacy. Another benefit of such vaccines would be a single visit to a healthcare practitioner for a vaccination. Vaccination would be cheaper and simpler.

With such objectives in mind, a CMR Q fever vaccine was developed at the RML in the late 1970s. Initial testing showed that CMR did not cause adverse reactions in mice at doses several times larger than doses of phase I cellular vaccine that caused severe adverse reactions *(81)*. Studies have established the efficacy of *C. burnetii* phase I CMR vaccine after injection into laboratory rodents challenged by the intraperitoneal or aerosol routes *(105,106)*. CMR vaccine has also been shown to reduce the shedding of *C. burnetii* when used to vaccinate sheep *(107)*.

The most thoroughly tested Q fever vaccine in use today is Q-Vax. This is a formalin-killed, Henzerling strain phase I cellular vaccine produced and licensed for use in Australia *(99)*. This vaccine has been very effective in preventing clinical Q fever in occupationally at-risk individuals. When a single subcutaneous dose (30 µg) of this vaccine was given to over 2000 abattoir workers screened for prior immunity, the protective efficacy was 100% *(99)*. The duration of protection was more than 5 yr. A comparative study in cynomolgus monkeys demonstrated that Q-Vax and CMR vaccines were equally efficacious and immunogenic after aerosol challenge *(108)*. Efficacious Q fever vaccines would be of benefit to those occupationally at risk for Q fever, those residing in areas endemic for Q fever, and soldiers or civilians who may be exposed as the result of a bioterrorist or biowarfare attack.

4.2. Diagnostics

4.2.1. Serum-Based

Diagnosis of Q fever based on clinical signs and symptoms is difficult because the illness has no unique, characteristic features that distinguish it from other febrile illnesses, such as influenza and pneumonia caused by mycoplasma or chlamydia infection. Because of the nonspecific clinical presentation of acute Q fever, human *C. burnetii* infections are often mistaken for viral illnesses *(62)*. Because cultivating *C. burnetii* or working with the native microorganism can be hazardous to laboratory personnel, the diagnosis of Q fever is usually based on serological testing. Although specific cellular immune responses may be suppressed in cases of acute Q fever, humoral immune responses appear to continue unabated during infection *(109,110)*. Because of the relative ease of assaying serum samples for antibodies, serological profiles of patients with Q fever have been established *(104,110)*. Thus, clinicians frequently encounter situations where a presumptive diagnosis of acute Q fever, based on nonspecific signs, a history of animal exposure, and serology (if available), is considered likely enough to warrant treatment.

The two antigenic forms of *C. burnetii* that are important for serologic diagnosis of Q fever are the phase I (e.g., virulent microorganism with smooth LPS [S-LPS]) and phase II (e.g., avirulent microorganism with rough LPS [R-LPS]) whole-cell antigens *(111,112)*. Infection of humans produces characteristic serologic profiles by various antibody tests. Whereas the complement fixation assay (CFA) is generally regarded as the most specific serological assay for Q fever, the indirect fluorescent antibody assay (IFA), the microagglutination assay, and the enzyme immunoassay (EIA) can provide positive results earlier in the course of an infection *(113)*. Recent results showed good correlation between the IFA and EIA when testing sera from acute Q fever patients and patients diagnosed with other bacterial diseases *(114)*. Determination of antibodies against phase I and phase II *C. burnetii* may help distinguish between acute and chronic Q fever *(110)*.

The primary tests used today for the serodiagnosis of Q fever are the IFA and EIA. In the IFA, patient sera are serially diluted in microtiter plate wells and then transferred to microscope slides whose Teflon-templated wells are previously coated with the relevant diagnostic antigen. A secondary antibody which recognizes human immunoglobulin and is covalently attached to a fluorescent molecule is added to the wells. Antigens are observed under an epifluorescence microscope. The well containing the highest dilution of patient serum showing specific, bright green fluorescence on at least some of the organisms in the field is the diagnostic end point. The reciprocal of the corresponding serum dilution is the end point titer. The dilution after the end point will typically show all organisms as dull gray ovoids. Both phase I and phase II antigens, in crude yolk sac form and dotted separately onto the slides, are used. The IFA is generally used when equipment or space are limited or when small numbers of samples are tested. The IFA is not considered the optimal test for epidemiologic surveys of Q fever because the antibodies decay rapidly, the slides require some experience to read correctly, and it is not easily adapted for testing large numbers of specimens *(115)*. The IFA has been shown to be sensitive when used to test patient sera 3 and 4 wk after the onset of acute Q fever (50 and 70%, respectively) *(116)*. The specific IgM titer to phase

II antigens can be detected 7 d after infection *(110,112)* but may be found for less than 17 wk *(112,117)*. The use of crude suspensions or homogenates of phase I and II organisms, unpurified from their yolk sac growth medium, routinely function very well in this test. This is a large advantage, in that such preparations are often more available commercially or are readily attainable from research labs.

In the EIA, patient sera are serially diluted in the wells of a microtiter plate coated with diagnostic antigen. An antibody conjugate, composed of antibody that recognizes human immunoglobulin coupled to an enzyme (horseradish peroxidase or alkaline phosphatase), is added. After the enzyme substrate is added, a colormetric change in the wells resulting from the interaction of enzyme and substrate indicates the relative amount of patient immunoglobulin reacting with diagnostic antigen and is measured spectrophotometrically. The well containing the highest dilution of serum for which the optical density exceeds a previously determined level corresponds to the endpoint. The reciprocal of that dilution is the end point titer. An EIA for the detection of *C. burnetii*-specific IgM was first described by Field and Hunt *(118)* for the detection of Q fever in abattoir workers. The EIA is highly sensitive, easy to perform, has great potential adaptability for automation, can be applied in epidemiologic surveys *(115,118,119)*, and has been shown to be of value for the diagnosis of acute and chronic Q fever *(120)*. A disadvantage is the requirement for a more highly purified cellular antigen for EIA, in contrast to IFA. Such purified antigens are not usually commercially available.

We validated an EIA for the serodiagnosis of acute Q fever using 152 serum samples from human volunteers with no evidence of previous Q fever to establish diagnostic titers *(104)*. These samples were used to determine diagnostic titers corresponding to a false-positive rate of 1%. Fifty-one serum samples from patients with acute Q fever with known times since the onset of disease were then used to evaluate the sensitivity of the assay. Our objective in validating this serological assay was to determine diagnostic titers to specific phase I and II antigens that maximized both sensitivity and specificity.

A fourfold rise in titer between acute and convalescent sera is an accepted practice to support a clinical diagnosis. However, sera may not be acquired during acute disease and a single sample drawn at some point after disease onset is frequently the only sample available on which to confirm a clinical diagnosis. Furthermore, if the initial serum sample was collected in early convalescence, a fourfold rise in titer may not occur *(114)*. In either event, diagnostic titers must be established that could support a clinical diagnosis of Q fever using a single serum sample. Therefore, we wanted to establish diagnostic titers based on statistical analysis of the differences between titers observed in patients with clinically confirmed acute Q fever and those with no history of prior *C. burnetii* infection.

Minimum diagnostic antiphase II IgM and IgG titers of 512 and 1024 and antiphase I IgM and IgG titers of 128 and 64, respectively, were determined. Because of differences in equipment, personnel, and methods, minimum diagnostic EIA titers in other laboratories will be different. We have also noted that patients with a clinical diagnosis of Q fever also have two or more positive tests.

When sera from patients with acute Q fever was tested, IgM and IgG responses to phase II microorganisms were sensitive (84 and 80%, respectively) and specific (>99%) using titrations of early (19–30 d after disease onset) convalescent-phase sera. Fifty-seven and 58% of intermediate (67–75 d after disease onset) and late convalescent (98–107 d after disease onset) sera, respectively, had positive IgM antiphase II antibody. In contrast, sensitivities of the IgG and IgM responses to phase I *C. burnetii* were highest when the late and intermediate sera, respectively, were tested. All patient sera collected 5.5 yr after disease onset had positive IgG response against phase I and II diagnostic antigen. Determination of a significant antibody response to phase I *C. burnetii* could help clinicians distinguish the acute from the chronic forms of the disease *(110)*. Including phase I antigen in a test battery for acute Q fever may also help determine whether the infection is recent. Because a higher proportion of early convalescent-phase sera had titers for phase II than phase I microorganisms in this study, the presence of antibody to phase II *C. burnetii* and the absence of antibody (IgG) to phase I *C. burnetii* supports a diagnosis of acute Q fever infection occurring within the preceding 6 mo. Whereas the IgM antiphase I response measured by EIA persists for up to 35 wk (Waag, unpublished data), the duration of the antiphase I IgG response after infection is unknown. The persistence of a late IgM response has also been noted using complement fixation and IFA *(112)*. Therefore, a positive IgM titer may not necessarily indicate a current case of Q fever.

Acute Q fever may be distinguished from chronic Q fever serologically. In sera from patients with acute Q fever, the magnitude of antiphase II titers exceeds those of antiphase I titers *(110)*. However, in chronic Q fever patients, the antiphase I titers exceed those to phase II *C. burnetii*. Elevated serum IgA titers to *C. burnetii* antigens are rare, but specific phase II and I IgA titers may be observed as the illness progresses from the acute to the chronic stage *(110)*.

In a study to evaluate the specificity of the EIA as compared with the IFA test and to assess the use of EIA as an alternative diagnostic test for Q fever in humans, 95 acute and convalescent serum samples from patients diagnosed with Q fever, rickettsial infections, or Legionnaires' disease and with a fourfold rise in IFA titer were tested blindly using an EIA *(114)*. Results showed that the agreement between the EIA and IFA test for the diagnosis of Q fever was excellent. However, the specificity of the EIA was markedly improved by using the phase I whole cell as an additional diagnostic antigen. Prior studies suggested that the EIA was more sensitive than the IFA in detecting specific antibodies to *C. burnetii (120,122)*. The study *(114)* concluded that because of its many advantages such as high sensitivity, convenient technical features, and potential for automation, the EIA may be efficiently used as an alternative to the IFA test for the diagnosis of *C. burnetii* infection in humans.

4.2.2. Basic and Applied Genomics

C. burnetii was recently removed from the Rickettsial family and transferred to the gammaproteobacteria, order *Legionellales*, family Coxiellaceae, genus Coxiella *(123)*. The phylogenetic similarity between this organism and Legionella species was established in part through rRNA sequence comparisons *(124)*. The rDNA exists in a single copy *(125)*. There is general similarity between *Coxiella* and *Legionella* and *Franciscella* at the DNA level. *Coxiella* DNA has a relatively high G + C content, 42–43 mol% *(126)*. The genome has been sequenced by The Institute for Genomic Research (TIGR) *(127)*. The Nine Mile strain in phase I was sequenced and contained 1911 Kbp, which places its size well above the genome sizes of the rickettsias, chlamydias, mycoplasmas, and leptospiras *(127)*. Prior to this work by TIGR, a German group formed the physical map of the genome *(128)*. They reported that the Nine Mile genome was larger, at more than 2103 Kbp, and found that the genome sizes of several other *Coxiella* isolates vary considerably. Another independent group has discovered that the genomes of two Nine Mile phase I strain descendants have undergone spontaneous chromosomal deletions *(129)*. The Nine Mile phase II strain, which has a severely truncated LPS, has deleted approx 27 kb of DNA, in a region spanning O-antigen synthesis genes and other LPS biosynthesis functions *(129)*. This strain arose by sequential passages in embryonated eggs, and is avirulent in humans and animals. Another isolate, termed RSA 514 "Crazy," was isolated from a pregnant guinea pig several months after being innoculated with the Nine Mile phase I strain. "Crazy" has undergone a deletion in the same region as phase II, but surprisingly its DNA deletion is larger *(129)*. The "Crazy" LPS length is intermediate between phase I and II, and its virulence characteristics are also intermediate *(24)*. The mechanism of deletion of these DNA regions remains speculative; however, crossovers between reiterated regions has been a suggested route *(129)*.

A large number of isolates and strains of *C. burnetii* are available but remain largely uncharacterized. Little is known about their comparative pathogenicities because only a few careful studies have been done *(24,26)*. These have been shown to sort into three or four different plasmid types *(see* below) and into three or more LPS types *(24,26)*. For purposes of categorization, typing, and epidemiology, the DNA regions encoding plasmid and lipopolysaccharide functions are obvious sequences to exploit.

Previously, an autonomous replication sequence, *ars,* which could be the chromosomal origin of replication, was isolated using origin search and rescue techniques in *E. coli* strains *(130)*. This *ars* region was found to contain at least two perfect DnaA protein boxes, which are sites for the binding of DnaA protein to initiate DNA replication. *E. coli* plasmids recombined with this *ars* region can be used to genetically transform *Coxiella* by homologous recombination events following electroporation of the shuttle plasmids *(131)*. It is not known whether the organism possesses any natural recombination mechanisms such as transformation or conjugation (but *see* plasmids, below). Illegitimate recombination, less than ideal selection mechanisms, and the lack of an efficient plating or plaquing system for screening large numbers of potential transformants make targeted genetic manipulations difficult in this organism *(132)*.

The *C. burnetii* prototype strain Nine Mile contains a resident plasmid QpH1 that remains cryptic (function unknown) *(133)*. QpH1 contains 37329 bp and a G + C content of 39.3 mol % *(134)*. The resident plasmid structure and size varies from biotype to biotype *(57,135)*. At least five different plasmid types have been identified to date *(135)*. These appear to differ in the arrangement of genes and in surface proteins, which they encode, and also differ in size, varying from 34 to more than 50 kb *(135)*. The QpRS plasmid, which was obtained from the Priscilla (goat abortion) strain, contains 39,280 bp and has a G + C content of 39.7% *(136)*. Two other plasmid types, named QpDG, from the Dugway rodent strain *(137)*, and QpDV, from strain R1140 *(135)*, have been identified. In addition, in the Scurry strain of *C. burnetii,* all of the plasmid sequence present has been integrated into the chromosome *(137)*. Later sequencing work showed that the Scurry chromosome contains only 17,965 bp of sequence homologous to QpH1; this represents a conservation of only six open reading frames

(ORFs) *(138)*. Apparently the remainder of the plasmid sequences found in QpH1, QpRS, and the others, and not found in the chromosome-integrated element, is necessary for the autonomous plasmid replication *(135)*. The plasmid QpH1 contains ORFs that possess similarities, at the amino acid level, with proteins known to have DNA replication roles *(134)*. ORFs believed to correspond to (a) a replication protein from *Pseudomonas putida*; (b) DNA helicase I from *E. coli*; (c) the stability of plasmid (SopA) from *E. coli*; and (d) replication protein B (Rep B) from *Agrobacterium sp*, were identified *(134)*. The plasmid contains elements that can functionally complement conjugative plasmid instability in *E. coli,* suggesting that the encoded protein(s) have something to do with segregating two or more copies of plasmids to each daughter cell during cell division *(139)*. This protein, termed Q fever organism stability of plasmid (Qsop), and another described as replication origin associated (Roa307) *(140)* were considered to be involved with plasmid inheritance to daughter *Coxiella* cells.

The plasmids may serve as a primary method for biotyping (distinguishing) various members of the genus. Genetic variation within the genus is also evident by the fact that genome size varies between isolates; much, if not most, of the variation is a result of chromosomal and not plasmid differences *(128)*. Furthermore, spontaneous chromosomal deletions are known to occur in at least one strain (e.g., Nine Mile; refs. *129* and *141*). Continuous passage in laboratory hosts that do not possess competent immune systems, such as embryonated egg yolk sacs, may allow *Coxiella* cells with the deleted region to accumulate *(23,129)*. The consequence of the DNA deletion is the loss of *O*-antigen genes, which in turn explains antigenic phase variation and a loss of virulence owing to the truncated LPS *(24,129)*.

4.2.3. Nucleic Acid-Based Detection

Polymerase chain reaction (PCR) methods are specific and sensitive. If "real time" PCR via 5' exonuclease (hydrolysis probe degradation) methods are used, the lack of need for gel analysis lowers the labor expense but raises the reagent expense, as fluorescent probes are expensive. The newer instrumentation and reporter methods brings to life the use of assays handling much larger numbers of samples. Therefore, this method is seen as a powerful technique for detection of pathogens.

Numerous PCR-based assays employing conventional gel-based systems have been developed and published for use on the Q pathogen *(142–153)*. Of these, by far the most popular and useful have been those that employ the insertion sequence IS1111 as a target (Trans PCR; refs. *129, 146, 150, 153*, and *154*). There are at least 19 copies of this gene, presumably a transposon, in each *C. burnetii* Nine Mile strain chromosome *(127)*; no *Coxiella* isolate tested to date lacks multiple copies of this element. The original Trans PCR assay, developed by Willems et al. *(146)*, generates a 687-bp product and detects a DNA quantity equivalent to less than one genome *(146)*. The protocol, which in modified form is still in use today by the Centers for Disease Control and Prevention (CDC) Rickettsiology Unit, calls for denaturation at 94°C, annealing 75–65°C in six consecutive steps of 2°C, followed by extension at 77°C. It is a gel-based assay. The Trans PCR assay, or slight variations of it, has been used successfully to detect *Coxiella* in cow's milk, in organs including placentas, in heart valves, in blood specimens, in ovine genital swabs, and in fecal samples *(146,150,153)*. For human blood samples, citrated or ethylenendiaminetetraacidic acid (EDTA) blood is used, and the leukocyte layer is retained for use in PCR assays *(154)*.

The superoxide dismutase gene has also been successfully targeted in samples of barn straw and hay *(155)*, animal genital swabs and fecal samples, milk *(153)*, and heart valves from humans *(145)*. Other genes or sequences used for PCR identification have been isocitrate dehydrogenase *(152)*, rRNA sequences *(148)*, com 1 outer membrane protein in human serum samples *(151)*, QpH1-QpRS *(143,155)*, and the *htpAB* (heat shock) genetic locus in paraffin-embedded clinical samples *(149)*.

4.2.4. Culturing as a Diagnostic Tool

The development of a microculture technique for *C. burnetii* encouraged the use of culture to aid in diagnosis and assessment of Q fever *(19,20,156)*. This method also aids the isolation of new strains and isolates and could be used to make significant contributions to the phylogenetic study of the genus. However, it remains a technique that is time-consuming and subjective in interpretation of positive and negative results. If fluorescent antibody methods are used to detect the organism, care must be used to keep red cell and debris, especially hemoglobin, out of the assays *(154)*. For this reason, it is probably wise to confirm fluorescence as being authentically associated with intracellular microorganisms, rather than residual specimen background (nonspecific) fluorescence. This is done by use of a standard stain method such as Stamp's *(157)* or Gimenez *(158)*. Alternatively, trypsinization, recovery, and thorough washing of the cells in the initial shell vial monolayer, followed by replating in a new shell vial and further culture for a day or two, significantly reduces the troublesome background fluorescence. The infected cells will carry over in the passage and replating, but most of the original background material adhering to the surface of the monolayer will not (H.A. Thompson, unpublished). This modification has the additional advantage of extending the culture time, which appears to be necessary for samples that initially have fewer than 100–1000 organisms (H.A. Thompson, unpublished). However, this extends to 8–9 d the amount of time needed to get a culture result and does not eliminate the need for a second coverslip culture for staining by standard methods for confirmation that observed fluorescence is correlated with the presence of intracellular vacuoles containing organisms. Even with these precautions, the method could miss clinical specimens that contain smaller numbers of viable organisms.

In our limited experience, we have found this technique to be useful in a research application, but do not recommend it as a sole method on which to base clinical decisions.

4.3. Disinfection

Even before the life cycle incorporating an endospore-like body *(28)* was elucidated, the resistance of *C. burnetii* to environmental degradation was well-known *(159–161)*. The ability of this microorganism to survive in the environment has resulted in infections in humans and animals. As this microorganism infects a wide range of hosts (including domestic ungulates and humans), control measures are exceedingly complex. Previously, it was assumed that methods of chemical disinfection sufficient to inactivate *Bacillus* spores would also kill *C. burnetii*. However, experiments showed that formaldehyde gas without humidity control was not able to completely sterilize a large room containing *C. burnetii*, although *Bacillus* spores were inactivated *(37)*. To evaluate the efficacy of chemical disinfectants, *C. burnetii* was suspended in Lysol, ethyl alcohol, sodium hypochlorite, formalin, chloroform, Alcide, Enviro-Chem, ethylene oxide, and Roccal for selected periods of time at room temperature and the microorganism resuspended in growth medium after separation from the disinfectant solution by centrifugation *(37)*. To determinine the presence of viable *C. burnetii*, treated samples were injected into fertilized hen eggs. Yolk sacs were harvested and injected into mice and the presence of viable microorganisms determined by seroconversion. *C. burnetii* was completely inactivated within 30 min by exposure to 70% ethyl alcohol, 5% chloroform, or 5% Enviro-Chem *(37)*. (The latter chemical, a formulation of two quaternary ammonium compounds, is now known as Micro-Chem Plus and is available through National Chemical Laboratories, Philadelphia, PA.) Formaldehyde gas was also an effective sterilizing agent when administered in a humidified (80% relative humidity) environment. Previous work had shown that 1% aqueous formalin was effective but only after 72 h of exposure *(38)*. Overnight exposure to 12% ethylene oxide at 24°C sterilized filters seeded with viable *C. burnetii (37)*. Experiments were conducted with purified *C. burnetii*. If samples contain additional organic material, disinfection is more difficult.

The determination of effective milk pasteurization procedures took into account the frequent presence of the Q fever organism in cow's milk. A temperature of 143°F (61.7°C) was required to kill 10^8 organisms within 1 cc of raw milk in a time period of 20 min *(39)*. Another report was in general agreement, reporting 63°C for 30 min *(38)*. When experimental or diagnostic circumstances indicate inactivation by heat, we incubate aqueous suspensions of the organism at 80°C for 1 h.

γ-irradiation can be an effective method to sterilize biological preparations *(162)*. Crucial to the decision of whether samples will be sterilized by γ-irradiation without degradation are considerations of dose, temperature, complexity, and size of the genome, and nature of the suspending medium. Scott et al. *(163)* conducted experiments to determine the minimun lethal dose of γ-irradiation for *C. burnetii*. Virulent *C. burnetii*, either as a 50% yolk sack suspension or purified whole cells, was exposed to varying doses of γ-irradiation. Viability was assessed by amplifying any viable microorganisms in chick embro yolk sacs followed by seroconversion after injection into mice. The amount of γ-irradiation required to reduce infectivity by 90% was 8.9×10^4 rads for the yolk sac suspension and 6.4×10^4 rads for the purified specimen *(163)*. The sterilizing dose was calculated to be 6.6×10^5 rads. We use an irradiation dose of 2.1×10^6 rads for sterilizing serum samples.

An important consideration is that useful biological specimens are not degraded after activation by irradiation. γ-irradiation (1×10^6 rads) was shown to have very little effect on the antibody-binding capacity of *C. burnetii* antigen, on the antigen-binding capability of anti-*C. burnetii* antibody, on the morphological appearance of *C. burnetii* by electron microscopy, or on the distribution of a major surface antigen *(163)*.

5. CONCLUSION

Although many of the disease manifestations of *Coxiella* infection are mild, it is obvious that this organism is nonetheless a very definite biothreat when considering intentional release. It has potential, especially in a cocktail with a Category A agent such as anthrax, to significantly confuse and complicate the response to an outbreak, and would undoubtedly heighten terror. Because of its high infectivity and exterior stability, it would make a logical copartner for a formidable release. Given our present population profile in the United States, a significant proportion, perhaps as high as 20%, would probably suffer moderate to severe manifestations 2–4 wk after inhaling as few as 10 organisms. Its inclusion in a release, as a dehydrated embryonated egg slurry would not be difficult to attain. Another aspect that must be considered, but for which no data are present, is the effect of Q fever disease on a concomitant anthrax infection and intoxication within the same patient. Would underlying Q fever lower the human LD_{50} for anthrax? It is not believable that the organism's effects would be insignificant in such a combination. Because this organism is not hard to grow in embryonated eggs, and in bulk form is stable perhaps indefinitely in ultracold freezers, its co-use in any intentional aerosol release by organized terrorists should be anticipated. It is fortunate that *Coxiella's* antibiotic susceptibilities are likely to make it treatable with the same regimen of antimicrobials that are deemed efficacious for anthrax.

What specific measures would succeed in adding to our abilities for managing Q fever outbreaks, be they intentional or natural? It is clear that we need much better diagnostics, especially in the DNA-based approaches. The Trans PCR is still done as a conventional, gel-based assay in most labs. A second area needing exploitation is much better culture methods for *Coxiella,* because a means of assessing the presence and quantity of viable organisms is essential for managing this disease. New methods that assess for viable cells and process large numbers of samples much more rapidly are needed. It is likely that a better understanding of the organism's metabolic pathways, its recently deleted or decayed genes, and its pathogenic qualities will be forthcoming from the TIGR genome study *(127)*. And, in turn, this increased understanding may lead to breakthroughs in culture, detection, and treatment.

ACKNOWLEDGMENTS

The authors dedicate this review to the memory of Louis Mallavia, (Washington State University, 1967–1998), whose contributions to Q fever research continue to serve as a beacon for all of us still engaged with this fascinating and difficult organism. We would like to thank the Bioterrorism Preparedness and Response Program for support to H.A. Thompson.

REFERENCES

1. Derrick, E. H. (1937) Q fever, a new entity: clinical features, diagnosis and laboratory investigations. *Med. J. Aust.* **2,** 281–299.
2. Marmion, B. P. (1999) Q fever; Your questions answered: MediMedia Communications and CSL limited. 32pp.
3. Dyer, R. E. (1938) A filter-passing infectious agent isolated from ticks. IV. Human infection. *Public Health Rep.* **53,** 2277–2283.
4. Davis, G. and Cox, H. (1938) A filter-passing infectious agent isolated from ticks. I. Isolation from Dermacentor andersoni, reactions in animals, and filtration experiments. *Public Health Rep.* **53,** 2259–2267.
5. Cox, H. (1938) A filter-passing infectious agent isolated from ticks. III. Description of organism and cultivation experiments. *Public Health Rep.* **53,** 2270–2276.
6. Cox, H. R. and Bell, E. J. (1939) The cultivation of Rickettsia diaporica in tissue culture and in tissues of developing chick embryos. *Public Health Rep.* **54,** 2171–2178.
7. Burnet, F. M. and Freeman, M. (1937) Experimental studies on the virus of "Q" fever. *Med. J. Aust.* **2,** 299–305.

8. Cox, H. R. (1939) Studies of a filter-passing infectious agent isolated from ticks. V. Further attempts to cultivate in cell-free media. Suggested classification. *Public Health Rep.* **54,** 1822–1827.

9. Derrick, E. H. (1939) *Rickettsia burnetii*: the cause of "Q" fever. *Med. J. Aust.* **1,** 14.

10. Philip, C. B. (1948) Comments on the name of the Q fever organism. *Public Health Rep.* **63,** 58.

11. Huebner, R. J. (1947) Report of an outbreak of Q fever at the National Institute of Health. II. Epidemiological features. *Am. J. Public Health* **37,** 431–440.

12. Spicknall, C. G., Huebner, R. J., Finger, J. A., and Blocker, W. P. Report of an outbreak of Q fever at the National Institute of Health. I. Clinical features.

13. Topping, N. H, Shephard, C. C., and Irons, J. V. (1947) Epidemiolgic studies of an outbreak among stock handlers and slaughterhouse workers. *JAMA* **133,** 813–815.

14. Cox, H. R. (1941) Cultivation of rickettsiae of the Rocky Mountain spotted fever, typhus and Q fever groups in the embryonic tissues of developing chicks. *Science* **94,** 399–403.

15. Luoto, L. and Huebner, R. J. (1950) Q fever studies in Southern California. IX. Isolation of Q fever organisms from parturient placentas of naturally infected dairy cows. *Public Health Rep.* **65,** 541–544.

16. Welsh, H. H., Lennette, E. H., Abinanti, F. R., and Winn, J. F. Q fever in California. IV. Occurrence of *Coxiella burnetii* in the placenta of naturally infected sheep. *Public Health Rep.* **66,** 1473–1477.

17. Waag, D. M., Williams, J. C., Peacock, M. G., and Raoult, D. (1991) Methods for isolation, amplification, and purification of *Coxiella burnetii*, in *Q fever: The Biology of Coxiella burnetii.* (Williams, J. C. and Thompson, H. A., eds.), CRC, Boca Raton, FL, pp. 73–115.

18. Thompson, H. A. (1988) Relationship of the physiology and composition of *Coxiella burnetii* to the Coxiella-host cell interaction, in *Biology of Rickettsial Diseases.* Vol. II. (Walker, D. H., ed.), CRC, Boca Raton, FL, pp. 51–78.

19. Raoult, D., Vestris, G., and Enea, M. (1990) Isolation of 16 strains of *Coxiella burnetii* from patients by using a sensitive centrifugation cell culture system and establishment of the strains in HEL cells. *J. Clin. Microbiol.* **28,** 2482–2484.

20. Musso, D. and Raoult, D. (1995) *Coxiella burnetii* blood cultures from acute and chronic Q-fever patients. *J. Clin. Microbiol.* **33,** 3129–3132.

21. Schramek, S. and Mayer, H. (1982) Different sugar compositions of lipopolysaccharides isolated from phase I and pure phase II cells of *Coxiella burnetii. Infect. Immun.* **38,** 53–57.

22. Amano, K. and Williams, J. C. (1984) Chemical and immunological characterization of lipopolysaccharides from phase I and phase II *Coxiella burnetii. J. Bacteriol. 160,* 994–1002.

23. Stoker, M. G. P. and Fiset, P. (1956) Phase variation of the Nine Mile and other strains of *Rickettsia burnetii. Can. J. Microbiol.* **2,** 310–321.

24. Moos, A. and Hackstadt, T. (1987) Comparative virulence of intra- and interstrain lipopolysaccharide variants of *Coxiella burnetii* in the guinea pig model. *Infect. Immun.* **55,** 1144–1150.

25. Schramek, S., Radziejewska-Lebrecht, J., and Mayer, H. (1985) 3-C-branched aldoses in lipopolysaccharide of phase I *Coxiella burnetii* and their role as immunodominant factors. *Eur. J. Biochem.* **148,** 455–461.

26. Amano, K., Williams, J. C., Missler, S. R., and Reinhold, V. N. (1987) Structure and biological relationships of *Coxiella burnetii* lipopolysaccharides. *J. Biol. Chem.* **262,** 4740–4747.

27. Zuber, M., Hoover, T. A., and Court, D. L. (1995) Analysis of a *Coxiella burnetti* gene product that activates capsule synthesis in *Escherichia coli*: requirement for the heat shock chaperone DnaK and the two-component regulator RcsC. *J. Bacteriol.* **177,** 4238–4244.

28. McCaul, T. F. and Williams, J. C. (1981) Developmental cycle of *Coxiella burnetii*: structure and morphogenesis of vegetative and sporogenic differentiations. *J. Bacteriol.* **147,** 1063–1076.

29. Samuel, J. E. (2000) Developmental cycle of *Coxiella burnetii*, in *Procaryotic Development.* (Brun, Y. V. and Shimkets, L. J., eds.), ASM, Washinton, DC, pp. 427–440.

30. Seshadri, R., Hendrix, L. R., and Samuel, J. E. (1999) Differential expression of translational elements by life cycle variants of *Coxiella burnetii*. *Infect. Immun.* **67,** 6026–6033.

31. Heinzen, R. A. and Hackstadt, T. (1996) A developmental stage-specific histone H1 homolog of *Coxiella burnetii*. *J. Bacteriol.* **178,** 5049–5052.

32. Hackstadt, T., Baehr, W., and Ying, Y. (1991) Chlamydia trachomatis developmentally regulated protein is homologous to eukaryotic histone H1. *Proc. Natl. Acad. Sci. USA* **88,** 3937–3941.

33. Heinzen, R. A., Howe, D., Mallavia, L. P., Rockey, D. D., and Hackstadt, T. (1996) Developmentally regulated synthesis of an unusually small, basic peptide by *Coxiella burnetii*. *Mol. Microbiol.* **22,** 9–19.

34. McCaul, T. F., Banerjee-Bhatnagar, N., and Williams, J. C. (1991) Antigenic differences between *Coxiella burnetii* cells revealed by postembedding immunoelectron microscopy and immunoblotting. *Infect. Immun.* **59,** 3243–3253.

35. Samuel, J. E., Kiss, K., and Varghees, S. (2003) Molecular pathogenesis of *Coxiella burnetii* in a genomics era. *Ann. NY Acad. Sci.* **990,** 653–673.

36. Heinzen, R. A., Hackstadt, T., and Samuel, J. E. (1999) Developmental Biology of *Coxiella burnetii*. *Trends Microbiol.* **7,** 149–154.

37. Scott, G. H. and Williams, J. C. Susceptibility of *Coxiella burnetii* to chemical disinfectants. *Ann. NY Acad. Sci.* **590,** 291–296.

38. Ransom, S. E. and Huebner, R. J. (1951) Studies on the resistance of *Coxiella burnetii* to chemical and physical agents. *Am. J. Hyg.* **53,** 110–119.

39. Enright, J. B., Sadler, W. W., and Thomas, R. C. Thermal inactivation of *Coxiella burnetii* and its relation to the pasteurization of milk. Public Health Service Publication No. 517, Public Health Reports. Vol. 72, No. 10. Washington, DC, United States Government Printing Office (Public Health Monograph No. 47), 30pp.

40. Donahue, J. P. and Thompson, H. A. (1980) Protein synthesis in cell-free extracts of *Coxiella burnetii*. *J. Gen. Microbiol.* **121,** 293–302.

41. Hackstadt, T. and Williams, J. C. (1981) Biochemical stratagem for obligate parasitism of eukaryotic cells by *Coxiella burnetii*. *Proc. Natl. Acad. Sci. USA* **78,** 3240–3244.

42. Thompson, H. A. (1991) Metabolism in *Coxiella burnetii*, in *Q-Fever: The Biology of Coxiella burnetii*. (Williams, J. C. and Thompson, H. A., eds.), CRC, Boca Raton, FL, pp. 131–156.

43. Kosatsky, T. (1984) Household outbreak of Q-fever pneumonia related to a parturient cat. *Lancet* **2,** 1447–1449.

44. Langley, J. M., Marrie, T. J., Covert, A., Waag, D. M., and Williams, J. C. (1988) Poker players' pneumonia. An urban outbreak of Q fever following exposure to a parturient cat. *N. Engl. J. Med.* **319,** 354–356.

45. Laughlin, T., Waag, D., Williams, J., and Marrie, T. (1991) Q fever: from deer to dog to man. *Lancet* **337,** 676, 677.

46. Pinsky, R. L., Fishbein, D. B., Greene, C. R., and Gensheimer, K. F. (1991) An outbreak of cat-associated Q fever in the United States. *J. Infect. Dis.* **164,** 202–204.

47. Baca, O. G. and Paretsky, D. (1983) Q fever and *Coxiella burnetii*: a model for host-parasite interactions. *Microbiol. Rev.* **47,** 127–149.

48. Welsh, H. H., Lennette, E. H., Abinanti, F. R., and Winn, J. F. (1958) Air-borne transmission of Q fever: the role of parturition in the generation of infective aerosols. *Ann. NY Acad. Sci.* **70,** 528–540.

49. DeLay, P. D., Lennette, E. H., and Deome, K. B. (1959) Q fever in California. II. Recovery of *Coxiella burnetii* from naturally infected airborne dust. *J. Immunol.* **65,** 211–220.
50. Lennette, E. H. and Welsh, H. H. (1951) Q fever in California. X. Recovery of *Coxiella burnetii* from the air of premises harboring infected goats. *Am. J. Hyg.* **54,** 44–49.
51. Marrie, T. J. (1990) Epidemiology of Q fever, in *Q Fever: The Disease.* Vol. 1. (Marrie, T. J., ed.), CRC, Boca Raton, FL, pp. 49–70.
52. Huebner, R. J., Jellison, W. L., Beck, M. D., Parker, R. R., and Shepard, C. C. (1948) Q fever studies in Southern California. I. Recovery of Rickettsia burneti from raw milk. *Public Health Rep.* **63,** 214–222.
53. Tigertt, W. D., Benenson, A. S., and Gochenour, W. S. (1961) Airborne Q fever. *Bacteriol. Rev.* **25,** 285–293.
53a. Marrie, T. J., Stein, A., Janigan, D., and Raoult, D. (1996) Route of infection determines the clinical manifestations of acute Q fever. *J. Infect. Dis.* **173,** 484–487.
54. Fishbein, D. B. and Raoult, D. (1992) A cluster of *Coxiella burnetii* infections associated with exposure to vaccinated goats and their unpasteurized dairy products. *Am. J. Trop. Med. Hyg.* **47,** 35–40.
55. Marrie, T. J., Durant, H., Williams, J. C., Mintz, E., and Waag, D. M. (1988) Exposure to parturient cats: a risk factor for acquisition of Q fever in Maritime Canada. *J. Infect. Dis.* **158,** 101–108.
56. Hendrix, L. R., Samuel, J. E., and Mallavia, L. P. (1991) Differentiation of *Coxiella burnetii* isolates by analysis of restriction-endonuclease-digested DNA separated by SDS-PAGE. *J. Gen. Microbiol.* **137(Pt 2),** 269–276.
57. Samuel, J. E., Frazier, M. E., and Mallavia, L. P. (1985) Correlation of plasmid type and disease caused by *Coxiella burnetii. Infect. Immun.* **49,** 775–779.
58. Yu, X. and Raoult, D. (1994) Serotyping *Coxiella burnetii* isolates from acute and chronic Q fever patients by using monoclonal antibodies. *FEMS Microbiol. Lett.* **117,** 15–19.
59. (1986) Q fever among slaughterhouse workers—California. *Morbd. Mortal. Wkly. Rep.* **35,** 223–226.
60. McIntire, M. S., Wiebelhaus, H. A., and Youngstown, J. A. (1958) Serological survey of packaging house workers in Omaha for Q fever. *Nebr. Med.* **43,** 206–209.
61. Pavilanis, V., Duval, L., and Faley, R. A. (1958) An epidemic of Q fever at Princeville, Quebec. *Can. J. Public Health* **49,** 520–529.
62. Rauch, A. M., Tanner, M., Pacer, R. E., Barrett, M. J., Brokopp, C. D., Schonberger, L. B. (1987) Sheep-associated outbreak of Q fever. Idaho. *Arch. Intern. Med.* **147,** 341–344.
63. Sawyer, L. A., Fishbein, D. B., and McDade, J. E. (1987) Q fever: current concepts. *Rev. Infect. Dis.* **9,** 935–946.
64. Tigertt, W. D. and Benenson, A. S. (1956) Studies on Q fever in man. *Trans. Assoc. Am. Phys.* **69,** 98–104.
65. Derrick, E. H. (1973) The course of infection with *Coxiella burnetii. Med. J. Aust.* **1,** 1051–1057.
66. Marrie, T. J. (1990) Acute Q fever, in *Q Fever, The Disease.* Vol. 1. (Marrie, T. J., ed.), CRC, Boca Raton, FL, pp. 125–160.
67. Ferrante, M. A. and Dolan, M. J. (1993) Q fever meningoencephalitis in a soldier returning from the Persian Gulf War. *Clin. Infect. Dis.* **16,** 489–496.
68. Smith, D. L., Ayres, J. G., Blair, I., et al. (1993) A large Q fever outbreak in the West Midlands: clinical aspects. *Respir. Med.* **87,** 509–516.
69. Marrie, T. J. (1995) *Coxiella burnetii* (Q fever) pneumonia. *Clin. Infect. Dis.* **21(Suppl 3),** S253–264.
70. Fournier, P.-E., Marrie, T. J., and Raoult, D. (1998) Minireview: diagnosis of Q fever. *J. Clin. Microbiol.* **36,** 1823–1834.
71. Smith, D. L., Wellings, R., Walker, C., et al. (1991) The chest x-ray report in Q fever: a report on 69 cases from the 1989 West Midlands outbreak. *Br. J. Radiol.* **64,** 1101–1108.

72. Tselentis, Y., Gikas, A., Kofteridis, D., et al. (1995) Q fever in the Greek Island of Crete: epidemiologic, clinical, and therapeutic data from 98 cases. *Clin. Infect. Dis.* **20,** 1311–1316.

73. Heard, S. R., Ronalds, C. J., and Heath, R. B. (1985) *Coxiella burnetii* infection in immunocompromised patients. *J. Infect.* **11,** 15–18.

74. Raoult, D., Levy, P. Y., Dupont, H. T., et al. (1993) Q fever and HIV infection. *Aids 7,* 81–86.

75. Yebra, M., Marazuela, M., Albarran, F., and Moreno, A. (1988) Chronic Q fever hepatitis. *Rev. Infect. Dis.* **10,** 1229, 1230.

76. Ghassemi, M., Agger, W. A., Vanscoy, R. E., and Howe, G. B. (1999) Chronic sternal wound infection and endocarditis with *Coxiella burnetii. Clin. Infect. Dis.* **28,** 1249–1251.

77. Tobin, M. J., Cahill, N., Gearty, G., et al. (1982) Q fever endocarditis. *Am. J. Med.* **72,** 396–400.

78. Westlake, P., Price, L. M., Russell, M., and Kelly, J. K. (1987) The pathology of Q fever hepatitis. A case diagnosed by liver biopsy. *J. Clin. Gastroenterol.* **9,** 357–363.

79. Koster, F. T., Williams, J. C., and Goodwin, J. S. (1985) Cellular immunity in Q fever: specific lymphocyte unresponsiveness in Q fever endocarditis. *J. Infect. Dis.* **152,** 1283–1289.

80. Waag, D. M. and Williams, J. C. (1988) Immune modulation by *Coxiella burnetii*: characterization of a phase I immunosuppressive complex differentially expressed among strains. *Immunopharmacol. Immunotoxicol.* **10,** 231–260.

81. Williams, J. C. and Cantrell, J. L. (1982) Biological and immunological properties of *Coxiella burnetii* vaccines in C57BL/10ScN endotoxin-nonresponder mice. *Infect. Immun.* **35,** 1091–1102.

82. Koster, F. T., Williams, J. C., and Goodwin, J. S. (1985) Cellular immunity in Q fever: modulation of responsiveness by a suppressor T cell-monocyte circuit. *J. Immunol.* **135,** 1067–1072.

83. Mege, J. L., Maurin, M., Capo, C., and Raoult, D. (1997) *Coxiella burnetii*: the 'query' fever bacterium. A model of immune subversion by a strictly intracellular microorganism. *FEMS Microbiol. Rev.* **19,** 209–217.

84. Waag, D. M., Kende, M., Damrow, T. A., Wood, O. L., and Williams, J. C. (1990) Injection of inactivated phase I *Coxiella burnetii* increases non-specific resistance to infection and stimulates lymphokine production in mice. *Ann. NY Acad. Sci.* **590,** 203–214.

85. Capo, C., Zaffran, Y., Zugun, F., Houpikian, P., Raoult, D., J.L. M. (1996) Production of interleukin-10 and transforming growth factor beta by peripheral blood mononuclear cells in Q fever endocarditis. *Infect. Immun.* **64,** 4143–4147.

86. Perez-Fontan, M., Huarte, E., Tellez, A., Rodriguez-Carmona, A., Picazo, M. L., and Martinez-Ara, J. (1988) Glomerular nephropathy associated with chronic Q fever. *Am. J. Kidney Dis.* **11,** 298–306.

87. Akporiaye, E. T. and Baca, O. G. (1983) Superoxide anion production and superoxide dismutase and catalase activities in *Coxiella burnetii. J. Bacteriol.* **154,** 520–523.

88. Turco, J., Thompson, H. A., and Winkler, H. H. (1984) Interferon-gamma inhibits growth of *Coxiella burnetii* in mouse fibroblasts. *Infect. Immun.* **45,** 781–783.

89. Scott, G. H., Williams, J. C., and Stephenson, E. H. (1987) Animal models in Q fever: pathological responses of inbred mice to phase I *Coxiella burnetii. J. Gen. Microbiol.* **133(Pt 3),** 691–700.

90. Humphres, R. C. and Hinrichs, D. J. (1981) Role of antibody in *Coxiella burnetii* infection. *Infect. Immun.* **31,** 641–645.

91. Kishimoto, R. A., Rozmiarek, H., and Larson, E. W. (1978) Experimental Q fever infection in congenitally athymic nude mice. *Infect. Immun.* **22,** 69–71.

92. Smadel, J. E., Snyder, M. J., and Robins, F. C. (1948) Vaccination against Q fever. *Am. J. Hyg.* **47,** 71–78.

93. Ormsbee, R. A., Bell, E. J., Lackman, D. B., and Tallent, G. (1964) The influence of phase on the protective potency of Q fever vaccine. *J. Immunol.* **92,** 404–412.

94. Fiset, P. (1956) Vaccination against Q fever. First international conference on vaccines against viral and rickettsial diseases, 1956. Vol. 147. Pan American Health Organization, Washington DC.

95. Stoker, M. G. P. (1957) Q fever down the drain. *Br. Med. J.* **1,** 425–427.

96. Bell, F. J., Lackman, D. B., Meis, A., and Hadlow, W. J. (1964) Recurrent reaction at site of Q fever vaccination in a sensitized person. *Milit. Med.* **124,** 591–595.

97. Benenson, A. S. (1959) Q fever vaccine: efficacy and present status, in *Med Sci Pub No. 6.* (Smadel, J. E., ed.), US Government Printing Office, Washington, DC, pp. 47–60.

98. Lackman, D. B., Bell, E. J., Bell, J. F., and Picken, E. G. (1962) Intradermal sensitivity testing in man with a purified vaccine for Q fever. *Am. J. Public Health* **52,** 87–93.

99. Ackland, J. R., Worswick, D. A., and Marmion, B. P. (1994) Vaccine prophylaxis of Q fever. A follow-up study of the efficacy of Q-Vax (CSL) 1985-1990. *Med. J. Aust.* **160,** 704–708.

100. Ormsbee, R. A., Bell, E. J., and Lackman, D. B. (1962) Antigens of *Coxiella burnetii.* I. Extraction of antigens with nonaqueous organic solvents. *J. Immunol.* **88,** 741–749.

101. Brezina, R. and Urvolgyi, I. (1961) Extraction of *Coxiella burnetii* phase I antigen by means of trichloracetic acid. *Acta Virol.* **5,** 193.

102. Genig, V. A. (1968) A live vaccine 1/M-44 against Q fever for oral use. *J. Hyg. Epidemiol. Microbiol. Immunol.* **12,** 265–273.

103. Johnson, J. W., McLeod, C. G., Stookey, J. L., Higbee, G. A., Pedersen, C. E., Jr. (1977) Lesions in guinea pigs infected with *Coxiella burnetii* strain M-44. *J. Infect. Dis.* **135,** 995–998.

104. Waag, D., Chulay, J., Marrie, T., England, M., and Williams, J. (1995) Validation of an enzyme immunoassay for serodiagnosis of acute Q fever. *Eur. J. Clin. Microbiol. Infect. Dis.* **14,** 421–427.

105. Williams, J. C., Damrow, T. A., Waag, D. M., and Amano, K. (1986) Characterization of a phase I *Coxiella burnetii* chloroform-methanol residue vaccine that induces active immunity against Q fever in C57BL/10 ScN mice. *Infect. Immun.* **51,** 851–858.

106. Waag, D. M., England, M. J., and Pitt, M. L. (1997) Comparative efficacy of a *Coxiella burnetii* chloroform:methanol residue (CMR) vaccine and a licensed cellular vaccine (Q-Vax) in rodents challenged by aerosol. *Vaccine* **15,** 1779–1783.

107. Brooks, D. L., Ermel, R. W., Franti, C. E., et al. (1986) Q fever vaccination of sheep: challenge of immunity in ewes. *Am. J. Vet. Res.* **47,** 1235–1238.

108. Waag, D. M., England, M. J., Tammariello, R. F., et al. (2002) Comparative efficacy and immunogenicity of Q fever chloroform:methanol residue (CMR) and phase I cellular (Q-Vax) vaccines in cynomolgus monkeys challenged by aerosol. *Vaccine* **20,** 2623–2634.

109. Dupuis, G., Peter, O., Peacock, M., Burgdorfer, W., and Haller, E. (1985) Immunoglobulin responses in acute Q fever. *J. Clin. Microbiol.* **22,** 484–487.

110. Peacock, M. G., Philip, R. N., Williams, J. C., and Faulkner, R. S. (1983) Serological evaluation of O fever in humans: enhanced phase I titers of immunoglobulins G and A are diagnostic for Q fever endocarditis. *Infect. Immun.* **41,** 1089–1098.

111. Dupuis, G., Peter, O., Luthy, R., Nicolet, J., Peacock, M., and Burgdorfer, W. (1986) Serological diagnosis of Q fever endocarditis. *Eur. Heart J.* **7,** 1062–1066.

112. Peter, O., Dupuis, G., Burgdorfer, W., and Peacock, M. (1985) Evaluation of the complement fixation and indirect immunofluorescence tests in the early diagnosis of primary Q fever. *Eur. J. Clin. Microbiol.* **4,** 394–396.

113. Williams, J. C., Thomas, L. A., and Peacock, M. G. (1986) Humoral immune response to Q fever: enzyme-linked immunosorbent assay antibody response to *Coxiella burnetii* in experimentally infected guinea pigs. *J. Clin. Microbiol.* **24,** 935–939.

114. Uhaa, I. J., Fishbein, D. B., Olson, J. G., Rives, C. C., Waag, D. M., and Williams, J. C. (1994) Evaluation of specificity of indirect enzyme-linked immunosorbent assay for diagnosis of human Q fever. *J. Clin. Microbiol.* **32,** 1560–1565.

115. Roges, G. and Edlinger, E. (1986) Immunoenzymatic test for Q-fever. *Diag. Microbiol. Infect. Dis.* **4,** 125–132.

116. Dupont, H. T., Thirion, X., and Raoult, D. (1994) Q fever serology: cutoff determination for microimmunofluorescence. *Clin. Diagn. Lab. Immunol.* **1,** 189–196.

117. Hunt, J. G., Field, P. R., and Murphy, A. M. (1983) Immunoglobulin responses to *Coxiella burnetii* (Q fever): single-serum diagnosis of acute infection, using an immunofluorescence technique. *Infect. Immun.* **39,** 977–981.

118. Field, P. R., Hunt, J. G., and Murphy, A. M. (1983) Detection and persistence of specific IgM antibody to *Coxiella burnetii* by enzyme-linked immunosorbent assay: a comparison with immunofluorescence and complement fixation tests. *J. Infect. Dis.* **148,** 477–487.

119. Behymer, D. E., Ruppanner, R., Brooks, D., Williams, J. C., and Franti, C. E. (1985) Enzyme immunoassay for surveillance of Q fever. *Am. J. Vet. Res.* **46,** 2413–2417.

120. Embil, J., Williams, J. C., and Marrie, T. J. (1990) The immune response in a cat-related outbreak of Q fever as measured by the indirect immunofluorescence test and the enzyme-linked immunosorbent assay. *Can. J. Microbiol.* **36,** 292–296.

121. Guigno, D., Coupland, B., Smith, E. G., Farrell, I. D., Desselberger, U., and Caul, E. O. (1992) Primary humoral antibody response to *Coxiella burnetii*, the causative agent of Q fever. *J. Clin. Microbiol.* **30,** 1958–1967.

122. Peter, O., Dupuis, G., Peacock, M. G., and Burgdorfer, W. (1987) Comparison of enzyme-linked immunosorbent assay and complement fixation and indirect fluorescent-antibody tests for detection of *Coxiella burnetii* antibody. *J. Clin. Microbiol.* **25,** 1063–1067.

123. *Bergey's Manual of Systematic Bacteriology.* 2nd Ed. Vol. I. (2001) Boone, D. R. and Costenholz, R., eds. Taxonomie Outline of the Archaea and Bacteria. pp. 157–160.

124. Weisburg, W. G., Dobson, M. E., Samuel, J. E., et al. (1989) Phylogenetic diversity of the Rickettsiae. *J. Bacteriol.* **171,** 4202–4206.

125. Afseth, G. and Mallavia, L. P. (1997) Copy number of the 16S rRNA gene in *Coxiella burnetii. Eur. J. Epidemiol.* **13,** 729–731.

126. Tyerar, F., Weiss, E., Millar, D., Bozeman, F., and Ormsbee, R. A. (1973) DNA base composition of rickettsia. *Science* **180,** 415–417.

127. Seshadri, S., Paulsen, I. T., Eisen, J. A., et al. (2003) The complete genome sequence of the Q-fever pathogen *Coxiella burnetii. Proc. Natl. Acad. Sci. USA* **100,** 5455–5460.

128. Willems, H., Jager, C., and Baljer, G. (1998) Physical and genetic map of the obligate intracellular bacterium *Coxiella burnetii. J. Bacteriol.* **180,** 3816–3822.

129. Hoover, T. A., Culp, D., Vodkin, M. H., Williams, J. C., and Thompson, H. A. (2002) Chromosomal deletions explain phenotypic characteristics of phase II and RSA 514 (crazy) *Coxiella burnetii* Nine Mile strains. *Infect. Immun.* **170,** 6726–6733.

130. Suhan, M., Chen, S.-Y., Thompson, H. A., Hoover, T. A., Hill, A., and Williams, J. C. (1994) Cloning and characterization of an autonomous replication sequence from *Coxiella burnetii. J. Bacteriol.* **176,** 5233–5243.

131. Suhan, M., Chen, S.-Y., and Thompson, H. A. (1996) Transformation of *Coxiella burnetii* to ampicillin resistance. *J. Bacteriol.* **178,** 2701–2708.

132. Thompson, H. A., Chen, S.-Y., Suhan, M. L., and Watson, V. (1999) Genetic transformation of *Coxiella burnetii:* origins, vectors, and recombination, in *Rickettsiae and Rickettsial Diseases at the Turn of the Third Millenium.* (Raoult, D. and Brouqui, P., eds.), Elsevier, Paris, pp. 74–91.

133. Samuel, J. E., Frazier, M. E., Kahn, M. L., Thomashow, L. S., and Mallavia, L. P. (1983) Isolation and characterization of a plasmid from phase I *Coxiella burnetii. Infect. Immun.* **41,** 488–493.

134. Thiele, D., Willems, H., Haas, M., and Krauss, H. (1994) Analysis of the entire nucleotide sequence of the cryptic plasmid QpH1 from *Coxiella burnettii. Eur. J. Epidemiol.* **10,** 413–420.

135. Willems, H., Lautenschlager, S., Radomski, K. U., Jager, C., and Baljer, G. (1999) Coxiella burnetii plasmid types, in *Rickettsiae and Rickettsial Diseases at the Turn of the Third Millenium.* (Raoult, D. and Brouqui, P., eds.), Elsevier, Paris, pp. 92–102.

136. Lautenschlager, S., Willems, H., Jager, C., and Baljer, G. (2000) Sequencing and characterization of the cryptic plasmid QpRS from *Coxiella burnetii. Plasmid* **44,** 85–88.

137. Savinelli, E. A. and Mallavia, L. P. (1990) Comparison of *Coxiella burnetii* plasmids to homologous chromosomal sequences present in a plasmidless endocarditis-causing isolate. *Ann. NY Acad. Sci.* **590,** 523–533.

138. Willems, H., Ritter, M., Jager, C., and Thiele, D. (1997) Plasmid-homologous sequences in the chromosome of plasmidless *Coxiella burnetii* Scurry Q217. *J. Bacteriol.* **179,** 3293–3297.

139. Lin, Z. and Mallavia, L. P. (1994) Identification of a partition region carried by the plasmid QpH1 of *Coxiella burnetii. Mol. Microbiol.* **13,** 513–523.

140. Lin, Z., Howe, D., and Mallavia, L. P. (1995) Roa307, a protein encoded on *Coxiella burnetii* plasmid QpH1, shows homology to proteins encoded in the replication origin region of bacterial chromosomes. *Mol. Gen. Genet.* **248,** 487–490.

141. Vodkin, M. H. and Williams, J. C. (1986) Overlapping deletion in two spontaneous phase variants of *Coxiella burnetii. J. Gen. Microbiol.* **132(Pt 9),** 2587–2594.

142. Harris, R. J., Storm, P. A., Lloyd, A., Arens, M., and Marmion, B. P. (2000) Long-term persistence of *Coxiella burnetii* in the host after primary Q fever. *Epidemiol. Infect.* **124,** 543–549.

143. Frazier, M., Mallavia, L., Samuel, J., and Baca, G. (1990) DNA probes for the identification of *Coxiella burnetii* strains, in *Rickettsiology: Current Issues and Perspectives.* (Hechemy, K., Paretsky, D., Walker, D., and Mallavia, L., eds.). *Ann. NY Acad. Sci.* **590,** 445–458.

144 Mallavia, L. P., Whiting, L. L., Minnick, M. F., Heinzen, R., Reschke, D., Foreman, M., Baca. O. G., et al. (1990) Strategy for detection and differentiation of *Coxiella burnetii* strains using the polymerase chain reaction, in *Rickettsiology: Current Issues and Perspectives.* (Hechemy, K., Paretsky, D., Walker, D., and Mallavia, L., eds.). *Ann. NY Acad. Sci.* **590,** 572–581.

145 Stein, A. and Raoult, D. (1992) Detection of *Coxiella burnetii* by DNA amplification using polymerase chain reaction. *J. Clin. Microbiol.* **30,** 2462–2466.

146 Willems, H., Thiele, D., Frolich-Ritter, R., and Krauss, H. (1994) Detection of *Coxiella burnetii in* cow's milk using the polymerase chain reaction (PCR). *J. Vet. Med. B.* **41,** 580–587.

147 Thiele, D. and Willems, H. (1994) Is plasmid based differentiation of *Coxiella burnetii* in 'acute' and 'chronic' isolates still valid? *Eur. J. Epidemiol.* **10,** 427–434.

148 Thiele, D., Willems, H., and Krauss, H. (1994) The 16S/23S ribosomal spacer region of *Coxiella burnetii. Eur. J. Epidemiol.* **10,** 421–426.

149. Yuasa, Y., Yoshiie, K., Tkasaki, T., Yoshida, H., and Oda, H. (1996) Retrospective survey of chronic Q fever in Japan by using PCR to detect *Coxiella burnetii* DNA in paraffin-embedded clinical samples. *J. Clin. Microbiol.* **34,** 824–827

150. Lorenz, H., Jager, C., Willems, H., and Baljer, G. (1998) PCR detection of *Coxiella burnetii* from different clinical specimens, especially bovine milk, on the basis of DNA preparation with silica matrix. *App. Env. Microbiol.* **64,** 4234–4237.

151 Zhang, G., Nguyen, S., To, H., Ogawa, M., Hotta, A., Yamaguchi, T., Kim, H., et al. (1998) Clinical evaluation of a new PCR assay for detection of *Coxiella burnetii* in human serum samples. *J. Clin. Microbiol.* **36,** 77–80.

152. Nguyen, S. V. and Hirai, K. (1999) Differentiation of *Coxiella burnetii* isolates by sequence determination and PCR-restriction fragment length polymorphism analysis of isocitrate dehydrogenase gene. *FEMS Microbiol. Lett.* **180,** 249–254.

153. Berri, M., Laroucau, K., and Rodolakis, A. (2000) The detection of *Coxiella burnetii* from ovine genital swabs, milk and fecal samples by the use of a single touchdown polymerase chain reaction. *Vet. Microbiol.* **72,** 285–293.

154. Fournier, P.-E., Marrie, T. J., Raoult, D. (1998) Diagnosis of Q fever. *J. Clin. Microbiol.* **36,** 1823–1834.

155. Rustscheff, S., Norlander, L., Macellaro, A., Sjosted, A., Vene, S., and Carlsson, M. (2000) A case of fever acquired in Sweden and isolation of the probable etiological agent, *Coxiella burnetii* from an indigenous source. *Scand. J. Infect. Dis.* **32,** 605–607.

156. Raoult, D., Torres, H., and Drancourt, M. (1991) Shell vial assay: evaluation of a new technique for determining antibiotic susceptibility, tested in 13 isolates of *Coxiella burnetii. Antimicrob. Agents Chemother.* **35,** 2070–2077.

157. Office Intenational Des Epizooties, Manual of Standards, Diagnostic Tests and Vaccines 2000; Part 3, Q Fever. 4th edition.

158. Gimenez, D. F. (1964) Staining rickettsiae in yolk sac cultures. *Stain Technol.* **39,** 135–140.

159. Ormsbee, R. A. (1970) Q fever rickettsia, in *Viral and Rickettsial Infections of Man.* (Horsfall, F. L. and Tamm, I., eds.), J.B. Lippincott, Philadelphia, PA, pp. 1144–1160.

160. Babudieri, B. (1959) Q fever: a zoonosis. *Adv. Vet. Sci.* **5,** 81–182.

161. Malloch, R. A. and Stoker, M. G. P. (1952) Studies on the susceptibility of *Rickettsia burnetii* to chemical disinfectants, and on techniques for detecting small numbers of viable organisms. *J. Hyg.* **50,** 502–514.

162. Jordan, R. T. and Kempe, L. L. (1956) Inactivation of some animal viruses with gamma irradiation from cobalt-60. *Proc. Soc. Exp. Biol. Med.* **91,** 212–215.

163. Scott, G. H., McCaul, T. F., and Williams, J. C. (1989) Inactivation of *Coxiella burnetii* by gamma irradiation. *J. Gen. Microbiol.* **135(Pt 12),** 3263–3270.

10

Glanders

New Insights Into an Old Disease

David M. Waag and David DeShazer

1. BACKGROUND

Glanders is a disease of antiquity, although occasional cases can still be found. This disease is naturally found in equines, who occasionally transmit the infection to humans *(1)*. Glanders is one of the oldest diseases ever described. Disease symptoms were recorded by Hippocrates around the year 425 BC, and the disease was given the name "melis" by Aristotle in approx 350 BC. Glanders is suggested as the cause of the sixth plague of Egypt, as described in the Bible *(2)*. However, this disease was not studied in a systematic matter until the early part of the 19th century. Through much of recorded history, glanders has been a world problem. Because of the serious problem posed by glanders in the French cavalry horses, the first veterinary school was established by King Louis XV at Lyons, France, in the mid-1800s. Unfortunately, many early investigators became infected during the course of their studies and died of glanders *(3)*.

Up until the early 20th century, horses and mules were vital means of transportation. These animals, on occasion, were housed under crowded conditions and the contagion of glanders was passed from infected to uninfected animals. As an example, during the American Civil War, thousands of horses on both the Union and Confederate sides were corralled at remount stations and glanders was found in epidemic proportions. Interestingly, there were no recorded simultaneous epidemics of human glanders. After the Civil War, horses that were no longer needed were sold by the Army to civilians at bargain prices, and glanderous horses were dispersed to become sources of infection. At this time, the etiologic agent of glanders was unknown and would not be discovered for another 17 yr. In 1882, the causative agent *Burkholderia mallei* was isolated from the liver and spleen of a glanderous horse by Loeffler and Schutz in Germany *(4–6)*. Only when horses were replaced by motorized transport in the early 20th century did the incidence of glanders decrease. Factors that eliminated glanders in the Western world were the development of an effective skin test and a process of identification and slaughter of infected animals. These control measures finally led to the eradication of glanders in the United States in 1934. The disease is now excluded from the United States by quarantine. Although developed nations are currently free of glanders, South

From: *Infectious Diseases: Biological Weapons Defense: Infectious Diseases and Counterterrorism*
Edited by: L. E. Lindler, F. J. Lebeda, and G. W. Korch © Humana Press Inc., Totowa, NJ

and Central America, the Middle East, and parts of the former Soviet Union have endemic foci of infection *(7)*.

B. mallei is a nonmotile, Gram-negative bacillus that is an obligate animal pathogen *(8)*, unlike the closely related *Burkholderia pseudomallei*, which can be isolated from tropical soil. Laboratory studies on this Category B pathogen *(9)* are performed at biosafety level 3. Although growth requirements for the organism are not complex, glycerol (4%) can be added to the medium to enhance growth. Since its discovery, this microorganism has been placed in several genera, including *Bacillus*, *Corynebacterium*, *Mycobacterium*, *Loefflerella*, *Pfeifferella*, *Malleomyces*, *Actinobacillus,* and *Pseudomonas (10)* and was placed in its current genus in 1992 *(11)*. In Gram stains, the cells characteristically exhibit bipolar staining. This microorganism is not particularly hardy in the environment. Although *B. mallei* can survive in contaminated tap water for up to 1 mo *(12)*, the bacteria normally die rapidly when dried or heated *(10)*.

2. DISEASE

2.1. Horses

B. mallei is an obligate animal pathogen, whose natural hosts are horses, donkeys, and mules *(11,13,14)*. However, many animal species can be infected naturally, including lions and dogs that are fed infected horse meat *(15)*, and experimentally, including mice, hamsters, guinea pigs, rabbits, and monkeys *(1)*. Although the primary route of equine infection is somewhat controversial, it is thought that horses are infected by eating feed or drinking water contaminated with the nasal discharges of infected animals *(16)*. Surprisingly, considering this route, the pathologic changes in the gut and associated lymphatic tissues are fewer than one would expect *(10)*. The major pathological changes occur in the lungs and airways of infected animals. The disease course can be acute or chronic, and the host factors dictating which form of the disease will occur are unknown. Generally, donkeys and mules develop the acute form of glanders, and horses become chronically infected.

Acute glanders is characterized by high fever, shivering, depression, and rapid emaciation *(17)*. There is ulceration of the nasal septum and turbinate bones with mucopurulent to hemorrhagic nasal discharge (called "snot" from the Dutch name for the disease). Submaxillary lymph nodes are swollen, lobulated, painless, and seldom rupture. Also noted are edema of the glottis and obstruction of the air passages by the nasal discharge. Nodules are distributed throughout the spleen, liver, and other internal organs. Diagnosis generally relies on the isolation of *B. mallei*, which is relatively numerous in affected tissues. Death as a result of bronchopneumonia and septicemia generally occurs within 3–4 wk.

Chronically infected horses generally display a long disease course with the cycle of symptoms worsening and then improving to where few outward symptoms are displayed. Clinical signs of chronic glanders may be categorized as nasal, pulmonary, and cutaneous *(17)*. Nasal symptoms include an intermittent cough, and a thick, mucopurulent chronic nasal discharge from one or both nostrils, with or without ulceration of the nasal septum. Pulmonary signs include lung lesions with a structure similar to a tubercle. Nodules are 0.5–1 cm in diameter, with a purulent center surrounded by epithelioid and giant cells *(18)*. Nodules can be found in other organs, especially the liver and spleen. The whole lesion may be encased in fibrous tissue. When clinical signs develop, they include intermittent cough, nasal discharge, and malaise. Nodules appear in the submucosa of the nasal cavity, particularly on the nasal septum and the turbinates. Lungs are invariably infected *(17)*. Thrombosis can be found in the large venous vessels of nasal mucous membranes *(19)*.

Chronic glanders also has a cutaneous form, known as farcy. In this disease, nodules form along the lymphatics between affected lymph nodes. Lymph vessels become thickened and nodules often ulcerate and rupture, discharging a thick exudate that may be a source of infection. Intermittent periods of healing and recrudescence may also occur in chronically infected animals. Most horses suffering from farcy also have glanders nodules in the lungs *(20)*. Poor diet, overwork, and lack of rest are factors that can cause a chronic infection to become acute, followed by the swift demise of the animal *(21)*. Attempts to isolate *B. mallei* from chronically infected animals are usually unsuccessful.

2.2. Humans

Humans are accidental hosts of *B. mallei*. The majority of natural cases have been the result of occupational contact with infected animals (stablemen, veterinarians, and slaughterhouse employees) *(10)*. Whereas equines are generally infected orally, the primary routes of infection in humans are by skin abrasions and the mucosae of the nose and lungs *(22)*. Because there have been no documented glanders epidemics in humans in spite of epidemics in horses, it can be surmized that *B. mallei* is much less infectious for humans in a natural setting *(23)*. The disease is not contagious, although human-to-human transmission has been reported *(24)*. The presence of glanders-associated nodules at autopsy among people who had contact with infected equines suggest that subclinical infection is not rare *(25)*. However, in a laboratory setting, this microorganism can be very infectious *(24,26–32)*. In a laboratory specially constructed for research on this organism, one-half of workers were infected within 1 yr *(29)*. Besides *Francisella tularensis*, *B. mallei* is regarded as the most dangerous microorganism to handle in the laboratory *(33)*. The organism may be far more infectious than its natural history would indicate, and clinical infections tend to be very serious. Laboratory-acquired infections have been by aerosol exposure and the cutaneous route and generally result in an acute glanders infection. Culturing the microorganism from infected patients is rare but can be accomplished during terminal stages of disease and in the presence of purulent cutaneous lesions.

Glanders in humans can have a varied clinical picture. The disease may present as an acute fulminating septicemia of sudden onset with a significant degree of prostration; an acute pulmonary infection with nasal mucopurulent discharge and pneumonia; an acute suppurative infection with multiple eruptions of the skin; a chronic suppurative infection characterized by remission and exacerbation; a latent infection characterized by recrudescence; and a subclinical infection consisting of encapsulated nodules, which are generally discovered at autopsy *(8,10,20,25)*. Cases of human glanders are equally divided between acute and chronic forms of disease. Symptoms associated with acute glanders consist of fever, malaise, myalgia, fatigue, inflammation, and swelling of the face and limbs and the development of painful nodules involving the face, arms, and legs *(23,34)*. These nodules develop into pustular eruptions of the skin. Physical findings on initial presentation are usually unremarkable but frequently include fever and splenomegaly. If the infection was by aerosol, chest radiographs characteristically show evidence of lung abscesses (22). The septicemic form of disease is usually fatal in 7–10 d, if untreated. In cases of aerosol-acquired glanders, an incubation period of 10–14 d is followed by fever, myalgia, fatigue, headache, chest pain, photophobia, and diarrhea. Chronic cases are characterized by coryza and multiple subcutaneous abscesses, enlarged lymph nodes, nodules which may ulcerate in respiratory and alimentary mucosa, necrotic foci in bones, and nodules in the viscera (18). Meningitis may develop in cases of chronic glanders (23). Patients may become symptomatic after apparent recovery. The disease may be active for months or years, but, without treatment, is almost always fatal. In the chronic form of the disease, the most frequent clinical finding is multiple abscesses in the SC and intramuscular areas, usually involving the arms or legs (8).

The lack of human glanders cases in recent times has, until recently, hampered a comprehensive clinical evaluation of this disease in humans. The clinical course of infection of patients infected by the cutaneous, nasal, and alimentary routes will be illustrated by case studies.

2.2.1. Cutaneous Route of Infection

In March 2000, a microbiologist was infected while working with *B. mallei* ATCC 23344 in the laboratory (31,35). The patient presented with a painful enlarged axillary lymph node and was febrile (38.6°C). The infection was not controlled by cephalosporin treatment and the patient became increasingly fatigued, suffering from night sweats, malaise, rigors, and weight loss. One month after infection, symptoms resolved after a course of clarithromycin. Symptoms returned, 4 d after completion of the therapy, and the patient developed severe abdominal pain. Multiple blood cultures were negative for bacteria. A computerized tomography (CT) scan performed approx 2 mo after infection revealed multiple abscesses in the spleen and liver. The patient was hospitalized and given intravenous tobramycin and doxycycline. Aspiration of a liver lesion yielded small, Gram-negative bipolar-staining rods. By determining motility and performing cellular fatty acid analysis and 16S ribosomal sequencing, researchers identified the microorganism from the liver abscess as *B. mallei*. The patient was treated with imipenem and doxycycline and symptoms improved markedly. A repeat CT scan showed slight regression of the splenic and liver abscesses. The patient was discharged from the hospital and treated with oral doxycycline and azithromycin. Additional CT scans showed further resolution of the lesions in the spleen and liver. The disease was not spread to members of the patient's family, coworkers, or healthcare workers.

2.2.2. Nasal Route of Infection

In cases of aerosol-acquired glanders, reported by Kazantseva and Matkovskii in 1970, the incubation period ranged from 3 to 5 d. Symptoms included general intoxication, chills, temperature 39–40°C, dry cough, rhinitis, purulent rash on face, skin ulcers, muscle abscesses, and pneumonia (36). Sanford reported an incubation period of 10–14 d followed by fever, myalgia, fatigue, headache, chest pain, photophobia, and diarrhea (22). Pathological findings in the chronic suppurative form of the disease included multiple subcutaneous and im abscesses, often involving the arms or legs.

Almost 60 yr ago, there were six cases of human glanders in a US Army laboratory (29). Four individuals were exposed to a strain of relatively low virulence and two were exposed to a strain of higher virulence. These numbers represent almost 50% of workers in that laboratory. The low virulence strain was being washed from agar plates during the preparation of vaccines and presumably the workers were infected by the aerosol route. The strain of higher virulence was being grown in liquid culture with oxygen or air bubbled through the medium for aeration. On one or two occasions, the containers were opened immediately after aeration ceased, presumably infecting the individuals. *B. mallei* was not isolated from any patient. Five of six patients developed a significant rise in their agglutinating titers and all the patients infected with the less virulent strain became positive by the complement fixation test. Five patients also responded positively after skin testing with mallein (0.1 mL of a 1:10,000 dilution of commercial mallein). Clinical laboratory analysis showed a persistent leukopenia and a relative lymphocytosis. Radiographs of four patients were similar, showing circular, well-defined, early lung abscesses. Lesions had the appearance of a diffuse and infiltrating pneumonitis in one patient infected with the more virulent *B. mallei* strain. Both patients infected with the more virulent strain complained of pain consistent with pleural irritation. All patients were treated with sulfadiazine for a course of 20 d. A single course of treatment proved insufficient in one patient infected with the lower virulence strain as symptoms reappeared and a second course was given. The earlier sulphadiazine treatment was initiated in these cases, the sooner regression of pulmonary lesions was noted.

2.2.3. Alimentary Route of Infection

In 1913, the first of two papers was published as a fascinating first-person account of glanders *(27)*. The route of infection was presumed to be oral, as the initial pain was abdominal, and the author had no recollection of accidental inoculation and no lesions of the respiratory tract were ever documented. The author, a veterinarian, acquired glanders after culturing abscess material from a horse and injecting cultured bacteria into a guinea pig. The first symptom noted was a severe headache and a temperature of 102°F followed in a few days by acute pain between the diaphragm and liver, which the author ascribed to the formation of adhesions in the peritoneal cavity. Also noted was pain in the intercostal mucsles on the right side. Three weeks after infection and after a slight blow to the left hand, a painful swelling and redness were noted and accompanied by a temperature of 102°F. Pus was obtained from the lesion and a bacillus was cultured. The patient noted lines of inflammation ascending the wrist and forearm, finally reaching the axilla. Over the next 3 mo, the patient endured several surgeries on his hand and forearm to drain and pack the lesions with disinfectant-soaked gauze. The patient was then given five doses of "vaccine" prepared from killed microorganisms, which had no positive effect. Four and one-half months after infection, the axillary area was surgically cleaned. However, the infection progressed from the wrist to the forearm and the left arm was amputated below the elbow 11.5 mo after the onset of disease in an effort to control the infection. Shortly after surgery, the author experienced a painful swelling of his right wrist and pain in his left ankle. Fourteen months after the original infection, the author was given 10 doses of "vaccine," which the author thought beneficial. In June 1913, almost 2 yr after contracting glanders, the last of the lesions healed. The author had undergone surgery 45 times. At the conclusion of his first report, the author states that he made a complete recovery.

Unfortunately, the recovery was not complete and a second paper recorded his continuing battle against glanders *(37)*. Reappearance of glanders 7 mo after the last attack coincided with an attack of malaria and lasted 21 mo. The initial lesion involved the shoulder, and progressed to the knee. Abscesses reoccurred on the extremities and head and the temperature reached 104°F. A feature of this second attack was bone necrosis, observed in seven bones. Numerous abscesses were surgically drained (37 operations) and the abscess cavities swabbed with antiseptic solutions. Hepatomegaly and splenomegaly were noted. Approximately 2 mo after reoccurrence of glanders, pain in the head, eyes, and nose required morphine. The left nostril began bleeding and large clots formed. Bleeding likely occurred from ulcers forming in the nasal mucosa. Abdominal pain and diarrhea were attributed by the author as the result of swallowing infected pus and exudate. Nine months after reappearance of glanders, the author was injected 12 times with escalating doses of a killed *B. mallei* "vaccine." The author stated that this procedure was ineffective. Two years were required to recover from this second bout of glanders.

2.3. Animal Models

One of the objectives of the US Army Medical Research Institute of Infectious Diseases (USAMRIID) glanders research program is to develop animal models for testing vaccines and therapeutics that simulate, as closely as possible, the disease seen in humans. We were aided in this endeavor by a prior study of the susceptibility of various animal species to glanders *(1)*. Goats, dogs, ferrets, moles, cats, and hamsters were found to be highly susceptible; monkeys, sheep, camels, and white mice were slightly susceptible; while cattle, hogs, rats, and birds were resistant.

Golden hamsters are a traditional animal model used to study glanders because of their uniform susceptibility to infection (LD_{50} approx 10 microorganisms when challenged intraperitoneally or by aerosol with the most virulent strains). Infection in hamsters is characterized by an acute sepsis and the development of exudative granulomas with pronounced necrosis *(38,39)*. Bacteria were found intra- and extracellularly in all tissues studied. Although no difference in susceptibility to infection could be correlated with sex of the hamster, adult male hamsters were sometimes preferred because of the development of the Strauss reaction, where the scrotal sac becomes enlarged because of peritonitis. Interestingly, in a study using BALB/c mice, investigators observed spheroplast-like structures in electron micrographs of impression smears made from liver, spleen, and lymph nodes. The involvement of spheroplasts in the persistence of glanders remains unclear. Destruction of the white pulp in the spleen could contribute to the host's inability to control infection. The authors hypothesized that persistence of these microorganisms in the cells of the reticuloendothelial system leads to granuloma formation, and disorders in protein (amyloidosis) and carbohydrate metabolism.

The virulence of the strain of *B. mallei* can affect the clinical presentation after infection *(1)*. Strains of low virulence tended to produce subacute or chronic forms of the disease, whereas strains of high virulence produced acute fulminating infections. Cultivating *B. mallei* in vitro for 1–3 mo resulted in a decrease in virulence, but one to two passages through hamsters restored full virulence. Guinea pigs were found to be variably susceptible to infection after intraperitoneal injection of 6.9×10^5 organisms, some animals becoming acutely infected, although others were chronically infected. However, the most virulent strains produced only acute glanders. Male guinea pigs inoculated intraperitoneally with *B. mallei* developed the Strauss reaction. Rabbits and white rats were resistant to infection with the organism. Although inbred mouse strains were not available at the time of the study, black and white mice were identified as intermediately susceptible, with a minimum lethal dose of 4.5×10^5.

Development of glanders in monkeys was also studied *(1)*. Six rhesus monkeys were given graded doses of the virulent *B. mallei* strain C4. The animal given the largest dose (1.5 million organisms, subcutaneously) developed an abscess at the site of inoculation 4 d after injection. The abscess was 2 cm in diameter, drained spontaneously after 4 d, and healed completely after 3 wk. During this time, there was a daily temperature elevation of 1–3°C, a rapid sedimentation rate, and a marked increase in the white blood cell count with a moderate relative lymphocytosis. There was a loss of about 1 lb. of body weight and the animal appeared moderately ill. Specific agglutination and complement fixation tests became positive within 8–14 d after vaccination and the titers rose progressively to a maximum 4 wk later. Agglutination titers reached 2560; complement fixation titers reached 640; intradermal skin tests with mallein were negative 4 and 6 wk after inoculation. The animal regained normal health and vigor after the abscess healed and appeared completely normal 2 mo after inoculation. At necropsy, cultures of all organs were negative. Monkeys infected with lower doses of *B. mallei* showed no clinical or laboratory evidence of infection and displayed no pathological changes or positive bacterial cultures on autopsy.

At USAMRIID, animal models have been developed for determining the efficacy of putative vaccines and therapeutic agents *(39–41)*. We recently re-established mice and hamsters as experimental models for vaccine and therapeutic efficacy testing. Histopathology studies of hamsters inoculated intraperitoneally with *B. mallei* have shown early lesions in spleens, mediastinal and mesenteric lymph nodes, mediastinum, liver, and bone marrow. At later timepoints, lesions also developed in the lung, submandiblar lymph nodes, and brain. Intraperitoneal infection in hamsters is characterized by a pyogranulomatous inflammation. Pyogranulomas were initially seen in the lymph nodes, spleen, bone marrow, and ultimately were widely disseminated throughout the body. In the later stages of the disease, the inflammation and necrosis virtually destroyed the organs and tissues in which they are present. The findings suggested that intraperitoneal bacteria were rapidly transported to mediastinal lymph nodes by the transdiaphragmatic lymphatics and ultimately seeded other tissues hematogenously. Bacteria were cultured from the blood, spleen, liver, and lungs. Because of the high susceptibility of hamsters to glanders infection, we do not think that hamsters are an ideal model of human disease.

Although the exquisite sensitivity of the hamster to *B. mallei* (LD_{50} <10 colony-forming units [CFU]) makes it unlike human susceptibility *(39)*, the BALB/c mouse model may more closely simulate human infection *(40)*. Mice infected intraperitoneally were characterized by a pyogranulomatous inflammation and pathological changes in mediastinal lymph nodes, spleen, liver, peripheral lymph nodes, and bone marrow. Necrosis was not as frequently present as in hamsters. The inflammation involved most lymphoreticular tissues early in the disease, but was more localized. A mouse model of glanders in which *B. mallei* was acquired by aerosol exposure was established at

USAMRIID. Mice were sequentially killed at 6 h postinoculation and daily for 4 d after infection with 10 LD_{50} of virulent *B. mallei*. The characteristic change was pyogranulomatous inflammation. Histopathologic changes were initially seen at 6 h after exposure in the nasal cavities of all mice, which rapidly progressed to the lung, trachea, spleen, liver, submandibular lymph node, and the brain. Pathological changes generally reached maximal severity at day 3. Lesions found in the nasal cavity included an acute inflammatory cell infiltrate, erosion, and ulceration of both respiratory and olfactory epithelium and a marked serocellular exudate. Involvement of the olfactory tract and olfactory lobe of the brain was present in all mice at day 4. The authors hypothesized that the infection extended into the cranial vault from the nasal olfactory mucosa through channels in the cribriform plate into which the olfactory nerves extend. The severity of the nasal infection and its extension into the cranial vault was particularly worrisome because of the poor distribution of systemic antibiotics to the nasal sinuses. Infection and ulceration of the nasal mucosa are also characteristic of human disease. The presence of encephalitis in human glanders cases has not been characterized, possibly because of the scarcity of glanders cases. At this point, it remains conjectural whether glanders can cause encephalitis in humans, but the ulcerations and necrotic nasal lesions found in infected humans makes this a distinct possibility *(42)*.

We have noted that hamsters are exquisitely sensitive to *B. mallei*, regardless of the route of infection (LD_{50} <10 CFU). In the BALB/c mouse model, however, mice were much more susceptible to infection by the aerosol route than the intraperitoneal route (LD_{50} approx 10^3 and 10^6, respectively). The dose needed to infect a human by any route is unknown.

3. MECHANISMS OF VIRULENCE

The identification of suitable vaccine candidates for preventing equine and human glanders will require a better understanding of *B. mallei* virulence determinants and pathogenesis. Some virulence factors of this pathogen have been characterized (*see* Subheadings 3.1.–3.5.). The recently completed genome of *B. mallei* ATCC 23344 (http://www.tigr.org/) revealed putative gene products that were similar to virulence factors in other Gram-negative bacteria, including a type II secretion system, a type III secretion system, type IV pili, autotransporter proteins, iron acquisition proteins, fimbriae, quorum sensing systems, and various of transcriptional regulators *(43–45)*. The roles of these putative proteins as virulence factors need to be examined by constructing defined mutations and examining the relative virulence of the resulting mutants in an animal model of *B. mallei* infection.

3.1. Capsule

Polysaccharide capsules are highly hydrated polymers that mediate the interaction of bacteria with their immediate surroundings *(46)*. As a result, these surface structures often play integral roles in the interaction of pathogens with their hosts *(47)*. There are several reports, especially in the older literature, that indicate *B. mallei* does not possess a capsule *(10,48–50)*. On the other hand, numerous studies demonstrate that *B. mallei* does make a capsule and that it is important for virulence *(12,29,39,40,51–54)*. In 1991, Popov et al. detected a capsular structure on the surface of *B. mallei* by transmission electron microscopy (TEM) *(52)*. In these studies, guinea pigs were infected intraperitoneally with *B. mallei*, the peritoneal cavities were washed, and the peritoneal exudates were examined by TEM. Three hours after infection, approx 33% of the bacteria outside of phagocytic cells possessed an extracellular formation considered to be a capsule. Bacteria that did not possess this capsular material appeared to be more readily engulfed by phagocytic cells, suggesting that the capsule may protect the pathogen from being phagocytized *(52)*. A similar study in 1995 confirmed this observation and also demonstrated the presence of a capsule in *B. pseudomallei (53)*. Another report demonstrated that encapsulated bacteria engulfed in vivo by mononuclear phagocytes appear undamaged inside phagosomes, phagolysosomes, and in the cytoplasm *(54)*. Interestingly, Fritz et al. also observed encapsulated *B. mallei* in the cytoplasm of phagocytic cells *(39)*. Taken together, these studies suggest that the *B. mallei* capsule may prevent phagocytosis early in infection and may block the microbicidal action of phagocytes after internalization. It is possible that the capsule confers resistance of the bacteria to lysosomal enzymes and allows *B. mallei* to persist long enough to escape from the phagosome and/or phagolysosome by an unknown mechanism. Note that the chemical structure of the capsule described in these studies is unknown.

Subtractive hybridization has been used to identify genetic determinants present in *B. mallei (51)* and *B. pseudomallei (55)*, but not in *Burkholderia thailandensis*, a non-pathogenic soil microbe *(56–58)*. In both species, subtractive hybridization products were mapped to a genetic locus encoding proteins involved in the biosynthesis, export, and translocation of a capsular polysaccharide *(51)*. The *B. mallei* capsule gene cluster exhibited 99% nucleotide identity to a *B. pseudomallei* capsule gene cluster that encodes a homopolymeric surface polysaccharide with the following structure: -3)-2-*O*-acetyl-6-deoxy-β-D-*manno*-heptopyranose-(1- *(51,55)*. There was a significant decrease in the G + C content of these polysaccharide gene clusters as compared to the rest of the *B. mallei* and *B. pseudomallei* genomes *(51,55)*. Nucleotide sequences acquired via lateral gene transfer often contain a G + C content that differs from that of the rest of the recipient genome *(59)*. It is tempting to speculate that the capsule genes were acquired via lateral transfer after the divergence of *B. mallei* and *B. pseudomallei* from *B. thailandensis*. Based on genetic and biochemical criteria, polysaccharide capsules can be classified into four distinct groups *(60)*. The *B. mallei* and *B. pseudomallei* capsule gene clusters most closely resemble group 3 gene clusters because of their gene arrangement and because they lack the *kpsF* and *kpsU* homologs that are present in group 2 gene clusters *(51,55)*.

Figure 1 shows an immunogold electron micrograph of *B. mallei* ATCC 23344 reacted with polyclonal capsular antibodies. The capsule forms a thick (approx 200 nm) and evenly distributed surface layer around the bacteria (*see* Fig. 1). A capsule-negative mutant, termed *B. mallei* DD3008, is avirulent in Syrian hamsters and BALB/c mice *(51)*. There was a greater than 5 log difference in the LD_{50}s of *B. mallei* ATCC 23344 and *B. mallei* DD3008 in hamsters and a greater than 3 log difference in mice. There were no deaths or signs of clinical illness in the animals challenged with *B. mallei* DD3008, including those animals that received doses as high as 10^6 CFU. The animal studies demonstrate that the capsular polysaccharide is a major virulence factor of *B. mallei*.

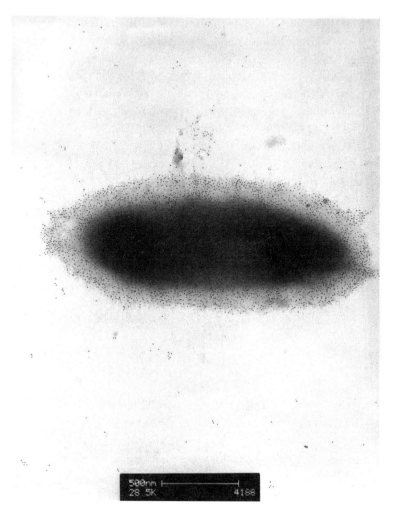

Fig. 1. Capsular polysaccharide of *B. mallei* ATCC 23344. The primary antibody was polyclonal rabbit antiserum directed against the capsular polysaccharide of *B. pseudomallei* and the secondary antibody was a goat anti-rabbit IgG gold conjugate (5 nm). Bar represents 500 nm.

3.2. Antigen 8

Russian scientists have described an extracellular capsule-like substance on the surface of *B. mallei* and *B. pseudomallei*, which they termed antigen 8 (Ag8), which is considered to be a pathogenicity factor because of its antiphagocytic and immunosuppressive properties *(61–63)*. Ag8 is a glycoprotein composed of 10% protein and 90% carbohydrate and has a molecular mass of approx 800 kDa *(61)*. In *B. mallei* cultures, Ag8 production cannot be detected until the second half of exponential growth phase and production is maximal during stationary phase *(63)*. The carbohydrate moiety of Ag8, a homogeneous polymer of 6-d-D-mannoheptose *(62)*, is identical in structure to the capsular polysaccharide of *B. pseudomallei* and *B. mallei* (*see* Subheading 3.1.). Further studies are necessary to determine if Ag8 and capsule are the same molecule or if they are distinct molecular entities.

3.3. Lipopolysaccharide

B. pseudomallei strains deficient in lipopolysaccharide (LPS) *O*-antigen are sensitive to killing by 30% normal human serum (NHS), and are less virulent than wildtype strains in animal models of melioidosis *(64)*. Similarly, *B. mallei* strains that are deficient in LPS *O*-antigen are killed by 30% NHS *(65)*. Previous studies revealed that *B. mallei* LPS *O*-antigens cross-react with polyclonal antibodies raised against *B. pseudomallei* LPS *O*-antigens *(51,65,66)* and that the LPS *O*-antigen gene clusters of these species are 99% identical at the nucleotide level *(64,65)*. In fact, the *B. mallei* LPS *O*-antigen is similar to that previously described for *B. pseudomallei* LPS *O*-antigen, a heteropolymer of repeating D-glucose and L-talose (65,67,68). However, changes are apparent in the *O*-acetylation pattern of the *B. mallei* L-talose residue compared to the pattern in *B. pseudomallei*. Similar to the *B. pseudomallei* LPS *O*-antigen, the *B. mallei* LPS *O*-antigen contained an *O*-acetyl or *O*-methyl substitution at the 2' position of the talose residue. On the other hand, the *B. mallei* LPS *O*-antigen is devoid of an *O*-acetyl group at the 4' position of the talose residue *(65)*. Thus, the structure of *B. mallei* LPS *O*-antigen is best described as -3)-β-D-glucopyranose-(1,3)-6-deoxy-α-L-talopyranose-(1- in which the talose residue contains 2-*O*-methyl or 2-*O*-acetyl substituents *(65)*.

3.4. Pathoadaptive Mutations

Comparative genomic analysis of closely related bacteria has revealed that gene loss and gene inactivation are common themes in host-adapted pathogens *(69–72)*. These mutations, termed pathoadaptive mutations, improve fitness by modifying traits that interfere with survival in host tissues *(69)*. *B. mallei* is a host-adapted parasite of equines whereas *B. pseudomallei* is an opportunistic parasite of numerous hosts *(33)*. The genomic sequences of *B. mallei* ATCC 23344 (http://www.tigr.org/) and *B. pseudomallei* K96243 (http://www.sanger.ac.uk/) are completed and can be directly compared. Although the genes conserved between these species are approx 99% identical, *B. pseudomallei* contains approx 1 megabase (Mb) of DNA that is not present in *B. mallei*. *B. pseudomallei* may have acquired this DNA through lateral transfer after the divergence of these two species from a common progenitor *(59)*. Alternatively, this DNA was present in the common progenitor and was subsequently deleted in *B. mallei (71)*. In addition, *B. mallei* has numerous insertion sequences and several of these are present within genes (gene inactivation). Gene loss and gene inactivation probably played important roles in the evolution of *B. mallei* by eliminating factors that were not required (or were inhibitory) for a successful host–parasite interaction. Thus, it appears that pathoadaptive mutations have played an important role in the evolutionary adaptation of *B. mallei* to a parasitic mode of existence.

3.5. Notables

3.5.1. Exopolysaccharide

A survey of phenotypic traits that are present in *B. mallei* and *B. pseudomallei*, but absent in *B. thailandensis*, may allow the identification of new virulence determinants. One candidate virulence factor that fits these criteria is a capsule-like exopolysaccharide *(73)*. This exopolysaccharide is a linear tetrasaccharide repeating unit consisting of three galactose residues, one bearing a 2-linked *O*-acetyl group, and a 3-deoxy-D-manno-2-octulosonic acid residue: -3)-β-D-Galp2Ac-(1,4)-α-D-Galp-(1,3)-β-D-Galp-(1,5)-β-Kdo- *(74)*. The genes encoding the exopolysaccharide have not been identified in *B. mallei* and *B. pseudomallei*, and its role in the pathogenesis is currently unknown.

3.5.2. R68.45 and RP4

The broad-host-range (BHR) plasmids R68, R68.45, and RP1 lead to a decrease in virulence of *Pseudomonas aeruginosa* for mice and an increased susceptibility to human serum bactericidal activity *(75)*. The reason for the decreased virulence and serum resistance in plasmid-bearing strains is unknown but may be caused by plasmid-encoded proteins altering the bacterial surface *(75)*. Verevkin et al. studied the effect of plasmids R68.45 and RP4 on the virulence of *B. mallei (76)*. They found that the transfer (*tra*) systems of these plasmids played a profound role in the virulence of *B. mallei* for hamsters *(76)*. Plasmid-free strains of *B. mallei* exhibited a LD_{50} of less than 10 bacteria in hamsters. In comparison, the LD_{50} of *B. mallei* strains harboring R68.45 and RP4 was greater than 10^8 and 10^5, respectively. After successive transfers in vitro, plasmid-bearing strains were isolated that could no longer transfer (conjugate) these plasmids to other bacteria. The hamster LD_{50} values for the bacteria containing R68.45 (*tra*–) and RP4 (*tra*–) was similar to the value for plasmid-free strains *(76)*. Thus, a *tra* gene(s) present on R68.45 and RP4 considerably alters the virulence of *B. mallei* for hamsters. The gene(s) involved in this process are unknown, but an understanding of this phenomenon may lead to the identification of new vaccines, therapeutics, and virulence factors.

3.5.3. Auxotrophy

Auxotrophic mutants of *B. mallei* deficient in the synthesis of different amino acids and nitrous bases were obtained by using the alkylating agent nitrosoguanidine *(77)*. *B. mallei* mutants containing one to six markers of auxotrophy were similar to wildtype strains regarding to their morphological and biochemical properties. There was a decrease in hamster virulence for most of the auxotrophic mutants but there was no correlation between the acquisition of certain markers of auxotrophy and virulence *(77)*. The auxotrophic mutants probably could not persist in the animal host because of their inability to synthesize essential compounds required for growth. Whereas the mutated proteins cannot be considered virulence factors, auxotrophic mutants could be used in genetic mapping studies or as attenuated vaccines.

4. MOLECULAR GENETICS OF *B. MALLEI*

B. mallei has not been extensively studied in the Western Hemisphere since the 1940s, and relatively little is known about the genetics and molecular biology of this organism. However, the potential use of this pathogen as a biological weapon *(78,79)* has led to a resurgence in research on *B. mallei*. In collaboration with scientists at USAMRIID, The Institute for Genomic Research (TIGR) determined the genomic sequence of *B. mallei* ATCC 23344, a strain isolated in December 1944 from postmortem cultures of knee fluid, skin pustules, and blood of a Chinese soldier who died of a glanders-melioidosis type of infection in Burma *(11,33,80)*. The 5.8-Mb genome consists of two circular chromosomes with an average G + C content of 68% (http://www.tigr.org/).

4.1. Antibiotic Resistance Markers Used for Genetic Manipulation

Genetic manipulation of bacteria often involves the use of antibiotic-resistant markers to select for the acquisition of plasmids, transposons, and mutant alleles, and to select against donor strains after conjugation. *B. mallei* is sensitive to many commonly used antibiotics in vitro *(81,82)*, and numerous antibiotic-resistant markers have been used to positively select genetic elements in *B. mallei*; these include gentamicin, kanamycin, streptomycin, tetracycline, chloramphenicol, trimethoprim, and zeocin *(51,65,76,83–93)*. However, the continued use of tetracycline-resistance determinants is not recommended given the fact that doxycycline appears to be useful for the clinical management of human glanders *(31)*. *B. mallei* is inherently resistant to polymyxin B and ampicillin in vitro, and these antibiotics can be used to select against donor strains after conjugative transfer of plasmids to *B. mallei (51,81,82,89)*. Spontaneous naladixic acid-, chloramphenicol-, rifampicin-, or streptomycin-resistant mutants of *B. mallei* can also be used for counterselection *(76,89,90,92,94)*.

4.2. Conjugation

Conjugation is the transfer of DNA containing an origin of transfer (*oriT*) from one bacterium to another through the use of transfer (*tra*) genes. Conjugation is the most common method for introducing DNA into *B. mallei (51,65,76,84–90,92–94)*. Conjugative BHR plasmids, nonconjugative BHR plasmids, suicide plasmids, and chromosomal DNA have all been transferred to *B. mallei* by conjugation. Conjugative BHR plasmids contain both an *oriT* and *tra* genes and are self-transmissible, but nonconjugative BHR plasmids and suicide plasmids contain only an *oriT* and require *tra* genes provided *in trans* to be transmitted. Helper plasmids that harbor the RP4 *tra* genes, such as pTH10 and pRK2013 *(95)*, have been used to mobilize nonconjugative plasmids and suicide plasmids into *B. mallei*. *Escherichia coli* SM10 and S17-1, two strains that have the RP4 *tra* genes stably integrated on the chromosome *(96)*, have also been used to mobilize nonconjugative plasmids and suicide plasmids into *B. mallei*.

4.2.1. BHR Plasmids

BHR plasmids can replicate in a wide variety of bacterial species and are useful for cloning and expressing genes in bacteria outside of the Enterobacteriaciae. The following conjugative and nonconjugative BHR plasmids have been transferred to *B. mallei*: RP4 *(76,84,86,88,90,92)*, RP1::Tn*10 (94)*, RSF1010 *(84,88,90)*, pBS222 *(90)*, pBS221 *(90)*, pBS227 *(90)*, pBS231 *(90)*, pBS70 *(90)*, pBS79 *(90)*, pBHR1 *(93)*, R68.45 *(76)*, pTH10 *(87,88)*, pSa *(84)*, and R15 *(84)*. The frequency of plasmid transfer (transconjugants per recipient) varied from 10^{-8} to 10^{-2} and all plasmids replicated autonomously in *B. mallei*. The plasmid antibiotic resistance markers are expressed and the plasmids are stably maintained in *B. mallei* in the presence of the appropriate antibiotics. R388, a BHR plasmid of the W incompatibility group, is one of the few exceptions as it is not stably maintained in *B. mallei (94)*. The BHR plasmids transferred to *B. mallei* included representatives from several incompatibility (Inc) groups, including IncPα, IncPβ, IncQ, IncN, IncW, and several unknown Inc groups. Thus, various of commonly available BHR plasmids can be used for genetic studies on *B. mallei*.

4.2.2. Suicide Plasmids

Suicide plasmids are vectors that have a narrow-host-range and are unable to replicate in a wide range of bacteria because of the absence of specific host factors or proteins. Plasmids based on ColE1 or R6K are considered to be suicide plasmids in *B. mallei* because they do not replicate and are not stably maintained in this species unless they recombine into the chromosome *(51,65,84,85,89)*.

4.2.2.1. pSUP202

The first study that explored the use of suicide plasmids in *B. mallei* was published in 1995 *(84)*. Abaev et al. demonstrated that suicide plasmids could be maintained in *B. mallei* if they contained a selectable antibiotic resistance marker and a DNA insert that allowed homologous recombination with the bacterial chromosome. The frequency of integration into the bacterial chromosome was directly dependent on the size of the homologous DNA insert cloned in the suicide plasmid *(84)*. *B. mallei* DNA inserts of various sizes were cloned into the suicide vector pSUP202, mobilized into *B. mallei*, and transconjugants were selected. The frequency of transconjugants formed when pSUP202 contained DNA inserts of 100, 700, 1500, and 3000 bp was 10^{-8}, 10^{-7}, 10^{-5}, and 10^{-5}, respectively. The transconjugants were relatively stable and could be maintained in the absence of antibiotic selection *(84)*. No transconjugants formed when pSUP202 alone was mobilized into *B. mallei*, which demonstrated the importance of homologous recombination with the bacterial chromosome for maintenance of this suicide plasmid *(84)*.

4.2.2.2. pGSV3

The suicide plasmid pGSV3 was used in *B. mallei* to construct mutant strains that contained plasmid disruptions of capsular polysaccharide genes and to clone genes flanking the site(s) of pGSV3 integration *(51,65)*. Nine internal gene fragments from the *B. mallei* capsular polysaccharide locus were cloned into pGSV3, and the recombinant derivatives were used to construct mutant strains that contained plasmid disruptions in *yggB*, *yafJ*, *manC*, *wcbB*, *wcbL*, *wcbM*, *wcbP*, *wcbQ*, and *wcbR* *(51)*. These mutants were useful for identifying the boundary of the capsule gene cluster and for characterizing genes involved in capsule biosynthesis, export, and translocation. With the availability of the *B. mallei* genome sequence (http://www.tigr.org/), it should be relatively straightforward to PCR-amplify internal gene fragments, clone them into pGSV3, and generate plasmid disruptions in virtually any nonessential open reading frame. The phenotypes of the resulting mutants can be studied and the functions of the mutated genes can be determined.

Another useful feature of suicide plasmids like pGSV3 is that the DNA flanking the plasmid integration site can be easily cloned without having to construct and screen a genomic library. This process has been termed "self-cloning" or "plasmid rescue" and it involves isolating chromosomal DNA from a transconjugant strain, digesting it with an appropriate restriction endonuclease, ligating it, and transforming it into *E. coli* (where the suicide plasmid can replicate). This method was used to clone all of the genes involved in capsular polysaccharide biosynthesis *(51)*.

4.2.2.3. pKAS46

Allelic exchange (gene replacement) is a process in which a wildtype gene is replaced with a gene that has been modified in vitro by a point mutation, insertion, or deletion *(97)*. Two homologous recombination events, one on each side of the introduced genetic mutation, are required for the acquisition of the mutant allele. The suicide plasmids used for allelic exchange contain counter-selectable genetic markers that allow for positive selection of mutants that have obtained the desired mutation and have lost the plasmid vector *(97)*. Burtnick et al. used the allelic exchange vector pKAS46 to construct a mutant strain that contained both a deletion of the acid phosphatase gene *(acpA)* and a zeocin resistance cassette *(89)*. It was not possible to use the *rpsL* (streptomycin sensitivity) counterselectable marker of pKAS46 because spontaneous streptomycin-resistant mutants of *B. mallei* were streptomycin-dependent. However, they were able to identify a single double-crossover event by selecting for a transconjugant containing zeocin resistance and lacking acid phosphatase activity *(89)*. Further studies will be required to identify the optimal allelic exchange vector/bacterial strain combination for allelic exchange in *B. mallei*, particularly if allelic exchange vectors based on *rpsL* (streptomycin sensitivity) cannot be used as a counter-selectable marker in this species.

4.2.2.4. pTnMod-OGm'

Transposons are mobile DNA elements that promote their own movement from one DNA location to another through the use of a transposase *(98)*. The integration of a transposon into a gene results in an insertional mutation, and transposon mutagenesis has been used extensively to study the physiology and pathogenesis of bacteria. Dennis et al. recently described the construction of modular, self-cloning minitransposons for use in the genetic analysis of Gram-negative bacteria *(99)*. Tn5 minitransposons function in a wide range of Gram-negative bacteria and exhibit virtually no preference for a specific target DNA sequence *(99–101)*. We used the Tn5 minitransposon TnMod-OGm' *(99)* to construct insertional mutations in *B. mallei* ATCC 23344 (DeShazer, unpublished results). This minitransposon was delivered to *B. mallei* via the suicide plasmid pTnMod-OGm' *(99)* and gentamicin resistant transconjugants occured with a frequency of 3×10^{-4} (per recipient cell). The minitransposon inserted randomly into the *B. mallei* chromosome and DNA flanking the TnMod-OGm' insertions were isolated by self-cloning.

TnMod-OGm' is modular in nature and reporter genes, such as β-galactosidase *(lacZ)*, can be added to increase its functionality *(99)*. Burtnick et al. used a TnMod-OGm' derivative that contained a promoterless and truncated alkaline phosphatase gene *('phoA)* to mutagenize *B. mallei* G8PN, a strain that harbored a mutation eliminating endogenous phosphatase activity *(89)*. Because alkaline phosphatase is only active if it is secreted past the inner membrane, *'phoA* can be used as a reporter gene to identify periplasmic, outer membrane, and secreted proteins. Six *phoA*+ *B. mallei* strains were identified and the gene products included putative periplasmic and outer membrane proteins *(89)*. It appears that TnMod-OGm' and its derivatives will be useful for the genetic analysis of *B. mallei*.

4.3. Transformation

4.3.1. Cryotransformation

In 1992, Abaev et al. *(83)* published a report describing cryotransformation of *B. mallei* with the BHR plasmids RSF1010 and pES154. Cryotransformation, a method for generating an artificial state of competence in a bacterial suspension by freezing it in liquid nitrogen and thawing, resulted in 80–200 transformants per µg of RSF1010 and 50–80 transformants per µg of pES154. RSF1010 was stably maintained in *B. mallei* in the absence of antibiotic selection, but pES154, a recombinant derivative of RSF1010, was not maintained without antibiotic selection *(83)*. Both RSF1010 and pES154 replicated autonomously in *B. mallei* and could be reisolated using a plasmid alkaline lysis procedure. This study clearly demonstrated that nonconjugative, BHR plasmids can be introduced into *B. mallei* by cryotransformation and that RSF1010 can be used as a cloning vector in this microbe.

4.3.2. Chemical Transformation

In an attempt to achieve a state of chemical competence, Abaev et al. *(83)* treated *B. mallei* with solutions containing calcium ions, magnesium ions, or a combination of rubidium and magnesium ions. They demonstrated that treating *B. mallei* with rubidium chloride (RbCl) and magnesium chloride (MgCl$_2$) in 3-[morpholino] propane sulfonic acid (MOPS) buffer created a state of competence whereas treatment with calcium ions or magnesium ions alone was ineffective. Three BHR plasmids were compared; RSF1010, pBS222, and pBS355. Chemical transformation resulted in 12 transformants per µg of RSF1010, 38 transformants per µg of pBS222, and 15 transformants per µg of pBS355 *(83)*. Thus, chemical transformation of *B. mallei* was attained, but it was somewhat less efficient than cryotransformation. The incompatibility groups of pBS222 and pBS355 are unknown, but both were stably maintained in *B. mallei* in the absence of antibiotic selection *(83)*.

4.4. Transduction

Transduction is a process in which bacterial DNA is transferred from one bacterium to another via a bacteriophage. Specialized transducing bacteriophages transfer DNA close to the bacteriophage attachment site, but generalized transducing bacteriophages can transfer essentially any region of the bacterial chromosome and are useful for genetic manipulation of bacteria. There are several reports in the literature describing bacteriophages that infect *B. mallei (91,93,102–104)*, but only one of these describes transduction of *B. mallei (91)*. *B. pseudomallei* and *B. thailandensis* strains spontaneously produce bacteriophages that infect *B. mallei*, and Manzeniuk et al. examined 17 *B. pseudomallei* bacteriophages for their ability to transduce the antibiotic-resistance markers of Tn5 (kanamycin) and Tn7 (trimethoprim and streptomycin). They found that five bacteriophages, PP16, PP25, PP32, PP61, and PP64, were able to transduce the Tn7 antibiotic-resistance markers *(91)*. However, only 59% of the transductants contained both the trimethoprim and streptomycin resistance determinants, suggesting that only part of Tn7 was transduced. Interestingly, no kanamycin resistant transductants were identified with any of the bacteriophages. Taken together, Manzeniuk et al. demonstrated that genetic material could be transferred to *B. mallei* by transduction,but it seemed unlikely that any of the bacteriophages they described would be useful as generalized transducing bacteriophages. Further studies are necessary to identify and characterize generalized transducing bacteriophages for transferring genetic markers between *B. mallei* strains.

4.5. High-Frequency Recombination Donor Strains

Genetic analysis of bacteria often involves the construction of donor strains that can mobilize chromosomal DNA to recipients by conjugation. These donor strains are often referred to as high-frequency recombination (Hfr) strains because the chromosomal

DNA they transfer can recombine with a recipient strain's chromosomal DNA. As a result, Hfr donor strains and are useful for mapping chromosomal genes. The conjugative plasmid pTH10 is useful for creating Hfr strains because it is temperature-sensitive for maintenance and it can integrate into a bacterial chromosome by Tn*1*-mediated homologous recombination at a nonpermissive temperature *(105)*. Ageeva et al. conjugated pTH10 to *B. mallei* and it conferred resistance to tetracycline, kanamycin, and ampicillin and sensitivity to bacteriophage PRD-1 *(105)*. However, initial attempts to construct a *B. mallei* Hfr donor strain with a temperature-independent drug resistance phenotype was unsuccessful because of the inability of *B. mallei* to grow above 40°C *(87)*. An alternative method, resistance to bacteriophage PRD-1, was used to select *B. mallei* strains in which pTH10 integrated into the chromosome. Approximately 3% of the PRD-1-resistant strains lacked plasmid DNA, were impaired in conjugative transfer, and displayed resistance to kanamycin, suggesting that pTH10 integrated into the genome. The plasmid pTH10 was reintroduced into these strains and the resulting transconjugants were able to transfer chromosomal markers to four distinct *B. mallei* auxotrophic mutants *(87)*. Thus, it is possible to create *B. mallei* Hfr donor strains and such strains may be useful for mapping unmarked mutations in future studies.

4.6. Insertion Sequence Elements

Insertion sequence (IS) elements are small, mobile DNA elements that can mediate insertions, deletions, and chromosomal rearrangements *(106)*. *B. mallei* ATCC 23344 harbors greater than 87 copies of IS*407*A, a 1236-bp member of the IS*3* family *(51)*. The *B. mallei* ATCC 23344 genome (http://www.tigr.org/) also contains 14 copies of IS*Bm*1 *(51)* and a previously uncharacterized IS*1562*-like element (107). Spontaneous IS*407*A insertion mutations have been detected in *B. mallei* gene clusters that encode surface polysaccharides, particularly after repeated subculture of the organism in vitro *(51,65,93)*. *B. mallei* DD420 contained an IS*407*A insertion in *wcbF*, resulting in a strain that was deficient in capsular polysaccharide production *(51)*. Similarly, NCTC 120 and DB110795 harbored IS*407*A insertions in *wbiE* and *wbiG*, respectively *(65,93)*. These strains did not produce LPS *O*-antigen and were resistant to infection with the *B. mallei*-specific bacteriophage E125 *(93)* and sensitive to the killing action of 30% normal human serum *(65)*. Serial subculture of *B. mallei* in laboratory medium results in a loss of virulence for animals *(1,25,50,79)*, and it is tempting to speculate that IS*407*A is responsible, directly or indirectly, for this phenomenon. In addition, a comparative genomic analysis suggests that IS elements have mediated more deletions and rearrangements in *B. mallei* than in *B. pseudomallei*.

5. B. MALLEI AS A BIOLOGICAL WEAPON

B. mallei has been used as a biowarfare agent. Over the years, there have been rumors and documented cases of its use against enemy personnel and resources. In the American Civil War, Union Colonel Samuel Ringwald told General George B. McClellan that as the Confederates abandoned Manasses, VA, they "carefully left behind…a number of horses infected with that horrible and contagious disease, the glanders" *(108)*.

During World War I, the Germans had plans to conduct covert operations in the United States against horses and mules destined for service in Europe. In 1916 a clandestine biological weapons laboratory was set up in Chevy Chase, MD, to produce *B. mallei* for the inoculation of draft animals, horses and mules that the Allies purchased in the United States for use by their military forces in Europe *(109)*. In addition, the Germans sent *B. mallei* cultures to Romania in 1916 to infect sheep being shipped to Russia; in 1917 they tried to infect Norwegian reindeer and to infect mules used by British forces in Mesopotamia; they infected sheep, cattle, and horses, being shipped from Argentina to Britain and to the Indian Army; they infected horses being shipped from Argentina to France and Italy; and they tried to infect advancing allied forces with glanders and cholera organisms during the German retreat in October 1918 *(110)*.

In his book *Biohazard*, Dr. Alibek alleges that development of an offensive capability using *B. mallei* was an important part of the Soviet bioweapons program *(78)*. Among his allegations, Dr. Alibek states that a Soviet scientist conducting weapon trials at the Aral Sea proving grounds died of glanders in 1942. In the 1930s, 20 workers were reported to have acquired glanders during experiments. In the 1980s or 1990s, Russian scientists at Obolensk were said to have developed a multidrug-resistant strain of *B. mallei*. Finally, Dr. Alibek claimed to have been told by a senior officer of a *B. mallei* attack against the mujaheddin in Afghanistan between 1982 and 1984. The Soviets viewed *B. mallei* as an excellent battlefield weapon. When sprayed from the air, this microorganism could immobilize or incapacitate forces hiding in rugged terrain or otherwise inaccessible to conventional munitions.

6. DEFENSIVE STRATEGIES

6.1. Vaccines

There currently is no evidence for immunity against glanders by virtue of previous infection or vaccination *(49,111)*. Infections in horses that seemed to symptomatically recover from glanders would recrudesce when the animals were challenged with *B. mallei*. Numerous attempts to vaccinate horses and laboratory animals against glanders were unsuccessful during 1895–1928. Farasa, a vaccine tested between 1910 and 1920, was prepared by treating whole cells with urea or glycerin *(49)*. Vaccination resulted in some resistance to infection, but animals still contracted glanders. Horses were infected with virulent *B. mallei* and attenuated vaccine (Konev II) and were challenged by scarification with virulent organisms *(16)*. A majority of the controls died from glanders within 3 mo. A majority of the vaccinated horses got glanders, but in a chronic form. One surviving horse, which had been vaccinated, was challenged with increasing doses of *B. mallei* and was clinically healthy. Attempts to transfer immunity through serum were unsuccessful *(16,49)*.

Others have used a vaccine prepared from a suspension of dried glanders bacilli (2 mg/mL) obtained from the New York City Board of Health *(111)*. Guinea pigs received three weekly injections. However, none were resistant to challenge. Seventeen glanders-free horses received three or four doses of vaccine. Doses escalated from 1 to 12 mL. Two horses were infected with *B. mallei* via the nasal mucous membranes 1 week after the last dose. Both contracted glanders and one died of acute disease in 21 d. The remainder were exposed to natural infection. Four animals developed disease within 8 mo. In vaccinated animals, agglutination titers fell to normal levels within 6 mo. Complement fixation (CF) titers disappeared within 3 mo (injections with mallein resulted in a similar serological profile.) Of 13 horses vaccinated, 9 contracted glanders naturally. Authors concluded that control and eradication of glanders was dependent on the elimination of infected horses and prevention of infected horses from entering stables that were free from disease.

In a recent study, Amemiya et al. found that nonviable *B. mallei* failed to protect mice from a parenteral live challenge *(112)*. They examined heat-killed *B. mallei*, irradiation-inactivated *B. mallei*, and an irradiation-inactivated *B. mallei* capsule mutant in the BALB/c model of glanders, and found a mixed T-cell helper (Th)1- and Th2-like immune response to all of the nonviable cell preparations. Splenocytes from the vaccinated mice responded similarly to the different nonviable *B. mallei* cells, and they were found to express interleukin (IL)-2, interferon-γ, measurable amounts of IL-4 and IL-5, and IL-10 under the same conditions. Generally, all of the nonviable cell preparations induced high levels of IgG and moderate amounts of IgM. Further examination of the immunoglobulin subclasses revealed that nonviable *B. mallei* cells induced a much higher level of IgG1than IgG2a. These later results were independent of the nonviable cell type used or concentration of cells used to vaccinate the mice or the adjuvant used in the study. It was suggested that nonviable *B. mallei* cell preparations did not protect mice in the study because of the induction of a mixed cytokine response and increased IgG1 vs IgG2a subclass response *(112)*.

Although unsuccessful attempts to find a vaccine against glanders were initiated more than 100 yr ago, we are hopeful that by using modern approaches to identify virulence factors and by studying the ways putative vaccines modulate the immune system, we can develop a glanders vaccine that is able to induce sterile immunity. Our initial attempts to protect mice by using an irradiation-killed whole cell preparation have resulted in an increased time to death, compared to controls, but spleens of survivors were not sterile (David M. Waag, unpublished data). The most desirable vaccine for glanders will be a recombinant protein or a biochemically purified preparation that when administered gives long-term sterile immunity.

6.2. Diagnostics

6.2.1. Culture and Serum-Based

Diagnostic tools for glanders were developed in the early 20th century so that infected animals could be identified and culled. These tools were especially needed for the diagnosis of chronic glanders because isolating the etiologic agent was more difficult. The use of mallein was initiated as a diagnostic tool in the United States and Canada in 1905 *(10)*. It was developed in Russia in 1891 by Gelman and Kalning and was composed of a filtrate of bacteria cultured for 4–8 mo *(49)*. Mallein causes an inflammatory, purulent reaction within 48 h of injection into the eyelid of infected horses. The CF test was initially used in the diagnosis of glanders in 1909 *(113)*.

In equines, chronic glanders is diagnosed serologically and/or by skin testing with mallein. CF antibodies are detectable 4–12 wk after infection. In the United States, where glanders has been eradicated, the CF test is used for glanders screening *(13)*. The mallein test is performed only on those animals that are positive for CF antibodies. However, only 20% of mallein reactors were seropositive by the CF test *(16)*. Studies have shown that mallein will induce a transient appearance of CF antibodies *(13)*.

Therefore, it is recommended that CF tests follow mallein tests for a minimum of 6 wk. If the test is equivocal, a skin test with mallein is performed. Horses sensitized to *B. pseudomallei* may exhibit a positive mallein reaction *(10)* and their sera may cross-react with virulent *B. mallei (49)*.

Mallein has been used in the diagnosis of glanders in humans, although the test does not become positive until 3–4 wk after infection, and, therefore, may have little value *(25)*. There are no specific serodiagnostic tests for glanders in humans. The indirect hemagglutination and CF tests have been used *(114,115)*. However, the CF test may not detect chronic cases of glanders *(16)*. We developed an enzyme-linked immunosorbent assay (ELISA) for human glanders by using irradiation-killed *B. mallei* whole cells. This test is able to discriminate glanders from anthrax, brucellosis, tularemia, Q fever, and spotted fever (unpublished data). However, because of the antigenic similarity between *B. mallei* and *B. pseudomallei*, the ELISA is currently unable to distinguish between cases of melioidosis and glanders. Background reactivity of normal sera is high *(22)*. Currently, we are attempting to refine our serodiagnostic reagents to increase the sensitivity of our assay and reduce the nonspecific activity.

Gram stains of lesion exudates may reveal small Gram-negative bacteria, but microorganisms are generally very difficult to find, even in acute abscesses *(22)*. Blood cultures are frequently negative until terminal stages of the disease *(22)*.

6.2.2. Nucleic Acid and Bacteriophage-Based

The high level of nucleotide identity between *B. mallei* and *B. pseudomallei* makes it challenging to use nucleic acid-based assays to discriminate between *B. mallei* and *B. pseudomallei (116,117)*. However, the availability of the genomic sequences of these organisms should facilitate the rational design of oligodeoxyribonucleotide primers and molecular probes for nucleic acid-based diagnostic assays. The use of a combination of diagnostic assays may be necessary to discriminate these species, including nucleic acid-based assays, phenotypic assays (colony morphology, motility, and carbohydrate utilization), ELISA, intact cell MALDI-TOF, and bacteriophage susceptibility.

In 1957, Smith and Cherry described eight lysogenic *B. pseudomallei* strains that produced bacteriophages that were more active on *B. mallei* than on *B. pseudomallei (104)*. In fact, bacteriophage E attacked *B. mallei* strains exclusively. Manzenyuk et al. found that 91% of their *B. pseudomallei* strains were lysogenic and that three bacteriophages, PP19, PP23, and PP33, could be used in combination for identifying *B. mallei (103)*. A *B. mallei*-specific bacteriophage, termed φE125, was recently isolated and characterized *(93)*. Bacteriophage φE125 was spontaneously produced by *B. thailandensis* E125, a strain isolated in 1991 from soil in northeastern Thailand *(118)*. The host range of φE125 was examined using 139 bacterial strains, including 13 strains of *B. mallei*, 50 strains of *B. pseudomallei*, and 32 strains of *B. thailandensis*. Bacteriophage φE125 formed plaques on 10 of 13 *B. mallei* strains but did not form plaques on any of the *B. pseudomallei* or *B. thailandensis* strains examined *(93)*. φE125 plaque formation was also evaluated on 15 additional species of *Burkholderia*, 4 species of *Pandoraea*, 2 species of *Pseudomonas*, *Ralstonia solanacearum*, *Stenotrophomonas maltophilia*, *Salmonella typhimurium*, *Serratia marcescens*, and *E. coli*. None of these bacteria formed plaques with bacteriophage φE125. Bacteriophage φE125, in conjunction with other methods, may be a useful diagnostic tool for identifying *B. mallei*.

6.3. Antibiotics

There are numerous reports in the scientific literature describing the in vitro suscep-tibilities of *B. mallei* to antibiotics *(81,82,119–132)*. Generally, these studies demon-strate that most *B. mallei* strains are susceptible to the following antibiotics: amikacin, netilmicin, gentamicin, streptomycin, tobramycin, azithromycin, piperacillin, imipenem, ceftazidime, tetracycline, oxytetracycline, minocycline, doxycycline, ciprofloxacin, norfloxacin, ofloxacin, erythromycin, sulfadiazine, and amoxicillin-clavulanate. Because it is likely that *B. mallei* is a facultative intracellular pathogen, aminoglycosides and other antibiotics incapable of penetrating host cells probably will not be useful in vivo *(81,82,133)*. Most *B. mallei* strains exhibit resistance to amoxicillin, ampicillin, penicillin G, carbenicillin, oxacillin, cephalothin, cephalexin, cefotetan, cefuroxime, cefazolin, ceftriaxone, metronidazole, and polymyxin B. A class A β-lactamase gene *(penA)* has recently been identified in *B. mallei* ATCC 23344 and the encoded β-lactamase is probably responsible for resistance to penicillins and cepha-losporins *(134)*.

Experimental chemotherapy of glanders has been performed in equines, hamsters, guinea pigs, and monkeys *(121–123,126–128,133,135,136)*. Miller et al. demonstrated that sodium sulfadiazine was effective for treating acute glanders in hamsters *(127)*. Penicillin and streptomycin, on the other hand, were not useful chemotherapeutic agents in this experimental model of glanders. Doxycycline and ciprofloxacin were also examined in the hamster model of glanders *(133)*. Doxycycline therapy was superior to ciprofloxacin therapy, but relapse did occur in some of the treated animals 4–5 wk after challenge. In a separate study, hamsters infected subcutaneously or by aerosol with *B. mallei* were treated with ofloxacin, biseptol, doxycycline, and minocycline *(123)*. Whereas all of the antimicrobials exhibited some activity in animals challenged subcu-taneously, ofloxacin was superior. None of the antimicrobials demonstrated appreciable activity against a high dose of *B. mallei* delivered by aerosol, but doxycycline provided 70% protection against a low dose delivered by this route *(123)*. The results of other studies demonstrate that a combination of antimicrobials are therapeutically useful in *B. mallei*-infected hamsters *(126,136)*. Muhammad et al. treated 13 draught equines diagnosed with glanders using Ringer's-lactate-dextrose + dimethyl sulfoxide and norfloxacin *(128)*. The animals showed a dramatic improvement in clinical signs for 2–3 wk, but this was followed by a relapse. The same result occurred after a second round of treatment *(128)*. It is difficult to directly compare the results of different experimen-tal chemotherapy studies because of the number of variables involved (animal model, route of infection, challenge dose, antibiotic, treatment dose, duration of treatment, and length of follow-up). However, these studies suggest that a prolonged course of therapy with a combination of antimicrobials (doxycycline, ciprofloxacin, and ofloxacin) may provide the best chance of recovery from experimental glanders.

The majority of human glanders cases occurred before the antibiotic era and the mortality rate was above 90% *(137)*. There have been several cases of human glanders since the 1940s, primarily in laboratory workers, that have been successfully treated with antibiotics *(29,31,131,138,139)*. Six cases were successfully treated with sulfadi-azine in 1944–1945 *(29)* and two additional cases were successfully treated with sul-fadiazine in 1949–1950 *(138)*. Streptomycin was used to treat a patient infected with

B. mallei and *Mycobacterium tuberculosis (139)*. Treatment with streptomycin reportedly cured the glanders but had little effect on the tuberculosis of the bone in this patient. In a recent case of laboratory-acquired glanders, the patient received imipenem and doxycycline intravenously for 1 mo followed by oral azithromycin and doxycycline for 6 mo *(31)*. This treatment regimen was successful and there was no relapse of disease.

6.4. Disinfection

Long ago it was recognized that an important element in preventing the spread of glanders in livestock was disinfecting stalls, water buckets, and hay manger in areas occupied by glanderous horses. Before initiating *B. mallei* studies at USAMRIID, we needed to determine which chemical disinfectants were efficacious for surface decontamination. Solutions of sodium hypochlorite, ethyl alcohol, Micro-Chem™, Zephiran™, Lysol™, and formaldehyde (1 and 5%) were tested. Sodium hypochlorite (12.5%), ethyl alcohol (70%), and Micro-Chem (5%) were most efficacious (D. R. Brown, unpublished results). The chemical disinfectant routinely used in our laboratories is 5% Micro-Chem.

γ-irradiation is effective for sterilizing suspensions of this microorganism. In experiments to determine an appropriate dose of gamma irradiation necessary to inactivate *B. mallei*, microorganisms were exposed to irradiation doses ranging from 0.26 through 3.0 Mrads. Even at the lowest irradiation dose, *B. mallei* was completely inactivated (D. R. Brown, unpublished results). We routinely use an inactivation dose of 2.1 Mrads and plate the bacterial suspension on solid medium to confirm sterility.

7. CONCLUSIONS

There has been a renewed interest in *B. mallei* over the past decade because of its potential use as a biological weapon *(9,78,79)*. Future studies on the genomics, proteomics, and molecular biology of this intriguing pathogen should lead to a better understanding of the factors required for virulence in animal models of infection. These factors may be useful as vaccines for the prevention of human and equine glanders. In addition, further studies on the host response to infection with *B. mallei* should allow a more complete understanding of the pathogenesis of glanders. Equines are the only natural reservoir for *B. mallei*, and the worldwide eradication of glanders is theoretically possible but would require the diagnosis and slaughter of infected animals. The worldwide eradication of glanders would require significant funding, coordination, and cooperation from countries with infected equines.

REFERENCES

1. Miller, W. R., Pannell, L., Cravitz, L., Tanner, W. A., and Rosebury, T. (1948) Studies on certain biological characteristics of *Malleomyces mallei* and *Malleomyces pseudomallei*. II. Virulence and infectivity for animals. *J. Bacteriol.* **55,** 127–135.
2. Marr, J. S. and Malloy, C. D. (1996) An epidemiologic analysis of the ten plagues of Egypt. *Caduceus* **12,** 7–23.
3. Wilkinson, L. (1981) Glanders: medicine and veterinary medicine in common pursuit of a contagious disease. *Med. Hist.* **25,** 363–384.
4. Loeffler, F. (1886) The etiology of glanders (in German). *Arb. Kaiserl. Gesundh.* **1,** 141–198.

5. Schadewaldt, H. (1975) 100 years in the mirror of the German Medical Weekly. The discovery of the bacillus for glanders (in German). *German Med. Weekly* **100,** 2292–2295.

6. Struck, D. (1882) A preliminary report on work by the Imperial Health Care Office leading to the discovery of the glanders bacillus (in German). *German Medical Weekly* **52,** 707, 708.

7. Benenson, A. S. (1995) *Control of Communicable Diseases Manual.* American Public Health Association, Washington, D.C.

8. Sanford, J. P. (1990) Pseudomonas species (including melioidosis and glanders), in *Priciples and Practice of Infectious Diseases,* 3rd ed. (Mandell, G. L., Douglas, Jr., R. G., and Bennett, J. E., eds.), Churchill Livingstone, New York, pp. 1692–1696.

9. CDC. (2000) Biological and chemical terrorism: strategic plan for preparedness and response. *MMWR* **49(No. RR-4),** 1–14.

10. Steele, J. H. (ed.) (1979) Glanders, in *CRC Handbook Series in Zoonoses.* CRC, Boca Raton, FL, pp. 339–362.

11. Yabuuchi, E., Kosako, Y., Oyaizu, H., et al. (1992) Proposal of *Burkholderia* gen. nov. and transfer of seven species of the genus *Pseudomonas* homology group II to the new genus, with the type species *Burkholderia cepacia* (Palleroni and Holmes 1981) comb. nov. *Microbiol. Immunol.* **36,** 1251–1275.

12. Miller, W. R., Pannell, L., Cravitz, L., Tanner, W. A., and Ingalls, M. S. (1948) Studies on certain biological characteristics of *Malleomyces mallei* and *Malleomyces pseudomallei*. I. Morphology, cultivation, viability, and isolation from contaminated speciments. *J. Bacteriol.* **55,** 115–126.

13. Hagebock, J. M., Schlater, L. K., Frerichs, W. M., and Olson, D. P. (1993) Serologic responses to the mallein test for glanders in solipeds. *J. Vet. Diagn. Invest.* **5,** 97–99.

14. Pitt, T. L. (1990) *Pseudomonas mallei* and *Pseudomonas pseudomallei*, in *Topley & Wilson's Principles of Bacteriology, Virology and Immunity*, 8th ed. (Parker, M. T. and Collier, L. H., eds.), BC Decker, Philadelphia, PA, pp. 265–268.

15. Parker, M. (1990) Glanders and melioidosis, in *Topley & Wilson's Principles of Bacteriology, Virology and Immunity*, 8th ed. (Parker, M. T. and Collier, L. H., eds.), BC Decker, Philadelphia, PA, pp. 392–394.

16. Vyshelesskii, S. N. (1974) Glanders (Equina). *Trudy Vsessoiuznyi Institut Eksperimental'noi Veterinarii (in Russian)* **42,** 67–92.

17. Schlater, L. K. (1992) Glanders, in *Current Therapy in Equine Medicine*. (Robinson, N. E., ed.), W.B. Suanders, St. Louis, MO, pp. 761, 762.

18. Smith, G. R. and Easman, C. S. F. (1990) Bacterial diseases, in *Topley & Wilson's Principles of Bacteriology, Virology and Immunity*. (Parke, r. M. T. and Collie, r. L. H., eds.), B.C. Decker, Philadelphia, PA, pp. 392–397.

19. Arun, S., Neubauer, H., Gurel, A., et al. (1999) Equine glanders in Turkey. *Vet. Rec.* **144,** 255–258.

20. Smith, G. R., Pearson, A. D., and Parker, M. T. (1990) Pasteurella infections, tularemia, glanders and melioidosis, in *Topley and Wilson's Principles of Bacteriology, Virology and Immunity*, 8th ed. (Smith, G. R. and Easman, C. S. F., eds.), B.C. Decker, Philadelphia, PA, pp. 392–397.

21. Huidekeoper, R. S. (1907) General diseases, in *Diseases of the Horse*. (Melvin, A. D., ed.), Government Printing Office, Washington, DC, pp. 532–545.

22. Sanford, J. P. (1991) Melioidosis and Glanders, in *Harrison's Principles of Internal Medicine,* 12th ed. (Wilson, J. D., Braunwald, E., Isselbacher, K. J., et al., eds.), McGraw-Hill, New York, pp. 606–609.

23. Hornick, R. B. (1982) Diseases due to *Pseudomonas mallei* and *Pseudomonas pseudomallei*, in *Infections in Children*. (Wedgewood, R. J., ed.), Harper & Row, Philadelphia, PA, pp. 910–913.

24. Robins, G. D. (1906) A study of chronic glanders in man. *Studies from the Royal Victoria Hospital* **2,** 1–98.
25. Redfearn, M. S. and Palleroni, N. J. (1975) Glanders and melioidosis, in *Diseases Transmitted from Animals to Man.* (Hubbert, W. T., McCulloch, W. F., and Schnurrenberger, P. R., eds.), Charles C. Thomas, Springfield, IL, 110–128.
26. Alibasoglu, M., Yesildere, T., Calislar, T., Inal, T., and Calsikan, U. (1986) Malleus outbreak in lions in the Istanbul Zoo (in German). *Berl. Munch. Tierarztl. Wschr.* **99,** 57–63.
27. Gaiger, S. H. (1913) Glanders in man. *J. Comp. Pathol. Ther.* **26,** 223–236.
28. (1924) Glanders. Foreign letter from Prague. *J. Am. Med. Assoc.* **82,** 646.
29. Howe, C. and Miller, W. R. (1947) Human glanders: report of six cases. *Ann. Intern. Med.* **26,** 93–115.
30. Hunter, D. H. (1936) Saints and martyrs. *Lancet* **231,** 1131–1134.
31. Srinivasan, A., Kraus, C. N., DeShazer, D., et al. (2001) Glanders in a military microbiologist. *N. Engl. J. Med.* **354,** 256–258.
32. Stewart, J. C. (1904) Pyaemic glanders in the human subject. *Ann. Surg.* **40,** 109–113.
33. Redfearn, M. S., Palleroni, N. J., and Stanier, R. Y. (1966) A comparative study of *Pseudomonas pseudomallei* and *Bacillus mallei. J. Gen. Microbiol.* **43,** 293–313.
34. Steele, J. H. (1973) The zoonoses: an epidemiologist's viewpoint. *Prog. Clin. Pathol.* **5,** 239–286.
35. CDC. (2000) Laboratory-acquired human glanders-Maryland, May 2000. *MMWR* **49,** 532–535.
36. Kantseva, A. P. and Matkovskii, V. S. (1970) Specific lung disorders is especially dangerous and some little studied infections (in Russian). *Voennomeditsinkij Zhurnal* **7,** 82–86.
37. Gaiger, S. H. (1916) Glanders in man. A second attack after apparent recovery. *J. Comp. Path.* **29,** 26–46.
38. Ferster, L. N. and Kurilov, V. (1982) Characteristics of the infectious process in animals susceptible and resistant to glanders (in Russian). *Arkh. Patol.* **44,** 24–30.
39. Fritz, D. L., Vogel, P., Brown, D. R., and Waag, D. M. (1999) The hamster model of intraperitoneal *Burkholderia mallei* (glanders). *Vet. Pathol.* **36,** 276–291.
40. Fritz, D. L., Vogel, P., Brown, D. R., DeShazer, D., and Waag, D. M. (2000) Mouse model of sublethal and lethal intraperitoneal glanders (*Burkholderia mallei*). *Vet. Pathol.* **37,** 626–636.
41. Fritz, D., Miller, L., England, M., and Waag, D. (2001) Mouse model of aerosolized glanders (*Burkholderia mallei*). *Vet. Pathol.* **38,** 591.
42. Rosenbloom, M., Leikin, J. B., Vogel, S. N., and Chaudry, Z. A. (2002) Biological and chemical agents: a brief synopsis. *Am. J. Ther.* **9,** 5–14.
43. Finlay, B. B. and Falkow, S. (1997) Common themes in microbial pathogenesis revisited. *Microbiol. Mol. Biol. Rev.* **61,** 136–169.
44. Henderson, I. R. and Nataro, J. P. (2001) Virulence functions of autotransporter proteins. *Infect. Immun.* **69,** 1231–1243.
45. Zhu, J., Miller, M. B., Vance, R. E., Dziejman, M., Bassler, B. L., and Mekalanos, J. J. (2002) Quorum-sensing regulators control virulence gene expression in *Vibrio cholerae. Proc. Natl. Acad. Sci.* **99,** 3129–3134.
46. Roberts, I. S. (1996) The biochemistry and genetics of capsular polysaccharide production in bacteria. *Annu. Rev. Microbiol.* **50,** 285–315.
47. Moxon, E. R. and Kroll, J. S. (1990) The role of bacterial polysaccharide capsules as virulence factors. *Curr. Top. Microbiol. Immunol.* **150,** 65–85.
48. Jennings, W. E. (1963) Glanders, in *Diseases Transmitted from Animals to Man*, 5th ed. (Hull, T. G., ed.), Charles C. Thomas, Springfield, IL, pp. 264–292.
49. Kovalev, G. K. (1971) Glanders (Review) (in Russian). *Zh. Mikrobiol. Epidemiol. Immunobiol.* **48,** 63–70.

50. Minett, F. C. (1959) Glanders (and melioidosis), in *Infectious Diseases of Animals. Diseases due to Bacteria.* (Stableforth, A. W., ed.), Academic Press, New York, pp. 296–318.
51. DeShazer, D., Waag, D. M., Fritz, D. L., and Woods, D. E. (2001) Identification of a *Burkholderia mallei* polysaccharide gene cluster by subtractive hybridization and demonstration that the encoded capsule is an essential virulence determinant. *Microb. Pathogen.* **30,** 253–269.
52. Popov, S. F., Mel'nikov, B. I., Lagutin, M. P., and Kurilov, V. Y. (1991) Capsule formation in the causative agent of glanders (in Russian). *Mikrobiol. Zh.* **53(1),** 90–92.
53. Popov, S. F., Kurilov, V. Y., and Yakovlev, A. T. (1995) *Pseudomonas pseudomallei* and *Pseudomonas mallei*-capsule-forming bacteria (in Russian). *Zh. Mikrobiol. Epidemiol. Immunobiol.* **(5),** 32–36.
54. Popov, S. F., Tikhonov, N. G., N. N. P, Kurilov, V. Y., and Dement'ev, I. P. (2000) The role of capsule formation in *Burkholderia mallei* for its persistence *in vivo* (in Russian). *Zh. Mikrobiol. Epidemiol. Immunobiol.* **(3),** 73–75.
55. Reckseidler, S. L., DeShazer, D., Sokol, P. A., and Woods, D. E. (2001) Detection of bacterial virulence genes by subtractive hybridization: identification of capsular polysaccharide of *Burkholderia pseudomallei* as a major virulence determinant. *Infect. Immun.* **69,** 34–44.
56. Brett, P. J., DeShazer, D., and Woods, D. E. (1997) Characterization of *Burkholderia pseudomallei* and *Burkholderia pseudomallei*-like strains. *Epidemiol. Infect.* **118,** 137–148.
57. Brett, P. J., DeShazer, D., and Woods, D. E. (1998) *Burkholderia thailandensis* sp. nov., description of a *Burkholderia pseudomallei*-like species. *Int. J. Syst. Bacteriol.* **48,** 317–320.
58. Smith, M. D., Angus, B. J,. Wuthiekanun, V., and White, N. J. (1997) Arabinose assimilation defines a nonvirulent biotype of *Burkholderia pseudomallei*. *Infect. Immun.* **65,** 4319–4321.
59. Ochman, H., Lawrence, J. G., and Groisman, E. A. (2000) Lateral gene transfer and the nature of bacterial innovation. *Nature* **405,** 299–304.
60. Whitfield, C. and Roberts, I. S. (1999) Structure, assembly and regulation of expression of capsules in *Escherichia coli*. *Mol. Microbiol.* **31,** 1307–1319.
61. Khrapova, N. P., Tikhonov, N. G., and Prokhvatilova, Y. V. (1998) Detection of glycoprotein of *Burkholderia pseudomallei*. *Emerging Infect. Dis.* **4,** 336, 337.
62. Piven, N. N., Smirnova, V. I., Viktorov, D. V., et al. (1996) Immunogenicity and heterogeneity of *Pseudomonas pseudomallei* surface antigen 8 (in Russian). *Zh. Mikrobiol. (Moscow)* **4,** 75–78.
63. Samygin, V. M., Khrapova, N. P., Spiridonov, V. A., and Stepin, A. A. (2001) Antigen 8 biosynthesis during cultivation of *Burkholderia pseudomallei* and *B. mallei* (in Russian). *Zh. Mikrobiol. Epidemiol. Immunobiol.* **4,** 50–52.
64. DeShazer, D., Brett, P. J., and Woods, D. E. (1998) The type II O-antigenic polysaccharide moiety of *Burkholderia pseudomallei* lipopolysaccharide is required for serum resistance and virulence. *Mol. Microbiol.* **30,** 1081–1100.
65. Burtnick, M. N., Brett, P. J., and Woods, D. E. (2002) Molecular and physical characterization of *Burkholderia mallei* O antigens. *J. Bacteriol.* **184,** 849–852.
66. Pitt, T. L., Aucken, H., and Dance, D. A. (1992) Homogeneity of lipopolysaccharide antigens in *Pseudomonas pseudomallei*. *J. Infect.* **25,** 139–146.
67. Knirel, Y. A., Paramonov, N. A., Shashkov, A. S., et al. (1992) Structure of the polysaccharide chains of *Pseudomonas pseudomallei* lipopolysaccharides. *Carbohydrate Res.* **233,** 185–193.
68. Perry, M. B., MacLean, L. L., Schollaardt, T., Bryan, L. E., and Ho, M. (1995) Structural characterization of the lipopolysaccharide O antigens of *Burkholderia pseudomallei*. *Infect. Immun.* **63,** 3348–3352.

69. Day, W. A. J., Fernandez, R. E., and Maurelli, A. T. (2001) Pathoadaptive mutations that enhance virulence: genetic organization of the *cadA* regions of *Shigella* spp. *Infect. Immun.* **69,** 7471–7480.

70. Maurelli, A. T., Fernandez, R. E., Bloch, C. A., Rode, C. K., and Fasano, A. (1998) "Black holes" and bacterial pathogenicity: a large genomic deletion that enhances the virulence of *Shigella* spp. and enteroinvasive *Escherichia coli. Proc. Natl. Acad. Sci.* **95,** 3943–3948.

71. Mira, A., Ochman, H., and Moran, N. A. (2001) Deletional bias and the evolution of bacterial genomes. *Trends Genet.* **17,** 589–596.

72. Parkhill, J., Wren, B. W., Thomson, N. R., et al. (2001) Genome sequence of *Yersinia pestis,* the causative agent of plague. *Nature* **413,** 523–527.

73. Steinmetz, I., Rohde, M., and Brenneke, B. (1995) Purification and characterization of an exopolysaccharide of *Burkholderia (Pseudomonas) pseudomallei. Infect. Immun.* **63,** 3959–3965.

74. Nimtz, M., Wray, V., Domke, T., Brenneke, B., Haussler, S., and Steinmetz, I. (1997) Structure of an acidic exopolysaccharide of *Burkholderia pseudomallei. Eur. J. Biochem.* **250,** 608–616.

75. Wretlind, B., Becker, K., and Haas, D. (1985) IncP-1 R plasmids decrease the serum resistance and the virulence of *Pseudomonas aeruginosa. J. Gen. Microbiol.* **131,** 2701–2704.

76. Verevkin, V. V., Volozhantsev, N. V., Myakinina, V. P., and Svetoch, E. A. (1997) Effect of the TRA-system of RP4 and R68.45 plasmids on virulence of the glanders agent (in Russian). *Vestn. Ross. Akad. Med. Nauk.* **6,** 37–40.

77. Shipovskaia, N. P., Merinova, L. K., and Riapis, L. A. (1983) Properties of auxotrophic mutants of *Pseudomonas mallei* (in Russian). *Zh. Mikrobiol. Epidemiol. Immunobiol.* **4,** 36–39.

78. Alibek, K. and Handelman, S. (1999) *Biohazard: The Chilling True Story of the Largest Covert Biological Weapons Program in the World.* Random House, New York.

79. Neubauer, H., Meyer, H., and Finke, E. J. (1997) Human glanders. *Revue Internationale Des Services De Sante Des Forces Armees* **70,** 258–265.

80. Evans, D. H. (1966) Colonial variation in *Actinobacillus mallei. Can. J. Microbiol.* **12,** 609–616.

81. Heine, H. S., England, M. J., Waag, D. M., and Byrne, W. R. (2001) *In vitro* antibiotic susceptibilities of *Burkholderia mallei* (causative agent of glanders) determined by broth microdilution and E-test. *Antimicrob. Agents Chemother.* **45,** 2119–2121.

82. Kenny, D. J., Russell, P., Rogers, D., Eley, S. M., and Titball, R. W. (1999) In vitro susceptibilities of *Burkholderia mallei* in comparison to those of other pathogenic *Burkholderia* spp. *Antimicrob. Agents Chemother.* **43,** 2773–2775.

83. Abaev, I. V., Akimova, L. A., Shitov, V. T., Volozhantsev, N. V., and Svetoch, E. A. (1992) Transformation of pathogenic pseudomonads by plasmid DNA (in Russian). *Mol. Gen. Mikrobiol. Virusol.* **3–4,** 17–20.

84. Abaev, I. V., Astashkin, E. I., Pachkunov, D. M., Stagis, I. I., Shitov, V. T., and Svetoch, E. A. (1995) *Pseudomonas mallei* and *Pseudomonas pseudomallei*: introduction and maintenance of natural and recombinant plasmid replicons (in Russian). *Mol. Gen. Mikrobiol. Virusol.* **1,** 28–36.

85. Abaev, I. V., Pomerantseva, O. M., Astashkin, E. I., et al. (1997) The creation of genomic DNA libraries of *Pseudomonas mallei* and *Pseudomonas pseudomallei* (in Russian). *Mol. Gen. Mikrobiol. Virusol.* **1,** 17–22.

86. Ageeva, N. P. and Merinova, L. K. (1986) The effect of mating conditions on the effectiveness of transmitting RP4 plasmids in *Pseudomonas mallei* (in Russian). *Mikrobiol. Zh.* **48(5),** 3–6.

87. Ageeva, N. P., Merinova, L. K., and Peters, M. K. (1989) The use of the plasmid pTH10 for isolating the donor strains of *Pseudomonas mallei* (in Russian). *Mol. Gen. Mikrobiol. Virusol.* **4,** 14–18.

88. Anishchenko, M. A. and Merinova, L. K. (1992) Mobilization using incompatibility group P1 plasmids in strains of *Pseudomonas pseudomallei* and *Pseudomonas mallei* as potential vectors for DNA cloning (in Russian). *Mol. Gen. Mikrobiol. Virusol.* **5–6,** 13–16.

89. Burtnick, M. N., Bolton, A. J., Brett, P. J., Watanabe, D., and Woods, D. E. (2001) Identification of the acid phosphatase (*acpA*) gene homologues in pathogenic and non-pathogenic *Burkholderia* spp. facilitates Tn*phoA* mutagenesis. *Microbiology* **147,** 111–120.

90. Filonov, A. E., Manzeniuk, I. N., and Svetoch, E. A. (1996) Conjugative transfer and expression of R plasmids of the genus *Pseudomonas* in the cells of *Pseudomonas mallei* C-5 (in Russian). *Antibiot. Khimioter.* **41(3),** 20–24.

91. Manzeniuk, O. I., Volozhantsev, N. V., Astashkin, E. I., and Svetoch, E. A. (1993) Transduction of *Pseudomonas mallei* bacteria (in Russian). *Mol. Gen. Mikrobiol. Virusol.* **4,** 37–40.

92. Peters, M. K., Shipovskaia, N. P., and Merinova, L. K. (1983) A study of the possibility of conjugated transmission of the RP4 plasmid from *Pseudomonas aeruginosa* by strains of *Pseudomonas mallei* and *Pseudomonas pseudomallei* (in Russian). *Mikrobiol. Zh.* **45(3),** 11–14.

93. Woods, D. E., Jeddeloh, J. A., Fritz, D. F., and DeShazer, D. (2002) *Burkholderia thailandensis* E125 harbors a temperate bacteriophage specific for *Burkholderia mallei*. *J. Bacteriol.* **184,** 4003–4017.

94. Merinova, L. K., Antonov, V. A., Zamaraev, V. S., and Viktorov, D. V. (2000) Mobilization of a cryptic plasmid from the melioidosis pathogen in heterologous species of microorganisms (in Russian). *Mol. Gen. Mikrobiol. Virusol.* **2,** 37–40.

95. Figurski, D. H. and Helinski, D. R. (1979) Replication of an origin-containing derivative of plasmid RK2 dependent on a plasmid function provided *in trans. Proc. Natl. Acad. Sci.* **76,** 1648–1652.

96. Simon, R., Priefer, U., and Puhler, A. (1983) A broad host range mobilization system for *in vivo* genetic engineering: tranposon mutagenesis in gram negative bacteria. *Bio/Technology* **1,** 784–791.

97. Reyrat, J.-M., Pelicic, V., Gicquel, B., and Rappuoli, R. (1998) Counterselectable markers: untapped tools for bacterial genetics and pathogenesis. *Infect. Immun.* **66,** 4011–4017.

98. Berg, C. M., Berg, D. E., and Groisman, E. A. (1989) Transposable elements and the genetic engineering of bacteria, in *Mobile DNA*. (Berg, D. E. and Howe, M. M., eds.), American Society for Microbiology, Washington, DC, pp. 879–925.

99. Dennis, J. J. and Zylstra, G. J. (1998) Plasposons: modular self-cloning minitransposon derivatives for rapid genetic analysis of Gram-negative bacterial genomes. *Appl. Environ. Microbiol.* **64,** 2710–2715.

100. Berg, D. E. (1989) Transposon Tn*5*, in *Mobile DNA*. (Berg, D. E. and Howe, M. M., eds.), American Society for Microbiology, Washington, DC, pp. 185–210.

101. De Lorenzo, V., Herrero, M., Jakubzik, U., and Timmis, K. N. (1990) Mini-Tn*5* transposon derivatives for insertion mutagenesis, promoter probing, and chromosomal insertion of cloned DNA in gram-negative eubacteria. *J. Bacteriol.* **172,** 6568–6572.

102. Grishkina, T. A. and Merinova, L. K. (1993) Spontaneous phage production in *Pseudomonas pseudomallei* and in a range of hosts of melioidosis phages among representatives in the genus *Pseudomonas* (in Russian). *Mikrobiol. Z.* **55(4),** 43–47.

103. Manzeniuk, O. I., Volozhantsev, N. V., and Svetoch, E. A. (1994) Identification of *Pseudomonas mallei* bacteria with the help of *Pseudomonas pseudomallei* bacteriophages (in Russian). *Mikrobiologiia* **63(3),** 537–544.

104. Smith, P. B. and Cherry, W. B. (1957) Identification of *Malleomyces* by specific bacteriophages. *J. Bacteriol* **74,** 668–672.

105. Harayama, S., Tsuda, M., and Lino, T. (1980) High frequency mobilization of the chromosome of *Escherichia coli* by a mutant of plasmid RP4 temperature-sensitive for maintenance. *Mol. Gen. Genet.* **180,** 47–56.

106. Mahillon, J. and Chandler, M. (1998) Insertion sequences. *Microbiol. Mol. Biol. Rev.* **62,** 725–774.

107. Berge, A., Rasmussen, M., and Bjorck, L. (1998) Identification of an insertion sequence located in a region encoding virulence factors of *Streptococcus pyogenes. Infect. Immun.* **66,** 3449–3453.

108. Sharrer, G. T. (1995) The great glanders epizootic, 1861–1866. *Agricultural History* **69,** 79–97.

109. Witcover, J. (1989) *Sabotage at Black Tom: Imperial Germany's Secret War in America, 1914–1917.* Algonquin Books of Chapel Hill, Chapel Hill, NC.

110. Carus, W. S. (1998) Bioterrorism and biocrimes: the illicit use of biological agents in the 20th century. National Defense University: Center for Counterproliferation Research.

111. Mohler, J. R. and Eichhorn, A. (1914) Immunization tests with glanders vaccine. *J. Comp. Path.* **27,** 183–185.

112. Amemiya, K., Bush, G. V., DeShazer, D., and Waag, D. M. (2002) Nonviable *Burkholderia mallei* induces a mixed Th1- and Th2-like cytokine response in BALB/c mice. *Infect. Immun.* **70,** 2319–2325.

113. Schutz, K. and Schubert, O. (1909) Die Ermittelung der Rotzkrankheit mit Hilfe der Komplementablekungsmethod (in German). *Arch. Wiss. Prakt. Tierhlk.* **35,** 44–83.

114. Gangulee, P. C., Sen, G. P., and Sharma, G. L. (1966) Serological diagnosis of glanders by haemagglutination test. *Indian Vet. J.* **43,** 386–391.

115. Sen, G. P., Singh, G., and Joshi, T. P. (1968) Comparative efficacy of serological tests in the diagnosis of glanders. *Indian Vet. J.* **45,** 286–293.

116. Bauernfeind, A., Roller, C., Meyer, D., Jungwirth, R., and Schneider, I. (1998) Molecular procedure for rapid detection of *Burkholderia mallei* and *Burkholderia pseudomallei. J. Clin. Microbiol.* **36,** 2737–2741.

117. Tyler, S. D., Strathdee, C. A., Rozee, K. R., and Johnson, W. M. (1995) Oligonucleotide primers designed to differentiate pathogenic pseudomonads on the basis of the sequencing of genes coding for 16S-23S rRNA internal transcribed spacers. *Clin. Diag. Lab. Immunol.* **2,** 448–453.

118. Trakulsomboon, S., Dance, D. A. B., Smith, M. D., White, N. J., and Pitt, T. L. (1997) Ribotype differences between clinical and environmental isolates of *Burkholderia pseudomallei. J. Med. Microbiol.* **46,** 565–570.

119. Al-Ani, F. K., Al-Rawashdeh, O. F., Ali, A. H., and Hassan, F. K. (1998) Glanders in horses: clinical, biochemical and serological studies in Iraq. *Vet. Arhiv.* **68,** 155–162.

120. Al-Izzi, S. A. and Al-Bassam, L. S. (1989) *In vitro* susceptibility of *Pseudomonas mallei* to antimicrobial agents. *Comp. Immunol. Microbiol. Infect. Dis.* **12,** 5–8.

121. Batmanov, V. P. (1991) Sensitivity of *Pseudomonas mallei* to fluoroquinolones and their efficacy in experimental glanders (in Russian). *Antibiot. Khimioter.* **36,** 31–34.

122. Batmanov, V. P. (1994) Sensitivity of *Pseudomonas mallei* to tetracyclines and their effectiveness in experimental glanders (in Russian). *Antibiot. Khimioter.* **39,** 33–37.

123. Iliukhin, V. I., Alekseev, V. V., Antonov, I. V., Savchenko, S. T., and Lozovaia, N. A. (1994) Effectiveness of treatment of experimental glanders after aerogenic infection (in Russian). *Antibiot. Khimioter.* **39,** 45–48.

124. Ipatenko, N. G. (1972) Bacteriostatic and bactericidal action of some antibiotic on the glanders bacillus, *Bacillus (Actinobacillus) mallei* (in Russian). *Trudy Moskovskoi Veterinarnoi Akademii* **61,** 142–148.

125. Kovalev, G. K. and Gnetnev, A. M. (1975) Antibiotic sensitivity of the causative agent of glanders (in Russian). *Antibiotiki* **20,** 141–144.

126. Manzeniuk, I. N., Dorokhin, V. V., and Svetoch, E. A. (1994) The efficacy of antibacterial preparations against *Pseudomonas mallei* in *in-vitro* and *in-vivo* experiments (in Russian). *Antibiot. Khimioter.* **39,** 26–30.

127. Miller, W. R., Pannell, L., and Ingalls, M. S. (1948) Experimental chemotherapy in glanders and melioidosis. *Am. J. Hyg.* **47,** 205–213.

128. Muhammad, G., Khan, M. Z., and Athar, M. (1998) Clinico-microbiological and therapeutic aspects of glanders in equines. *J. Equine Sci.* **9,** 93–96.

129. Nagy, G. and Zalay, L. (1967) Antibiotic sensitivity and biochemical properties of *Bact. mallei* strains used in diagnostic preparations. *Acta Vet. Acad. Sci. Hung.* **17,** 285–286.

130. Stepanshin, I. G., Manzeniuk, I. N., Svetoch, E. A., and Volkovoi, K. I. (1994) *In vitro* development of fluoroquinolone resistance in the glanders pathogen (in Russian). *Antibiot. Khimioter.* **39,** 30–33.

131. Tezok, F. (1958) Three glanders strains isolated from three patients in 1956 and differing with regard to sensitivity to antibiotics. *Internat. Congr. Microbiol. Abstr.* **VII,** 344.

132. Yolv, Y. (1967) Effect of certain antibiotics, sulphonamides and other substances on the reproduction of *Pfeifferella (Actinobacillus) mallei in vitro. Vet. Med. Nauki. Sofia* **4,** 55–59.

133. Russell, P., Eley, S. M., Ellis, J., et al. (2000) Comparison of efficacy of ciprofloxacin and doxycycline against experimental melioidosis and glanders. *J. Antimicrob. Chemother.* **45,** 813–818.

134. Tribuddharat, C., Moore, R. A., Baker, P., and Woods, D. E. (2003) *Burkholderia pseudomallei* class a beta-lactamase mutations that confer selective resistance against ceftazidime or clavulanic acid inhibition. *Antimicrob. Agents Chemother.* **47,** 2082–2087.

135. Batmanov, V. P. (1993) Treatment of experimental glanders with combinations of sulfazine or sulfamonomethoxine with trimethoprim (in Russian). *Antibiot. Khimioter.* **38,** 18–22.

136. Manzeniuk, I. N., Manzeniuk, O. I., Filonov, A. V., Stepanshin, I. G., and Svetoch, E. A. (1995) Resistance of *Pseudomonas mallei* to tetracyclines: assessment of the feasibility of chemotherapy (in Russian). *Antibiot. Khimioter.* **40,** 40–44.

137. Howe, C. (1950) Glanders, in *The Oxford Medicine.* (Christian, H. A., ed.), Oxford University Press, New York, pp. 185–202.

138. Ansabi, M. and Minou, M. (1951) Two cases of chronic human glanders treated with sulfamides (in French). *Ann. Inst. Pasteur* **81,** 98–102.

139. Womack, C. R. and Wells, E. B. (1949) Co-existent chronic glanders and multiple cystic osseous tuberculosis treated with streptomycin. *Am. J. Med.* **6,** 267–271.

11

Medical Countermeasures for Filoviruses and Other Viral Agents

Alan Schmaljohn and Michael Hevey

1. INTRODUCTION

Many viruses were considered historically and have been reconsidered recently as potential agents of great harm, through intentional release as weapons of biological warfare or bioterrorism. Two such lists, of which several circulate, are shown in Table 1. Another variation, a recent prioritization of concerns by the National Institute of Allergy and Infectious Disease (NIAID), is shown in Table 2. The discerning reader may note that regarding certain viral agents, different listings may appear wildly or illogically discordant. Conflicting perspectives will not be resolved herein: a consideration of the particular threat characteristics, diseases, vaccines, and treatments for even these truncated rosters of viral agents is well beyond the scope of this chapter. It suffices to note that priorities and concerns are drawn from imprecise and sometimes disputed information about these viruses in myriad areas, including the medical consequences of infection in terms of morbidity and mortality; the feasibility and ease of agent production; the minimal viral dose required to cause disease; the stability of the virus in storage and in aerosol form; the contagiousness or limited transmissibility of the virus via contacts of infected persons; the current availability of medical countermeasures; the ease by which individuals or groups may acquire the virus; and credible intelligence information indicating past or present weaponization. Variola virus, causative agent of smallpox, is considered separately in this volume. Here, emphasis is on the filoviruses Marburg virus (MARV) and Ebola virus (EBOV); these are among the most frightening of natural viral threat agents, not as contagious as variola virus, but more deadly, and uncontrolled by any currently available vaccine or therapy. Genetically engineered viruses are not considered here, nor are agents that have serious but solely indirect effects on humans through their impacts on agriculture or environment.

2. A BRIEF GUIDE TO VIRAL AGENTS OF CONCERN

2.1. A World Aswarm With Viral Zoonoses

Table 3 shows a cursory guide to most of the agents in Tables 1 and 2. Diseases are listed in order of their primary manifestation in natural circumstances. Almost all are zoonoses—that is, diseases communicable from animals to humans under natural cir-

From: *Infectious Diseases: Biological Weapons Defense: Infectious Diseases and Counterterrorism*
Edited by: L. E. Lindler, F. J. Lebeda, and G. W. Korch © Humana Press Inc., Totowa, NJ

Table 1
Viral Agents of Listed Concern, CDC, and State Department

DHHS 42 CFR Part 72, Appendix A, select agents (viruses)[a]	Australia group: list of biological agents (viruses) for export control[b]
	Chikungunya virus
Crimean-Congo hemorrhagic fever virus	Congo-Crimean hemorrhagic fever virus
	Dengue fever virus
Eastern equine encephalitis virus	Eastern equine encephalitis virus
Ebola viruses	Ebola virus
Equine morbillivirus	
	Hantaan virus
Herpes B virus	
	Japanese encephalitis virus
	Junin virus
Lassa fever virus	Lassa fever virus
South American haemorrhagic fever viruses (Junin, Machupo, Sabia, Flexal, Guanarito)	
	Lymphocytic choriomeningitis virus
	Machupo virus
Marburg virus	Marburg virus
Monkeypox virus	Monkeypox virus
Nipah and Hendra Complex viruses	
Rift Valley fever virus	Rift Valley fever virus
Tick-borne encephalitis complex (flavi) viruses (Central European tick-borne encephalitis, Far eastern tick-borne encephalitis [Russian Spring and Summer encephalitis, Kyasanur Forest disease, Omsk hemorrhagic fever])	Tick-borne encephalitis virus (Russian Spring-Summer encephalitis virus)
Variola major virus (smallpox virus)	Variola virus
Venezuelan equine encephalitis virus	Venezuelan equine encephalitis virus
	Western equine encephalitis virus
	White pox
	Yellow fever virus
	Warning list: Kyasanur Forest, Louping ill, Murray Valley encephalitis, Omsk hemorrhagic fever, Oropouche, Powassan, Rocio, and St. Louis encephalitis viruses
	Also 15 viruses listed as animal pathogens

[a]CDC Select Agent (www.cdc.gov) Federal Register / Vol. 67, No. 164 / Friday, August 23, 2002/ Proposed Rules.
[b]Department of State Australia Group (www.state.gov) lists of viral agents subject to control.

cumstances. With a few exceptions, human infections are unnecessary or irrelevant to the maintenance of these viruses in nature; nonetheless, some are readily transmissible between humans, either in mosquito–human cycles or by close and unprotected contact with infected persons. Wholly human viral diseases (e.g., polioviruses, certain herpes-

Table 2
NIAID Category A, B, and C Priority Viral Pathogens

A	B	C

Variola major (smallpox) and other pox viruses
Viral hemorrhagic fevers
  Arenaviruses
    • LCM, Junin, Machupo, Guanarito viruses
    • Lassa fever
  Bunyaviruses
    • Hantaviruses
    • Rift Valley fever
  Flaviviruses
    • Dengue
  Filoviruses
    • Ebola
    • Marburg
	Viral encephalitides
	  • West Nile Virus
	  • LaCrosse
	  • California encephalitis
	  • VEE
	  • EEE
	  • WEE
	  • Japanese encephalitis virus
	  • Kyasanur Forest virus
	Food and Waterborne Pathogens
	  • Viruses (Caliciviruses, Hepatitis A)
		Emerging infectious disease threats, such as Nipah virus and additional hantaviruses.
		NIAID priority areas:
		  • Tickborne hemorrhagic fever viruses (Crimean-Congo hemorrhagic fever virus)
		  • Tickborne encephalitis viruses
		  • Yellow fever
		  • Influenza
		  • Rabies

(From http://www.niaid.nih.gov/dmid/biodefense/bandc_priority.htm, updated 06/13/02.)

viruses, measles, mumps, rubella, and so on) are sufficiently controlled by vaccination or are so ubiquitous that they are not usually considered in discussions of bioterrorism or biowarfare. Smallpox is a noteworthy exception: it is highly contagious, incapable of natural existence except by transmission in humans, and was eradicated as a natural disease.

2.2. The Diversity of Viral Hemorrhagic Fevers

The term "viral hemorrhagic fever" (VHF) is often used as a collective term to refer to those acute viral diseases typified by a significant incidence of vascular dysfunction and severe, life-threatening diseases in humans *(1)*. However, VHFs should be regarded cautiously as a term of convenience, a colloquially useful but taxonomically meaningless *(2)* catchall for hazardous viruses unfamiliar even to many virologists. Among the VHF are viruses of many genera and at least four families *(Filoviridae, Bunyaviridae, Flaviviridae, Arenaviridae)*. In terms of genetics, ecology, physical structure, and even disease pathogenesis, the agents of VHFs have relatively little in common with one another. For different VHF viruses, pathogenetic events leading to hemorrhagic symptoms may be precipitated by various of mechanisms: viral damage to liver, platelet depletion, direct viral damage to vascular epithelium, disseminated intravascular coagulation, indirect consequences of cytokine activation, and perhaps by other mechanisms. All of these mechanisms have been implicated with filoviruses, yet hemorrhage and dehydration do not necessarily account for the terminal shock in fatal cases *(3,4)*.

2.3. Natural vs Unnatural Infections

Significantly, in terms of the risks they pose, most of the agents of Tables 1 and 2 are known or suspected (from experimental infections of animals, laboratory accidents, nosocomial infections, and so on) to be infectious in an aerosol form. For some viruses, dose and route of infection (e.g., inhalation) may dramatically alter the disease course, increasing morbidity and mortality. This difference is especially problematic with viruses that cause encephalitis, such as the alphaviruses Venezuelan, eastern, and western equine encephalitis viruses, and is also of concern with members of the *Flaviviridae*, such as tick-borne encephalitis virus, the paramyxoviruses Hendra and Nipah (*Henipavirus* genus), and some of the *Bunyaviridae*, such as Rift Valley fever virus *(5)*. In the case of alphaviruses, altered pathogenesis has been attributed to the capacity of virus to infect olfactory nerves, leading to encephalitis more rapidly than would occur with natural infection such as a mosquito bite. A corollary problem is this: vaccine-induced immune responses that protect against parenteral infection may be in some cases significantly less effective against aerosol infections *(6)*, adding a level of complexity to vaccine design.

2.4. Clinical and Laboratory Diagnosis

As implied in Table 3, isolated cases of viral disease may present initially in ways very similar to other medical events that lead patients to family doctors or emergency rooms. Neither encephalitis nor hemorrhagic fevers are universal manifestations of the natural viral diseases that tend toward these pathologies, and the disease courses in humans exposed to these agents by aerosol routes is generally unknown. The small diagnostic advantage of a careful patient history (e.g., foreign travel, exposure to rodents) would be lost in the event of malicious domestic release of hazardous viruses. Nevertheless, one might expect that insightful physicians would be the first to recognize unusual symptoms or case-clusters and relay the alarm to diagnostic centers, as happened in the United States in the examples of hantavirus pulmonary syndrome *(7)*, and West Nile virus *(8)*. An improved and integrated knowledge management system (e.g., monitoring increased hospital admissions, mortalities, and unusual diagnoses in a more global fashion) has been proposed and may prove beneficial. However, in an initial outbreak and before case-definition criteria can be established, laboratory evaluations will be essential to identify a new or unexpected viral disease.

The reader is referred to other sources *(1)* for discussion of samples to be taken and to whom they might be submitted for analysis. In brief, frozen serum, whole blood, or tissues will usually suffice for viral isolation, for polymerase chain reaction (PCR) detection of viral genomes, and/or for serological studies (acute and convalescent serum samples are preferred in the latter case). Other embedded or fixed tissues may be useful for diagnosis by immunohistochemistry or in situ hybridization. Propelled by the recent increase in concern about bioterrorism, advances have been made in rapid and miniaturized diagnostic technologies with specific application for exotic viral disease agents. State and local laboratories may soon be equipped to receive samples that until now could only be sent to specialized laboratories, similarly to the Centers for Disease Control and Prevention (CDC).

Table 3
Viral Agents Affecting Humans and Frequently Considered as Potential Agents of Biological Warfare or Bioterrorism

Virus	Disease[a]	Natural transmission[b] to humans	Countermeasures[c]
Filoviridae family			
Ebola virus	Hemorrhagic fever	Blood, body fluids, and ?	NONE
Marburg virus	Hemorrhagic fever	Blood, body fluids, and ?	NONE
Alphavirus genus			
Venezuelan equine encephalitis virus	Fever, encephalitis	Mosquito	Vaccine (IND, l-a, k)
Eastern equine encephalitis virus	Fever, encephalitis	Mosquito	Vaccine (IND, k)
Western equine encephalitis virus	Fever, encephalitis	Mosquito	Vaccine (IND, k)
Chikungunya virus	Fever, arthralgia	Mosquito	Vaccine (IND, l-a)
Bunyaviridae family			
Congo-Crimean hemorrhagic fever virus	Hemorrhagic fever	Tick, blood, body fluids	Ribavirin
Hantaan, Seoul, Puumala viruses	Hemorrhagic fever, renal syndrome	Rodents, rodent excreta	Ribavirin
Sin Nombre virus, Andes viruses	Fever, respiratory distress syndrome	Rodents, rodent excreta	Ribavirin
Rift Valley fever virus	Fever, encephalitis, hemorrhagic fever	Mosquito, abattoir	Vaccine (IND, k),
ribavirin			
Arenavirus genus			
Lassa fever virus	Hemorrhagic fever	Rodents, rodent excreta	Ribavirin
Junin virus	Hemorrhagic fever	Rodents, rodent excreta	Vaccine (IND, l-a)
ribavirin			
Machupo virus	Hemorrhagic fever	Rodents, rodent excreta	Ribavirin
Flavivirus genus			
Tick-borne encephalitis viruses	Fever, encephalitis	Tick	Vaccine (European
license, k)			
Yellow fever virus	Fever, hemorrhagic fever	Mosquito	Vaccine licensed, l-a
Japanese encephalitis virus	Fever, encephalitis	Mosquito	Vaccine licensed, k
Dengue fever virus	Fever, hemorrhagic fever	Mosquito	Vaccine (IND, l-a)
Paramyxoviridae family			
Nipah and Hendra viruses	Fever, encephalitis	From outbreaks in pigs, horses; origin in bats	NONE?

(continued)

Table 3 (continued)

Virus	Disease[a]	Natural transmission[b] to humans	Countermeasures[c]
Orthopoxvirus genus			
Variola virus	Smallpox	Highly contagious, respiratory spread	Vaccine licensed, 1-a, cidofovir
Monkeypox virus	Smallpox-like	Close contact with infected small mammals, humans	Vaccine licensed, 1-a, cidofovir

[a]Diseases are listed in order of their primary manifestation.

[b]Natural Transmission refers to the manner in which humans become infected.

[c]Countermeasures include vaccines with FDA status of IND (i.e., vaccines with increasing human safety data, animal efficacy data, but insufficient human efficacy data and no supported application for licensure). Whereas newer approaches have shown great promise in laboratory studies, existing vaccines for human use are variations of classical killed (k) or live-attenuated (1-a) formulations. In general, ribavirin is not licensed for the above indications, but is inferred from in vitro data and incomplete clinical data to favor survival. Similarly, cidofovir (Vistide®) is licensed for treatment of cytomegalovirus (CMV) retinitis in patients with AIDS, but also shows considerable promise in limiting orthopoxvirus replication and ameliorating disease.

2.5. Countermeasures and Resources

Table 3 shows a cursory overview of the current status of vaccines and viral therapeutics for many viral agents. In brief, US-licensed vaccines exist for only a few agents, and vaccine supplies may be inadequate for immediate mass vaccinations. For other agents, vaccines may exist under Investigational New Drug (IND) status—that is, vaccines shown to be efficacious and safe in laboratory animals, manufactured for human testing, and tested (with Food and Drug Administration [FDA] oversight) for safety in scores and sometimes thousands of persons. For some agents (filoviruses, *see* Section 3), candidate vaccines are only now proceeding toward the first human trials. Among the vaccines that remain in IND status, reasons for nonlicensure are several and different for each vaccine but generally revolve historically around a paucity of financial commitment (public or private) to the high costs of unambiguously demonstrating both safety and efficacy in humans, as required for US licensure. In addition, some of the IND vaccines were thought likely to be replaced by improved products, further undermining any willingness to incur the costs of licensure.

Ribavirin is effective in vitro against arenaviruses and hantaviruses, and clinical studies have shown a trend toward efficacy against these viruses *(9,10)*. Licensed for human use in combination therapy of hepatitis C and also as a treatment option for respiratory syncytial virus, ribavirin has known side effects (anemia, possible teratogenicity) to be weighed against the gravity of the viral infection. The drug is ineffective against the causes of other viral hemorrhagic fevers (flaviviruses, filoviruses), and ineffective against alphaviruses. Thus, general recommendations are to begin treating suspected cases of viral hemorrhagic fevers with ribavirin until a diagnosis of arenavirus or bunyavirus infection has been ruled out, at which time drug therapy is to cease *(1)*.

Therapeutic administration of antibodies is generally unavailable and sometimes contraindicated. Whereas antibodies are relevant to immune clearance of many of the viruses shown in Tables 1 and 2 (especially alphaviruses, bunyaviruses, and flaviviruses) and may mitigate or prevent disease if given prophylactically or shortly after exposure, the usefulness of providing additional antibodies to symptomatic, immunocompetent patients is unclear. Nonetheless, additional research and testing may lead to future availability of therapeutic antibodies for certain of the agents.

For more comprehensive discussions of countermeasures and associated issues, the reader is referred to refs. *1* and *5*. For the most recent advances in vaccination or treatment, Web-based resources will likely remain most current, for example, those of the CDC (http://www.cdc.gov/), the Infectious Diseases Society of America (http://www.idsociety.org/bt/toc.htm), and the Johns Hopkins University's Center for Civilian Biodefense Strategies (http://www.hopkins-biodefense.org/).

3. FILOVIRUSES: FROM THE GENERAL TO THE PARTICULAR

Here, the particular case of filoviruses (EBOV and MARV) is both important and immensely illustrative. These characteristically filamentous viruses, which otherwise could be disregarded on account of their relatively insignificant global impact on human health, are among the most fearsome of biological threats. Although EBOV has achieved greater public notoriety, it is MARV that was allegedly weaponized in massive quantities by the former Soviet Union *(11,12)*.

3.1. Filovirus Background and Epidemiology

The first documented and characterized filovirus outbreak was in 1967, imported in Ugandan nonhuman primates to the German city from which MARV derives its name *(4)*. All initial cases were associated with laboratory workers engaged in processing kidneys from African green monkeys for cell-culture production. EBOVs were first recognized in 1976 and have been split into four species based on nucleotide sequence homology and other characteristics. In a somewhat fluid taxonomic state (e.g., *see* changes from ref. *2* to http://ictvdb.bio2.columbia.edu/), MARV is assigned a single species, and the four Ebola species are Zaire Ebola virus (ZEBOV), Ivory Coast Ebola virus, Sudan Ebola virus, and Reston Ebola virus.

Historically, confirmed filovirus outbreaks have been infrequent and unpredictable and so few in total number as to be amenable to listing in a single table (*see* Table 4). Whether the result of the many factors that may cause viral emergence into human populations *(13)* or because of increased surveillance, EBOV and/or MARV outbreaks are now so frequent that they may be thought of as endemic diseases in equatorial Africa *(14,15)*. Nonetheless, filoviruses continue to defy sound epidemiological description, and their natural reservoir remains unknown. A 1999–2000 outbreak of MARV in the Democratic Republic of Congo, involving more than 70 cases and fatality rates of around 75%, was linked to underground mining *(14)*, supporting but not proving a suspicion that bats may be a natural carrier of the virus *(16)*. With EBOV outbreaks, index cases have been difficult to identify, and epidemiological investigations have been frustrated by innumerable political, cultural, and other barriers to rigorous study *(17)*.

Filoviral infections in humans are typically acquired by close contact with fluids or tissues from infected patients or monkeys, by accidental exposure to infected sharps, and by iatrogenic spread in poorly equipped hospitals.

3.2. Filovirus Clinical Presentation

The initial symptoms of filoviral infection in humans can be so nonspecific as to be easily confused with numerous other diseases (*see* Table 5). Categorized as viral hemorrhagic fevers, the diseases caused by MARV and EBOV are not always hemorrhagic, and they manifest in somewhat different ways in different individuals *(3)*.

The clinical presentation for MARV was most extensively described in the first Marburg, Germany, outbreak in 1967 *(4,18)*. Because EBOV outbreaks have occurred mostly in remote areas of the Third World, comparable data on clinical presentation in a large cohort have not been reported. In the 1967 MARV outbreak, disease typically began after a 3- to 9-d incubation period with sudden marked prostration, headache, and muscle ache. Fever followed within a few hours, accompanied by nausea, frequent vomiting, and watery diarrhea (usually without observed blood or mucous contamination). Confusion and mental impairment were observed in many patients during acute disease. A characteristic nonitching, macular, papular rash began 5–8 d after initial symptoms, beginning on the face and then progressing to the trunk and extremities. An early lymphopenia was followed by leukocytosis with atypical lymphocytes. Thrombocytopenia was observed in all patients, and severe hemorrhagic diathesis in 30–50% of patients. Also observed in all patients, and peaking after 6–9 d of illness, were elevated liver enzymes, with nearly normal bilirubin levels. Deaths occurred on the 8th

Table 4
Filovirus Outbreaks Documented Through 2001

Location	Year	Virus	Cases (mortality)	Origin, epidemiology
Germany, Yugoslavia	'67	MARV	31 (23%)	Imported monkeys (Uganda)
Zimbabwe	'75	MARV	3 (33%)	Unknown. Two S. African contacts
Northern Zaire	'76	ZEBOV	318 (88%)	Unknown, then iatrogenic
Southern Sudan	'76	SEBOV	284 (53%)	Unknown. Close contacts.
Tandala, Zaire	'77	ZEBOV	1 (100%)	Unknown.
Southern Sudan	'79	SEBOV	34 (65%)	Unknown. Same site as 1976.
Kenya	'80	MARV	2 (50%)	Unknown. Physician survived.
Kenya	'87	MARV	1 (100%)	Unknown. Expatriate traveler.
United States	'89	REBOV	0 (0%)	Imported monkeys (Philippines), four asymptomatic human infections
Italy	'92	REBOV	0 (0%)	Imported monkeys (Philippines)
Ivory Coast	'94	CIEBOV	1 (0%)	chimpanzee contact
Kikwit, Zaire	'95	ZEBOV	315 (77%)	Unknown. Close contacts.
Gabon	'94–'96	ZEBOV	>43 dead	Unknown.
Dem. Republic of Congo (former Zaire)	'99–'00	MARV	99 (68%)	Diamond mine?. Multiple genotypes, multiple point sources.
Uganda	'00-'01	SEBOV	approx 400 (62%)	Unknown. From Sudan via troops?

to 16th day of illness with the immediate cause of death being cardiovascular failure, or cerebral coma. On autopsy, focal necroses appeared in almost all organs including brain and kidney, were most conspicuous in the liver and lymphatic system, but were absent from skeletal muscle. In patients displaying neurological symptoms, glial nodule encephalitis in the gray and white matter of all portions of the brain was observed. In those patients who did recover, the convalescent period was prolonged, with rapid fatigue a common hallmark months after infection. In recovering individuals, infectious virus or viral RNA may persist in some sites, and notably in semen, for weeks or months. The overall clinical picture is very similar with EBOV, although it should also be appreciated that there is considerable variation among individuals in both clinical presentation and course of disease *(3,19)*.

3.3. *Medical Treatment*

The medical and public health management of viral hemorrhagic fevers, including those caused by filoviruses, were recently reviewed in greater detail than will be pro-

Table 5
Viral Hemorrhagic Fevers: Case Definitions That May Warrant a Cascade of Reporting, Infection Control, Laborartory Diagnosis, and Initiation of Available Treatments

Symptoms possibly signaling viral hemorrhagic fevers	Ebola virus: case definitions used during kikwit outbreak
Patient presents with: Fever >101°F (38.3°C) of <3 wk duration *and*	Probable case defined as a person with: 1) Unexplained fever and contact with another probable case-patient, *or*
At least two of the following: hemorrhagic or purple rash, epistaxis, hematemesis, hemoptysis, blood in stools, or petechiae in nondependent areas *and*	2) Unexplained fever plus 3 or more of 10 symptoms (abdominal pain, anorexia, asthenia, simple [nonbloody] diarrhea, d ysphagia, dyspnea, headache, hiccups, myalgia and arthralgias, and nausea and vomiting, *or*
No predisposing factors for hemorrhage and no established alternative diagnoses	3) Unexplained acute hemorrhagic signs or symptoms, such as melena, hematemesis, petechiae, or epistaxis
http://www.idsociety.org/bt/toc.htm	Bwaka et al. *(3)*

vided here *(1)*. Briefly, the only medical care that can be recommended for filoviruses is palliative management of symptoms. In the 1967 MARV outbreak, case fatality rate was 22% (7 of 32) despite state-of-the-art critical care to manage hemostasis, electrolyte balance, and organ failure in patients *(4)*. A 1999–2000 outbreak of MARV in the Democratic Republic of Congo appeared to involve more than 70 cases and fatality rates of around 75%; only minimal or no medical care was available to victims of that outbreak *(14)*. The Zaire species of EBOV has caused fatality rates of approx 80% in major outbreaks, also with little medical intervention until late in the outbreak *(20)*. In the example of the 1995 ZEBOV outbreak in Kikwit, case-fatality rates during the lengthy outbreak declined from 93 to 69% *(21)*, coincident with more aggressive parenteral hydration of patients and decreased needlestick hazard *(3)*.

When MARV or EBOV is diagnosed or strongly suspected, additional precautions for both patients and medical staff are indicated. These may include airborne agent precautions, personal protection equipment, particular attention to hand hygiene, appropriate handling of medical equipment, environmental decontamination, and patient cohorting if multiple cases occur *(1)* (*see also* www.idsociety.org). Generally, the barrier nursing practices and universal precautions instituted in the clinic because of human immunodeficiency virus should provide sufficient protection and have been sufficient to arrest natural outbreaks, but the alarming clinical course and the unfamiliarity of filoviral disease can be expected to create tension or outright fear in medical staff. Laboratory specimens should be double-bagged and the exterior of the outer bag decontaminated before transport to the laboratory. Excreta and other contaminated materials should be autoclaved or decontaminated by the liberal application of hypochlorite or phenolic disinfectants. Clinical laboratory personnel are at risk for exposure and should employ a biosafety cabinet (if available) and barrier precautions when handling specimens. More specific and authoritative guidance is provided elsewhere *(1)*.

3.4. Diagnosis

Clinical diagnosis of viral hemorrhagic fevers can be problematic, especially with isolated and unexpected cases. Viral hemorrhagic fever may be among the suspected diagnoses in any patient presenting with a severe febrile illness and evidence of vascular involvement (postural hypotension, petechiae, easy bleeding, flushing of face and chest, nondependent edema), but especially in one who has traveled to an area where the virus is known to occur, or where information suggests that a biological attack may have occurred. General VHF criteria are presented in Table 5, as are the particular case definitions used during the 1995 ZEBOV outbreak in Kikwit. In the latter outbreak, around 85% of confirmed, hospitalized patients had weakness and diarrhea, but only 41% showed signs of bleeding, and only 15% were observed to have rashes (3). The nonpruritic, maculopapular rash was seldom identifed on black-skinned patients, who comprised the majority of patients in Kikwit. Fever was "almost always" noted (93%) but also went through periods of normality, especially in the last 2 d before death. Thrombocytopenia and leukopenia were common.

While diagnosis of MARV or EBOV infection may be suspected on clinical and epidemiological grounds, laboratory confirmation is also required; virus isolation, PCR, serology, immunohistochemistry, and/or electron microscopy can suffice. Most patients will have readily detectable viremia for days after onset of symptoms (22). Both the CDC (Atlanta, GA) and the US Army Medical Research Institute of Infectious Diseases (Frederick, MD) have diagnostic laboratories functioning at the highest containment level for virus isolation. Because natural outbreaks of these agents generally occur in remote, technologically undeveloped areas of the world, there has usually been a significant lag period between the first cases and confirmation of viral agent. Recently, the importance of interactive partnerships among US agencies—to refine and expedite future diagnostic capabilities for potential bioterrorism agents—has been recognized with the establishment of a Laboratory Response Network (*see* http://www.bt.cdc.gov/).

3.5. Filovirus Vaccines

As of 2003, no vaccine for either MARV or EBOV had entered human testing in the United States, although several promising vaccine candidates and approaches were identified recently (23–26). Earlier efforts to demonstrate the feasibility of vaccination against MARV were only partially successful, as inoculation with formalin-inactivated viruses only protected about half the test animals (guinea pigs or nonhuman primates) from fatal disease (27). Experiences with EBOV vaccines were similar to those with MARV, reinforcing the difficulties of classical approaches. Of the many new vaccine technologies, two recombinant DNA approaches—a defective (e.g., single infectious cycle) alphavirus called a replicon (24) and a defective adenovirus (28)—have been reported efficacious in nonhuman primates, animals that are highly susceptible to lethal infection and thought to be the most rigorous tests of filoviral vaccines. These vaccines are expected to be among the first manufactured for testing of safety and immunologic potency in human subjects.

Because outbreaks are too unpredictable and it would be unethical to include placebo control groups if vaccines were thought efficacious, filovirus vaccines represent cases in which the required efficacy demonstrations for licensure of human vaccines will likely be based on nonhuman data. To accommodate such special circumstances, the FDA recently established a process known colloquially as the "animal rule," by which vaccines may be licensed for human use under circumstances where human efficacy trials are not feasible or ethical (Federal Register: Vol. 64 (192), October 5, 1999, pp. 53,960–53,970). Briefly, the rule describes conditions for a drug or biological product under which it may be "reasonable to expect the effect of the product in animals to be a reliable indicator of its efficacy in humans." Notably, this rule does not exempt the separate requirement to establish vaccine safety in humans.

Minimally, a single vaccine for MARV and EBOV will require components of both; additional vaccine complexity may be required to protect against all medically relevant species and strains of both filovirus types. That is, no cross-protection between MARV and EBOV has been observed in any animal model, nor is any shared immunity expected from available data. In the glycoprotein, independently identified as an important vaccine antigen for both MARV and EBOV, amino acid identity between MARV (Musoke strain) and EBOV (Zaire strain) is only 30%. Polyclonal antibodies (immune sera) against MARV do not cross-react unless minimally with ZEBOV, nor are anti-EBOV antibodies known to cross-react with MARV. The genetic and antigenic diversity among EBOV species is even greater than among MARV isolates.

3.6. Challenges and Opportunities in the Development of Vaccines, Other Countermeasures

Vaccines represent one vitally important approach toward mitigating the medical consequences of viral diseases, accounting for most of the 99% or greater declines (from baseline 20th century figures) in smallpox, measles, mumps, rubella, and paralytic polio *(29)*. However, the discovery, development, manufacture, licensure, and use of virus vaccines present some difficult challenges that are only exacerbated in the case of vaccines against highly hazardous viral agents (*see* Table 6).

Regarding the prospects for alternative countermeasures, physical protection (including HEPA-filtered breathing apparatus) can be of significant if limited value. Discovery and development of new antiviral compounds would provide an important and complementary alternative to vaccination. This too has proven a daunting task in the past, but new technologies and new efforts have led (e.g., in the case of HIV) to more rapid advances than previously imagined. Antibody technologies are also evolving rapidly, so that specific antibody therapies may someday be added to the treatments for several viral agents.

4. PERSPECTIVES AND FUTURE DIRECTIONS

Numerous viral agents have been discussed as possible new threats to US and global health. Fortunately, substantial progress has been made already toward countermeasures against virtually the entire array of such viruses. In most cases, feasibility of vaccination has been proven in laboratory studies, protective antigens identified, and presumptive correlates of immunity defined. Moreover, a preliminary pathway to vaccine production has been illuminated in many cases, and candidate vaccines have been tested for safety in human volunteers. For some of the agents, an antiviral drug is available that may improve patient outcomes. Even with the deadly MARV and EBOV viruses, where no therapeutic interventions are available and the most promising vaccines are still being refined experimentally, the first countermeasures appear imminent. The United States and other nations are better prepared than ever before to

Table 6
Some Challenges in Vaccine Development for Emerging, Zoonotic, and Hazardous Viruses, Including Those of Special Concern as Possible Agents of Bioterrorism

Generic challenges in making vaccines against hazardous viruses	Special challenges for vaccines to protect against bioweapons
Biocontainment: increased costs, few capable laboratories	Operational or emergency need for rapid onset of immunity
Little or no commercial market: most often requires public funding	Requirement for immunity against aerosol as well as parenteral infection
Antigenic and biologic variations in agents: new research in some areas required	Possibility of unnaturally high doses
Animal models of disease are inadequate for many agents	Possibility of extraordinarily virulent, selected types
Paucity of data on human disease: focal or episodic outbreaks limit data collection	Specter of admixed agents as weapons, altering diagnosis, pathogenesis, treatment
Paucity of immunologic and pathogenetic data to guide vaccine design	Specter of genetically modified agents that circumvent vaccine
Few or no suitable study sites for vaccine efficacy trials in humans	Specter of benign agents or vectors engineered as weapons
Requirement for licensed vaccine, not "experimental" precursor, e.g., IND product	
Medical and political decisions on risk/benefit, vaccination versus vaccine stockpiling, long-term costs	

recognize, treat, and manage the public health consequences of previously unfamiliar viruses.

Nevertheless, a great deal remains to be done, especially in the areas of vaccines and antiviral drugs. Many of the first-generation vaccines prepared against exotic viral agents are not ideally suited for the 21st century. Vaccine stockpiles, where they exist, are highly limited. Existing antiviral drugs are only moderately suitable for some viruses, and ineffective against many others; safe, effective, broad-spectrum antiviral compounds remain highly elusive. Potential antibody-based therapies have not been fully researched nor developed. Fortunately, new national funding has provided unprecedented momentum to discover, improve, develop, and manufacture viral vaccines using a set of rapidly evolving vaccine technologies. Similarly, the recognized need for therapeutic interventions, including antiviral drugs, is coincident with both a boost in priority and an explosion of technological advances. The interplay between basic biological research, molecular biology, unexpected medical breakthroughs, as well as computational fields (genomics, proteomics, knowledge management) are likely to result in the rapid evolution of potential countermeasures for all viruses, including those considered present and future threats. Possibly, the most important and difficult challenges will lie in the coherent conversion of the anticipated new potentials (born of scientific ingenuity) into truly available countermeasures.

REFERENCES

1. Borio, L., et al. (2002) Hemorrhagic fever viruses as biological weapons: medical and public health management. *JAMA* **287(18),** 2391–2405.
2. van Regenmortel, M. H. V., et al. (eds.) (2000) *Seventh Report of the International Committee on Taxonomy of Viruses.* Academic Press.
3. Bwaka, M. A., et al. (1999) Ebola hemorrhagic fever in Kikwit, Democratic Republic of the Congo: clinical observations in 103 patients. *J. Infect. Dis.* **179(Suppl. 1),** S1–7.
4. Slenczka, W. G. (1999) The Marburg virus outbreak of 1967 and subsequent episodes. *Curr. Top. Microbiol. Immunol.* **235,** 49–75.
5. Sidell, F. R., et al. (1997) Medical aspects of chemical and biological warfare, in *Textbook of Military Medicine, Part I. Warfare, Weaponry, and the Casualty.* Washington, D.C.
6. Hart, M. K., et al. (1997) Venezuelan equine encephalitis virus vaccines induce mucosal IgA responses and protection from airborne infection in BALB/c, but not C3H/HeN mice. *Vaccine* **15(4),** 363–369.
7. Nichol, S. T., et al. (1993) Genetic identification of a hantavirus associated with an outbreak of acute respiratory illness. *Science* **262(5135),** 914–917.
8. Lanciotti, R. S., et al. (1999) Origin of the West Nile virus responsible for an outbreak of encephalitis in the northeastern United States. *Science* **286(5448),** 2333–2337.
9. Huggins, J. W., et al. (1991) Prospective, double-blind, concurrent, placebo-controlled clinical trial of intravenous ribavirin therapy of hemorrhagic fever with renal syndrome. *J. Infect. Dis.* **164(6),** 1119–1127.
10. McCormick, J. B., et al. (1986) Lassa fever. Effective therapy with ribavirin. *N. Engl. J. Med.* **314(1),** 20–26.
11. Alibek, K. and Handelman, S. (1999) Biohazard: the chilling true story of the largest covert biological weapons program in the world, told from the inside by the man who ran it. 1st ed. Random House, New York, p. 319.
12. Miller, J., Engelberg, S., and Broad, W. J., (2001) *Germs: Biological Weapons and America's Secret War.* Simon & Schuster, New York, p. 382.
13. Morse, S. S. (1995) Factors in the emergence of infectious diseases. *Emerg. Infect. Dis.* **1(1),** 7–15.
14. Bertherat, E., Talarmin, A., and Zeller, H. (1999) Democratic Republic of the Congo: between civil war and the Marburg virus. International Committee of Technical and Scientific Coordination of the Durba Epidemic. *Med. Trop.* **59(2),** 201–204.
15. Georges-Courbot, M. C., Leroy, E., and Zeller, H. (2002) Ebola: a virus endemic to central Africa? *Med. Trop.* **62(3),** 295–300.
16. Swanepoel, R., et al. (1996) Experimental inoculation of plants and animals with Ebola virus. *Emerg. Infect. Dis.* **2(4),** 321–325.
17. Leirs, H., et al. (1999) Search for the Ebola virus reservoir in Kikwit, Democratic Republic of the Congo: reflections on a vertebrate collection. *J. Infect. Dis.* **179(Suppl 1),** S155–163.
18. Martini, G. A. and Siegert, R. (1971) Marburg Virus Disease. Springer-Verlag, Berlin, vii, p. 230.
19. Leroy, E. M., et al. (2000) Human asymptomatic Ebola infection and strong inflammatory response. *Lancet* **355(9222),** 2210–2215.
20. Peters, C. J. and LeDuc, J. W. (1999) An introduction to Ebola: the virus and the disease. *J. Infect. Dis.* **179(Suppl 1),** ix–xvi.
21. Sadek, R. F., et al. (1999) Ebola hemorrhagic fever, Democratic Republic of the Congo, 1995: determinants of survival. *J. Infect. Dis.* **179(Suppl 1),** S24–27.
22. Rodriguez, L. L., et al. (1999) Persistence and genetic stability of Ebola virus during the outbreak in Kikwit, Democratic Republic of the Congo, 1995. *J. Infect. Dis.* **179(Suppl 1),** S170–176.

23. Bavari, S., et al. (2002) Lipid raft microdomains: a gateway for compartmentalized trafficking of ebola and marburg viruses. *J. Exp. Med.* **195(5),** 593–602.

24. Hevey, M., et al. (1998) Marburg virus vaccines based upon alphavirus replicons protect guinea pigs and nonhuman primates. *Virology* **251(1),** 28–37.

25. Hevey, M., et al. (2001) Marburg virus vaccines: comparing classical and new approaches. *Vaccine* **20(3-4),** 586–593.

26. Wilson, J. A., Bosio, C. M., and Hart, M. K., (2001) Ebola virus: the search for vaccines and treatments. *Cell. Mol. Life Sci.* **58(12-13),** 1826–1841.

27. Ignatyev, G. M. (1999) Immune response to filovirus infections. *Curr. Top. Microbiol. Immunol.* **235,** 205–217.

28. Sullivan, N. J., et al. (2000) Development of a preventive vaccine for Ebola virus infection in primates. *Nature* **408(6812),** 605–609.

29. Ten great public health achievements—United States, 1900–1999. Morb. Mortal. Wkly. Rep,. **48(12),** 241–243.

SELECTED WEB RESOURCES

http://www.cdc.gov/ Centers for Disease Control and Prevention

http://www.idsociety.org/bt/toc.htm Infectious Diseases Society of America, Bioterrorism Information and Resources

http://www.hopkins-biodefense.org/index.html Center for Civilian Biodefense Strategies, the Johns Hopkins University, Bloomberg School of Public Health*

http://ictvdb.bio2.columbia.edu/ Recent updates from International Committee on Viral Taxonomy:

http://www.vnh.org/MedAspChemBioWar/ Textbook of Military Medicine: Medical Aspects of Chemical and Biological Warfare, Office of the Surgeon General, Department of the Army

http://www.vnh.org/MedAspChemBioWar/chapters/chapter_28.htm Viral Encephalitides Textbook of Military Medicine: Medical Aspects of Chemical and Biological Warfare: Chapter 28 Viral Encephalitides Jonathan F. Smith, PH.D.; Kelly Davis, D.V.M.; Mary Kate Hart, PH.D.; George V. Ludwig, PH.D.; David J. McClain, M.D.; Michael D. Parker, PH.D.; and William D. Pratt, D.V.M., PH.D.

http://www.vnh.org/MedAspChemBioWar/chapters/chapter_29.htm Textbook of Military Medicine: Medical Aspects of Chemical and Biological Warfare: Chapter 29 Viral Hemorrhagic Fevers, Peter B. Jahrling PH.D.

---

* This is now affiliated with the Center for Biosecurity of the University of Pittsburgh Medical Center (UPMC), www.upmc-biosecurity.org.

12

Medical Defense Against Protein Toxin Weapons

Review and Perspective

Charles B. Millard

1. PROTEIN TOXIN WEAPONS

The term "toxin weapon" has been used to describe poisons, classically of natural origin but increasingly accessible by modern synthetic methods, which are suitable for delivery on a battlefield in a form that causes death or severe incapacitation at relatively low concentrations (reviewed in ref. *1*). Several of the most important toxin weapons are proteins, and these molecules are the focus of this chapter. Recent technological changes have increased the importance of protein toxins for biological warfare (BW): (a) progress in biotechnology has made large-scale production and purification feasible for a larger number of protein toxins; (b) molecular biology techniques, especially the polymerase chain reaction, have enabled the identification, isolation and comparison of extended families of previously obscure natural toxins; and (c) gene manipulation and microbiology have greatly expanded the accessible delivery vehicles for protein toxins to include, for example, natural or genetically modified bacteria and engineered viruses.

Advances in biotechnology notwithstanding, if we consider only those protein toxins with characteristics suitable for direct use as mass-casualty weapons in the absence of replicating, biological delivery systems, then only a small subset of known proteins are of immediate concern *(1)*. The list of practicable toxin weapons is small because: (a) proteins are not volatile and generally do not persist long in the environment; (b) simple, physical protection offers an effective natural defense against foreign proteins; and (c) relatively sophisticated research, development, testing, and evaluation is required to establish conclusively that each specific protein toxin is a viable open-air, aerosol weapon.

Although small in number, toxin weapons should not be neglected. Similarly to chemical weapons or noninfectious biological agents such as anthrax spores, toxins offer the aggressor a tactical weapon to strike at the enemy in a controlled manner that is difficult or impossible with infectious agents, for example by the selective contamination of key terrain or high-value targets. Aerosolized protein toxins can be used both as lethal agents and as severe incapacitating agents, thereby greatly burdening medical

From: *Infectious Diseases: Biological Weapons Defense: Infectious Diseases and Counterterrorism*
Edited by: L. E. Lindler, F. J. Lebeda, and G. W. Korch © Humana Press Inc., Totowa, NJ

care and logistical systems. Moreover, unlike chemical nerve agents and anthrax spores, there are no effective postexposure treatments widely available for the most dangerous protein toxins.

In what forms can we expect to encounter protein toxin weapons? Most predictions of the potential medical threat posed by direct delivery of protein toxin weapons are predicated on military doctrine that assumes a trained, equipped, and healthy population in control of its own food and water supplies. For a prepared military force, the primary threat in an open-air battlefield environment is stable, respirable aerosols of the most toxic molecules by weight (reviewed in ref. *1*). Closed-air delivery of respirable aerosols, for example, within a building or other enclosed space, poses a secondary threat that would be expected to cause far fewer casualties but may expand the set of potential toxin weapons to include those with lower toxicity or those lacking outdoor stability.

An accurate assessment of which protein toxins are effectively "most toxic" by aerosol delivery must consider complex biological and environmental variables. As a first approximation, the most potent toxins (typically bacterial proteins) are those that are lethal for 50% of test animals (i.e., toxin LD_{50}) at amounts less than 25 ng/kg by intravenous or intra-peritoneal exposure routes *(1–4)*. Aerosol lethality is a function of both toxin concentration and exposure time, and this is reported as an LCt_{50} value with units of mg/min/m^{-3}.[1] Direct comparison among published toxin LD_{50} or LCt_{50} values can be easily confounded by numerous experimental variables, including the method of aerosol exposure, time of exposure, breathing patterns, and other interspecies variations among animal models, as well as physical differences in the purity, stability, or potency of the toxin employed. Furthermore, lethality data alone are unsatisfactory for gaging the severe incapacitation caused by lung injury that may be enhanced by aerosol delivery routes for proinflammatory toxins.

Some bacterial protein toxins are notoriously potent food poisons *(5)*. Sabotage of food or beverage supplies with protein toxins is unlikely to produce mass casualties against a military force but could have a significant disruptive effect upon unprepared populations. Fortunately, the threat of intentional poisoning is significantly mitigated by modern food-processing practices, dilution, and routine public health measures such as monitoring, rapid communication, and other controls.

Protein toxins are not expected to pose a significant mass-casualty threat by percutaneous or ocular delivery routes because the stratified epithelial tissues of skin and cornea provide barriers that limit penetration of foreign proteins, provided that the tissue has not been compromised by injury or other means. Protein toxins may cause incapacitating ocular inflammation by direct or indirect effects on exposed cornea and conjunctiva, but these effects generally are reversible.

From even a brief assessment of the medical threat posed by protein toxin weapons, it is apparent that respiratory protective equipment, for example, a gas mask or respirator, and immediate decontamination offer the best defense. However, if natural or other physical barriers and rapid decontamination fail to prevent internalization of a protein toxin, then survival may depend on the availability of adequate medical countermea-

---

[1]A detailed discussion of the pathogenesis of toxin bioaersols, including selected toxin aerosol LCt_{50} values, is presented elsewhere in this volume by Pitt and LeClaire.

sures, including vaccines, other pretreatments, or antidotes. The purpose of this chapter is to provide a review of selected medical products under development for protection against protein toxins of military significance and to offer a perspective on the critical role of protein engineering[2] in the iterative process of optimizing those medical products. In addition to medical countermeasures, the status of protein engineering of toxins also is discussed.

2. OVERVIEW OF MEDICAL COUNTERMEASURES

2.1. *Vaccines*

Vaccination, the intentional induction of a lasting, protective immune response mediated by antibodies, offers one of the most powerful, flexible, and safe methods known to achieve medical protection from protein toxins. Ideal vaccines to protect against BW protein toxins would safely induce lasting levels of high-avidity IgG antibodies within the alveolar lining fluid, as well as IgA antibodies secreted into the mucous membranes lining the lung airway, such that toxins are neutralized before reaching their biological targets.

There is a general, progressive strategy that has been employed for developing vaccines to protect against protein toxin threats. Initially, an inactivated "toxoid" vaccine is prepared from biological homogenates or crude toxin preparations. Toxoid vaccines provide a generally safe and effective solution, as exemplified by the enduring use of tetanus toxoid vaccines worldwide *(6)*. Yet, toxoid vaccines are susceptible to production, safety, or storage limitations that stem from use of denaturants, crosslinking agents, residual live toxin, or from the partial reversion of inactivated toxoid back to active toxin. To improve on toxoid vaccines, effective "neutralizing epitopes" are identified within toxin structures, and this information is applied to develop recombinant immunogens with enhanced safety and ease of production.

Protein engineering, especially recombinant DNA technology for site-specific substitutions and commercial protein expression systems, has contributed to the development of a number of new, recombinant vaccine candidates that were inaccessible previously because of small quantities or inherent toxicity of natural immunogens. Recombinant immunogens are generally well-defined and suited to current Good Manufacturing Practices. However, the limited immune system responses to purified, recombinant proteins or polypeptide subunits, compared to responses to natural infections or attenuated vaccines, must be overcome by careful selection of epitopes and the use of adjuvants or other activators *(7)*.

As a more-detailed structural concept of the toxin and vaccine candidate emerges, protein engineering methods may permit cycles of vaccine improvement, for example, to achieve better presentation of the neutralizing epitopes or enhanced stability. Engineering may result in production of new immunogens based on inactivated holotoxins, polypeptide subunits, or independent polypeptide domains.

Because of the importance of the aerosol threat in BW, traditional vaccination strategies for some toxins may benefit from additional protection of critical target organs,

---

[2]Protein engineering is the deliberate modification of polypeptide structure to achieve a desired form or function.

especially the portals of toxin entry such as the respiratory tract. Alternate vaccine-delivery methods, including transdermal, intranasal, inhalation, or oral routes for vaccine priming or boosting, may permit more effective administration of engineered vaccines to induce stronger mucosal antibody responses. This approach includes the application of novel devices or adjuvant-device combinations that also may facilitate simultaneous delivery of multiple immunogens *(8)*. Along with nontraditional routes of vaccine delivery, it may be possible to enhance protection of target organs by the use of adjunct therapeutics.

Despite the power of vaccination to protect against protein toxin weapons, there will continue to be a limited number of military or first responder scenarios in which there is insufficient time for vaccines to elicit a protective immune response. Additionally, it may be impractical or undesirable to vaccinate large, healthy populations against the relatively remote threat of all potential toxins. The vaccine candidates currently available have been developed for use in limited, volunteer military forces comprising mostly healthy young adults subject to regular medical screening and care. Additional optimization studies may be required to ensure safe administration to larger, more diverse civilian populations.

Other limitations may arise with complete reliance on vaccination as a medical solution for toxin weapons. As the clinical use of toxins themselves as medical therapies (so-called "medicotoxins") continues to expand, for example, the growing medical use of botulinum neurotoxin (BoNT) injections to control the cholinergic neuromuscular junction in various disease states (reviewed in ref. *9*), it will become increasingly difficult to justify the use of vaccination against toxin weapons for the general population. Once an individual is vaccinated against a toxin, the clinical administration of that specific molecule as a medicotoxin becomes much more difficult *(10)*.

Consequently, the development of antitoxin therapeutics as adjuncts to vaccines and, in some BW scenarios, as viable replacements for vaccination is an important component of medical defense against protein toxins. Therapeutic approaches include antibody-based biological therapeutics, as well as emerging biomedical research to discover cost-effective small-molecule antidotes.

2.2. Immunotherapeutics

The use of antibody molecules before an anticipated toxin exposure, or as a therapy immediately after exposure, is called "passive immunotherapy" or "antitoxin" therapy. Specific antibodies or processed binding fragments of antibodies (FAbs) can be prepared by various technologies, including vaccination of a suitable donor with toxin vaccine candidates or recombinant DNA-based protein expression systems. Purified immunotherapeutics subsequently can be administered to at-risk or exposed recipients as "bioscavengers" to bind and eliminate toxic molecules from the body before they reach critical target sites. The use of preformed antibodies to mitigate symptoms of BoNT toxin, for example, has been an accepted part of the routine clinical management of food-borne botulism in humans since the 1960s *(11)*.

Antitoxin antibodies historically have been captured from the polyvalent immune serum of vaccinated or hyperimmune animals and subsequently used to treat human patients exposed to protein toxins. Although processing to remove expendable portions of the antibody molecule that are distal to the essential antigen combining end ("despeciation") may reduce the human immune reaction, serious side effects such as anaphylaxis and serum sickness still may occur because the animal-derived products are recognized as foreign. Because of this immunological "rejection" of foreign protein by the human patient, animal-derived products become more dangerous if administered repeatedly; this greatly limits the utility of animal products as a pretreatment.

Antitoxin derived from human immune serum of vaccinated volunteers overcomes the major limitations imposed by immunological rejection of animal serum. For example, human antitoxin products would be expected to circulate longer and could be given by repeated injections, thus opening up the possibility of a safe pretreatment for toxin exposure. However, the production of suitable human immune serum in sufficient quantities for use in mass casualty scenarios may be impractical because the number of suitable immune human donors is small. Furthermore, the widespread use of human immune serum antitoxin carries the risk of transfer of unknown or undetectable human pathogens or adventitious agents from donor to recipient.

Although the flexibility and specificity of an antibody-based therapeutic is unquestionable, the application of this approach as a routine medical solution in a field situation poses several logistical and technical challenges: (a) the success depends critically on stability of the proper three-dimensional structure of the antibody therapeutic employed; (b) the therapeutic window for antibody use is narrow because symptoms of toxin exposure typically appear hours to days after exposure when the toxin already has bound its target or has been internalized to intracellular compartments inaccessible to antibody molecules; and (c) antibodies and FAbs are large molecules that bind reversibly with a limited stoichiometry and, therefore, it generally will require large amounts of therapeutic by weight to neutralize supralethal quantities of toxin.

2.3. Small-Molecule Experimental Therapeutics

Selective, low-molecular-weight drugs are unavailable at present for the most deadly protein toxin weapons, but active research programs are underway and have produced key resources in the past several years, including solved three-dimensional X-ray structures of toxin and toxin-inhibitor complexes, cloned toxin subunit genes, and specific, high-throughput toxin activity assays. In addition to antibody-based scavenger approaches, novel toxin therapeutics may be directed against one or more of the molecular steps required for intoxication. For those protein toxins that achieve very high potency by enzymatic catalysis, for example, it may be possible to develop selective, very high affinity or irreversible active-site inhibitors as effective toxin therapeutics.

In summary, four general approaches are being taken to develop pharmaceuticals to protect against protein toxin weapons: toxoid vaccines, engineered vaccines, immunotherapeutics, and small-molecule therapeutics. I will expand on the relative advantages and disadvantages of each approach through a review of past and ongoing research efforts to protect against three specific protein toxin weapons: BoNT, *Staphylococcus aureus* enterotoxins (SE), and ricin toxin from *Ricinus communis*. BoNT, SE, and ricin are chosen on the basis of the maturity of medical product candidates currently under development and also because each represents an important class of protein toxin: cholinergic toxins, immune system modulators, and ribosome inactivating toxins, respectively.

3. BoNT

Botulism is caused by a family of potent neurotoxins (BoNT) that are produced for unknown reasons by *Clostridium botulinum* bacteria from one of at least seven different serotypes (designated BoNT types /A through /G) *(12)*. Four of the serotypes (/A, /B, /E, and, less commonly, /F) are significant for human poisoning through contaminated food, wound infection, or infant botulism (reviewed in ref. *13)*. Although botulism is a relatively rare disease worldwide, the extreme toxicity of BoNT makes it a potential toxin weapon *(11,14)*.

Within the past few years, three-dimensional structures of holotoxins or isolated domains of toxins from *Clostridium* bacteria have been solved, and consequently, a more complete picture of toxin function is emerging *(15–18)*. Like the closely related tetanus neurotoxin (TeNT), the BoNT proteins are disulfide-bonded heterodimers composed of an approx 50 kD zinc metalloprotease "light chain" and an approx100 kD receptor-binding "heavy chain" (Hc). The Hc has been subdivided structurally and functionally into a C-terminal domain that binds the toxin to gangliosides and other receptors on the surface of peripheral cholinergic neurons (so-called Hc domain), and an N-terminal domain that is believed to enhance cell binding and translocation of the catalytic light chain across the vesicular membrane (reviewed in ref. *19; see* Fig. 1). Additionally, BoNT naturally is associated with numerous nontoxic "accessory proteins," some of which may stabilize the toxins in vivo *(20)*.

The mechanism by which BoNT traverses neuron cell membranes is incompletely understood, but it may involve a large conformational change in the toxin. A conformational change or partial unfolding of the light chain has been proposed to explain passage of the toxin catalytic portion through narrow transmembrane channels or pores formed by the amino terminal portion of the BoNT heavy chain *(21–24)*.

Once inside the neuron, the catalytic subunit of BoNT acts as a selective, zinc metalloprotease to cleave essential polypeptide components of the so-called "SNARE complex" required for normal neurotransmitter release or membrane fusion. BoNT/A, /C1, and /E cleave the polypeptide SNAP-25 (BoNT/C1 cleaves syntaxin), and BoNT/ B, /D, /F, and /G cleave synaptobrevin (reviewed in ref. *19)*. The exact mechanisms by which the soluble *N*-ethyl maleimide-sensitive factor attachment protein receptors (SNARE) complex mediates vesicle fusion or release of neurotransmitter acetylcholine (ACh) into the synaptic cleft remain controversial, but it is clear that the integrity of the complex is critical for normal cholinergic nerve transmission (reviewed in refs. *25–27)*.

By disrupting ACh exocytosis at the peripheral neuromuscular junction, BoNT causes cholinergic autonomic nervous system dysfunction in effected patients. Signs and symptoms of BoNT intoxication typically manifest 12–36 h after toxin exposure and include generalized weakness, lassitude, and dizziness. There may be decreased salivation and dry mouth or sore throat; motor symptoms reflect cranial nerve dysfunction, including dysarthria, dysphonia, and dysphagia, followed by symmetrical descending and progressive muscle paralysis *(13)*. Without adequate supportive care, death may occur abruptly as a result of respiratory failure. The molecular precision of BoNT renders it among the most toxic substances known by weight; internalized BoNT may cause fatal paralysis in animals at nanogram/kilogram levels *(3)*.

3.1. BoNT Toxoid Vaccines

Preparations of inactivated, partially purified BoNT have been used as vaccines to protect humans for many years *(28)*. BoNT from each of the serotypes /A–/E was prepared, inactivated with formalin, adsorbed to aluminum hydroxide, and blended to produce an effective pentavalent toxoid vaccine (PBT) *(29–33)*. The PBT vaccine currently is administered to at-risk laboratory workers under an Investigational New Drug (IND) protocol. An effective vaccination regimen has been found to comprise initial doses (0.5 mL) of 10 µg of toxin protein equivalent given at 0, 2, and 12 wk, followed by annual boosters. Annual boosters have been offered contingent on serum-neutralizing BoNT antibody levels, as measured by mouse neutralization assays. In human volunteers, the available PBT induces antibodies that neutralize the toxicity of BoNT/A and /B in mouse bioassays *(34)*. Protective titers for other serotypes have not been established as rigorously as for BoNT/A, but neither have the exposure threshold levels of toxin for which a laboratory worker may be at risk.

Additional BoNT toxoid vaccines have been produced and used safely in humans. The PHLS Center for Applied Microbiology and Research, Porton Down (Salisbury, Wiltshire, England) produced a monovalent BoNT/A vaccine. A monovalent toxoid vaccine for BoNT/F subsequently was developed after BoNT/F botulism outbreaks were diagnosed in 1980–1990 *(35)*. A tetravalent vaccine candidate (BoNT/A, /B, /E, and /F) has recently been produced for human use *(36)*.

Despite the effectiveness of BoNT toxoid vaccines, there are significant cost and technical barriers associated with their production. Because of the sporulating nature of *C. botulinum*, a dedicated, contained manufacturing facility currently is required to produce toxoid. Additionally, the natural yields of BoNT from *C. botulinum* are low relative to the quantities of toxin needed for vaccine starting material. Moreover, there is a small but significant number of minor adverse reactions associated with toxoid vaccine, perhaps because of the use of formalin in the manufacturing process (reviewed in ref. *37*). These concerns have led to the development of recombinant BoNT vaccines *(38–40)*.

3.2. Engineered BoNT Vaccines

Simpson et al. reported that TeNT Hc fragments could compete for neuron binding and, thereby, antagonize the neuromuscular blocking properties of native TeNT and, to a lesser extent, BoNT *(41,42)*. This observation led to the immunization of mice against TeNT with fragments of TeNT synthesized in *E. coli (38,43)*. A similar vaccine for BoNT/A based on the recombinant Hc became possible once the toxin gene was cloned and expressed *(39,40,44)* (*see* Fig. 1). Subsequent epitope mapping of BoNT/A identified two specific polypeptides, both from Hc ($H_{455-661}$ and $H_{1150-1289}$), that were capable of protecting mice from a supralethal challenge with the toxin *(45)*.

The US Army Medical Research Institute of Infectious Diseases (USAMRIID) developed recombinant BoNT Hc vaccine candidates for BoNT/A, /B, and /F that confer protection in mice against supralethal challenges with toxin *(46–50)*. This approach recently was extended to include BoNT Hc fragments from BoNT/C and /D *(51)*. Unlike the BoNT toxoids, the recombinant Hc vaccine candidates do not require treatment with denaturants and are not susceptible to reversion of catalytic activity. If no

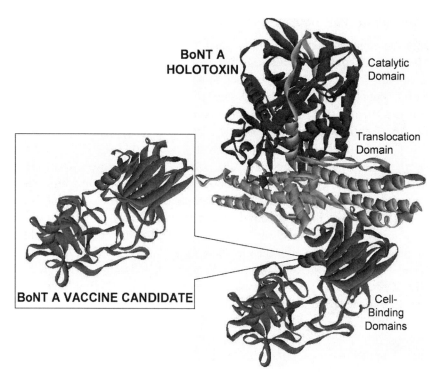

Fig. 1. Topology of recombinant BoNT Hc vaccine candidates with respect to the overall three-dimensional structure of the holotoxin. The figure shows a ribbon diagram of the BoNT/ A holotoxin structure solved by X-ray crystallography (PDB entry 3BTA) that includes the three functional domains colored separately. A hypothetical projection of the recombinant vaccine candidate structure based upon the known amino acid sequence is shown as inset.

serious safety issues are identified, then the BoNT Hc vaccine candidates will require final formulation with an appropriate adjuvant, and optimization of the stability of each vaccine during scale-up production and formulation *(37,50,52)*. Additionally, a strategy for effective delivery of multiple recombinant BoNT Hc subunit immunogens is needed to ensure protection against all relevant BoNT serotypes.

Although apparently safe and effective as vaccine candidates, an inherent limitation of the recombinant Hc fragment vaccines is their lack of cross-reactivity among BoNT serotypes. A separate Hc fragment immunogen is required for each BoNT serotype and, perhaps, for some different strains of each BoNT serotypes. Future protein engineering studies may employ detailed structural comparisons of essential residues within the Hc binding sites among the relevant BoNT serotypes to identify conserved epitopes *(53)*. The solved X-ray crystal structures of receptor-binding domains from TeNT and multiple BoNT serotypes, both free and bound with receptor analogs, should facilitate this approach by identifying critical, conserved binding features among serotypes *(18,54)*. Additional work is needed to explore the possibility of developing new vaccine candidates based on cross-reactive neutralizing epitopes within the translocation and catalytic domains of different BoNT serotypes *(55)*.

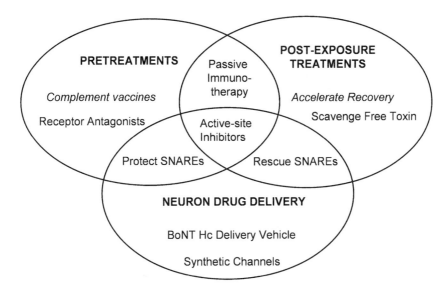

Fig. 2. Venn diagram depicting several complementary, mechanism-based research approaches being undertaken to develop novel therapeutics for protection against BoNT. Current therapeutics efforts include three primary research areas: (a) pretreatments; (b) postexposure antidotes; and (c) cholinergic neuron drug delivery systems for delivery therapeutics as appropriate.

3.3. Alternate Delivery of BoNT Vaccines

Several alternate vaccine-delivery routes for recombinant BoNT Hc immunogens have been explored recently in animal models including inhalation and oral vaccine delivery, as well as the use of self-replicating RNA virus or DNA-based vectors *(56–59)*. Proof-of-concept for the use of inactivated holotoxin as an oral immungen was reported by Simpson et al. *(60,61)*. However, it remains unproven whether these experimental delivery approaches offer any practical advantage for BW defense against BoNT compared with traditional, intramuscular vaccination. More data are needed describing the kinetics and biodistribution of BoNT after aerosol exposure in primates to evaluate whether there is a role for boosting mucosal immunity in protecting against supralethal BoNT exposures.

Protein engineering also may permit a combination of the toxoid and recombinant vaccine approaches. It has been shown that expression levels of BoNT can be increased in an *E. coli* system by amplifying specific transfer RNA (tRNA) genes for rare codons *(62)*. Additionally, progress also has been made on bacterial expression systems based on non-toxigenic strains of *C. botulinum (63)*. These results suggest the possibility that superior BoNT toxoid vaccines might be produced in *E. coli* or other protein expression systems by introducing active-site substitutions to selectively inactivate holotoxin, without the need for costly, dedicated production facilities or the risk of toxin reversion that limits older toxoid technology. Similarly, these tools may facilitate the future design of stable, multivalent, BoNT vaccines based on recombinant chimeras of multiple serotypes.

SE-A TOXIN VACCINE CANDIDATE

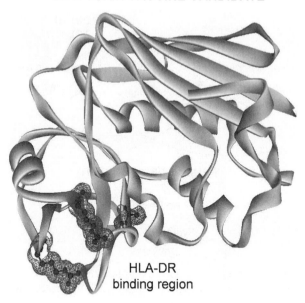

HLA-DR
binding region

Fig. 3. Position of the three inactivating substitutions used to produce the current recombinant SE vaccine candidates with respect to the overall toxin structure and HLA binding site. The figure shows a ribbon diagram of the SE/A triple substitution structure solved by X-ray crystallography (PDB entry 1DYQ). The side chains of the substituted amino acid residues (Arg70, Arg48, and Ala92) are displayed with VDW surfaces.

3.4. Immunotherapeutics

Current medical treatment for BoNT intoxication is likely to involve prolonged life-support for incapacitated survivors, including the continual use of mechanical ventilation *(11)*. The potential of BoNT as a mass casualty weapon, combined with the high cost and logistical burden of symptomatic medical treatment, has led to increased emphasis on the development of selective and cost-effective BoNT therapeutics. Some of the experimental approaches being explored in this actively growing research area are summarized in Fig. 2.

Animal and human studies suggest that the presence of preformed, neutralizing antibodies in the serum to bind and eliminate toxin before it reaches target cells can prevent or reduce BoNT intoxication. Several different antitoxin products for human use to protect against BoNT have been developed. A "trivalent" (serotypes /A, /B, and /E) equine antitoxin product, as well as a monovalent BoNT/E antitoxin, are licensed by Aventis Pateur Canada (formerly Connaught Laboratories, Ltd.) and approved for use in the United States. Biomed of Warsaw, Poland also produces a trivalent BoNT/A/ B/E anti-toxin. Additionally, an experimental, despeciated equine heptavalent (serotypes /A-/G) product was developed at USAMRIID and currently is administered under an IND protocol for limited use.

Several efforts have been undertaken to produce a human antibody-based therapeutic since the widespread clinical recognition of infant botulism in the late 1970s *(11)*. In 1981–1982, the US Army, the California Department of Health Services, and the

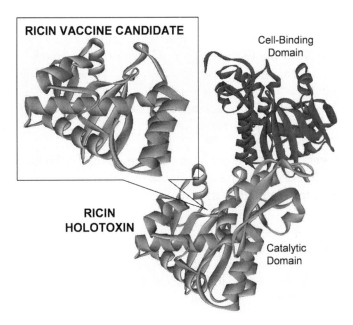

Fig. 4. Topology of recombinant ricin vaccine candidates with respect to the overall three-dimensional structure of the holotoxin. The figure shows a ribbon diagram of the ricin holotoxin structure solved by X-ray crystallography (PDB entry 2AAI). The holotoxin includes two subunits, RTA (light gray), and RTB (dark gray). The hypothetical structure of the domain (RTA1-198) used for recombinant vaccine candidates is projected from the toxin structure based on the known amino acid sequence.

University of Minnesota collaborated to produce a human botulism immune globulin (BIG) antiserum from different pools of plasma obtained from human donors who had been vaccinated previously with the PBT vaccine. Subsequently, a human antitoxin (BIG-IV) was developed and distributed for treating infant botulism under a United States Food and Drug Administration (FDA)-authorized IND protocol *(11)*. Intravenous administration of BIG significantly reduces the hospital stay of infants diagnosed with botulism, but it is not clear to what extent the success of BIG with infant botulism will also apply to treating patients exposed to BoNT by aerosol. Moreover, because of the obvious logistical barriers in production of antiserum in humans, the available BIG supplies are not expected to meet the mass casualty demands of a BW attack.

There are several ongoing biotechnological approaches aimed at expanding the availability of anti-toxins for human use. It is beyond the scope of this chapter to review all promising technologies underway, but we offer two examples currently being explored: the design and production of human recombinant monoclonal antibodies (MAbs) and the production of transgenic animals capable of producing human antibodies.

Preliminary studies showed that MAbs produced in rodents could neutralize large amounts of BoNT toxin, at least 10–100 times the BoNT toxin LD_{50} doses *(45,64)*. Subsequent work by Marks et al. generated phage antibody libraries from mice vaccinated with the Hc neutralizing epitope identified in earlier studies or from human volunteers previously vaccinated with PBT *(65,66)*. The technology permits recombinant expression of human antibodies for potential use as therapeutics. Rapidly evaluating a relatively large number of unique MAbs from these libraries has opened up the possibility of achieving a multiplicative increase in toxin neutralization by combining high-affinity antibodies with nonoverlapping binding sites. Using this approach under optimal conditions, it has been possible to neutralize very large amounts of BoNT/A, thereby providing protection in animal models against greater than 10,000–100,000 times the toxin LD_{50} doses *(67)*. The medical product expected from this research will be well-defined "oligoclonal" mixtures of selected human MAbs specific for toxin serotypes.

An alternative approach to achieve large-scale production of high-affinity therapeutic antibodies for BoNT or other toxins is the use of human artificial chromosome vectors to introduce the entire, unrearranged sequences for human Ig light- and heavy-chain genes into livestock. Kuroiwa et al. demonstrated that a human artificial chromosome vector can be inserted into bovine fetal fibroblast cells, thereby allowing for the production of cloned cattle carrying the human antibody genes *(68)*. Such animals could be used to produce large quantities of human polyclonal antisera against BoNT or other toxins without the side effects and logistical burden inherent in the past clinical use of despeciated antisera.

3.5. Small-Molecule Experimental Therapeutics

There currently is no safe and effective small-molecule therapeutic for preventing or reversing BoNT intoxication. During the past several years, however, a more-detailed understanding of the complex steps involved in BoNT intoxication, including neuron binding, translocation, and catalysis, has opened up the possibility for rational development of therapeutic intervention at the molecular level.

Ongoing research has focused on BoNT active-site inhibitors, including peptide-based captopril derivatives and other classes of zinc metalloprotease inhibitors *(69–72)*. Most of the inhibitors reported to date are either nonselective or bind with affinity that is too low to be useful as a therapeutic. Iterative inhibitor design is improving the situation and recently a β-amino thiol inhibitor of BoNT B was reported with a *Ki* of 20 nM *(73,74)*. Technical challenges to this approach include the use of peptide derivatives as drugs, the difficulty in delivering drugs within the nervous system, and the likely need to develop specific inhibitors for each serotype of BoNT.

With the goal of arriving at therapeutics that will antagonize multiple serotypes of BoNT, small molecules that act indirectly to overcome the presynaptic blockade of neurotransmitter release also have been explored. Toosendanin, a triterpenoid derivative from the bark of *Melia toosendan*, has limited efficacy in antagonizing the effects of BoNT intoxication in cell-based systems, as well as in a preliminary nonhuman primate study *(75–77)*. The mechanism of action for Toosendanin remains unclear, although it appears to act as a complex presynaptic blocking agent that can alter the quantal release of ACh by modulating calcium channel activity *(78,79)*. However, toxicity is expected to limit its usefulness as a drug because Toosendanin itself blocks presynaptic ACh release under conditions close to those found to show efficacy against BoNT.

The potassium channel blocker, 3,4-diaminopyridine (3,4-DAP) also can antagonize the effects of BoNT in vivo, provided that the drug concentration is maintained at plasma concentrations of about 30 μM during the entire clinical course of intoxication

(80,81). The results were comparable when 3,4-DAP was given 1, 2, 3, or 7 d after BoNT/A intoxication, but the compound was also essentially ineffective in antagonizing the paralytic actions of BoNT/B or BoNT/F. As with Toosendanin, one expects that the general toxicity of 3,4-DAP, coupled with the requirement of prolonged drug administration at relatively high levels, preclude routine therapeutic use.

Other experimental approaches being explored as future BoNT therapeutics include receptor antagonists as pretreatments that selectively block toxin receptor binding, as well as therapies that reverse intoxication by replacing target molecules destroyed by the toxin. An example of the latter is the replacement of SNARE proteins by gene therapy to rescue BoNT-intoxicated neurons *(82)*.

4. *STAPHYLOCOCCUS AUREUS* ENTEROTOXINS

Whereas BoNT achieves its potency by dampening an amplified extracellular signal of nerve cells via enzymatic catalysis, the *S. aureus* enterotoxins (SE) operate by inappropriately amplifying an extracellular signal of key immune cells. The SE belong to an extended family of stable 23–29 kD protein toxins that includes SE serotypes /A, /B, /Cn, /D, /E, and /H, and streptococcal pyrogenic exotoxins serotypes /A-/C; /F-/H, and /J, as well as toxic shock syndrome toxin (TSST-1) *(83)*. Based on their common ability to cause severe illness in animals by inducing a physiological overreaction of the host-immune response, these toxins have been categorized collectively as "superantigens" (SAgs); they are a major cause of human food poisoning and also contribute significantly to opportunistic bacterial infections in hospital patients (reviewed in refs. *84–88*).

The most important SAg in the context of BW is SE serotype /B (SE/B). SE/B is a two-domain, α–β-protein that contains discrete binding sites for the major histocompatibility complex (MHC) class II molecule and the Vβ regions of T-cell antigen receptors (TCRs) *(89–91)*. By binding to these two receptor molecules, and perhaps through other cell–surface interactions, SE/B is able to activate both antigen-presenting cells and a relatively large number of T lymphocytes to cause release of pyrogenic cytokines, chemokines, and other proinflammatory molecules (reviewed in ref. *92*).

The more common forms of SAg food poisoning can be managed with routine supportive care, but SE/B poses a formidable aerosol threat because of its high potency and stability. It is estimated that SE/B can produce human incapacitation and death at levels as low as 0.03 and 1.5 μg, respectively, by the aerosol route of exposure.[3] Primates are more sensitive than are many other animal species, perhaps partly because of higher affinity of the primate MHC class II receptors for SE/B. In a rhesus monkey model, exposure to lethal amounts of SE/B caused disabling emesis followed by a rapid drop in blood pressure, elevated temperature, skin rashes, toxic shock, multiple organ failure, and death (reviewed in ref. *93*).

4.1. SE Toxoid Vaccines

Almost 40 yr ago, it was shown that SE/B can be isolated from bacterial culture supernatants in highly purified form, and inactivated with neutral formaldehyde solu-

---

[3]These values are estimates for a 70-kg human based upon extrapolation of limited laboratory reports of accidental intoxication; the aerosol LD_{50} in primates is 20–30 μg/kg.

tions to produce an effective toxoid vaccine *(94)*. Anecdotal safety problems were reported during early animal studies of an SE/B toxoid vaccine, perhaps because there was not a standard methodology for making the toxoid *(95–97)*. Warren et al. systematically characterized different conditions of pH and formaldehyde concentration and suggested that conditions for crosslinking the toxin were critical for obtaining reproducible and immunogenic vaccine candidates; from these studies, an effective SE/B toxoid vaccine was later produced by incubating toxin with 1% formaldehyde at 37°C for 30 d at pH 7.5 *(98,99)*.

The SE/B toxoid combined with a suitable adjuvant or enhancer protected monkeys from an SE/B aerosol challenge of greater than 10 LD$_{50}$ *(100–102)*. Complexes of the SE/B toxoid with selected components of the meningococcal outer membrane (so-called "SE/B toxoid proteosomes"), for example, induced protective immunity intranasally or intramuscularly, and protected 100% of monkeys challenged with SE/B aerosol *(102,103)*. Nevertheless, the requirement of active toxin production as starting material, the possibility of toxoid reversion to yield active SE/B toxin, as well as minor reactogenicity associated with formaldehyde-inactivated vaccines, has prompted research to develop improved SE/B vaccines.

4.2. Engineered SE Vaccines

Comparative structural and biochemical studies carried out during the 1990s focused on the development of nontoxic, recombinant immunogens capable of eliciting a protective immune response against multiple SAg toxins *(83,104)*. Ulrich et al. at USAMRIID attempted to inactivate SE by modifying three structural regions of the toxin that are involved in HLA-DR1 binding: a polar pocket created by three β-strand elements of the β-barrel domain of the toxin, a hydrophobic reverse turn, and a disulfide-bonded loop *(104)*.

The polar binding pocket binding region in SE/B comprises three key residues of the toxin, Glu67, Tyr89, and Tyr115, that are postulated to form favorable interactions with Lys39 of the HLA-DR1 α-subunit by ion-pairing and hydrogen bonding *(90,105,106)*. Removing the anion at Glu67 (Glu→Gln substitution) resulted in an approx 100-fold reduction in binding affinity; substituting either Tyr89 or Tyr115 with Ala also reduced binding by 100-fold *(104,105)*.

A second critical binding region between SE/B and the HLA-DR molecule involves a hydrophobic reverse turn region comprising amino acid residues 44–47 that connects β-strands 1 and 2 of SE/B *(105,107)*. The backbone atoms of these residues are positioned to participate in attractive electrostatic interactions with the HLA-DR1 α-subunit; there also appears to be favorable hydrophobic packing between the toxin and the receptor mediated by SE/B Leu45.

Replacing Leu45 with a large, polar residue (Leu→Arg substitution) reduced binding of the toxin to HLA-DR1 to below detectable limits *(105)*. The Leu45Arg substitution may alter the volume and polarity of this small hydrophobic pocket of SE/B sufficiently to disrupt its binding with HLA-DR1. Vaccinating mice with Leu45Arg or with site-specific mutants designed to disrupt backbone contacts within the reverse turn region (Gln43Pro and Phe44Pro), protected against a supralethal (approx 30 times LD$_{50}$) challenge with SE/B; the Leu45Arg mutant also induced a greater IgG2a and IgG2b immune response in vaccinated mice than did either of the Pro mutants *(108)*.

Finally, a disulfide bonded loop region of the SE/B structure was implicated in receptor binding by analogy with TSST results, and substitution within this region (Tyr94→Ala) reduced binding of SE/B with HLA-DR1 *(104)*.

By combining substitutions in each of these three structural regions of SE/B (Tyr89Ala, Leu45Arg, and Tyr94Ala) within a single immunogen, a recombinant vaccine candidate (rSE/Bv) was produced that lacks detectable SAg activity. An analogous recombinant immunogen subsequently was developed for SE type A (SE/A) by introducing comparable substitutions: Asp70Arg, Leu48Arg, and Tyr92Ala. Figure 3 depicts the relative positions of the altered side chains within the solved, three-dimensional X-ray crystal structure of the SE/A immunogen *(109)*.

The rSE/Bv was tested in rodent[4] and nonhuman primate model systems for safety and efficacy. The vaccine elicited high antibody titers, and vaccinated mice survived supralethal challenges with SE/B toxin. When administered at a 20-μg dose, three-dose schedule, using alum as adjuvant, rSE/Bv protected nonhuman primates against greater than 20 LD_{50} of SE/B toxin. Moreover, in contrast with natural toxin, rSE/Bv showed no evidence of toxic SAg activity. In ex vivo assays conducted with human immune cells, rSE/Bv did not bind human MHC class II receptors; did not stimulate cytokine release; and did not elicit nonspecific T-cell cell mitosis. A suitable process has been developed to produce rSE/Bv in a high-level *E. coli* expression system under conditions compatible with current Good Manufacturing Practices *(111)*.

Additional structural and mutation studies have been undertaken to produce analogous vaccine candidates for protection against other SAgs *(83,105,112–114)*. Suggestive evidence has been presented that vaccination with SE/B and SE/A vaccine candidates may offer some protection against other SE toxin serotypes, raising the possibility of a single vaccine that can offer protection against multiple SAgs.

4.3. Experimental Therapeutics

There is no approved therapeutic for reversing the effects of SE intoxication; treatment is aimed at reducing the incapacitating symptoms, maintaining adequate hydration, and preventing or managing the clinical sequelae of systemic shock.

Several experimental approaches are underway to evaluate potential therapeutic approaches to SE. These include suppressing abnormal T-cell activation by preventing or disrupting abnormal TCR–MHC interactions; mitigating downstream cytokine or chemokine release caused by activated lymphocytes and macrophages after SAg exposure; and blocking the costimulatory molecules involved in activation or other effector functions of T cells *(115–117)*.

---

[4]Unlike the MHC receptors of humans and other primates, the α-chain of mouse MHC class II lacks key amino acid residues involved in high affinity toxin binding. For this reason, mouse models of SE/B exposure require addition of a potentiating molecule, such as lipopolysaccharide preparations from Gram-negative bacteria, along with the toxin to model the severe incapacitation observed in primates exposed to SE/B alone. Recently, it has become possible to test SE/B vaccine candidates in transgenic mice expressing human leukocyte antigen (HLA)-DR3 and human CD4 molecules, in the absence of murine major histocompatibility complex (MHC) class II molecules (see ref. *110.* DaSilva, L., et al. (2002) Humanlike immune response of human leukocyte antigen-DR3 transgenic mice to staphylococcal enterotoxins: a novel model for superantigen vaccines. *J. Infect. Dis.* **185(12),** 1754–1760.) This animal model eliminates the need for toxin potentiation with lipopolysaccharide.

5. RICIN TOXIN

Ricin is a disulfide-bonded, heterodimeric toxin from the seeds of *Ricinus communis* (castor bean plant) that has been recognized as a potential toxin weapon since World War I *(118)*. Although much less lethal by weight than BoNT or SE *(119–121)*, ricin is nevertheless a potent BW agent because sublethal doses cause incapacitating pulmonary damage and because the toxin is widely available; the castor bean plant is cultivated worldwide for several beneficial applications, and the toxin is easily extracted from common byproducts of the seeds *(122,123)*.

Entry of ricin into target cells is greatly enhanced by the ricin B-chain (RTB); RTB is a galactose-specific lectin that binds receptors on the surface of target cells, thereby promoting endocytosis and trafficking to the trans Golgi. The ricin A-chain (RTA) is a multidomain *N*-glycosidase that depurinates a specific adenosine of the essential 60S ribosomal RNA (rRNA) subunit (reviewed in ref. *124*). Once eukaryotic rRNA has been damaged in this way, the target cell cannot synthesize new protein and inevitably will die. Ricin is representative of a diverse class of "ribosome inactivating proteins" (RIPs) that includes the plant toxins abrin, modeccin and viscumin, as well as several potent bacterial toxins *(125,126)*.

Human poisoning by ricin aerosol exposure is not documented, but based on extrapolation from accidental, human sublethal exposures, the signs and symptoms are likely to include high fever, dyspnea, and coughing that is delayed for 4–8 h after exposure *(123,127,128)*. In nonhuman primates, aerosolized ricin causes a dose-dependent set of signs that is delayed from 8 to 24 h; anorexia and lethargy are frequently observed. In one study of rhesus monkeys exposed to approx 20–40 µg/kg of ricin aerosol, death occurred by acute respiratory distress about 36–48 h after exposure; necropsy revealed fibrinopurulent pneumonia, acute inflammation of trachea and airways, and massive pulmonary alveolar flooding *(129)*.

5.1. Ricin Toxoid Vaccines

Toxoid vaccine prepared from formalin-inactivated ricin holotoxin was developed during World War II and shown to enhance survival significantly in animals exposed to ricin *(118)*. An improved ricin toxoid vaccine based on denatured toxin adsorbed to Alhydrogel adjuvant was developed at USAMRIID in the 1990s and shown to be effective at protecting rhesus monkeys against ricin toxin aerosol exposures. All vaccinated monkeys survived a supralethal ricin aerosol challenge; however, as with earlier studies, vaccination did not protect completely against short-term (up to 14 d postexposure) bronchiolar and interstitial pulmonary inflammation. The general failure of toxoid vaccines to protect the respiratory tract of exposed animals from the cytotoxic effects of ricin underscores the need to develop effective recombinant vaccines and alternative vaccine-delivery systems that can elicit an enhanced mucosal immune response *(121,130)*.

5.2. Deglycosylated Ricin A-Chain Vaccine

RTA conjugated with tumor-specific antibodies has been used clinically as medicotoxin to target and kill tumors in animals and humans *(131,132)*. Supporting studies with RTA-antibody conjugates contributed to the development of a recombinant ricin vaccine because they demonstrated unequivocally that RTA is much less toxic than is the whole toxin when administered parenterally to animals in the absence of the RTB *(133,134)*.

During the early 1990s, researchers at USAMRIID demonstrated that purified RTA can act as an effective immunogen in animals to elicit antibodies that neutralize whole ricin toxin *(135,136)*. A suitable lot (meeting current Good Manufacturing Practices) of chemically degylosylated (dg) RTA subsequently was produced from the natural toxin and shown to protect against supralethal ricin aerosol challenges in two animal models.[5] However, technical limitations were raised regarding the use of RTA or dgRTA as a human vaccine candidate; both immunogens retain residual *N*-glycosidase activity and show significant aggregation during expression, purification, or upon prolonged storage in solution.

Recombinant vaccine candidates with active-site specific substitutions designed to reduce the *N*-glycosidase activity of RTA without disrupting the antigenic properties of the molecule have been proposed as vaccine candidates *(135,137–139)*. Some of these recombinant candidates also have been altered to remove a putative "vascular leak peptide" sequence reported to contribute to the toxicity observed with very high levels of RTA used in immunotoxin chemotherapy studies *(132,139)*. Active-site substitutions in RTA essentially eliminate the problem of residual toxic activity but do not address the important manufacturing problem of RTA instability and aggregation.

5.3. Engineered Ricin Vaccines

Olson recognized that the tendency of subunit-based RTA vaccines to self-aggregate under physiological conditions was related to hydrophobic domains exposed by the absence of the natural RTB subunit. Starting from a theoretical analysis of the functional architecture of the toxin compared with related single-chain RIPs *(140–142)*, it was hypothesized that reducing the hydrophobic surface of RTA by large-scale deletions might result in a better structural platform for presenting the neutralizing epitope than that of the parent molecule.

Along with a reduced hydrophobic surface, recombinant vaccine candidates were required to retain the surface loop that is believed to serve as a neutralizing immunological epitope for ricin toxin (RTA residues 97–106; ref. *137*). Candidates also were required to lack key amino acid residues of the RNA binding site that are essential for toxic *N*-glycosidase activity. From experimental trials with a range of recombinant RTA candidates, we found that immunogens based approximately on the *N*-terminal domain of RTA (residues 1–198) best satisfied the design criteria (Fig. 4).

Under physiological conditions, polypeptides based on RTA1-198 remain folded as judged by circular dichroism and infrared spectroscopy, are more stable thermodynamically than is RTA, and exhibit dynamic light scattering indicating monodisperse monomers without significant aggregation. Moreover, the single-domain immunogens show no detectable toxin activity and protect mice against supralethal exposure to ricin toxin by injection or by aerosol. In this case, protein engineering based partly on a functional analysis of protein domains has yielded ricin vaccine candidates that are superior to traditional approaches, including inactivated holotoxin or toxin subunit vaccines containing simple active-site mutations.

---

[5]Unpublished observations of Dr. R.W. Wannemacher, USAMRIID, Fort Detrick, MD 21010.

5.4. Experimental Therapeutics

There currently is no selective therapeutic pretreatment or antidote for ricin intoxication. Treatment is symptomatic and dependent on the route of exposure. Gastric lavage and similar treatment methods with activated charcoal to bind and remove free toxin have been proposed to treat ricin food poisoning. Such nonspecific clinical approaches are only of limited practical value in a mass casualty situation because the toxin acts almost immediately upon target tissues and there is a delay between time of exposure and the appearance of symptoms.

Proof-of-concept animal studies have demonstrated that prophylactic administration of a large quantity of heterologous immunoglobulin intraveneously can protect mice against inhalation challenge with ricin *(120)*. However, high-affinity human antibodies currently are unavailable for development as an immunotherapeutic. Moreover, because ricin acts immediately and directly on cells lining the respiratory tract during exposure, some pulmonary damage may occur prior to neutralization of the toxin by circulating antitoxin antibodies. Indeed, none of the presently available vaccine candidates has been shown to protect completely against the pulmonary lesions caused by inhalation of ricin.

Prophylactic, low-molecular-weight inhibitors of ricin as adjuncts to vaccination might overcome some of the limitations of using larger, more expensive immunotherapeutics. However, devising a suitable small-molecule inhibitor for ricin has proven challenging partly because of the large binding interface between the RTA and its target RNA substrate *(140)*. Current research is directed at systematically modifying specific substrate transition-state analogs and the highly soluble 8-methyl-9-oxoguanine derivates, which may form structural platforms for the development of future development as therapeutics *(143,144)*.

6. GENETICALLY ENGINEERED PROTEIN TOXINS

Although protein engineering has led to improved candidate vaccines and immunotherapeutics for some of the most important toxin threats, the same approach potentially may be misused to produce new BW threats. Our biological systems depend strongly on intrinsic complexity, synergism, and proper molecular compartmentalization and, therefore, offer a very large number of possible targets for future toxin weapons. In light of biotechnological advances and a very large number of possible targets, how does one approach the problem of medical protection against future protein toxins?

Progress is being made in the pharmaceutical industry toward identifying the set of all "druggable" human targets *(145)*. This approach attempts to systematically delineate the critical target molecules that participate in essential or amplified biological processes, as well as to discover therapeutic intervention to capitalize on general host responses that can protect against multiple threats. Many of these drug targets also will be toxin targets. However, even this powerful approach cannot be relied on to identify cases where the amplification step is carried by the toxin (e.g., enzymes like BoNT or ricin), nor can it be employed to anticipate unusual toxin-host synergisms or biological chain reactions involving otherwise normal cellular constituents such as those initiated by prion-like proteins. Even apparently innocuous proteins may act as deadly toxins if delivered by genetically engineered bacteria or viruses in unnatural amounts or combinations to the wrong organ, target cell, or compartment; examples of such adventitious "toxins" may include polypeptide hormones, growth factors, and cytokines or other immune system modulators *(146)*.

It is clear that if toxins are considered in the context of genetically engineered microbes, then it is not possible at present to delimit the complete set of potential protein toxins. However, if we assume that engineered protein toxin weapons initially will likely employ or modify existing natural toxin scaffolds or functions, then the problem becomes more tractable. Such future threats might involve, for example, the conversion of structural neighbors of known toxins into closely related toxins; novel chimeras comprising known toxin subunits or domains; or protein engineering and co-/posttranslational modifications employed to defeat natural immunity, approved vaccines, or detection systems.

Although the rational design of protein toxins remains largely impractical at present, biotechnology and understanding of protein structure have started to test this limit in two specific areas: (a) subunit combinations to create toxin chimeras, and (b) building upon common structural scaffolds to transfer function among polypeptide toxins. Growing interest in these areas is driven by potential benefits of medicotoxins, as well as the power of using toxins in basic biomedical research to selectively perturb biological systems.

6.1. Protein Toxin Chimeras

Many protein toxins operate by combining relatively diverse functions, such as binding receptors on target cells, promoting toxin internalization (membrane translocation), intracellular trafficking to target compartments, and subsequently exerting a toxic intracellular effect such as hydrolysis of an essential cellular component. The structure of natural toxins often exhibits a corresponding multiplicity, with functions partitioned among different polypeptide subunits or domains. During the past several years, it has become possible to attribute specific functions to toxin parts and, using protein engineering, to produce synthetic toxin chimeras composed of unnatural combinations of binding and catalytic subunits.

Toxin chimeras have been employed clinically to target and kill unwanted cell types or tumors. This application hitches the most deadly bacterial toxin subunits, often the catalytic domain of a multichain RIP toxin, to a binding subunit or antibody (so-called "immunotoxin") that targets a particular receptor. For example, the active subunit of diphtheria toxin has been conjugated with an epidermal growth factor-like domain to target cells expressing specific receptors *(147,148)*. Similarly, the neuron-binding domain of one toxin, such as TeNT or BoNT Hc, has been combined with the diphtheria toxin RIP subunit *(149)*. Neurons also have been targeted by chimeras of diphtheria toxin RIP subunit and modified substance P; the result is a directed protoxin that is activated by a specific posttranslational modification *(150)*.

It has been shown that there is a degree of permissiveness in the types of catalytic or functional subunits that can be delivered into mammalian cells by toxin binding and translocation processes. For example, the catalytic domains from two of the most deadly bacterial toxins known, TeNT and Shiga toxin, have been combined with the anthrax toxin ensemble to produce cytotoxins that will target a broader class of mammalian cell types *(151,152)*. Likewise, bacterial toxin translocation systems, for example, the pore-forming toxin streptolysin-*O*, are being developed as a means of intracellular delivery of relatively large (approx 100 kD) unrelated toxin subunits *(153)*.

Synthetic toxin chimeras are of interest in BW defense because, although they are expected to be less potent than parent molecules generally, the chimeras may result in confusing medical signs and symptoms. Chimeras also pose a challenging dilemma for medical diagnostics of BW casualties by reacting with detection systems for one toxin, while carrying the biological functionality of another.

6.2. Modification of Natural Toxin Scaffolds

Protein engineers currently lack understanding sufficient to permit *de novo* design and production of new toxins that are significantly more potent than the parent molecules. However, it has become increasingly feasible to engineer controlled modifications into existing protein toxin structures. The widespread appearance of diverse protein and polypeptide toxins in animal venoms has led to the manipulation of certain stable, natural protein scaffolds for the design or transfer of toxic function.

One permissive toxin scaffold is the "three-finger" fold employed by a number of single polypeptide chain animal toxins *(154)*. This toxin family fold is based on what is primarily a β-sheet protein core that is greatly stabilized by disulfide bonds coupled with highly variable surface loops that tolerate significant structural changes because of the stability of the protein core. Menez et al. applied structural and molecular biology to alter venom toxin binding specificity in the design and synthesis of a hybrid toxin that retains more than 50% identity to one toxin (toxin-α), while binding the natural target molecule, acetylcholinesterase, of a second toxin, fasciculin-II (FASII), with high affinity *(155)*. A model of residues essential for binding of FASII with acetylcholinesterase was proposed based on primary sequence and structural homologies among a large number of three-finger snake toxins, as well as the solved three-dimensional structure of the FASII-acetylcholinesterase complex *(156)*. Although the work is remarkable for demonstrating the transfer of function from one toxin (FASII) onto the sequence of another, the hybrid toxin is much less potent than FASII, underscoring the limitations of understanding protein–protein interactions from structural studies alone.

Another permissive protein toxin scaffold may be the disulfide-stabilized α–β-fold employed in large families of scorpion venoms (reviewed in ref. *157*). Zilberberg et al. applied site-directed mutagenesis to modify the binding specificity of a scorpion neurotoxin (Lqh α IT) *(158)*. Additionally, the potency of one long-chain scorpion toxin (BotIX) could be enhanced by the transferring select residues from a scorpion alpha toxin (Lqh α IT) *(159)*.

Small, structural mimics of natural protein toxins are also a concern for the future. The increasingly fine detail available for how polypeptide toxins bind to critical cell receptors or ion channels may result in the development of toxic, low-molecular-weight oligopeptides or peptide mimetics. Venoms from *Conus* hunting snails provide a natural example of how relatively small polypeptides can produce a large repertoire of stable, diverse and functionally synergistic toxins ("conotoxins" reviewed in ref. *160*). Peptide mimetics that carry some of the toxicity of the holotoxin, but with a much lower molecular weight and greater stability, may effectively enhance the potency of known toxins.

7. CONCLUSION

During the past decade, effective vaccine candidates for several of the most dangerous toxin weapons, including BoNT, SE/B, and ricin, have been designed, produced, or improved by protein engineering. Vaccination remains the foundation of effective medical protection against macromolecular threats, but it is clearly impractical and, in some scenarios, unethical to vaccinate against all possible threat molecules. Additionally, there are military operational requirements for which BW vaccination regimens that require weeks to months may be too slow or inflexible. Effective toxin therapies, such as engineered human antitoxins or small-molecule antagonists, are needed as adjuncts or replacements for vaccination.

Future directions include reducing the size and/or increasing the binding stoichiometry of antitoxin molecules. Protein engineering of catalytic scavengers has shown increasing promise as a potential medical countermeasure for low-molecular-weight toxins *(161,162)*, and it may become possible to develop catalysts that combine the binding specificity of antitoxins with protease activity to selectively catalyze the hydrolysis or inactivation of protein toxins. Design or development of irreversible protease inhibitors as prophylactic antitoxins also merits increased emphasis.

This review intentionally emphasizes how protein engineering can be applied in medical research to effectively shorten the timescale of evolving natural defenses against toxins. This approach holds out tremendous promise for protection against many known chemical and BW agents, provided the toxin does not change structure appreciably during the lifetime of the vaccine or therapy. A darker, competing view holds that biotechnology, combined with an open scientific literature, may have the same powerful accelerating effect on emergence or creation of novel threat agents to confound our engineered vaccines or, alternatively, to short-circuit natural immune processes.

A key resource for devising better medical protection remains analyzed, high-resolution structural biology data. Existing bioinformatics, computational chemistry, and structural biology tools for large-scale, comparative analysis of solved protein structures, and mechanisms can be applied to protein toxins *(163–165)*. Knowledge of the set of structural "building blocks" for natural protein toxins will emerge and may serve to improve medical products for simultaneous neutralization of multiple toxin weapons. We must remain cognizant, however, that the growing markets for beneficial medicotoxins against a range of human illnesses will continue to drive protein engineering of toxin chimeras, as well as new means to develop tolerance or defeat immunity to extend the clinically useful lifetime of toxin-based drugs. Consequently, researchers with a commitment to medical defense against BW agents should expect increasingly to wield, as well as to encounter, the double-edged sword of protein engineering.

ACKNOWLEDGMENTS

Ms. Ashley Merriman and Cadet Melissa Roy provided valuable research assistance. The opinions and assertions contained herein belong to the author and do not necessarily reflect the official views of the US Army or Department of Defense.

REFERENCES

1. Franz, D. R. (1997) Defense against toxin weapons, in *Medical Aspects of Chemical and Biological Warfare* (Sidell, F. R., Takafuji, E. T., and Franz, D. R., eds.), Office of the Surgeon General, Department of the Army, United States of America: Washington, D.C. pp. 603–620.
2. Gill, D. M. (1982) Bacterial toxins: a table of lethal amounts. *Microbiol. Rev.* **46(1),** 86–94.
3. Hatheway, C. L. (1990) Toxigenic clostridia. *Clin. Microbiol. Rev.* **3(1),** 66–98.
4. Paddle, B. M. (2003) Therapy and prophylaxis of inhaled biological toxins. *J. Appl. Toxicol.* **23(3),** 139–170.
5. Dack, G. M. (1956) *Food Poisoning.* Third ed. The University of Chicago Press, Chicago, p. 251.
6. Morgan, J. C. and Bleck, T. P. (2002) Clinical aspects of tetanus, in *Scientific and Therapeutic Aspects of Botulinum Toxin.* (Brin, M. F., Jankovic, J., and Hallett, M., eds.), Lippincott Williams & Wilkins, Philadelphia, PA, pp. 151–164.
7. Newman, M. J. and Powell, M. F. (1995) Immunological and formulation design considerations for subunit vaccines, in *Vaccin Design: The Subunit and Adjuvant Approach.* (Powell, M. F. and Newman, M. J., eds.), Plenum Press, New York, pp. 1–42.
8. Mikszta, J. A., et al. (2002) Improved genetic immunization via micromechanical disruption of skin-barrier function and targeted epidermal delivery. *Nat. Med.* **8(4),** 415–419.
9. Aoki, K. R. (2002) Physiology and pharmacology of therapeutic botulinum neurotoxins. *Curr. Prob. Dermatol.* **30,** 107–116.
10. Jankovic, J. (2002) Botulinum toxin: clinical implications of antigenicity and immunoresistance, in *Scientific and Therapeutic Aspects of Botulinum Toxin.* (Brin, M. F., Jankovic, J., and Hallett, M., eds.), Lippincott Williams & Wilkins, Philadelphia, PA, 409–415.
11. Arnon, S. S., et al. (2001) Botulinum toxin as a biological weapon: medical and public health management. *JAMA* **285(8),** 1059–1070.
12. Simpson, L. L. (1981) The origin, structure, and pharmacological activity of botulinum toxin. *Pharmacol. Rev.* **33(3),** 155–188.
13. Shapiro, R. L., Hatheway, C., and Swerdlow, D. L. (1998) Botulism in the United States: a clinical and epidemiologic review. *Ann. Intern. Med.* **129(3),** 221–228.
14. Franz, D. R., Parrott, C. D., and Takafuji, E. T. (1997) The U. S. Biological Warfare and Biological Defense Programs, in *Medical Aspects of Chemical and Biological Warfare* (Sidell, F. R., Takafuji, E. T., and Franz, D. R., eds.), Office of the Surgeon General, Department of the Army, United States of America, Washington, D.C., pp. 425–436.
15. Umland, T. C., et al. (1997) Structure of the receptor binding fragment HC of tetanus neurotoxin. *Nat. Struct. Biol.* **4(10),** 788–792.
16. Lacy, D. B., et al. (1998) Crystal structure of botulinum neurotoxin type A and implications for toxicity. *Nat. Struct. Biol.* **5(10),** 898–902.
17. Lacy, D. B. and Stevens, R. C. (1999) Sequence homology and structural analysis of the clostridial neurotoxins. *J. Mol. Biol.* **291(5),** 1091–1104.
18. Eswaramoorthy, S., Kumaran, D., and Swaminathan, S. (2001) Crystallographic evidence for doxorubicin binding to the receptor-binding site in *Clostridium botulinum* neurotoxin B. *Acta Crystallogr. D Biol. Crystallogr.* **57(Pt 11),** 1743–1746.
19. Montecucco, C. (1986) How do tetanus and botulinum toxins bind to neuronal membranes? *Trends Biochem. Sci.* **11,** 314–317.
20. Fujinaga, Y., et al. (1997) The haemagglutinin of *Clostridium botulinum* type C progenitor toxin plays an essential role in binding of toxin to the epithelial cells of guinea pig small intestine, leading to the efficient absorption of the toxin. *Microbiology* **143(Pt 12),** 3841–3847.

21. Koriazova, L. K. and Montal, M. (2003) Translocation of botulinum neurotoxin light chain protease through the heavy chain channel. *Nat. Struct. Biol.* **10(1),** 13–18.

22. Sheridan, R. E. (1998) Gating and permeability of ion channels produced by botulinum toxin types A and E in PC12 cell membranes. *Toxicon* **36(5),** 703–717.

23. Simpson, L. L. (1986) Molecular pharmacology of botulinum toxin and tetanus toxin. *Annu. Rev. Pharmacol. Toxicol.* **26,** 427–453.

24. Poulain, B., et al. (1991) Heterologous combinations of heavy and light chains from botulinum neurotoxin A and tetanus toxin inhibit neurotransmitter release in Aplysia. *J. Biol. Chem.* **266(15),** 9580–9585.

25. Hanson, P. I., Heuser, J. E., and Jahn, R. (1997) Neurotransmitter release—four years of SNARE complexes. *Curr. Opin. Neurobiol.* **7(3),** 310–315.

26. Brunger, A. T. (2001) Structure of proteins involved in synaptic vesicle fusion in neurons. *Annu. Rev. Biophys. Biomol. Struct.* **30,** 157–171.

27. Rizo, J. (2003) SNARE function revisited. *Nat. Struct. Biol.* **10(6),** 417–419.

28. Reames, H. R., et al. (1947) Studies on botulinum toxoids, types A and B III. Immunization in man. *J. Immunol.* **55,** 309–324.

29. Sterne, M. and Wentzel, L. M. (1950) A new method for the large-scale production of high-titre botulinum formol-toxoid types C and D. *J. Immunol.* **65,** 175–183.

30. Fiock, M. A., Cardella, M. A., and Gearinger, N. F. (1963) Studies of immunities to toxins of Clostridium botulinum. IX. Immunologic response of man to purified pentavalent ABCDE botulinum toxoid. *J. Immunol.* **90,** 697–702.

31. Cardella, M. A. (1964) Botulinum toxoids, in *Botulism, Proceedings of a Symposium.* U. S. Public Health Service Publication No. 999-FP-1. (Lewis, Jr., K. H. a. C., ed.), Public Health Service, Cincinnati, OH, pp. 113–130.

32. Anderson, J. H. and Lewis, G. E. (1981) Clinical evaluation of botulinum toxoids, in *Biomedical Aspects of Botulism.* (Lewis, G. E., ed.), Academic Press, New York, pp. 233–246.

33. Oguma, K., Fujinaga, Y., and Inoue, K. (1995) Structure and function of *Clostridium botulinum* toxins. *Microbiol. Immunol.* **39(3),** 161–168.

34. Siegel, L. S. (1988) Human immune response to botulinum pentavalent (ABCDE) toxoid determined by a neutralization test and by an enzyme-linked immunosorbent assay. *J. Clin. Microbiol.* **26(11),** 2351–2356.

35. Hatheway, C. (1976) Toxoid of *Clostridium botulinum* type F: purification and immunogenicity studies. *Appl. Environ. Microbiol.* **31,** 234–242.

36. Torii, Y., et al. (2002) Production and immunogenic efficacy of botulinum tetravalent (A, B, E, F) toxoid. *Vaccine* **20(19-20),** 2556–2561.

37. Byrne, M. P. and Smith, L. A. (2000) Development of vaccines for prevention of botulism. *Biochimie* **82(9-10),** 955–966.

38. Fairweather, N. F., Lyness, V. A., and Maskell, D. J. (1987) Immunization of mice against tetanus with fragments of tetanus toxin synthesized in *Escherichia coli. Infect. Immun.* **55(11),** 2541–2545.

39. Clayton, M. A., et al. (1995) Protective vaccination with a recombinant fragment of *Clostridium botulinum* neurotoxin serotype A expressed from a synthetic gene in *Escherichia coli. Infect. Immun.* **63(7),** 2738–2742.

40. LaPenotiere, H. F., Clayton, M. A., and Middlebrook, J. L. (1995) Expression of a large, nontoxic fragment of botulinum neurotoxin serotype A and its use as an immunogen. *Toxicon* **33(10),** 1383–1386.

41. Simpson, L. L. (1984) Fragment C of tetanus toxin antagonizes the neuromuscular blocking properties of native tetanus toxin. *J. Pharmacol. Exp. Ther.* **228(3),** 600–604.

42. Simpson, L. L. (1984) Botulinum toxin and tetanus toxin recognize similar membrane determinants. *Brain Res.* **305(1),** 177–180.

43. Helting, T. B. and Nau, H. H. (1984) Analysis of the immune response to papain digestion products of tetanus toxin. *Acta Pathol. Microbiol. Immunol. Scand. (C)* **92(1),** 59–63.

44. Thompson, D. E., et al. (1990) The complete amino acid sequence of the *Clostridium botulinum* type A neurotoxin, deduced by nucleotide sequence analysis of the encoding gene. *Eur. J. Biochem.* **189(1),** 73–81.

45. Dertzbaugh, M. T. and West, M. W. (1996) Mapping of protective and cross-reactive domains of the type A neurotoxin of *Clostridium botulinum. Vaccine* **14(16),** 1538–1544.

46. Middlebrook, J. L. (1995) Protection strategies against botulinum toxin. *Adv. Exp. Med. Biol.* **383,** 93–98.

47. Potter, K. J., et al. (1998) Production and purification of the heavy-chain fragment C of botulinum neurotoxin, serotype B, expressed in the methylotrophic yeast *Pichia pastoris. Protein Expr. Purif.* **13(3),** 357–365.

48. Byrne, M. P., et al. (1998) Purification, potency, and efficacy of the botulinum neurotoxin type A binding domain from *Pichia pastoris* as a recombinant vaccine candidate. *Infect. Immun.* **66(10),** 4817–4822.

49. Byrne, M. P., et al. (2000) Fermentation, purification, and efficacy of a recombinant vaccine candidate against botulinum neurotoxin type F from *Pichia pastoris. Protein Expr. Purif.* **18(3),** 327–337.

50. Potter, K. J., et al. (2000) Production and purification of the heavy chain fragment C of botulinum neurotoxin, serotype A, expressed in the methylotrophic yeast *Pichia pastoris. Protein Expr. Purif.* **19(3),** 393–402.

51. Woodward, L. A., et al. (2003) Expression of HC subunits from Clostridium botulinum types C and D and their evaluation as candidate vaccine antigens in mice. *Infect. Immun.* **71(5),** 2941–2944.

52. Bouvier, A., et al. (2003) Identifying and modulating disulfide formation in the biopharmaceutical production of a recombinant protein vaccine candidate. *J. Biotechnol.* **103(3),** 257–271.

53. Atassi, M. Z. (2002) Immune recognition and cross-reactivity of botulinum neurotoxins, in *Scientific and Therapeutic Aspects of Botulinum Toxin.* (Brin, M. F., Jankovic, J., and Hallett, M., eds.), Lippincott, Williams & Wilkins, Philadelphia, PA, pp. 385–408.

54. Swaminathan, S. and Eswaramoorthy, S. (2000) Structural analysis of the catalytic and binding sites of *Clostridium botulinum* neurotoxin B. *Nat. Struct. Biol.* **7(8),** 693–699.

55. Chaddock, J. A., et al. (2002) Expression and purification of catalytically active, non-toxic endopeptidase derivatives of *Clostridium botulinum* toxin type A. *Protein Expr. Purif.* **25(2),** 219–228.

56. Lee, J. S., et al. (2001) Candidate vaccine against botulinum neurotoxin serotype A derived from a Venezuelan equine encephalitis virus vector system. *Infect. Immun.* **69(9),** 5709–5715.

57. Park, J. B. and Simpson, L. L. (2003) Inhalational poisoning by botulinum toxin and inhalation vaccination with its heavy-chain component. *Infect. Immun.* **71(3),** 1147–1154.

58. Bennett, A. M., Perkins, S. D., and Holley, J. L. (2003) DNA vaccination protects against botulinum neurotoxin type F. *Vaccine 21(23),* 3110–3117.

59. Foynes, S., et al. (2003) Vaccination against type F botulinum toxin using attenuated *Salmonella enterica* var Typhimurium strains expressing the BoNT/F H(C) fragment. *Vaccine* **21(11-12),** 1052–1059.

60. Kiyatkin, N., Maksymowych, A. B., and Simpson, L. L. (1997) Induction of an immune response by oral administration of recombinant botulinum toxin. *Infect. Immun.* **65(11),** 4586–4591.

61. Simpson, L. L., Maksymowych, A. B., and Kiyatkin, N. (1999) Botulinum toxin as a carrier for oral vaccines. *Cell Mol. Life Sci.* **56(1-2),** 47–61.

62. Zdanovsky, A. G. and Zdanovskaia, M. V. (2000) Simple and efficient method for heterologous expression of clostridial proteins. *Appl. Environ. Microbiol.* **66(8),** 3166–3173.

63. Bradshaw, M., Goodnough, M. C., and Johnson, E. A. (1998) Conjugative transfer of the *Escherichia coli-Clostridium perfringens* shuttle vector pJIR1457 to *Clostridium botulinum* type A strains. *Plasmid* **40(3),** 233–237.

64. Pless, D. D., et al. (2001) High-affinity, protective antibodies to the binding domain of botulinum neurotoxin type A. *Infect. Immun.* **69(1),** 570–574.

65. Amersdorfer, P., et al. (1997) Molecular characterization of murine humoral immune response to botulinum neurotoxin type A binding domain as assessed by using phage antibody libraries. *Infect. Immun.* **65(9),** 3743–3752.

66. Amersdorfer, P., et al. (2002) Genetic and immunological comparison of anti-botulinum type A antibodies from immune and non-immune human phage libraries. *Vaccine* **20(11-12),** 1640–1648.

67. Nowakowski, A., et al. (2002) Potent neutralization of botulinum neurotoxin by recombinant oligoclonal antibody. *Proc. Natl. Acad. Sci. USA* **99(17),** 11,346–11,350.

68. Kuroiwa, Y., et al. (2002) Cloned transchromosomic calves producing human immunoglobulin. *Nat. Biotechnol.* **20(9),** 889–894.

69. Adler, M., et al. (1994) Evaluation of captopril and other potential therapeutic compounds in antagonizing botulinum toxin-induced muscle paralysis, in *Therapy with Botulinum Toxin* (Jankovic, J. and Hallett, M., eds.), Marcel Dekker, New York, pp. 63–70.

70. Adler, M., et al. (1998) Efficacy of a novel metalloprotease inhibitor on botulinum neurotoxin B activity. *FEBS Lett.* **429(3),** 234–238.

71. Schmidt, J. J., Stafford, R. G., and Millard, C. B. (2001) High-throughput assays for botulinum neurotoxin proteolytic activity: serotypes A, B, D, and F. *Anal. Biochem.* **296(1),** 130–137.

72. Schmidt, J. J. and Stafford, R. G. (2002) A high-affinity competitive inhibitor of type A botulinum neurotoxin protease activity. *FEBS Lett.* **532(3),** 423–426.

73. Anne, C., et al. (2003) Development of potent inhibitors of botulinum neurotoxin type B. *J. Med. Chem.* **46(22),** 4648–4656.

74. Anne, C., et al. (2003) Thio-derived disulfides as potent inhibitors of botulinum neurotoxin type B: implications for zinc interaction. *Bioorg. Med. Chem.* **11(21),** 4655–4660.

75. Zou, J., et al. (1985) The effect of toosendanin on monkey botulism. *J. Tradit. Chin. Med.* **5(1),** 29, 30.

76. Wang, Z. F. and Shi, Y. L. (2001) Toosendanin-induced inhibition of small-conductance calcium-activated potassium channels in CA1 pyramidal neurons of rat hippocampus. *Neurosci. Lett.* **303(1),** 13–16.

77. Xu, Y. and Shi, Y. (1993) Action of toosendanin on the membrane current of mouse motor nerve terminals. *Brain Res.* **631(1),** 46–50.

78. Shih, Y. L. (1986) Abolishment of non-quantal release of acetylcholine from the mouse phrenic nerve endings by toosendanin. *Jpn. J. Physiol.* **36(3),** 601–605.

79. Ding, J., Xu, T. H., and Shi, Y. L. (2001) Different effects of toosendanin on perineurially recorded Ca(2+) currents in mouse and frog motor nerve terminals. *Neurosci. Res.* **41(3),** 243–249.

80. Adler, M., et al. (1996) Effect of 3,4-diaminopyridine on rat extensor digitorum longus muscle paralyzed by local injection of botulinum neurotoxin. *Toxicon* **34(2),** 237–249.

81. Adler, M., Capacio, B., and Deshpande, S. S. (2000) Antagonism of botulinum toxin A-mediated muscle paralysis by 3, 4-diaminopyridine delivered via osmotic minipumps. *Toxicon* **38(10),** 1381–1388.

82. O'Sullivan, G. A., et al. (1999) Rescue of exocytosis in botulinum toxin A-poisoned chromaffin cells by expression of cleavage-resistant SNAP-25. Identification of the minimal essential C-terminal residues. *J. Biol. Chem.* **274(52),** 36,897–36,904.

83. Ulrich, R. G., Bavari, S., and Olson, M. A. (1995) Bacterial superantigens in human disease: structure, function and diversity. *Trends Microbiol.* **3(12),** 463–468.

84. Spero, L., Johnson-Winegar, A., and Schmidt, J. J. (1988) Enterotoxins of Staphylococci, in *Bacterial Toxins: Handbook of Natural Toxins* (Hardegree, M. C. and Tu, A. T. eds.), Marcel Dekker, New York, pp. 131–163.

85. Bohach, G. A., et al. (1996) The staphylococcal and streptococcal pyrogenic toxin family. *Adv. Exp. Med. Biol.* **391,** 131–154.
86. Sundberg, E. J., Li, Y., and Mariuzza, R. A. (2002) So many ways of getting in the way: diversity in the molecular architecture of superantigen-dependent T-cell signaling complexes. *Curr. Opin. Immunol.* **14(1),** 36–44.
87. Dinges, M. M., Orwin, P. M., and Schlievert, P. M. (2000) Exotoxins of *Staphylococcus aureus. Clin. Microbiol. Rev.* **13(1),** 16–34, table of contents.
88. Ulrich, R. G. (2000) Evolving superantigens of *Staphylococcus aureus. FEMS Immunol. Med. Microbiol.* **27(1),** 1–7.
89. Swaminathan, S., et al. (1988) Crystallization and preliminary X-ray study of staphylococcal enterotoxin B. *J. Mol. Biol.* **199(2),** 397.
90. Swaminathan, S., et al. (1992) Crystal structure of staphylococcal enterotoxin B, a superantigen. *Nature* **359(6398),** 801–806.
91. Swaminathan, S., et al. (1995) Residues defining V beta specificity in staphylococcal enterotoxins. *Nat. Struct. Biol.* **2(8),** 680–686.
92. Krakauer, T. (1999) Immune response to staphylococcal superantigens. *Immunol. Res.* **20,** 163–173.
93. Ulrich, R. G., et al. (1997) Staphylococcal enterotoxin B and related pyrogenic toxins, in *Medical Aspects of Chemical and Biological Warfare* (Sidell, F. R., Takafuji, E. T., and Franz, D. R., eds.), Office of the Surgeon General, Department of the Army, United States of America, Washington, D.C., pp. 621–630.
94. Schantz, E. J., et al. (1965) Purification of staphylococcal enterotoxin B. *Biochemistry* **4,** 1011–1016.
95. McGann, V. G. (1969) Evaluation of immunity against staphylococcal enterotoxin B. Commission on Epidemiological Survey, Annual Report to the Armed Forces.
96. McGann, V. G., et al. (1970) Immunological studies with microbial toxins. Research and Techology Work Unit Summary. Annual Progress Report. U. S. Army Medical Research Institute of Infectious Diseases, Fort Detrick, MD.
97. Denniston, J. C., et al. (1970) Hypersensitivity reaction to staphylococcal enterotoxin B. Commission on Eppidemiological Survey. Annual Report to the Armed Forces Epidemiological Board FY 1970. Fort Detrick, MD.
98. Warren, J. R., Spero, L., and Metzger, J. F. (1974) The pH dependence of enterotoxin polymerization by formaldehyde. *Biochim. Biophys. Acta* **365(2),** 434–438.
99. Warren, J. R., et al. (1975) Immunogenicity of formaldehyde-inactivated enterotoxins A and C1 of *Staphylococcus aureus. J. Infect. Dis.* **131(5),** 535–542.
100. Tseng, J., et al. (1993) Immunity and responses of circulating leukocytes and lymphocytes in monkeys to aerosolized staphylococcal enterotoxin B. *Infect. Immun.* **61(2),** 391–398.
101. Tseng, J., et al. (1995) Humoral immunity to aerosolized staphylococcal enterotoxin B (SEB), a superantigen, in monkeys vaccinated with SEB toxoid-containing microspheres. *Infect. Immun.* **63(8),** 2880–2885.
102. Lowell, G. H., et al. (1996) Immunogenicity and efficacy against lethal aerosol staphylococcal enterotoxin B challenge in monkeys by intramuscular and respiratory delivery of proteosome-toxoid vaccines. *Infect. Immun.* **64(11),** 4686–4693.
103. Lowell, G. H., et al. (1996) Intranasal and intramuscular proteosome-staphylococcal enterotoxin B (SEB) toxoid vaccines: immunogenicity and efficacy against lethal SEB intoxication in mice. *Infect. Immun.* **64(5),** 1706–1713.
104. Ulrich, R. G., Olson, M. A., and Bavari, S. (1998) Development of engineered vaccines effective against structurally related bacterial superantigens. *Vaccine* **16(19),** 1857–1864.
105. Ulrich, R. G., Bavari, S., and Olson, M. A. (1995) Staphylococcal enterotoxins A and B share a common structural motif for binding class II major histocompatibility complex molecules. *Nat. Struct. Biol.* **2(7),** 554–560.

106. Leder, L., et al. (1998) A mutational analysis of the binding of staphylococcal enterotoxins B and C3 to the T cell receptor beta chain and major histocompatibility complex class II. *J. Exp. Med.* **187(6)**, 823–833.

107. Olson, M. A. and Cuff, L. (1997) Molecular docking of superantigens with class II major histocompatibility complex proteins. *J. Mol. Recognit.* **10(6)**, 277–289.

108. Woody, M. A., et al. (1998) Differential immune responses to staphylococcal enterotoxin B mutations in a hydrophobic loop dominating the interface with major histocompatibility complex class II receptors. *J. Infect. Dis.* **177(4)**, 1013–1022.

109. Krupka, H. I., et al. (2002) Structural basis for abrogated binding between staphylococcal enterotoxin A superantigen vaccine and MHC-IIalpha. *Protein Sci.* **11(3)**, 642–651.

110. DaSilva, L., et al. (2002) Humanlike immune response of human leukocyte antigen-DR3 transgenic mice to staphylococcal enterotoxins: a novel model for superantigen vaccines. *J. Infect Dis.* **185(12)**, 1754–1760.

111. Coffman, J. D., et al. (2002) Production and purification of a recombinant Staphylococcal enterotoxin B vaccine candidate expressed in *Escherichia coli. Protein Expr. Purif.* **24(2)**, 302–312.

112. Bavari, S., Dyas, B., and Ulrich, R. G. (1996) Superantigen vaccines: a comparative study of genetically attenuated receptor-binding mutants of staphylococcal enterotoxin A. *J. Infect. Dis.* **174(2)**, 338–345.

113. Nilsson, I. M., et al. (1999) Protection against *Staphylococcus aureus* sepsis by vaccination with recombinant staphylococcal enterotoxin A devoid of superantigenicity. *J. Infect. Dis.* **180(4)**, 1370–1373.

114. Swietnicki, W., et al. (2003) Zinc Binding and dimerization of streptococcus pyogenes pyrogenic exotoxin C are not essential for T-cell stimulation. *J. Biol. Chem.* **278(11)**, 9885–9895.

115. Krakauer, T. and Buckley, M. (2003) Doxycycline is anti-inflammatory and inhibits staphylococcal exotoxin-induced cytokines and chemokines. *Antimicrob. Agents Chemother.* **47(11)**, 3630–3633.

116. Krakauer, T., Li, B. Q., and Young, H. A. (2001) The flavonoid baicalin inhibits superantigen-induced inflammatory cytokines and chemokines. *FEBS Lett.* **500(1-2)**, 52–55.

117. Krakauer, T. (2001) Suppression of endotoxin- and staphylococcal exotoxin-induced cytokines and chemokines by a phospholipase C inhibitor in human peripheral blood mononuclear cells. *Clin. Diagn. Lab. Immunol.* **8(2)**, 449–453.

118. Cope, A. C. (1946) Chapter 12: Ricin in Summary technical report of Division 9 on Chemical warfare and related problems: Parts I-II. National Defense Research Committee, Office of Scientific Research and Development, Washington DC, pp. 179–203.

119. Knight, B. (1979) Ricin—a potent homicidal poison. *Br. Med. J.* **1(6159)**, 350, 351.

120. Hewetson, J. F., et al. (1993) Protection of mice from inhaled ricin by vaccination with ricin or by passive treatment with heterologous antibody. *Vaccine* **11(7)**, 743–746.

121. Griffiths, G. D., et al. (1996) The inhalation toxicology of the castor bean toxin, ricin, and protection by vaccination. *J. Defense Sci.* **1(2)**, 227–235.

122. Crompton, R. and Gall, D. (1980) Georgi Markov—death in a pellet. *Med. Leg. J.* **48(2)**, 51–62.

123. Franz, D. R. and Jaax, N. K. (1997) Ricin toxin, in *Medical Aspects of Chemical and Biological Warfare* (Sidell, F. R., Takafuji, E. T., and Franz, D. R., eds.), Office of the Surgeon General, Department of the Army, United States of America, Washington, D.C., pp. 631–642.

124. Robertus, J. (1991) The structure and action of ricin, a cytotoxic *N*-glycosidase. *Semin. Cell Biol.* **2(1)**, 23–30.

125. Lord, J. M., Hartley, M. R., and Roberts, L. M. (1991) Ribosome inactivating proteins of plants. *Semin. Cell Biol.* **2(1)**, 15–22.

126. Obrig, T. G. (1994) Toxins that inhibit host protein synthesis. *Methods Enzymol.* **235,** 647–656.
127. Balint, G. A. (1974) Ricin: the toxic protein of castor oil seeds. *Toxicology* **2(1),** 77–102.
128. Brugsch, H. G. (1960) Toxic hazards: The castor bean. *Mass. Med. Soc.* **262(1039-1040).**
129. Wilhelmsen, C. L. and Pitt, M. L. (1996) Lesions of acute inhaled lethal ricin intoxication in rhesus monkeys. *Vet. Pathol.* **33(3),** 296–302.
130. Griffiths, G. D., Phillips, G. J., and Bailey, S. C. (1999) Comparison of the quality of protection elicited by toxoid and peptide liposomal vaccine formulations against ricin as assessed by markers of inflammation. *Vaccine* **17(20-21),** 2562–2568.
131. Ghetie, V. and Vitetta, E. (1994) Immunotoxins in the therapy of cancer: from bench to clinic. *Pharmacol. Ther.* **63(3),** 209–234.
132. Vitetta, E. S., Thorpe, P. E., and Uhr, J. W. (1993) Immunotoxins: magic bullets or misguided missiles? *Trends Pharmacol. Sci.* **14(5),** 148–154.
133. Soler-Rodriguez, A. M., et al. (1992) The toxicity of chemically deglycosylated ricin A-chain in mice. *Int. J. Immunopharmacol.* **14(2),** 281–291.
134. Lord, J. M., et al. (1987) Ricin: cytotoxicity, biosynthesis and use in immunoconjugates. *Prog. Med. Chem.* **24,** 1–28.
135. Lemley, P. V. and Creasia, D. A. (1995) Vaccine against ricin toxin, in U. S. Patent & Trademark Office. United States of America, Secretary of the Army, Washington, DC.
136. Lemley, P. V. and Wright, D. C. (1992) Mice are actively immunized after passive monoclonal antibody prophylaxis and ricin toxin challenge. *Immunology* **76(3),** 511–513.
137. Aboud-Pirak, E., et al. (1993) Identification of a neutralizing epitope on ricin a chain and application of its 3D structure to design peptide vaccines that protect against ricin intoxication, in 1993 Medical Defense Bioscience Review. U. S. Army Medical Research & Materiel Command, Baltimore, MD.
138. Griffiths, G. D., et al. (1998) Local and systemic responses against ricin toxin promoted by toxoid or peptide vaccines alone or in liposomal formulations. *Vaccine* **16(5),** 530–535.
139. Smallshaw, J. E., et al. (2002) A novel recombinant vaccine which protects mice against ricin intoxication. *Vaccine* **20(27-28),** 3422–3427.
140. Olson, M. A. (1997) Ricin A-chain structural determinant for binding substrate analogues: a molecular dynamics simulation analysis. *Proteins* **27(1),** 80–95.
141. Olson, M. A. and Cuff, L. (1999) Free energy determinants of binding the rRNA substrate and small ligands to ricin A-chain. *Biophys. J.* **76(1 Pt 1),** 28–39.
142. Olson, M. A. (2001) Electrostatic effects on the free-energy balance in folding a ribosome-inactivating protein. *Biophys. Chem.* **91(3),** 219–229.
143. Tanaka, K. S., et al. (2001) Ricin A-chain inhibitors resembling the oxacarbenium ion transition state. *Biochemistry* **40(23),** 6845–6851.
144. Miller, D. J., et al. (2002) Structure-based design and characterization of novel platforms for ricin and shiga toxin inhibition. *J. Med. Chem.* **45(1),** 90–98.
145. Hopkins, A. L. and Groom, C. R. (2002) The druggable genome. *Nat. Rev. Drug Discov.* **1(9),** 727–730.
146. Finkel, E. (2001) Australia. Engineered mouse virus spurs bioweapon fears. *Science* **291(5504),** 585.
147. Landgraf, R., et al. (1998) Cytotoxicity and specificity of directed toxins composed of diphtheria toxin and the EGF-like domain of heregulin beta1. *Biochemistry* **37(9),** 3220–3228.
148. vanderSpek, J. C. and Murphy, J. R. (2000) Fusion protein toxins based on diphtheria toxin: selective targeting of growth factor receptors of eukaryotic cells. *Methods Enzymol.* **327,** 239–249.
149. Francis, J. W., et al. (2000) Enhancement of diphtheria toxin potency by replacement of the receptor binding domain with tetanus toxin C-fragment: a potential vector for delivering heterologous proteins to neurons. *J. Neurochem.* **74(6),** 2528–2536.

150. Fisher, C. E., et al. (1996) Genetic construction and properties of a diphtheria toxin-related substance P fusion protein: in vitro destruction of cells bearing substance P receptors. *Proc. Natl. Acad. Sci. USA* **93(14),** 7341–7345.

151. Arora, N., et al. (1994) Cytotoxic effects of a chimeric protein consisting of tetanus toxin light chain and anthrax toxin lethal factor in non-neuronal cells. *J. Biol. Chem.* **269(42),** 26,165–26,171.

152. Arora, N. and Leppla, S. H. (1994) Fusions of anthrax toxin lethal factor with shiga toxin and diphtheria toxin enzymatic domains are toxic to mammalian cells. *Infect. Immun.* **62(11),** 4955–4961.

153. Walev, I., et al. (2001) Delivery of proteins into living cells by reversible membrane permeabilization with streptolysin-*O*. *Proc. Natl. Acad. Sci USA* **98(6),** 3185–3190.

154. Ohno, M., et al. (1998) Molecular evolution of snake toxins: is the functional diversity of snake toxins associated with a mechanism of accelerated evolution? *Prog. Nucleic Acid Res. Mol. Biol.* **59,** 307–364.

155. Le Du, M. H., et al. (2000) Stability of a structural scaffold upon activity transfer: X-ray structure of a three fingers chimeric protein. *J. Mol. Biol.* **296(4),** 1017–1026.

156. Harel, M., et al. (1995) Crystal structure of an acetylcholinesterase-fasciculin complex: interaction of a three-fingered toxin from snake venom with its target. *Structure* **3(12),** 1355–1366.

157. Meves, H., Simard, J. M., and Watt, D. D. (1986) Interactions of scorpion toxins with the sodium channel, in *Tetrodotoxin, Saxitoxin, and The Molecular Biology of the Sodium Channel* (Yao, C. Y. and Levinson, S. R., eds.), The New York Academy of Sciences, New York, NY, pp. 113–132.

158. Zilberberg, N., et al. (1996) Functional expression and genetic alteration of an alpha scorpion neurotoxin. *Biochemistry* **35(31),** 10,215–10,222.

159. Bouhaouala-Zahar, B., et al. (2000) A chimeric scorpion alpha-toxin displays *de novo* electrophysiological properties similar to those of alpha-like toxins. *Eur. J. Biochem.* **269(12),** 2831–2841.

160. Olivera, B. M., et al. (1985) Peptide neurotoxins from fish-hunting cone snails. *Science* **230(4732),** 1338–1343.

161. Broomfield, C. A., Lockridge, O., and Millard, C. B. (1999) Protein engineering of a human enzyme that hydrolyzes V and G nerve agents: design, construction and characterization. *Chem. Biol. Interact.* **119–120,** 413–418.

162. Sun, H., et al. (2002) Cocaine metabolism accelerated by a re-engineered human butyrylcholinesterase. *J. Pharmacol. Exp. Ther.* **302(2),** 710–716.

163. Lacy, D. B. and Stevens, R. C. (1998) Unraveling the structures and modes of action of bacterial toxins. *Curr. Opin. Struct. Biol.* **8(6),** 778–784.

164. Gerstein, M. (2000) Integrative database analysis in structural genomics. *Nat. Struct. Biol.* **7(Suppl.),** 960–963.

165. Gerstein, M., et al. (2003) Structural genomics: current progress. *Science* **299(5613),** 1663.

13

Antimicrobials for Biological Warfare Agents

Jon B. Woods

1. INTRODUCTION

Biological warfare (BW) agents also cause natural human or animal diseases. The natural forms of these agents can often be treated successfully by using specific antimicrobial agents (for example, *see* Tables 1 and 2). In many cases, the antimicrobial susceptibilities and perhaps the most efficacious therapy of the resultant infections are well-documented in the scientific literature. For some agents, however, natural susceptibilities and treatments are poorly documented, as is the case for human glanders. And although the development of antimicrobial resistance is a major concern, even for naturally acquired disease, it is far more of a concern for infectious agents developed as biological warfare agents, as recent advances in genetic engineering make intentional production of multiple antibiotic-resistant strains achievable at the microbiology graduate student level.

This chapter provides a broad overview of antibacterial and antiviral pharmacologic agents that can be used to treat infections caused by biological warfare agents. For a more detailed treatment of this subject area, the reader is referred to one of many excellent textbook chapters or review articles *(1–13)* that discuss antimicrobial susceptibilities and resistance patterns of BW agents. An outline of antimicrobial therapies for some of these agents can be found in Table 3.

Antimicrobial resistance is generally classified as either naturally occurring or acquired. Natural, or "intrinsic," resistance to an antimicrobial agent is a characteristic that is inherent to that particular organism. For instance, *Staphylococcus aureus* is naturally resistant to second- and third-generation cephalosporins. Naturally resistant organisms may lack the appropriate drug-susceptible target or possess natural barriers that prevent the agent from reaching the target. Acquired resistance results from a genetic change in an organism that renders a previously effective antimicrobial ineffective. These genetic changes can occur in the following ways: mutational resistance, in which random errors in genetic replication can lead to mutations that confer resistance to antimicrobials (e.g., the mechanism by which viruses acquire resistance to antiviral agents), orhorizontal transfer of resistance genes from one organism to another, which can occur by (a) direct transfer (conjugation) between bacteria of small circular pieces of DNA (plasmids); (b) bacteriophage transfer of DNA (transduction); and (c) direct transfer of naked DNA (transformation).

From: *Infectious Diseases: Biological Weapons Defense: Infectious Diseases and Counterterrorism*
Edited by: L. E. Lindler, F. J. Lebeda, and G. W. Korch © Humana Press Inc., Totowa, NJ

Table 1
Antibiotics

Antimicrobial	Examples	Mechanism of action	Resistance mechanisms
Aminoglycosides	Streptomycin, gentamicin, tobramycin, amikacin	Inhibit protein synthesis by binding to a portion of the 30S portion of the bacterial ribosome. Most of them are bacteriocidal (e.g., cause bacterial cell death).	Modifying enzymes (acetylation, adenylation, phosphorylation). Reduced permeability or energy-dependent uptake. Decreased ribosomal binding.
Bacitracin		Inhibits cell wall production by blocking the step in the process (recycling of the membrane lipid carrier) that is needed to add on new cell wall subunits.	Reduced permeability
β-lactam antibiotics	Penicillins: ampicillin, amoxicillin, ticarcillin Cephalosporins: ceftriaxone, cefoxitin, cephalexin, ceftazidime Monobactams: Aztreonam Carbepenems: imipenem, meropenem	Inhibits formation of the bacterial cell wall by blocking cross-linking of the cell wall structure at the penicillin-binding proteins (peptidoglycan synthetic enzymes).	Altered target (penicillin-binding protein). Reduced permeability. β-lactamase.
Chloramphenicol		Blocks transfer of amino acids to peptide chains at the 50S portion of the bacterial ribosome; inhibits protein synthesis.	Reduced permeability. Active efflux. Inactivating enzyme (acetylation).
Glycopeptides	vancomycin	Interferes with cell wall development by blocking the attachment of new cell wall subunits (muramyl pentapeptides).	Altered peptidoglycan precursor binding site.
Lincosamides	Clindamycin, lincomycin	Blocks transfer of amino acids to peptide chain at the 50S portion of the bacterial ribosome; inhibits protein synthesis.	Decreased ribosomal binding (methylation of ribosomal RNA). Reduced permeability. Modifying enzymes.

Class	Mechanism of Action	Mechanism of Resistance
Macrolides	Erythromycin, clarithromycin, azithromycin	Inhibits translocation of the 50S portion of the bacterial ribosome on messenger RNA; inhibits protein.	Reduced permeability. Modifying enzymes. Decreased ribosomal binding (methylation of ribosomal RNA)
Metronidazole		Damages nucleic acid structure.	Altered drug activation pathways.
Oxazolidonones	Linezolid, eperezolid	Inhibit protein synthesis at the 23S rRNA of the 50S subunit of the bacterial ribosome.	Altered target.
Quinolones	Ciprofloxacin, levofloxacin, ofloxacin, norfloxacin, nalidixic acid, sparfloxacin	Blocks DNA synthesis by DNA gyrase, topoisomerase intravenously.	Target alteration (DNA gyrase, topoisomerase intravenously). Reduced permeability. Active efflux.
Rifampin		Inhibits RNA synthesis by DNA-dependent RNA polymerase, and thus protein synthesis.	Reduced RNA polymerase binding.
Sulfonamides	Sulfamethoxazole, sulfacetamide, sulfadoxine	Competitive inhibition of synthesis of dihydrofolate from p-aminobenzoic acid at Dihydropteroate synthetase.	Altered dihydropteroate synthetase. Increased p-aminobenzoic acid. Reduced permeability.
Streptogramins	Quinupristin/dalfopristin	Blocks extrusion of newly synthesized peptide chains from the 50S portion of the bacterial ribosome.	Decreased ribosomal binding (methylation of ribosomal RNA). Reduced permeability. Modifying enzymes.
Tetracyclines	Tetracycline, oxytetracycline, doxycycline, minocycline	Inhibits binding of transfer RNA on the 30S portion of the bacterial ribosome; inhibits protein synthesis.	Drug detoxification. Permeability barriers. Active efflux. Altered target (ribosome).
Trimethoprim		Inhibits reduction of dihydrofolate to tetrahydrofolic acid at Dihydrofolate reductase.	Altered dihydrofolate reductase. Increased p-aminobenzoic acid. Reduced permeabilit

Table 2
Antiviral Agents (Non-HIV)

Antiviral	Mechanism of action	Mechanism of resistance
Acyclovir Valacyclovir Famciclovir Penciclovir Ganciclovir	Guanosine analogs; inhibit virus-specific DNA polymerase.	Modified thymidine kinase Modified DNA polymerase
Cidofovir	Cytosine analog; inhibits virus-specific DNA polymerase.	Modified DNA polymerase
Idoxuridine and trifluorothymidine	Thymidine analogs; inhibit virus-specific DNA polymerase.	Modified DNA polymerase
Lamividine	Deoxy-nucleoside analog; inhibits reverse transcriptase (e.g. HIV), inhibits the DNA polymerase of hepatitis B virus.	Modified reverse transcriptase Modified DNA polymerase
Ribavirin	Purine nucleoside analog; mechanism not entirely understood; competitive inhibition of host enzymes results in reduced intracellular concentrations of guanosine triphosphate and decreased synthesis of DNA; inhibition of the viral RNA polymerase complex.	Unknown
Foscarnet	Pyrophosphate analog of phosphonoacetic acid; noncompetitive inhibitor of viral DNA polymerase and reverse transcriptase.	Modified DNA polymerase
Amantadine and Rimantadine	High dose: inhibit an early stage of the infection involving fusion between the virus envelope and the membrane of secondary lysosomes. Low dose: inhibit virus assembly by interacting with hemagglutinin.	Modified transmembrane domain of the M2 protein
Oseltamivir and Zanamavir	Sialic acid analogs; inhibitors of the neuraminidases of influenza A and B.	Modified neuraminidase
Interferons	Glycoprotein cytokines; immunomodulating, antineoplastic, and antiviral properties.	

The basic antimicrobial resistance mechanisms are:

1. Enzymatic inactivation of the drug before it reaches its target.
2. Changes in the outer layers of the cell which prevent the drug from entering.
3. Active pumping of drug out of the cell ("efflux").
4. Modification of the drug's target rendering the drug ineffective.
5. Acquisition of an alternative metabolic pathway that renders the antibiotic's target redundant ("bypass").

Table 3
Summary of BW Agent Therapeutics, and Prophylaxis

Disease	Chemotherapy (Rx)	Chemoprophylaxis (Px)	Comments
Anthrax	Ciprofloxacin 400 mg intravenously q 12 h or doxycycline 200 mg intravenously, then 100 mg intravenously q 12 h and two or more additional antibiotics (26). Avoid penicillins as single agent.	Ciprofloxacin 500 mg PO bid for at least 60 d or doxycycline 100 mg PO bid for at least 60 d. May be able to shorten course to 4 wk If immunized (or initiate immunization).	Consider amoxicillin for prophylaxis in children or pregnant women if strain is susceptible. Avoid doxycycline in pregnancy.
Cholera	Oral rehydration therapy during period of high fluid loss. Tetracycline 500 mg q 6 h × 3 d or doxycycline 300 mg once, or 100 mg q 12 h × 3 d. Ciprofloxacin 500 mg q 12 h × 3 d Norfloxacin 400 mg q 12 h × 3 d	NA	Vaccine not recommended for routine protection in endemic areas (50% efficacy, short-term). Alternates for Rx: erythromycin, trimethoprim and sulfamethoxazole, and furazolidone Quinolones for tetra/doxy resistant strains.
Q Fever (acute)	Tetracycline 500 mg PO q 6 h × 5–7 d continued at least 2 d after afebrile or doxycycline 100 mg PO q 12 h × 5–7 d continued at least 2 d after afebrile.	Tetracycline 500 mg PO qid × 5 d (start 8-12 d postexposure) or doxycycline 100 mg PO bid × 5 d (start 8–12 d postexposure).	Fluoroquinolones may be a reliable alternative (147) for acute disease.
Mellioidosis/Glanders	Ceftazidime plus TMP-SMX IV until clinically well enough to switch to PO doxy+TMP-SMX × 20 wk.	Postexposure prophylaxis may be tried with TMP-SMX.	No large therapeutic human trials have been conducted owing to the rarity of naturally occurring disease.

(continued)

Table 3 (*continued*)

Disease	Chemotherapy (Rx)	Chemoprophylaxis (Px)	Comments
Plague	Streptomycin 30 mg/kg/d intramuscularly in 2 divided doses × 10–14 d or gentamicin 5 mg/kg or intravenously once daily × 10–14 d or ciprofloxacin 400 mg intravenously q 12 h until clinically improved then 750 mg PO bid for total of 10–14 d.	Doxycycline 100 mg PO bid × 7 d or duration of exposure. Ciprofloxacin 500 mg PO bid × 7 d.	Addition of chloramphenicol for plague meningitis is required 25 mg/kg intravenously, then 15 mg/kg qid × 14 d.
	Doxycycline 200 mg intravenously then 100 mg IV bid, until clinically improved then 100 mg PO bid for total of 10–14 d.	Tetracycline 500 mg PO qid × 7 d.	Alternate Rx: trimethoprim-sulfamethoxazole.
Brucellosis	Doxycycline 200 mg/d PO plus rifampin 600 mg/d PO × 6 wk. Ofloxacin 400/rifampin 600 mg/d PO × 6 wk.	Doxycycline 200 mg/d PO plus rifampin 600 mg/d PO × 6 wk.	Trimethoprim-sulfamethoxazole may be substituted for rifampin; however, relapse may reach 30%.
Tularemia	Streptomycin 7.5–10 mg/kg intramuscularly bid × 10–14 d.	Doxycycline 100 mg PO bid × 14 d.	
	Gentamicin 3–5 mg/kg/d intravenously × 10–14 d.	Tetracycline 500 mg PO qid × 14 d.	
	Ciprofloxacin 400 mg intravenously q 12h until improved, then 500 mg PO q 12 h for total of 10–14 d.	Ciprofloxacin 500 mg PO q 12 h for 14 d.	
	Ciprofloxacin 750 mg PO q 12 h for 10–14 d.		
Viral encephalitides	Supportive therapy: analgesics and anticonvulsants prn.	NA	
Viral hemorrhagic fevers	Ribavirin (CCHF/Lassa) (IND) 30 mg/kg intravenously initial dose; then 16 mg/kg intravenously q 6 h × 4 d; then 8 mg/kg intravenously q 8 h × 6 d.	Consider ribavirin.	
	Passive antibody for AHF, BHF, Lassa fever, and CCHF.		

| Smallpox | No current Rx other than supportive; Cidofovir (effective in vitro); animal studies ongoing. | Vaccine within up to 7 d of exposure is best prophylaxis (within 24 h best). Vaccinia immune globulin 0.6 mL/kg intramuscularly (within 3 d of exposure, best within 24 h). |

(Adapted from ref. *43*.)
*Drug recommendations in this table do not necessarily represent FDA-approved uses.

Antimicrobial susceptibility testing permits identification of acquired antimicrobial resistance. Susceptibility testing can be accomplished by conventional (phenotypic) or by molecular (genotypic) means. Conventional susceptibility testing measures the in vitro activity of the resistance phenotype, typically expressed as the minimum inhibitory concentration (MIC) of antimicrobial necessary to visibly inhibit growth of the organism in culture medium. Studies reporting on the mean susceptibilities of many different isolates or strains of an organism may report MIC90s—the antimicrobial MIC to which 90% of the tested strains are susceptible. For results of conventional susceptibility testing results to be reproducible, procedures for conducting such testing must be rigidly standardized. In the United States, the National Committee for Clinical Laboratory Standards (NCCLS) provides these standards; however, in other parts of the world, different standards exist, and thus published results from outside this country must be interpreted with that fact in mind. NCCLS also publishes guidelines for interpreting MIC data. These guidelines are determined for each infectious agent based on known human pharmacokinetics for each of the tested antimicrobials in addition to the results of clinical tests of multiple isolates of the organism to each of the antimicrobials. However, because clinical data are limited for some of the BW agents, guidelines for interpretation of susceptibility testing may not be well established. An excellent review of the most common susceptibility tests used in clinical microbiology labs was recently published *(14)*.

It is important to recognize that in vitro susceptibility testing may not predict in vivo efficacy. This may be especially true for intracellular organisms in the case of antimicrobials with poor intracellular penetration, such as gentamicin. Additionally, many antibiotics are rendered inactive by the low pH within phagolysosomes, where organisms like the *Brucellae* and *Coxiella burnetii* can survive.

With these caveats, there exists a well-developed literature for antimicrobial agents against commonly acquired bacterial agents and a growing literature for antiviral compounds. The information becomes sparser as one explores the options for chemotherapy of biological warfare agents. However, this should change, as funding is applied toward assessment of new countermeasures for these agents. The remainder of this chapter summarizes the current knowledge for antimicrobials against specific BW agents. Antimicrobial treatment recommendations made within this chapter are based on clinical experience and review of the existing literature and do not always represent Food and Drug Administration (FDA)-approved uses.

2. ANTIBIOTICS FOR THE BACTERIAL BW AGENTS

2.1. Bacillus anthracis

Naturally occurring strains of *B. anthracis* are generally susceptible to penicillins, first-generation cephalosporins, tetracyclines, rifampin, aminoglycosides, vancomycin, clindamycin, and fluoroquinolones; they are variably susceptible to second- and third-generation cephalosporins, macrolides, novobiocin, and chloramphenicol and resistant to sulfonamides and trimethoprim *(15–19)*. Researchers recently demonstrated that 20 strains of *B. anthracis* also displayed sensitivity to imipenem, meropenem, daptomycin, quinupristin-dalfopristin, linezolid, GAR936, BMS284756, ABT773, LY333328, and resistance to clofazamine *(18,19)*.

Only rare cases of penicillin resistance are reported in naturally occurring B. anthracis *(17,20–22)*. When present, penicillin resistance is often a result of production of β-lactamase. The *B. anthracis* isolate from the October 2001 anthrax letters showed an inducible β-lactamase in addition to a constitutive cephalosporinase. The importance of the β-lactamases is unknown, as these strains remain highly sensitive to β-lactam antibiotics by disc diffusion methods, with MICs of less than 0.06 µg/mL *(23)*. Researchers studying the chromosome of the penicillin-susceptible Sterne strain of anthrax demonstrated the presence of two genetic loci that seem to encode for β-lactamases: one with 93.8% identity to the type I β-lactamase gene of *B. cereus*; and another with 92.9% identity to the C-terminal end of the type II β-lactamase of *B. cereus (24)*. Except for *B. anthracis*, all members of the *B. cereus* group are resistant to penicillin caused by production of chromosomally encoded β-lactamases *(25)*. Interestingly, 20 strains of *B. anthracis* that were highly susceptible to β-lactam antibiotics by the disk diffusion method were demonstrated to be highly resistant to β-lactam antibiotics by the broth dilution method. In these studies, MICs to all penicillins and cephalosporins were generally 64 µg/mL or greater, although the strains remained susceptible to amoxicillin/clavulanate and carbepenems *(18,19)*. These broth dilution studies raise the theoretical concern that β-lactam sensitivity could be overcome with a large bacterial burden. For this reason, the Centers for Disease Control and Prevention has advised that monotherapy with a penicillin should be avoided and that a multiple drug regimen including doxycycline or ciprofloxacin and at least two other antibiotics be adopted for treating severe anthrax disease *(26)*. Other naturally occurring resistance mechanisms reported for *B. anthracis* include an inducible macrolide-lincosamide-streptogramin B resistance determinant *(27)* and spontaneous mutations for rifampin resistance *(28)*.

However, genetically engineered antibiotic resistance, may be of even greater concern than natural resistance to antibiotics. Several reports have been published demonstrating the use of recombinant plasmids for conferring antibiotic resistance in *B. anthracis*. One plasmid-containing strain was resistant to tetracycline, doxycycline, and minocycline. Interestingly, the authors report that despite MICs dramatically exceeding those for the initial strain, minocycline (but not tetracycline or doxycycline) continued to show clinical efficacy in animal models of anthrax disease *(29)*. In another study, a recombinant plasmid encoding for resistance to penicillin, tetracycline, chloramphenicol, rifampin, macrolides, and lincomycin was inserted into the STI-1 strain of *B. anthracis*. This plasmid-mediated resistance was stably inherited over several generations *(30)*. Other researchers have demonstrated that the Sterne strain of *B. anthracis* can be induced to develop resistance to macrolides and quinolones by successive subcultures containing subinhibitory concentrations of the antibiotics *(31)*. In a similar study, the Sterne strain was exposed to doxycycline but failed to develop resistance *(32)*.

There have been no controlled trials of antibiotics for treating human inhalational anthrax, and thus present treatment recommendations are based on anecdotal reports of human cases and the results of animal studies. Historically, inhalational anthrax has had very high mortality. The improved survival in the recent intentional inhalational anthrax cases in the United States was felt to be caused by aggressive initiation of treatment with fluoroquinolones plus one or more active antibiotics *(26)*. The present recommendations for treating inhalational anthrax in adults include ciprofloxacin 400 mg IV twice a day or doxycycline 100 mg IV twice a day plus one or two additional antibiotics. Intravenous antibiotics should be continued until the patient's clinical course allows switching to oral antibiotics, which are continued until at least 60 d of total antibiotics have been received *(23)*. The ideal combination of antibiotics for treating inhalational anthrax has not been determined. Clindamycin has been suggested as a good additional antibiotic in part because of its proven therapeutic benefit in the treatment of disease caused by other Gram-positive toxin-producing organisms such as *Streptococcus pyogenes*, *S. aureus*, and *Clostridium perfringens (33–35)*. Rifampin may represent another good choice for an additional antibiotic because of its excellent cerebrospinal fluid penetration compared to many of the other suggested antibiotics (e.g., tetracyclines, penicillins, quinolones, and clindamycin). Empiric antibiotic coverage of central nervous system anthrax may be prudent, because 50% of the 43 inhalational anthrax fatalities of the 1979 Sverdlovsk incident for whom autopsy data were available showed anthrax meningitis as a complication *(36)*. Because they have demonstrated inhibition of metalloproteases *(37)*, the tetracycline class of antibiotics may not only help eliminate the organism but, in theory, may inactivate one of the anthrax toxins, lethal factor, also a metalloprotease. Further studies are necessary to prove these hypotheses, as well as to obtain synergy data for various antibiotic combinations both in vitro and in vivo.

Doxycycline or ciprofloxacin are recommended as components of optimal therapy for inhalational anthrax during pregnancy and in pediatric patients despite relative contraindications for these classes of drugs in these patients. The risk of adverse effects of the drugs may be justified by the risk of antibiotic failure should other, less-effective drugs be used *(23)*. If the anthrax strain shows susceptibility to both drugs, the fluoroquinolones may represent a better choice of antibiotic than the tetracyclines during pregnancy. Although the tetracyclines can have a detrimental effect on the skeletal development and bone growth of the fetus or child, as well as increased risk of tetracycline-induced hepatitis in the mother, the limited human studies performed to date have failed to demonstrate increased adverse events with the use of ciprofloxacin during pregnancy *(38)*. Tetracyclines are not generally recommended for patients less than age 8 yr, as prolonged courses of tetracyclines can cause permanent discoloration and enamel hypoplasia in developing teeth, as well as decreased linear skeletal growth rate. However, the American Academy of Pediatrics (AAP) recommends tetracyclines for serious infections (e.g., Rocky Mountain spotted fever) for which other drugs might be less effective *(39)*. The dose of doxycycline for children weighing 45 kg or less is 2.2 mg/kg (up to 100 mg) every 12 h *(23)*. Likewise, the fluoroquinolones are not generally recommended in children less than age 17 yr out of concern for cartilage damage; however, this concern is based predominantly on the results of animal studies that have not been adequately substantiated in humans *(40)*. As was the case for the tetracyclines, the AAP notes that for serious infections that lack more effective therapy, the fluoroquinolones may be used in children *(39)*. The dose of ciprofloxacin for children is 10–15 mg/kg (up to 1 g/d) every 12 h *(23)*.

Recommendations for postexposure prophylaxis of inhalational anthrax exposure are derived almost entirely from results of nonhuman primate (NHP) studies. Friedlander showed that monkeys receiving penicillin, doxycycline, or ciprofloxacin within

24 h of exposure to eight times the lethal dose of inhaled *B. anthracis* spores all survived until antibiotics were discontinued 30 d later. Once the antibiotics were discontinued, however, 10–30% of animals on antibiotics alone subsequently developed inhalational anthrax and died. Only animals that received antibiotic (doxycycline) and two doses of anthrax vaccine (at days 0 and 15) survived *(41)*. Earlier studies in NHPs demonstrated that viable spores persisted within the animals' lungs up to 100 d after exposure to aerosolized *B. anthracis (42)*. Combining these data and extrapolating it to humans, recommendations for postexposure prophylaxis generally include at least 60 d of quinolone or doxycycline—unless the patient is up to date with anthrax vaccination or can receive at least three doses given at 2-wk intervals if not previously vaccinated, in which case the duration of prophylaxis can perhaps be shortened *(43)*.

2.2. Brucella *species*

Determining the antibiotic susceptibilities for bacteria belonging to the genus *Brucella* can be particularly challenging. The organisms are fastidious, requiring special medium supplemented with hemoglobin and vitamins to grow well in the clinical microbiology laboratory *(44)*. Like many other organisms suitable for use as biological weapons, the *Brucellae* are facultatively intracellular, surviving within the acid environment of phagolysosomes. Thus, in vitro antibiotic susceptibilities may not accurately reflect in vivo activity. This may be particularly true of standard disk diffusion antibiotic susceptibility determinations *(44)*. An excellent review of antibiotic chemotherapy for human brucellosis has been published *(45)*.

Brucellae are generally sensitive in vitro to tetracyclines, aminoglycosides, quinolones, rifabutin, rifampicin, and rifampin *(46–50)*. Penicillin G, ampicillin, and third-generation cephalosporins have demonstrated good in vitro activity against *Brucellae* (MIC90 2–4 µg/mL), although the antipseudomonal penicillins (e.g., carbenicillin and piperacillin) were less active *(46)*. Sulfonamide resistance has been reported in up to 38% of clinical isolates *(51)*, but its clinical significance is controversial because there have been reports of clinical resolution with combination therapies including sulfonamide treatment despite in vitro resistance *(52)*. Indeed, no strong correlation between in vitro antibiotic susceptibility and clinical relapse has been found *(53)*. One study showed that quinupristin-dalfopristin, linezolid, eperezolid, and mupirocin had little to no activity against 105 strains of *Brucellae (50)*. Mixed data exist for macrolides. In one study, 358 *B. melitensis* strains from human blood cultures were tested, with MIC90 (microgram/milliliter) values ranging from 0.5 to 1.00 for azithromycin *(54)*. However, erythromycin has typically demonstrated poor activity *(46,47)*. Vancomycin likewise has demonstrated poor activity *(46)*. Some researchers have suggested that minimum bacteriocidal concentrations (MBCs) may be more representative of in vivo antimicrobial effectiveness than MICs, and found that only the aminoglycosides were bacteriocidal for *Brucellae (55)*. In bacteriocidal studies, aminoglycosides, fluoroquinolones, and rifampin showed bactericidal activity at concentrations one to four times the MIC, but tetracyclines or macrolides did not kill *Brucellae* below eight times the MIC. Kill-time experiments indicated that of the antibiotics tested, streptomycin killed *Brucellae* most rapidly *(47)*.

The susceptibilities of intracellular *Brucellae* to antimicrobials have not been well established. *Brucellae* survive in phagolysosomes where some antibiotics, despite intracellular penetration, are inactivated by the acidic pH. Because quinolones have good bioavailability, penetrate intracellularly, and have good in vitro activity against *Brucellae (56)*, they have been closely evaluated for use in treatment of brucellosis. However, a large inoculum size and low pH have been demonstrated to increase MBCs for quinolones *(57)*. In another study, azithromycin, streptomycin, and quinolones were active against *Brucella melitensis* at pH 7.0 but not at pH 5.0, whereas rifampin and doxycycline remained active at pH 5.0 *(58)*.

Standard, 6-wk combination drug treatment regimens of clinical brucellosis with an aminoglycoside plus a tetracycline, an aminoglycoside plus rifampin, or a tetracycline plus rifampin generally have relapse rates ranging from 5 to 10% *(49,52)*. In most cases, relapse can likely be attributed to poor compliance with the required prolonged treatment courses. In other cases, however, improper antibiotic choice, antibiotic resistance, or antagonistic effects of antimicrobials used in combination therapy regimens may be to blame. In a prospective study of 20 patients addressing antibiotic synergy, no therapeutic failure or relapse occurred in the group treated with doxycycline plus streptomycin, whereas 20% of patients in the group treated with doxycycline plus rifampin had a therapeutic failure or relapse after the 6-wk course was completed. In this study, serum doxycycline levels were inversely proportional to serum rifampin levels, suggesting that therapeutic failures or relapses may result from the in vivo interaction of this antibiotic combination *(59)*. In vitro antibiotic synergy data to support this assumption are conflicting *(47,58)*.

Trials of monotherapy regimens have yielded mixed results. In one study, 1100 children with brucellosis received oral therapy with oxytetracycline, doxycycline, rifampin, or trimethoprim-sulfamethoxazole (TMP/SMX) either alone, in combination with each other, or combined with streptomycin or gentamicin injections. Relapse rates for oral monotherapy were less than 10%, except for TMP/SMX, which had a relapse rate of 30%. Combined oral therapy with rifampin plus oxytetracycline, rifampin plus TMP/SMX, and oxytetracycline plus TMP/SMX resulted in no relapses in patients treated for 8 wk. Oral monotherapy plus parenteral aminoglycoside resulted in very few relapses *(52)*, and other studies have confirmed that combination regimens that include aminoglycosides may result in fewer relapses *(60)*. In a study of 16 patients with severe brucellosis caused by *B. melitensis* treated with ciprofloxacin alone, clinical relapse was common (27%) despite rapid improvement in acute symptoms *(61)*. In addition, in vivo resistance to ciprofloxacin (with cross-resistance to other quinolones) has been reported to develop within the course of treatment *(62)*.

Given these conflicting results, there is no consensus on preferred therapy of uncomplicated brucellosis. The best efficacy has been demonstrated with intramuscular streptomycin (1 g/d for first 2–3 wk) combined with a tetracycline for 4–6 wk. Gentamicin is likely an adequate alternative to streptomycin, as it is more active in vitro and can be dosed once per day; however, comparative clinical studies have not been performed. For uncomplicated brucellosis in adults, however, most sources recommend a combined oral therapy with 100 mg doxycycline twice a day and 900 mg rifampin per day for 4–6 wk *(45,63)*. The oral antibiotic combination is recommended because of ease of administration as well as better compliance, despite better-proven efficacy of the aminoglycosides. The same combination can be used in children over age 8 yr using 1–2 mg/kg doxycycline (up to 100 mg) twice per day and 15–20 mg/kg rifampin per day (in one or two divided doses; maximum: 600–900 mg/d). In children age 8 yr or younger, the combination of TMP/SMX (30–60 mg of trimethoprim per kg per day) and rifampin can be used *(39,52)*.

Drug combinations including rifampin should be used in pregnancy *(63,64)*. Although doxycycline plus rifampin may be the best combination for treating the mother's disease, the tetracycline class of antibiotics may result in growth abnormalities in developing fetal teeth and bones. Thus, a combination of rifampin and TMP/ SMX or rifampin and fluoroquinolone may be more prudent during pregnancy should antibiotic susceptibilities allow.

Brucella osteomyelitis has been successfully treated with doxycycline plus rifampin for 6 wk or longer, combined with intramuscular streptomycin for the first 2–3 wk *(45)*. Given the limited availability of streptomycin, gentamicin may have to be substituted.

Various combinations of antibiotics have been used in the treatment of *Brucella* meningoencephalitis with limited success unless therapy is continued for extended periods—often up to 6 mo. Hall recommends a regimen containing rifampin and TMP/ SMX for at least 90 d *(45)*.

Brucella endocarditis responds poorly to antibiotics alone, and early removal of the infected valve is recommended in addition to prolonged courses of multiple antibiotics *(65)*. Hall has recommended at least 90 d of rifampin, TMP/SMX, and doxycycline, augmented by streptomycin for the first 30 d *(45)*.

Antibiotic prophylaxis after natural exposure to brucellosis (e.g., consumption of contaminated goat cheese) is not currently recommended because this route of exposure results in relatively low infection rates. However, a 3- to 6-wk course of one of the combined therapy recommendations made above should be considered for victims of intentional use of aerosolized *Brucella* as a weapon, inadvertent laboratory exposure, or needle stick injury involving the live veterinary vaccine *(43)*.

As was the case for *B. anthracis*, scientists have demonstrated that it is possible to intentionally produce resistance to multiple antibiotics in a viable *B. abortus* vaccine strain. Spontaneous induction of resistance to rifampicin was followed by addition of a hybrid plasmid encoding for rifampicin, tetracycline, doxycycline, ampicillin, and streptomycin resistance *(66)*. Given the difficulty in treating disease caused by naturally acquired *Brucella*, the existence of resistant organisms is quite concerning.

2.3. Francisella tularensis

Generally, the two known biovars of *F. tularensis* may differ very little in their response to antimicrobials, the exception being their susceptibility to the macrolides. Whereas biovar A (subspecies *tularensis*) typically remains susceptible to erythromycin in vitro, biovar B (subspecies *holarctica,* formerly *paleartica*) is often resistant *(67,68)*. Resistance to macrolides does not seem to confer cross-resistance to streptomycin or other aminoglycosides in *F. tularensis (67)*. Numerous published studies have demonstrated that *F. tularensis* is generally susceptible in vitro to aminoglycosides, tetracyclines, rifampin, and chloramphenicol *(67,69–72)*. Even strains that are resistant to streptomycin may remain susceptible to amikacin *(73)*. Susceptibility to β-lactam and monobactam antibiotics is variable *(72)*. In one study, all tested *F. tularensis* biovar B strains were resistant to penicillin, cephalexin, cefuroxime, ceftazidime, aztreonam, imipenem, and meropenem with MICs greater than 32 μg/mL *(70)*. *F.*

tularensis is usually resistant to vancomycin and sulfonamides *(67)*. As for other intracellular bacterial agents, standard in vitro antibiotic susceptibility methods may not yield results that correlate well with the clinical response. This may be particularly true for the cephalosporins, which if used for treatment, may result in poor clinical outcomes despite low MICs *(74)*. In one experimental in vitro cell system for antimicrobial susceptibility testing, only aminoglycosides, tetracyclines, and fluoroquinolones, rifampin, and telithromycin were bactericidal against intracellular *F. tularensis (71)*.

Historically, the mainstay treatment for naturally acquired tularemia has been streptomycin. In a recent excellent review of the published literature concerning antibiotic treatment of tularemia, the cure rate for streptomycin was calculated at 97% with no relapses documented *(74)*. For gentamicin, the cure rate was lower (86%) with relapse rates of 6%, and failure rates of 8%; however, the calculated success may not have reflected its true efficacy as some included cases had delayed initiation and shortened duration of therapy. Tetracycline led to cures in 88% of subjects, with relapse rates of 12%, and no failures; chloramphenicol cured 77% of subjects, with relapse rates of 21%, and failure rates of 2%; and tobramycin cured 50% of subjects, with no relapses and a failure rate of 33%. In one series, ceftriaxone was ineffective in all eight cases in which it was used despite in vitro MICs suggesting susceptibility *(75)*. Because quinolones have low MIC values and give a good intracellular penetration, they have been considered strong possibilities as treatment alternatives to the aminoglycosides *(76)*. The clinical data that have been published seem to confirm this hypothesis. In one series, all five cases in which a quinolone was used to treat tularemia, resulted in a cure *(76)*. In another small series of ulceroglandular tularemia in children, 15–20 mg/kg oral ciprofloxacin daily in two divided doses, when tolerated, resulted in cure *(77)*. For therapy lasting fewer than 10 d, relapse is much more likely *(78)*. In a study in which mice were infected intraperitoneally with *F. tularensis* then provided antibiotic treatment, the relapse rate was high with 5 d of doxycycline or ciprofloxacin but zero with 10 d of ciprofloxacin *(79)*.

The current recommendation from the Working Group on Civilian Biodefense for the treatment of tularemia in adults is 1 g of streptomycin given intramuscularly twice daily for at least 10 d *(80)*. A does of 2.5 mg/kg gentamicin three times a day (dose must be adjusted for renal function) likely represents a suitable alternative. If the aminoglycosides are not available, 400 mg IV ciprofloxacin twice a day for 10 d, 100 mg IV doxycycline twice a day for at least 14–21 d, or 15 mg/kg IV chloramphenicol four times a day for at least 14–21 d are alternatives.

The antibiotic recommendations for treating tularemia in children are the same as for adults, with the following caveats: chloramphenicol should not be used in children less than age 2 yr; doxycycline use should be avoided in children age 8 yr or younger, unless a suitable alternative is not available. For children weighing less than 45 kg, the doxycycline dose is 2.2 mg/kg (up to 100 mg) twice daily. Ciprofloxacin use should be avoided in children less than age 17 yr unless a suitable alternative is not available. The dose of ciprofloxacin in children is 15 mg/kg (up to 1 g) given twice daily. The recommendations for treating tularemia during pregnancy are the same as for other patients except that chloramphenicol should not be used. Therapy should be started using parenteral antibiotics, but can be switched to oral antibiotics to complete the course once the patient's clinical course has improved.

Postexposure antibiotic prophylaxis by using one of the following regimens can be effective if initiated within 24 h of exposure to aerosolized F. tularensis *(43)*: 500 mg ciprofloxacin orally every 12 h for 2 wk; 100 mg doxycycline orally every 12 h for 2 wk; 500 mg tetracycline orally every 6 h for 2 wk *(43)*. Antibiotic prophylaxis is not recommended after natural exposure (e.g., game meat consumption or tick bite) to *F. tularensis*.

Ken Alibek, a former deputy director of the Soviet Union's civilian biological warfare program, claims that virulent, streptomycin-resistant *F. tularensis* strains have been examined in BW agent studies in the Soviet Union *(81)*. Researchers have published reports of successful insertion of plasmids encoding for resistance to chloramphenicol and tetracycline into *F. tularensis*, with subsequent replication and stable inheritance *(82,83)*. Thus, in the event that tularemia is used as a BW agent, obtaining antibiotic susceptibilities is paramount to ensuring adequate treatment.

2.4. B. mallei

Perhaps because of the rarity of natural disease caused by *B. mallei*, antibiotic susceptibility data for this organism are limited. Minimum inhibitory concentrations for multiple antibiotics were determined in three recent in vitro studies: In the first study, 10 reference *B. mallei* strains and 7 veterinary strains were tested against 16 antibiotics *(84)*; in the second study, 11 reference strains were tested against 28 antibiotics *(85)*; and in the third study, *B. mallei* was isolated from pus samples obtained from 34 horses and tested against 16 antibiotics *(86)*. The *B. mallei* were demonstrated to be susceptible to quinolones, aminoglycosides, azithromycin, piperacillin, doxycycline, ceftazidime, and imipenem. Strains were variably susceptible to trimethoprim and sulfonamides, rifampin, carbenicillin, and quinupristin-dalfopristin, and generally resistant to ampicillin, second- and third-generation cephalosporins (except ceftazidime), aztreonam, colistin, nitrofurantoin, and chloramphenicol. The in vitro antibiotic susceptibilities of *B. mallei* seems to more closely resemble those of *B. pseudomallei* than those of other *Burkholderia* species *(84)*.

Minimal in vivo data on antibiotic efficacy exist for humans *(87)*. Animal studies suggest that *B. mallei* may respond to similar antibiotic treatment regimens as *B. pseudomallei*, for which much more human data exist *(88–90)*. In a study in which mice were infected intraperitoneally with *B. mallei*, postexposure treatment with either doxycycline or ciprofloxacin was efficacious *(88)*.

Given the rarity of human disease caused by this organism, no well-established recommendations for treatment have been made. However, given the similarities between *B. mallei* and *B. pseudomallei*, antibiotic regimens for melioidosis (*see* Subheading 2.5.) would likely be effective for glanders as well.

2.5. B. pseudomallei

In contrast to its close relative *B. mallei*, numerous *B. pseudomallei* antibiotic susceptibility pattern and treatment regimen studies have been published. *B. pseudomallei* is a complex organism with multiple mechanisms of antibiotic resistance. Numerous large studies of in vitro antibiotic susceptibilities *(91–98)* show that most naturally occurring strains of *B. mallei* are quite susceptible to imipenem and meropenem (MIC range: 0.5–1.0 µg/mL), and generally susceptible to third-generation cephalosporins, with ceftazidime being most active (MIC range: 1–8 µg/mL). Most strains are susceptible to piperacillin, and β-lactam-β-lactamase inhibitor combinations (e.g., ampicillin-sulbactam or ticarcillin-clavulanate), tetracyclines, and quinolones. Strains are variably susceptible to sulfonamides (including TMP/SMX), and chloramphenicol, and generally resistant to aminoglycosides, macrolides, aztreonam, rifampicin, first- and second-generation cephalosporins and penicillin. It is likely that the intrinsic high-level resistance of *B. pseudomallei* to both aminoglycosides and macrolides is at least in part caused by the presence of a multidrug efflux pump system *(99)*. Additionally, the organism contains at least one chromosomally encoded β-lactamase *(100)*. It is well-documented that antimicrobial resistance can develop during treatment of melioidosis. One potential mechanism of acquired resistance is alteration of the chromosomal β-lactamase after exposure to β-lactam antibiotics *(100)*. In a large clinical study of melioidosis, 7.1% of patients treated with a chloramphenicol-containing regimen developed strains highly resistant to chloramphenicol (MIC greater than or equal to 256 µg/mL) during treatment. These strains frequently show cross-resistance to tetracyclines, sulfamethoxazole, trimethoprim, and ciprofloxacin but increased susceptibility to β-lactams and aminoglycosides *(94)*. Another study documented acquired resistance to doxycycline and to TMP/SMX *(97)*.

Susceptibility data can vary significantly depending on the method used to obtain them. One study showed that the standard disk diffusion method resulted in a high degree of false-susceptibility results for aztreonam, ciprofloxacin, and temafloxacin when compared to the agar dilution method *(93)*. Another study showed a 67.9% false resistant rate for TMP/SMX by the standard disk diffusion test compared to broth microdilution *(101)*.

Melioidosis is difficult to treat and often requires prolonged, broad-spectrum antibiotic courses to cure. Even with aggressive intravenous antibiotic therapy, mortality remains as high as 40% *(102,103)*. Ceftazidime has become a mainstay of acute antimicrobial treatment of melioidosis and has demonstrated a 50% lower overall mortality than previous conventional treatments consisting of doxycycline, chloramphenicol, and TMP/SMX *(102)*. Other clinical studies comparing ceftazidime with amoxicillin/clavulanate showed equivalent mortalities but better compliance with the former and thus overall higher therapeutic failure rate for amoxicillin/clavulanate *(103)*. A small study in Thailand suggested that the combination of cefoperazone-sulbactam plus TMP/SMX might have similar efficacy to ceftazidime plus TMP/SMX as treatment for severe melioidosis *(104)*. Another comparative trial in Thailand showed equivalent survival for severe melioidosis when using 50 mg/kg per day imipenem or 120 mg/kg per day ceftazidime for a minimum of 10 d. A recent review of cases from northern Australia has also showed efficacy of the carbepenems (imipenem and meropenem) *(105)*. Still, survival for the unfortunate patients who develop melioidosis septic shock is dismal, despite antibiotic therapy. Preliminary studies addressing the possible benefit of granulocyte colony-stimulating factor (G-CSF) therapy in melioidosis septic shock are very encouraging *(106)*. Hospital survival for the patients who received 300 µg of G-CSF intravenously daily for 10 d in addition to antibiotics increased from 5 to 100% ($p < 0.0001$).

If patients survive the acute phase of melioidosis, they typically require prolonged maintenance therapy for a minimum of 12–20 wk to prevent relapse *(107,108)*. In one study, patients receiving the conventional oral combination of chloramphenicol, TMP/SMX, and doxycycline for 20 wk had a relapse rate of 4%, compared with 16% for amoxicillin/clavulanate, and a 23% relapse rate for conventional treatment lasting only 8 wk *(107)*. Another study showed a relapse rate of 22% by using the interesting combination of ciprofloxacin and azithromycin for 12 wk, compared to 3% with a combination of TMP/SMX and doxycycline for 20 wk *(108)*. Poor compliance with maintenance therapy may be the most significant risk factor for subsequent relapse, although acquired resistance also occurs commonly *(94)*. For this reason, patients should be carefully monitored for the emergence of antibiotic-resistant strains during treatment of melioidosis.

There seems to be no consensus regarding the optimal antibiotic therapy of severe melioidosis; however, most experts recommend regimens containing either ceftazidime or a carbepenem (imipenem or meropenem) intravenously as first line, with initial therapy lasting at least 10–14 d *(105,109–112)*. Most of these experts include TMP/SMX in the initial phase of treatment as well. A 10-d course of intravenous G-CSF warrants strong consideration for the patients meeting criteria for melioidosis septic shock. If the patient is clinically well enough to be discharged from the intensive care unit or if the absolute neutrophil count exceeds 75×10^6/mL, then G-CSF is discontinued before completing the 10-d course *(106)*. Computed tomography scan to locate internal abscesses may be necessary as some abscesses respond poorly to antibiotics alone (e.g., prostatic) and must be surgically drained. Once the patient has clinically improved then intravenous antibiotics can be discontinued and oral maintenance therapy initiated. A combination of TMP/SMX and doxycycline treatment for 20 wk may be the maintenance therapy of choice for melioidosis *(108)*.

Postexposure prophylaxis for aerosolized *B. pseudomallei* used as a biological weapon has not been documented. Oral TMP/SMX can be tried, perhaps for 10–14 d, although the necessary duration of therapy and resultant efficacy are unknown *(43)*.

2.6. Yersinia pestis

Numerous studies have been published that document the antibiotic susceptibilities of naturally occurring *Y. pestis (113–118)*. *Y. pestis* is typically susceptible in vitro to penicillins, many cephalosporins, imipenem, meropenem, aminoglycosides, amikacin, quinolones, and tetracyclines. It is variably susceptible to trimethoprim, chloramphenicol, and rifampin and is commonly resistant to macrolides, clindamycin, novobiocin, quinupristin-dalfopristin, and clofazamine *(119)*.

Although rarely reported, naturally occurring, highly antibiotic-resistant strains of *Y. pestis* do occur. In a recent report, a strain isolated from a boy in Madagascar acquired a plasmid that mediated resistance not only to streptomycin, chloramphenicol, and tetracycline but also to ampicillin, sulfonamides, kanamycin, spectinomycin, and minocycline. All of these resistance factors were located on a single conjugative plasmid that was highly transferable in vitro to other *Y. pestis* strains *(120)*. Another strain from Madagascar with plasmid-mediated resistance to streptomycin was reported in 2001 *(121)*.

Although streptomycin is the historical drug of choice for treating both bubonic and pneumonic plague, it is no longer manufactured in the United States and is difficult to acquire. Good data exist to show that streptomycin dramatically reduces mortality from plague *(122)*. However, no controlled clinical trials have been performed comparing its efficacy with other antibiotics yielding generally excellent MICs in vitro, such as other aminoglycosides (e.g., gentamicin), tetracyclines (e.g., doxycycline), chloramphenicol, quinolones, or third-generation cephalosporins. Good anecdotal data of successful treatment with gentamicin exists *(123)* and animal studies verify this *(124)*, thus it is generally felt that this aminoglycoside represents a suitable alternative to streptomycin for treating plague *(125)*. The tetracyclines, especially doxycycline, have likewise been successful for treating uncomplicated plague *(126)*. Animal studies generally confirm these results *(124,127,128)*; however, natural tetracycline resistance rates as high as 13% in clinical isolates have been reported *(117)*, and thus tetracyclines have not been recommended as first-line therapy for plague. Fluoroquinolones have generally very low MICs in vitro and look promising in animal studies *(124,127–129)*. β-lactam antibiotics are historically not recommended for use in plague because of concerns about ineffectiveness. However, there is little clinical evidence repudiating the potential efficacy of newer penicillins or cephalosporins, which generally yield low MICs for *Y. pestis*. In an experimental mouse model of plague, ceftriaxone was successful in treating even β-lactamase-producing strains *(130)*. However, concerns about the efficacy of β-lactams have arisen from another study in plague-infected mice *(124)*. The mice were injected intraperitoneally with *Y. pestis*, then antibiotic therapy was started either 24 or 48 h afterward and continued for 5 d. Ceftriaxone, ceftazidime, and ampicillin all had comparable efficacy to streptomycin if initiated within 24 h of exposure, but accelerated mortality if started at 48 h, at a time when mice had positive blood cultures for *Y. pestis*. Further exploration of this potential problem with β-lactams is warranted before any recommendations for their use in treatment of plague can be made. Adding chloramphenicol has been suggested for treating *Y. pestis* invasion into tissue spaces poorly reached by the aminoglycosides, as might be the case in meningitis, pleuritis, or endophthalmitis *(131)*.

The Working Group on Civilian Biodefense has published recommendations for the antibiotic treatment of pneumonic plague *(125)*. The group's preferred antibiotic for adults and children is parenteral streptomycin or gentamicin. The recommended dose for streptomycin is 1 g per dose for adults and 15 mg/kg (up to 1 g/dose) in children. The dose for gentamicin for adults is 5 mg/kg intramuscularly or intravenously once daily or 2 mg/kg loading dose followed by 1.7 mg/kg intravenously or intramuscularly three times per day. For children, the recommended gentamicin dose is 2.5 mg/kg given three times daily. Although aminoglycosides should be generally avoided in pregnancy, they remain the drugs of choice for pneumonic plague nonetheless. Because streptomycin has rarely been the cause of irreversible fetal deafness, gentamicin should be the first choice of aminoglycoside in pregnant women. Aminoglycoside levels must be adjusted for renal function. Alternative antibiotics for adults include 100 mg iv doxycycline twice daily, 400 mg iv ciprofloxacin twice daily, or 25 mg/kg iv chloramphenicol four times daily. The dose of doxycycline for children weighing less than 45 kg is 2.2 mg iv twice daily (up to 100 mg). The dose of ciprofloxacin for children is 15 mg/kg iv twice daily (up to 500 mg). Chloramphenicol should not be given to children less than age 2 yr. Antibiotics should be continued for at least 10 d for treating pneumonic plague.

The best evidence regarding antibiotic efficacy for post *Y. pestis* aerosol exposure prophylactic treatment likewise comes from animal studies. In one study, mice were exposed to aerosolized *Y. pestis* then given either ciprofloxacin or doxycycline as postexposure prophylaxis at 24 or 48 h, followed by 5 d of treatment. Ciprofloxacin prophylaxis and therapy were successful for up to 24 h after challenge but not after 48 h. Both doxycycline prophylaxis and therapy regimens were ineffective, but the doxycycline dose may have been too low for efficacy in the mice *(127)*.

The Working Group on Civilian Biodefense recommends either ciprofloxacin or doxycycline for postexposure prophylaxis of pneumonic plague *(125)*. The dose for doxycycline in adults is 100 mg orally twice daily, and for children less than 45 kg it is 2.2 mg/kg (up to 100 mg) orally twice daily. The dose for ciprofloxacin in adults is 500 mg orally twice daily, and for children it is 20 mg/kg (up to 500 mg) orally twice daily. Chloramphenicol probably represents a viable alternative, but the oral formulation of this antibiotic is only available outside the United States. Prophylactic antibiotics should be continued for at least 7 d after exposure.

As has been the case for most potential bacterial biological warfare agents, researchers have published accounts of intentional genetic manipulation of organisms to cause antibiotic resistance. Particularly concerning is a study in which *Y. pestis* was exposed to low concentrations of rifampicin and nalidixic acid and subsequently developed resistance to these agents *(132)*. The resistant strain remained fully virulent in mice being treated with rifampicin, nalidixic acid, or ciprofloxacin. Thus, in a biological warfare setting it is even more important to obtain antibiotic susceptibilities.

2.7. C. burnetii

Typical methods for determining antibiotic susceptibility cannot be used for *C. burnetii*, which is an obligate intracellular pathogen and thus requires living cell cultures for growth in the microbiology laboratory. The existing in vitro cell culture data suggest that the three known genetically distinct groups of *C. burnetii* may have different antibiotic susceptibilities *(133–136)*. Most strains are susceptible in the acute phase to tetracyclines, rifampin, TMP/SMX, and quinolones, with variable susceptibility to macrolides, and chloramphenicol, and resistance to penicillins, cephalosporins, aminoglycosides, and amikacin. Although doxycycline has remained the mainstay of therapy for acute Q-fever, many quinolones, including levofloxacin, ofloxacin, moxifloxicin, and ciprofloxacin likewise have demonstrated good in vitro efficacy *(137–139)*. Although erythromycin classically has been variably effective against *C. burnetii* in vitro, newer macrolides like clarithromycin and azithromycin show increased activity and may warrant clinical evaluation *(140,141)*.

Another concern with *C. burnetii* is its diminished susceptibility to antibiotics in chronically vs acutely infected cells *(142)*. This finding may help explain the clinical observation that chronic Q-fever infection responds poorly to antibiotics. One study demonstrated in vitro synergy of an ofloxacin or ciprofloxacin plus rifampin combination against persistently infected cells, whereas ciprofloxacin plus doxycycline was not synergistic *(142)*, perhaps pointing to the fact that some antibiotic combinations may be more effective at clearing chronic infection. *C. burnetii* multiplies within the acidic phagolysosomes of cells. Research has demonstrated that agents such as chloroquine, ammonium chloride, and amantidine, which alkalinize the lysomes, increase bacteriocidal activity of antibiotics against *Coxiella (143)*.

Treatment of acute Q-fever has historically been with a tetracycline, typically doxycycline. However, quinolones or macrolides may be effective as well. In a recently published study of 113 patients with acute Q-fever, the mean times to defervescence with clarithromycin and erythromycin treatment were 3.3 and 3.9 d, respectively, vs 2.9 d for doxycycline and 6.4 d for β-lactams *(144)*. In another study, 11 patients who received erythromycin had a rapid clinical improvement vs only 2 of 8 patients who received other antibiotics *(145)*. A small study showed that although the quinolones ofloxacin and pefloxacin were effective for treating acute disease, 14–21 d of therapy were required *(146)*. Recommended therapy for acute Q fever is doxycycline 200 mg/d for up to 14 d *(147)*. Fluoroquinolones are probably an acceptable alternative and may be the drug class of choice in cases of Q fever meningoencephalitis, as this class of drug enters the cerebrospinal fluid more reliably than the tetracyclines or macrolides *(148)*. Other possible treatment alternatives for uncomplicated, acute Q fever are macrolides and TMP/SMX.

Whereas most patients who develop acute Q-fever will recover even without antibiotics, some will go on to develop chronic infection, especially endocarditis. This is particularly true of patients with pre-existing valvular heart disease (especially those with prosthetic valves), who in one study had a 39% chance of developing Q fever endocarditis *(149)*. The same study showed that the combination of doxycycline plus hydroxychloroquine was more effective at preventing the progression to endocarditis than doxycycline alone. Another group of patients requiring special treatment is pregnant women, who in one study had fewer premature deliveries if treated with TMP/ SMX for the duration of the pregnancy *(150)*, although treatment failures have been reported *(151)*.

Successful management of chronic Q-fever endocarditis requires combination antibiotic therapy for extended durations, often years. In the past, various regimens consisting of single agents or various combinations of tetracycline, quinolones, rifampin, and sulfonamides have been tried with limited success, despite years of therapy. Although tetracyclines, fluoroquinolones, rifampin, or TMP/SMX used alone produce clinical improvement, relapse often occurs on antibiotic withdrawal. A combination of doxycycline plus quinolone proved more effective than any of the classic combinations (6% mortality), yet relapse rates were still more than 50% on antibiotic withdrawal. At least 3 yr of therapy were recommended *(152)*. More recently, a study demonstrated that a combination of doxycycline plus hydroxychloroquine sulfate for at least 18 mo may be even more effective than 4 yr of therapy with doxycycline plus quinolone *(153)*. In this study, mortality for both regimens was less than 5%, but relapse occurred in only 14.3% of those receiving the hydroxychloroquine-containing regimen vs 64.3% of those receiving the quinolone-containing regimen. Present treatment recommendations for chronic Q fever are either (a) 100 mg doxycycline twice a day plus 200 mg hydroxychloroquine three times per day for at least 18 mo; or (b) 100 mg doxycycline twice a day plus 200 mg ofloxacin three times per day for at least 3 yr *(147)*. Antibiotics should be continued until phase I *C. burnetii* IgG and IgA levels decrease to 1:200 or less *(154)*. Despite the use of antibiotics, hemodynamic instability may necessitate the removal of the infected valve. Antibiotics should be continued even if the infected valve is surgically removed.

Prophylaxis of inhalational exposure to *C. burnetii* is complicated by the fact that initiation of antibiotics should be delayed after exposure for maximal efficacy *(155)*. Human studies with *C. burnetii* demonstrated that postexposure prophylaxis within 24 h of inhaling the organism merely prolonged the incubation phase—disease onset was delayed but not attenuated *(43)*. Therefore, the current recommendation is to delay starting doxycycline prophylaxis until 8–12 d have elapsed since exposure *(43)*.

An outstanding review of Q fever and its treatment was published recently *(147)*.

3. ANTIVIRALS FOR THE VIRAL BW AGENTS

3.1. Introduction

Very few antiviral agents are available for chemotherapy of the viral infections of highest BW concern. Because all viruses depend on the hosts' cellular machinery for replication, susceptibilities to antivirals must be conducted in living tissue or cell cultures, a fact that makes susceptibility testing difficult to perform in many clinical microbiology laboratories. This close tie between the host and virus also makes it difficult to disrupt many viral processes without causing similar problems (i.e., side effects) for the host; because most viruses are genetically simple compared to bacteria, unique targets for antiviral medications may be quite limited.

3.2. Encephalitis Viruses (Togaviridae, Alphaviruses)

No effective antiviral chemotherapy has been identified for the alphaviruses, which include the Western, Eastern, or Venezuelan equine encephalitis viruses. Ribavirin, which has activity against several other RNA viruses, has demonstrated no detectable in vivo activity against encephalitic infections caused by Venezuelan or Eestern equine encephalitis viruses *(156)*, probably in part because of its poor penetration of the central nervous system. A recently published mouse study showed improved survival in Venezuelan equine encephalitis virus-infected mice treated with interferon-α *(157)*. However, further research is warranted before recommendations for antiviral treatment can be made for this class of viruses.

3.3. Hemorrhagic Fever Viruses

Generally, there are few effective treatments for viral hemorrhagic fevers (VHFs) other than supportive care. However, ribavirin has been used with some success in human disease caused by some arenaviruses and bunyaviruses. If started within 6 d of the onset of fever, intravenous ribavirin can decrease mortality from Lassa fever from 76 to 9%; the mortality only decreased to 47% if started after 7 d of fever *(158)*. Anecdotal observations of clinical efficacy of ribavirin in treatment of Argentine hemorrhagic fever *(159,160)* and Bolivian hemorrhagic fever *(161)* have been documented as well; however, further clinical studies are necessary to confirm this apparent finding. Three healthcare providers with severe Crimean Congo hemorrhagic fever (CCHF) were treated with oral ribavirin 4 g/d for 4 d, then 2.4 g/d for 6 d and all survived *(162)*. In rodents and monkeys infected with Rift Valley fever virus, ribavirin therapy reduced their mortality *(163)*. Ribavirin was also shown to be effective in human infection with Hantaan virus, the Hantavirus that causes hemorrhagic fever with renal syndrome (HFRS) in China *(164)*. However, a large open-label observational study of ribavirin in the United States as a treatment for Hantavirus pulmonary syndrome (HPS) did not yield results which could be used to interpret efficacy against Sin Nombre virus *(165)*. As a result, the National Institutes of Health has sponsored a double-blinded, placebo-controlled trial of intravenous ribavirin for presumed HPS. Ribavirin does not show any efficacy against filoviruses or flaviviruses *(166)*. Several other antiviral agents showed promise against Ebola infection in mouse models *(167,168)* but thus far have not demonstrated efficacy when tested in cynomolgus monkeys.

In May 2002, the Working Group on Civilian Biodefense published recommendations for the use of ribavirin for some of the VHF viruses *(169)*. The group recommends using ribavirin to treat only clinically evident viral hemorrhagic fever of unknown etiology or disease resulting from arenaviruses (e.g., Lassa, New World arenaviruses) or bunyaviruses (e.g., CCHF, Rift Valley fever, viruses causing HFRS). In these cases, ribavirin can be administered as a loading dose of 30 mg/kg IV (up to 2 g), then 16 mg/kg (up to 1 g) per dose intravenously every 6 h for 4 d, followed by 8 mg/kg IV (up to 500 mg) every 8 h for 6 d. The oral formulation of ribavirin can be used if the intravenous formulation is not available or in mass casualty situations in which intravenous use is impractical. The oral dose recommended for adults is 2 g once, followed by 1200 mg/d (for those weighing 75 kg or more) or 1000 mg/d (for those weighing less than 75 kg) divided into two daily doses (400 mg in the morning and 600 mg in the evening for those weighing less than 75 kg). For children, the oral loading dose is 30 mg/kg, then 15 mg/kg/d divided into two daily doses. Duration of oral treatment is 10 d. Although ribavirin is generally contraindicated during pregnancy, the risk of mortality owing to the VHF is higher in pregnancy and thus ribavirin is recommended for these patients *(169)*. The Working Group does not recommend antiviral postexposure prophylaxis for the VHF viruses. Rather, they recommend close medical surveillance of this group, and prompt initiation of ribavirin treatment should fever to 101°F or greater develop within 21 d of exposure to an arenavirus, bunyavirus, or unknown VHF virus.

3.4. Variola

Studies of antiviral efficacy against variola virus are limited, largely because this virus has not existed as a human disease for more than 20 yr. Antiviral susceptibility studies are difficult to perform as the virus is only available now for legitimate research in two places in the world, and also poses a serious health risk to the researchers who work with it. Studies performed to date indicate that many antiviral agents have in vitro activity against variola in cell culture. An excellent review of these studies was recently published by De Clerq *(170)*. The next step, testing the agents with the best in vitro activity for efficacy in an animal model of human disease, has been made very difficult by the fact that good animal models for variola do not exist. In a model of intranasal cowpox as a surrogate for human variola, disease can be prevented or cured with one subcutaneous injection of, or inhaled dose of, cidofovir *(167,171)*. No antiviral drug has demonstrated efficacy in human smallpox disease once symptoms have developed, albeit clinical trials have been very limited. *N*-methylistatin 3-thiosemicarbazone (Marboran) was shown to be useful in prophylaxis of smallpox and for treating complications of vaccinia vaccine complications *(172)* but was not effective treatment of disease, had many severe side effects, and is no longer available. Small trials demonstrated that adenine arabinoside and cytosine arabinoside, two nucleoside analogs, were also ineffective chemotherapy for smallpox *(173,174)*.

Because of the promising results in animal studies, cidofovir is under investigational new drug (IND) status for use both as a backup to the limited supplies of vaccinia immune globulin for treating adverse effects of vaccinia vaccination, as well as a potential therapy for smallpox disease. The IND dose for adults with normal renal function is 5 mg/kg iv in a single dose given as a 1- to 2-h infusion. Cidofovir must be accompanied by oral probenecid, 2 g per dose given 3 h before the cidofovir, then 2 h and 8 h after completing the cidofovir infusion (three doses). Intravenous hydration with saline accompanies the infusion, and the dose must be adjusted for renal insufficiency. The physician may decide to give a second dose of cidofovir 1 wk later if clinically warranted.

4. CONCLUSION

Among the many challenges facing medical researchers in the field of BW defense is the vexing problem of timely development of new antimicrobials against the BW agents of greatest concern. This effort must become a top research priority. Although the process to get new antimicrobials approved for human use can take years, an adversary may require only a few weeks or months to create antimicrobial-resistant organisms. Thus, future treatment regimens will likely have to include not only novel antimicrobials, but also immune modulators and vaccines. These countermeasures are discussed in other chapters of this book.

5. DISCLAIMER

The views expressed in this chapter are those of the author and do not reflect the official policy or position of the Department of the Army, the Department of the Air Force, the Department of Defense, or the United States Government. This chapter includes recommendations for the use of antimicrobial drugs in circumstances that have not been approved by the FDA; these recommendations do not reflect the official views of the FDA. Any drugs used for non-FDA approved uses must be administered under the direct supervision of a physician and preferably under IND status.

REFERENCES

1. Mandell, G., Bennett, J., and Dolin, R., (eds.) (2000) Mandell, Douglas, and Bennett's *Principles and Practice of Infectious Diseases*. 5th ed. Churchill Livingstone, New York, pp. 236–253.
2. Alvarez-Elcoro, S. and Enzler, M. (1999) The macrolides: erythromycin, clarithromycin, and azithromycin. *Mayo. Clin. Proc.* **74,** 613–634.
3. Patel, R. (1998) Antifungal agents. Part I. Amphotericin B preparations and flucytosine. *Mayo. Clin. Proc.* **73,** 1205–25.
4. Kasten, M. (1999) Clindamycin, metronidazole, and chloramphenicol. *Mayo. Clin. Proc.* **74,** 825–833.
5. Edson, R. and Terrell, C. (1999) The aminoglycosides. *Mayo. Clin. Proc.* **74,** 519–528.
6. Estes, L. (1998) Review of pharmacokinetics and pharmacodynamics of antimicrobial agents. *Mayo. Clin. Proc.* **73,** 1114–1122.
7. Virk, A. and Steckelberg, J. (2000) Clinical aspects of antimicrobial resistance. *Mayo. Clin. Proc.* **75,** 200–214.
8. Thompson, R. and Wright, A. (1998) General principles of antimicrobial therapy. *Mayo. Clin. Proc.* **73,** 995–1006.
9. Cockerill, F. (1998) Conventional and genetic laboratory tests used to guide antimicrobial therapy. *Mayo. Clin. Proc.* **73,** 1007–1021.
10. Smilack, J. (1999) The tetracyclines. *Mayo. Clin. Proc.* **74,** 727–729.

11. Hellinger, W. and Brewer, N. (1999) Carbapenems and monobactams: imipenem, meropenem, and aztreonam. *Mayo. Clin. Proc.* **74**, 420–434.

12. Wright, A. (1999) The penicillins. *Mayo. Clin. Proc.* **74**, 290–307.

13. Keating, M. (1999) Antiviral agents for non-human immunodeficiency virus infections. *Mayo. Clin. Proc.* **74**, 1266–1283.

14. Louie, M. and Cockerill, F. (2001) Susceptibility Testing: Phenotypic and Genotypic Tests for Bacteria and *Mycobacteria. Infect. Dis. Clin. N. Am.* **15**.

15. Doganay, M. and Aydin, N. (1991) Antimicrobial susceptibility of *Bacillus anthracis. Scand. J. Infect. Dis.* **23**, 333–335.

16. Odendaal, M., Pieterson, P., de, V. V., and Botha, A. (1991) The antibiotic sensitivity patterns of *Bacillus* anthracis isolated from the Kruger National Park. *Onderstepoort. J. Vet. Res.* **58**, 17–19.

17. Lightfoot, N. F., Scott, R. J., and Turnbull, P. C. (1990) Antimicrobial susceptibility of *Bacillus anthracis*: proceedings of the international workshop on anthrax. *Salisbury Med. Bull.* **68**, 95–98.

18. Heine, H., Dicks, R., and Andrews, G. (2001) In vitro activity of oratavancin (LY33328), levofloxacin, meropenem, GAR936 and linezolid against strains of *Bacillus anthracis*. 41st Interscience Conference on Antimicrobial Agents and Chemotherapy, Chicago, IL. 173.

19. Heine, H., Dicks, R., and Byrne, W. (2000) In vitro activity of daptomycin, sparfloxacin, quinupristin-dalfopristin and other antibiotics against *Bacillus anthracis*. 40th Interscience Conference on Antimicrobial Agents and Chemotherapy, Toronto. 167.

20. Lalitha, M. and Thomas, M. (1997) Penicillin resistance in *Bacillus anthracis. Lancet* **349**, 1522.

21. Patra, G., Vaissaire, J., Weber-Levy, M., Le, D. C., and Mock, M. (1998) Molecular characterization of Bacillus strains involved in outbreaks of anthrax in France in 1997. *J. Clin. Microbiol.* **36**, 3412–3414.

22. Bradaric, N. and Punda-Polic, V. (1992) Cutaneous anthrax due to penicillin-resistant *Bacillus anthracis* transmitted by an insect bite. *Lancet* **340**, 306, 307.

23. Inglesby, T., O'Toole, T., Henderson, D., et al. (2002) Anthrax as a biological weapon, 2002: updated recommendations for management. *JAMA* **287**, 2236–2252.

24. Chen, Y., Succi, J., and Koehler, T. M. (2001) Silent β-lactamase Genes in *Bacillus anthracis*. 4th International Conference on Anthrax. Annapolis, MD.

25. Penn, C. C. and Klotz, S. A. (1998) *Bacillus anthracis* and other aerobic spore formers, in *Infectious Diseases*. 2nd ed. (Blacklow, N. R., ed.), Saunders, Philadelphia, PA, pp. 1747–1750.

26. Centers for Disease Control and Prevention. (2001) Update: investigation of bioterrorism-related anthrax and interim guidelines for exposure management and antimicrobial therapy, October 2001. [erratum appears in *MMWR Morb. Mortal. Wkly. Rep.* (2001) **50(43)**, 962]. *MMWR Morb. Mortal. Wkly Rep.* **50**, 909–919.

27. Kim, H., Choi, E., and Kim, B. (1993) A macrolide-lincosamide-streptogramin B resistance determinant from *Bacillus anthracis* 590: cloning and expression of ermJ. *J. Gen. Microbiol.* **139**, 601–607.

28. Pomerantsev, A., Sukovatova, L., and Marinin, L. (1993) [Characterization of a Rif-R population of *Bacillus anthracis*]. *Antibiot. Khimioter.* **38**, 34–38.

29. Pomerantsev, A., Shishkova, N., and Marinin, L. (1992) [Comparison of therapeutic effects of antibiotics of the tetracycline group in the treatment of anthrax caused by a strain inheriting tet-gene of plasmid pBC16]. *Antibiot. Khimioter.* **37**, 31–34.

30. Stepanov, A. V., Marinin, L. I., Pomerantsev, A. P., and Staritsin, N. A. (1996) Development of novel vaccines against anthrax in man. *J. Biotechnol.* **44**, 155–160.

31. Brook, I., Elliott, T., Pryor, H., et al. (2001) In vitro resistance of *Bacillus anthracis* Sterne to doxycycline, macrolides and quinolones. *Int. J. Antimicrob. Agents* **18**, 559–562.

32. Choe, C., Bouhaouala, S., Brook, I., Elliot, T., and Knudson, G. (2000) In vitro development of resistance to ofloxacin and doxycycline in *Bacillus anthracis* Sterne. *Antimicrob. Agents Chemother.* **44**, 1766.

33. Stevens, D., Gibbons, A., Bergstrom, R., and Winn, V. (1988) The Eagle effect revisited: efficacy of clindamycin, erythromycin, and penicillin in the treatment of streptococcal myositis. *J. Infect. Dis.* **158,** 23–28.

34. Russell, N. and Pachorek, R. (2000) Clindamycin in the treatment of streptococcal and staphylococcal toxic shock syndromes. *Ann. Pharmacother.* **34,** 936–939.

35. Stevens, D., Bryant, A., and Hackett, S. (1995) Antibiotic effects on bacterial viability, toxin production, and host response. *Clin. Infect. Dis.* **20(Suppl. 2),** S154–157.

36. Abramova, F. A., Grinberg, L. M., Yampolskaya, O. V., and Walker, D. H. (1993) Pathology of inhalational anthrax in 42 cases from the Sverdlovsk outbreak of 1979. *Proc. Natl. Acad. Sci. USA* **90,** 2291–2294.

37. Hurewitz, A., Wu, C., Mancuso, P., and Zucker, S. (1993) Tetracycline and doxycycline inhibit pleural fluid metalloproteinases. A possible mechanism for chemical pleurodesis. *Chest* **103,** 1113–1117.

38. Loebstein, R., Addis, A., Ho, E., et al. Pregnancy outcome following gestational exposure to fluoroquinolones: a multicenter prospective controlled study. *Antimicrob. Agents Chemother.* **42,** 1336–1339.

39. AAP (2003) Redbook: Report of the Committee on Infectious Diseases. 26th ed. *Am. Acad. Peds.*, pp. 693–694.

40. Burkhardt, J., Walterspiel, J., and Schaad, U. (1997) Quinolone arthropathy in animals versus children. *Clin. Infect. Dis.* **25,** 1196–1204.

41. Friedlander, A., Welkos, S., Pitt, M., et al. (1993) Postexposure prophylaxis against experimental inhalation anthrax. *J. Infect. Dis.* **167,** 1239–1243.

42. Henderson, D. W., Peacock, S., and Belton, F. C. (1956) Observations on the prophylaxis of experimental pulmonary anthrax in the monkey. *J. Hyg.* **54,** 28–36.

43. Kortepeter, M., Christopher, G., Cieslak, T., et al. (eds.) (2001) *Medical Management of Biological Casualties Handbook.* 4th ed. United States Army Medical Research Institute of Infectious Diseases (USAMRIID), Fort Detrick, p. 34.

44. King, A. (2001) Recommendations for susceptibility tests on fastidious organisms and those requiring special handling. *J. Antimicrob. Chemother.* **48(Suppl. 1),** 77–80.

45. Hall, W. H. (1990) Modern chemotherapy for brucellosis in humans. [see comments]. *Rev. Infect. Dis.* **12,** 1060–1099.

46. Mortensen, J. E., Moore, D. G., Clarridge, J. E., and Young, E. J. (1986) Antimicrobial susceptibility of clinical isolates of *Brucella*. *Diag. Microbiol. Infect. Dis.* **5,** 163–169.

47. Mateu-de-Antonio, E. and Martin, M. (1995) In vitro efficacy of several antimicrobial combinations against *Brucella canis* and *Brucella melitensis* strains isolated from dogs. *Vet. Microbiol.* **45,** 1–10.

48. Bosch, J., Linares, J., Lopez de Goicoechea, M. J., Ariza, J., Cisnal, M. C., and Martin, R. (1986) In-vitro activity of ciprofloxacin, ceftriaxone and five other antimicrobial agents against 95 strains of *Brucella melitensis*. *J. Antimicrob. Chemother.* **17,** 459–461.

49. Memish, Z., Mah, M. W., Al Mahmoud, S., Al Shaalan, M., and Khan, M. Y. (2000) *Brucella bacteraemia*: clinical and laboratory observations in 160 patients. *J. Infect.* **40,** 59–63.

50. Trujillano-Martin, I., Garcia-Sanchez, E., Fresnadillo, M., Garcia-Sanchez, J., Garcia-Rodriguez, J., and Montes, M. I. (1999) In vitro activities of five new antimicrobial agents against *Brucella melitensis*. *Int. J. Antimicrob. Agents* **12,** 185, 186.

51. Kinsara, A., Al-Mowallad, A., and Osoba, A. (1999) Increasing resistance of *Brucellae* to co-trimoxazole. *Antimicrob. Agents Chemother.* **43,** 1531.

52. Lubani, M. M., Dudin, K. I., Sharda, D. C., et al. (1989) A multicenter therapeutic study of 1100 children with brucellosis. *Ped. Infect. Dis. J.* **8,** 75–78.

53. Ariza, J., Bosch, J., Gudiol, F., Linares, J., Viladrich, P. F., and Martin, R. (1986) Relevance of in vitro antimicrobial susceptibility of *Brucella melitensis* to relapse rate in human brucellosis. *Antimicrob. Agents Chemother.* **30,** 958–960.

54. Landinez, R., Linares, J., Loza, E., Martinez-Beltran, J., Martin, R., and Baquero, F. (1992) In vitro activity of azithromycin and tetracycline against 358 clinical isolates of *Brucella melitensis. Eur. J. Clin. Microbiol. Infect. Dis.* **11,** 265–267.

55. Rolain, J., Maurin, M., and Raoult, D. Bactericidal effect of antibiotics on *Bartonella* and *Brucella* spp.: clinical implications. *J. Antimicrob. Chemother.* **46,** 811–814.

56. Trujillano-Martin, I., Garcia-Sanchez, E., Martinez, I., Fresnadillo, M., Garcia-Sanchez, J., and Garcia-Rodriguez, J. (1999) In vitro activities of six new fluoroquinolones against *Brucella melitensis. Antimicrob. Agents Chemother.* **43,** 194, 195.

57. Garcia-Rodriguez, J., Garcia, S. J., and Trujillano, I. (1991) Lack of effective bactericidal activity of new quinolones against *Brucella* spp. *Antimicrob. Agents Chemother.* **35,** 756–759.

58. Akova, M., Gur, D., Livermore, D., Kocagoz, T., and Akalin, H. (1999) In vitro activities of antibiotics alone and in combination against *Brucella melitensis* at neutral and acidic pHs. *Antimicrob. Agents Chemother.* **43,** 1298–1300.

59. Colmenero, J. D., Fernandez-Gallardo, L. C., Agundez, J. A., Sedeno, J., Benitez, J., and Valverde, E. (1994) Possible implications of doxycycline-rifampin interaction for treatment of brucellosis. *Antimicrob. Agents Chemother.* **38,** 2798–2802.

60. Montejo, J. M., Alberola, I., Glez-Zarate, P., et al. (1993) Open, randomized therapeutic trial of six antimicrobial regimens in the treatment of human brucellosis. *Clin. Infect. Dis.* **16,** 671–676.

61. al-Sibai, M., Halim, M., el-Shaker, M., Khan, B., and Qadri, S. (1992) Efficacy of ciprofloxacin for treatment of *Brucella melitensis* infections. *Antimicrob. Agents Chemother.* **36,** 150–152.

62. Qadri, S. M., Akhtar, M., Ueno, Y., and al-Sibai, M. B. (1989) Susceptibility of *Brucella melitensis* to fluoroquinolones. *Drugs Under Exp. Clin. Res.* **15,** 483–485.

63. (1986) Joint FAO/WHO expert committee on brucellosis. *World Health Org. Tech. Rep. Ser.* **740,** 1–132.

64. Figueroa, D. R., Rojas, R. L., and Marcano, T. E. (1995) [*Brucellosis* in pregnancy: course and perinatal results]. *Ginecol. Obstet. Mex.* **63,** 190–195.

65. Jacobs, F., Abramowicz, D., Vereerstraeten, .P, Le, C. J., Zech, F., and Thys, J. (1990) *Brucella endocarditis*: the role of combined medical and surgical treatment. *Rev. Infect. Dis.* **12,** 740–744.

66. Gorelov, V., Gubina, E., Grekova, N., and Skavronskaia, A. (1991) [The possibility of creating a vaccinal strain of *Brucella abortus* 19-BA with multiple antibiotic resistance]. *Zh. Mikrobiol. Epidemiol. Immunobiol.* **9,** 2–4.

67. Vasi'lev, N., Oborin, V., Vasi'lev, P., Glushkova, O., Kravets, I., and Levchuk, B. (1989) [Sensitivity spectrum of *Francisella tularensis* to antibiotics and synthetic antibacterial drugs]. *Antibiot. Khimioter.* **34,** 662–665.

68. Kudelina, R. and Olsufiev, N. (1980) Sensitivity to macrolide antibiotics and lincomycin in *Francisella tularensis* holarctica. *J. Hyg. Epidemiol. Microbiol. Immunol.* **24,** 84–91.

69. Ikaheimo, I., Syrjala, H., Karhukorpi, J., Schildt, R., and Koskela, M. (2000) In vitro antibiotic susceptibility of *Francisella tularensis* isolated from humans and animals. *J. Antimicrob. Chemother.* **46,** 287–290.

70. Scheel, O., Hoel, T., Sandvik, T., and Berdal, B. P. (1993) Susceptibility pattern of Scandinavian *Francisella tularensis* isolates with regard to oral and parenteral antimicrobial agents. *APMIS* **101,** 33–36.

71. Maurin, M., Mersali, N., and Raoult, D. (2000) Bactericidal activities of antibiotics against intracellular *Francisella tularensis. Antimicrob. Agents Chemother.* **44,** 3428–2431.

72. Baker, C., Hollis, D., and Thornsberry, C. (1985) Antimicrobial susceptibility testing of *Francisella tularensis* with a modified Mueller-Hinton broth. *J. Clin. Microbiol.* **22,** 212–215.

73. Tynkevich, N., Pavlovich, N., and Ryzhko, I. (1990) [Comparative study of the effectiveness of amikacin and streptomycin in experimental tularemia]. *Antibiot. Khimioter.* **35,** 35–37.

74. Enderlin, G., Morales, L., Jacobs, R. F., and Cross, J. T. (1994) Streptomycin and alternative agents for the treatment of tularemia: review of the literature. *Clin. Infect. Dis.* **19,** 42–47.

75. Cross, J. T. and Jacobs, R. F. (1993) Tularemia: treatment failures with outpatient use of ceftriaxone. *Clin. Infect. Dis.* **17,** 976–980.

76. Syrjala, H., Schildt, R., and Raisainen, S. (1991) In vitro susceptibility of Francisella tularensis to fluoroquinolones and treatment of tularemia with norfloxacin and ciprofloxacin. *Eur. J. Clin. Microbiol. Infect. Dis.* **10,** 68–70.

77. Johansson, A., Berglund, L., Gothefors, L., Sjostedt, A., and Tarnvik, A. (2000) Ciprofloxacin for treatment of tularemia in children. *Ped. Infect. Dis. J.* **19,** 449–453.

78. Sawyer, W. D., Dangerfield, H. G., Hogge, A. L., and Crozier, D. (1966) Antibiotic prophylaxis and therapy of airborne tularemia. *Bacteriol. Rev.* **30,** 542–550.

79. Russell, P., Eley, S. M., Fulop, M. J., Bell, D. L., and Titball, R. W. (1998) The efficacy of ciprofloxacin and doxycycline against experimental tularaemia. *J. Antimicrob. Chemother.* **41,** 461–465.

80. Dennis, D. T., Inglesby, T. V., Henderson, D. A., et al. (2001) Tularemia as a biological weapon: medical and public health management. *JAMA* **285,** 2763–2773.

81. Alibek, K. (1999) *Biohazard.* Random House, New York, pp. 157, 160.

82. Pavlov, V., Mokrievich, A., and Volkovoy, K. (1996) Cryptic plasmid pFNL10 from Francisella novicida-like F6168: the base of plasmid vectors for *Francisella tularensis.* *FEMS Immunol. Med. Microbiol.* **13,** 253–256.

83. Kuoppa, K., Forsberg, A., and Norqvist, A. (2001) Construction of a reporter plasmid for screening in vivo promoter activity in *Francisella tularensis.* *FEMS Microbiol. Lett.* **205,** 77–81.

84. Kenny, D. J., Russell, P., Rogers, D., Eley, S. M., and Titball, R. W. (1999) In vitro susceptibilities of *Burkholderia mallei* in comparison to those of other pathogenic *Burkholderia* spp. *Antimicrob. Agents Chemother.* **43,** 2773–2775.

85. Heine, H. S., England, M. J., Waag, D. M., and Byrne, W. R. (2001) In vitro antibiotic susceptibilities of *Burkholderia mallei* (causative agent of glanders) determined by broth microdilution and E-test. *Antimicrob. Agents Chemother.* **45,** 2119–2121.

86. Al-Izzi, S. A. and Al-Bassam, L. S. (1989) In vitro susceptibility of *Pseudomonas mallei* to antimicrobial agents. *Comp. Immunol. Microbiol. Infect. Dis.* **12,** 5–8.

87. Srinivasan, A., Kraus, C., De, S. D., et al. (2001) Glanders in a military research microbiologist. *N. Engl. J. Med.* **345,** 256–258.

88. Russell, P., Eley, S., Ellis, J., et al. (2000) Comparison of efficacy of ciprofloxacin and doxycycline against experimental melioidosis and glanders. *J. Antimicrob. Chemother.* **45,** 813–818.

89. Batmanov, V., Iliukhin, V., Lozovaia, N., and Iakovlev, A. (1996) [Recovery rate in chemotherapy of glanders]. *Antibiot. Khimioter.* **41,** 30–34.

90. Manzeniuk, I., Dorokhin, V., and Svetoch, E. (1994) [The efficacy of antibacterial preparations against *Pseudomonas mallei* in in-vitro and in-vivo experiments]. *Antibiot. Khimioter.* **39,** 26–30.

91. Eickhoff, T. C., Bennett, J. V., Hayes, P. S., and Feeley, J. (1970) *Pseudomonas pseudomallei*: susceptibility to chemotherapeutic agents. *J. Infect. Dis.* **121,** 95–102.

92. Kenny, D., Russell, P., Rogers, D., Eley, S., and Titball, R. (1999) In vitro susceptibilities of *Burkholderia mallei* in comparison to those of other pathogenic *Burkholderia* spp. *Antimicrob. Agents Chemother.* **43,** 2773–2775.

93. Sookpranee, T., Sookpranee, M., Mellencamp, M. A., and Preheim, L. C. (1991) *Pseudomonas pseudomallei*, a common pathogen in Thailand that is resistant to the bactericidal effects of many antibiotics. *Antimicrob. Agents Chemother.* **35,** 484–489.

94. Dance, D. A., Wuthiekanun, V., Chaowagul, W., and White, N. J. (1989) The antimicrobial susceptibility of *Pseudomonas pseudomallei*. Emergence of resistance in vitro and during treatment. *J. Antimicrob. Chemother.* **24,** 295–309.

95. Cheong, Y. M., Joseph, P. G., and Koay, A. S. (1987) In-vitro susceptibility of *Pseudomonas pseudomallei* isolated in Malaysia to some new cephalosporins and a quinolone. *SE Asian J. Trop. Med. Public Health* **18,** 94–96.

96. McEniry, D. W., Gillespie, S. H., and Felmingham, D. (1988) Susceptibility of *Pseudomonas pseudomallei* to new β-lactam and aminoglycoside antibiotics. *J. Antimicrob. Chemother.* **21,** 171–175.

97. Jenney, A. W., Lum, G., Fisher, D. A., and Currie, B. J. (2001) Antibiotic susceptibility of *Burkholderia pseudomallei* from tropical northern Australia and implications for therapy of melioidosis. *Int. J. Antimicrob. Agents* **17,** 109–113.

98. Koay, A. S., Rohani, M. Y., and Cheong, Y. M. (1997) In-vitro susceptibility of *Burkholderia pseudomallei* to cefoperazone-sulbactam combination. *Med. J. Malaysia* **52,** 158–160.

99. Moore, R. A., DeShazer, D., Reckseidler, S., Weissman, A., and Woods, D. E. (1999) Efflux-mediated aminoglycoside and macrolide resistance in *Burkholderia pseudomallei*. [see comments]. *Antimicrob. Agents Chemother.* **43,** 465–470.

100. Godfrey, A. J., Wong, S., Dance, D. A., Chaowagul, W., and Bryan, L. E. (1991) *Pseudomonas pseudomallei* resistance to β-lactam antibiotics due to alterations in the chromosomally encoded β-lactamase. *Antimicrob. Agents Chemother.* **35,** 1635–1640.

101. Lumbiganon, P., Tattawasatra, U., Chetchotisakd, P., Wongratanacheewin, S., and Thinkhamrop, B. (2000) Comparison between the antimicrobial susceptibility of *Burkholderia pseudomallei* to trimethoprim-sulfamethoxazole by standard disk diffusion method and by minimal inhibitory concentration determination. *J. Med. Assoc. Thailand* **83,** 856–860.

102. White, N. J., Dance, D. A. , Chaowagul, W., Wattanagoon, Y., Wuthiekanun, V., and Pitakwatchara, N. (1989) Halving of mortality of severe melioidosis by ceftazidime. [see comments]. *Lancet* **2,** 697–701.

103. Suputtamongkol, Y., Rajchanuwong, A., Chaowagul, W., et al. (1994) Ceftazidime vs. amoxicillin/clavulanate in the treatment of severe melioidosis. *Clin. Infect. Dis.* **19,** 846–853.

104. Chetchotisakd, P., Porramatikul, S., Mootsikapun, P., Anunnatsiri, S., and Thinkhamrop, B. (2001) Randomized, double-blind, controlled study of cefoperazone-sulbactam plus cotrimoxazole versus ceftazidime plus cotrimoxazole for the treatment of severe melioidosis. *Clin. Infect. Dis.* **33,** 29–34.

105. Currie, B., Fisher, D., Howard, D., et al. (2000) Endemic melioidosis in tropical northern Australia: a 10-year prospective study and review of the literature. *Clin. Infect. Dis.* **31,** 981–986.

106. Stephens, D., Fisher, D., and Currie, B. (2002) An audit of the use of granulocyte colony-stimulating factor in septic shock [in process citation]. *Intern. Med. J.* **32,** 143–148

107. Rajchanuvong, A., Chaowagul, W., Suputtamongkol, Y., Smith, M. D., Dance, D. A., and White, N. J. (1995) A prospective comparison of co-amoxiclav and the combination of chloramphenicol, doxycycline, and co-trimoxazole for the oral maintenance treatment of melioidosis. *Trans. Royal Soc. Trop. Med. Hyg.* **89,** 546–549.

108. Chetchotisakd, P., Chaowagul, W., Mootsikapun, P., Budhsarawong, D., and Thinkamrop, B. (2001) Maintenance therapy of melioidosis with ciprofloxacin plus azithromycin compared with cotrimoxazole plus doxycycline. *Am. J. Trop. Med. Hyg.* **64,** 24–27.

109. Samuel, M. and Ti, T. (2001) Interventions for treating melioidosis. *Cochrane Database Sys. Rev.* CD001263.

110. Apisarnthanarak, A. and Little, J. (2002) The role of cefoperazone-sulbactam for treatment of severe melioidosis. *Clin. Infect. Dis.* **34,** 721–723.

111. Simpson, A., Suputtamongkol, Y., Smith, M., et al. (1999) Comparison of imipenem and ceftazidime as therapy for severe melioidosis. *Clin. Infect. Dis.* **29,** 381–387.

112. Currie, B. J., Fisher, D. A., Anstey, N. M., and Jacups, S. P. (2000) Melioidosis: acute and chronic disease, relapse and re-activation. *Trans. Royal Soc. Trop. Med. Hyg.* **94,** 301–304.
113. Chanteau, S., Ratsitorahina, M., Rahalison, L., et al. (2000) Current epidemiology of human plague in Madagascar. *Microb. Infect.* **2,** 25–31.
114. Frean, J. A., Arntzen, L., Capper, T., Bryskier, A., and Klugman, K. P. (1996) In vitro activities of 14 antibiotics against 100 human isolates of *Yersinia pestis* from a southern African plague focus. *Antimicrob. Agents Chemother.* **40,** 2646, 2647.
115. Lyamuya, E. F., Nyanda, P., Mohammedali, H., and Mhalu, F. S. (1992) Laboratory studies on *Yersinia pestis* during the 1991 outbreak of plague in Lushoto, Tanzania. *J. Trop. Med. Hyg.* **95,** 335–338.
116. Smith, M. D., Vinh, D. X., Nguyen, T. T., Wain, J., Thung, D., and White, N. J. (1995) In vitro antimicrobial susceptibilities of strains of Yersinia pestis. *Antimicrob. Agents Chemother.* **39,** 2153, 2154.
117. Rasoamanana, B., Coulanges, P., Michel, P., and Rasolofonirina, N. (1989) Sensibilite de *Yersinia pestis* aux antibiotiques: 277 souches isolees a Madagascar entre 1926 et 1989. *Archives de l Institut Pasteur de Madagascar* **56,** 37–53.
118. Galenko, G., Akiev, A., and Tarasova, V. (1992) [Antibiotic sensitivity of plague microbe strains from foreign countries]. *Antibiot. Khimioter.* **37,** 23, 24.
119. Heine, H. (2002) In *Unpublished data,* Y. pestis *MIC Data.* (J. B. W., ed.), Fort Detrick, MD.
120. Galimand, M., Guiyoule, A., Gerbaud, G., et al. (1997) Multidrug resistance in *Yersinia pestis* mediated by a transferable plasmid. *N. Engl. J. Med.* **337,** 677–680.
121. Guiyoule, A., Gerbaud, G., Buchrieser, C., et al. (2001) Transferable plasmid-mediated resistance to streptomycin in a clinical isolate of *Yersinia pestis. Emerg. Infect. Dis.* **7,** 43–48.
122. (1994) Human plague—United States, 1993–1994. *MMWR Morb. Mortal. Wkly. Rep.* **43,** 242–246.
123. Welty, T., Grabman, J., Kompare, E., et al. (1985) Nineteen cases of plague in Arizona. A spectrum including ecthyma gangrenosum due to plague and plague in pregnancy. *W. J. Med.* **142,** 641–646.
124. Byrne, W. R., Welkos, S. L., Pitt, M. L., et al. (1998) Antibiotic treatment of experimental pneumonic plague in mice. *Antimicrob. Agents Chemother.* **42,** 675–681.
125. Inglesby, T., Dennis, D., Henderson, D., et al. (2000) Plague as a biological weapon: medical and public health management. Working Group on Civilian Biodefense. *JAMA* **283,** 2281–2290.
126. Crook, L. D. and Tempest, B. (1992) Plague. A clinical review of 27 cases. *Arch. Int. Med.* **152,** 1253–1256.
127. Russell, P., Eley, S. M., Green, M., et al. (1998) Efficacy of doxycycline and ciprofloxacin against experimental *Yersinia pestis* infection. [see comments]. *J. Antimicrob. Chemother.* **41,** 301–305.
128. Bonacorsi, S. P., Scavizzi, M. R., Guiyoule, A., Amouroux, J. H., and Carniel, E. (1994) Assessment of a fluoroquinolone, three beta-lactams, two aminoglycosides, and a cycline in treatment of murine *Yersinia pestis* infection. [erratum appears in *Antimicrob. Agents Chemother.* (1994) 38(7), 1694]. *Antimicrob. Agents Chemother.* 38, 481–486.
129. Ryzhko, I., Shcherbaniuk, A., Tsuraeva, R., et al. (1997) [A comparative study of fluoroquinolones and 3rd-generation cephalosporins in the prevention and treatment of experimental plague caused by *Yersinia pestis* strains typical and serologically atypical with respect to F1]. *Antibiot. Khimioter.* **42,** 12–16.
130. Ryzhko, I., Samokhodkina, E., Tsuraeva, R., Shcherbaniuk, A., and Pasiukov, V. [Experimental evaluation of prospects for the use of β-lactams in plague infection caused by pathogens with plasmid resistance to penicillins]. *Antibiot. Khimioter.* **43,** 11–15.
131. Becker, T. M., Poland, J. D., Quan, T. J., White, M. E., Mann, J. M., and Barnes, A. M. (1987) Plague meningitis—a retrospective analysis of cases reported in the United States, 1970–1979. *W. J. Med.* **147,** 554–557.

132. Ryzhko, I., Shcherbaniuk, A., Samokhodkina, E., et al. (1994) [Virulence of rifampicin and quinolone resistant mutants of strains of plague microbe with Fra+ and Fra- phenotypes]. *Antibiot. Khimioter.* **39,** 32–36.

133. Yeaman, M. R. and Baca, O. G. (1991) Mechanisms that may account for differential antibiotic susceptibilities among *Coxiella burnetii* isolates. *Antimicrob. Agents Chemother.* **35,** 948–954.

134. Raoult, D., Torres, H., and Drancourt, M. (1991) Shell-vial assay: evaluation of a new technique for determining antibiotic susceptibility, tested in 13 isolates of *Coxiella burnetii. Antimicrob. Agents Chemother.* **35,** 2070–2077.

135. Yeaman, M. R and Baca, O. G. (1990) Unexpected antibiotic susceptibility of a chronic isolate of *Coxiella burnetii. Ann. NY Acad. Sci.* **590,** 297–305.

136. Yeaman, M. R,. Mitscher, L. A., and Baca, O. G. (1987) In vitro susceptibility of *Coxiella burnetii* to antibiotics, including several quinolones. *Antimicrob. Agents Chemother.* **31,** 1079–1084.

137. Gikas, A., Spyridaki, I., Psaroulaki, A., Kofterithis, D., and Tselentis, Y. (1998) In vitro susceptibility of *Coxiella burnetii* to trovafloxacin in comparison with susceptibilities to pefloxacin, ciprofloxacin, ofloxacin, doxycycline, and clarithromycin. *Antimicrob. Agents Chemother.* **42,** 2747, 2748.

138. Rolain, J., Maurin, M., and Raoult, D. (2001) Bacteriostatic and bactericidal activities of moxifloxacin against *Coxiella burnetii. Antimicrob. Agents Chemother.* **45,** 301, 302.

139. Maurin, M. and Raoult, D. (1997) Bacteriostatic and bactericidal activity of levofloxacin against *Rickettsia rickettsii, Rickettsia conorii,* 'Israeli spotted fever group rickettsia' and *Coxiella burnetii. J. Antimicrob. Chemother.* **39,** 725–730.

140. Keysary, A., Itzhaki, A., Rubinstein, E., Oron, C., and Keren, G. (1996) The in-vitro anti-rickettsial activity of macrolides. *J. Antimicrob. Chemother.* **38,** 727–731.

141. Maurin, M. and Raoult, D. (1993) In vitro susceptibilities of spotted fever group rickettsiae and *Coxiella burnetti* to clarithromycin. *Antimicrob. Agents Chemother.* **37,** 2633–2637.

142. Yeaman, M. R., Roman, M. J., and Baca, O. G. (1989) Antibiotic susceptibilities of two *Coxiella burnetii* isolates implicated in distinct clinical syndromes. *Antimicrob. Agents Chemother.* **33,** 1052–1057.

143. Maurin, M., Benoliel, A. M., Bongrand, P., and Raoult, D. (1992) Phagolysosomal alkalinization and the bactericidal effect of antibiotics: the *Coxiella burnetii* paradigm. *J. Infect. Dis.* **166,** 1097–1102.

144. Gikas, A., Kofteridis, D., Manios, A., Pediaditis, J., and Tselentis, Y. (2001) Newer macrolides as empiric treatment for acute Q fever infection. *Antimicrob. Agents Chemother.* **45,** 3644–3646.

145. Perez-del-Molino, A., Aguado, J. M., Riancho, J. A., Sampedro, I., Matorras, P., and Gonzalez-Macias, J. (1991) Erythromycin and the treatment of *Coxiella burnetii* pneumonia. *J. Antimicrob. Chemother.* **28,** 455–459.

146. Bertrand, A., Janbon, F., Jonquet, O., and Reynes, J. (1988) [*Rickettsiaceae* infections and fluoroquinolones]. *Pathol. Biol. (Paris)* **36,** 493–495.

147. Maurin, M. and Raoult, D. (1999) Q fever. *Clin. Microbiol. Rev.* **12,** 518–553.

148. Drancourt, M., Raoult, D., Xeridat, B., Milandre, L., Nesri, M., and Dano, P. (1991) Q fever meningoencephalitis in five patients. *Eur. J. Epidemiol.* **7,** 134–138.

149. Fenollar, F., Fournier, P., Carrieri, M., Habib, G., Messana, T., and Raoult, D. Risks factors and prevention of Q fever endocarditis. *Clin. Infect. Dis.* **33,** 312–316.

150. Raoult, D., Fenollar, F., and Stein, A. (2002) Q fever during pregnancy: diagnosis, treatment, and follow-up. *Arch. Intern. Med.* **162,** 701–704.

151. Raoult, D. and Stein, A. (1994) Q fever during pregnancy—a risk for women, fetuses, and obstetricians. *N. Engl. J. Med.* **330,** 371.

152. Levy, P. Y., Drancourt, M., Etienne, J., et al. (1991) Comparison of different antibiotic regimens for therapy of 32 cases of Q fever endocarditis. *Antimicrob. Agents Chemother.* **35,** 533–537.

153. Raoult, D., Houpikian, P., Tissot Dupont, H., Riss, J. M., Arditi-Djiane, J., and Brouqui, P. (1999) Treatment of Q fever endocarditis: comparison of 2 regimens containing doxycycline and ofloxacin or hydroxychloroquine. *Arch. Int. Med.* **159,** 167–173.
154. Raoult, D. (1993) Treatment of Q fever. *Antimicrob. Agents Chemother.* **37,** 1733–1736.
155. Tigertt, W. D. and Benenson, A. S. (1956) Studies on Q fever in man. *Trans. Assoc. Am. Phys.* **69,** 98–104.
156. Canonico, P. G., Kende, M., Luscri, B. J., and Huggins, J. W. (1984) In-vivo activity of antivirals against exotic RNA viral infections. *J. Antimicrob. Chemother.* **14(Suppl A),** 27–41.
157. Lukaszewski, R. and Brooks, T. (2000) Pegylated alpha interferon is an effective treatment for virulent venezuelan equine encephalitis virus and has profound effects on the host immune response to infection. *J. Virol.* **74,** 5006–5015.
158. McCormick, J., King, I., Webb, P., et al. (1986) Lassa fever. Effective therapy with ribavirin. *N. Engl. J. Med.* **314,** 20–26.
159. Enria, D. A., Briggiler, A. M., Levis, S., Vallejos, D., Maiztegui, J. I., and Canonico, P. G. (1987) Tolerance and antiviral effect of ribavirin in patients with Argentine hemorrhagic fever. *Antivir. Res.* **7,** 353–359.
160. Enria, D. A. and Maiztegui, J. I. (1994) Antiviral treatment of Argentine hemorrhagic fever. *Antivir. Res.* **23,** 23–31.
161. Kilgore, P. E., Ksiazek, T. G., Rollin, P. E., et al. (1997) Treatment of Bolivian hemorrhagic fever with intravenous ribavirin. *Clin. Infect. Dis.* **24,** 718–722.
162. Fisher-Hoch, S., Khan, J., Rehman, S., Mirza, S., Khurshid, M., and McCormick, J. (1995) Crimean Congo-haemorrhagic fever treated with oral ribavirin. *Lancet* **346,** 472–475.
163. Kende, M., Lupton, H., Rill, W., Levy, H., and Canonico, P. (1987) Enhanced therapeutic efficacy of poly(ICLC) and ribavirin combinations against Rift Valley fever virus infection in mice. *Antimicrob. Agents Chemother.* **31,** 986–990.
164. Yang, Z. Q., Zhang, T. M., Zhang, M. V., et al. (1991) Interruption study of viremia of patients with hemorrhagic fever with renal syndrome in the febrile phase. *Chin. Med. J.* **104,** 149–153.
165. Mertz, G. J., Hjelle, B. L., and Bryan, R. T. (1997) Hantavirus infection. *Adv. Int. Med.* **42,** 369–421.
166. Huggins, J. (1989) Prospects for treatment of viral hemorrhagic fevers with ribavirin, a broad-spectrum antiviral drug. *Rev. Infect. Dis.* **11(Suppl. 4),** S750–761.
167. Bray, M., Driscoll, J., and Huggins, J. W. (2000) Treatment of lethal Ebola virus infection in mice with a single dose of an *S*-adenosyl-L-homocysteine hydrolase inhibitor. *Antivir. Res.* **45,** 135–147.
168. Huggins, J., Zhang, Z. X., and Bray, M. (1999) Antiviral drug therapy of filovirus infections: S-adenosylhomocysteine hydrolase inhibitors inhibit Ebola virus in vitro and in a lethal mouse model. *J. Infect. Dis.* **179(Suppl. 1),** S240–247.
169. Borio, L., Inglesby, T., Peters, C., et al. (2002) Hemorrhagic fever viruses as biological weapons: medical and public health management. *JAMA* **287,** 2391–2405.
170. De Clercq, E. (2001) Vaccinia virus inhibitors as a paradigm for the chemotherapy of poxvirus infections. *Clin. Microbiol. Rev.* **14,** 382–397.
171. Bray, M., Martinez, M., Kefauver, D., West, M., and Roy, C. (2002) Treatment of aerosolized cowpox virus infection in mice with aerosolized cidofovir. *Antivir. Res.* **54,** 129–142.
172. Bauer, D. (1965) Clinical experience with the antiviral drug marboran (1-methylisatin 3-thiosemicarbazone). *Ann. NY Acad. Sci.* **130,** 110–117.
173. Koplan, J. P., Monsur, K. A., Foster, S. O., et al. (1975) Treatment of *Variola major* with adenine arabinoside. *J. Infect. Dis.* **131,** 34–39.
174. Monsur, K., Hossain, M., Huq, F., Rahaman, M., and Haque, M. (1975) Treatment of *Variola major* with cytosine arabinoside. *J. Infect. Dis.* **131,** 40–43.

14

Nonspecific Immunomodulator Therapy

CpG

D. G. Cerys Rees, Arthur M. Krieg, and Richard W. Titball

1. INTRODUCTION—IMMUNOMODULATOR THERAPY: CpG

This chapter focuses on the immunomodulatory effects of synthetic cytosine and guanosine (CpG) DNA and its possible use as a generic therapy against infectious diseases. For many years, research into the development of medical countermeasures against microorganisms that could be used as a biological weapon has focused on the development of vaccines given preexposure and which induce pathogen-specific immune responses. Such vaccines are often highly effective. However, in some situations it may not be possible to immunize populations using vaccines, for example, if an attack is not anticipated, or if there is insufficient time (many vaccine regimes take weeks to generate an effective immune response). Also, for many of these pathogens, licensed vaccines are not available. The possibility of countermeasures that can protect against a range of biological warfare (BW) agents has been a goal of researchers for many years. Such countermeasures would be given shortly before or after exposure to the agents. This could also potentially overcome the limitations of the antimicrobials currently available; there are few available antibiotics effective against the bacterial BW agents and still less antiviral therapies (*see* Chapter 13).

The effects of different CpG classes and sequences are described, along with details of their effects on specific immune cells. In addition, protective data to a range of organisms, bacterial, viral and protozoal are described. These data reveal the broad range of effects of this type of therapy and suggests its possible use as a generic therapy. This would be of particular use as a medical countermeasure in the event of the deliberate release of a biological agent.

2. ANCIENT RECOGNITION SYSTEMS

The ability of multicellular organisms to defend against invasion by pathogens depends on their ability to mount effective immune responses. The innate (or natural) immune system is a highly conserved ancient system, evolved over hundreds of millions of years of evolution occurring in species from insects to humans *(1,2)*. This innate system has been shown to recognize a broad spectrum of pathogens without a need for prior exposure. The innate immune system has evolved to protect the host in

From: *Infectious Diseases: Biological Weapons Defense: Infectious Diseases and Counterterrorism*
Edited by: L. E. Lindler, F. J. Lebeda, and G. W. Korch © Humana Press Inc., Totowa, NJ

the early phase of an infectious challenge and relies on a set of germline-encoded receptors and molecules that recognize conserved molecular patterns found only in microorganisms. These invariant molecular structures found in pathogens (and other microorganisms) are the main targets of innate immune recognition and are defined as pathogen-associated molecular patterns (PAMPs). Host organisms have developed a range of receptors, with a broad range of specificities to detect these PAMPs; these are referred to as pattern recognition receptors (PRRs). PRRs are strategically expressed on those cells most likely to encounter pathogens in the early stages of infection, for example, surface epithelia and effector cells of the innate immune system such as dendritic cells, monocytes, macrophages, and natural killer (NK) cells.

2.1. Pattern Recognition Receptors

To date, several different families of proteins that form PRRs have been identified, these include: C-type lectins, including collectins, scavenger receptors, integrins and the recently identified Toll-like receptor (TLR) family.

The TLRs have been identified as crucial sensors of infection, which upon microbial recognition, induce activation of the immune and inflammatory responses. The Toll family of PRRs is a highly conserved group of proteins occurring in species as diverse as insects and humans *(1)*. Much of the work on Toll receptors has been on the fruitfly *Drosophila*. In this species, Toll proteins show exquisite specificity for the molecular pattern to which they respond. Toll itself has been shown to be responsible for mediating responses to fungi and Gram-positive bacteria and that different Toll receptors lead to production and activation of specific antimicrobial proteins to kill pathogens. It is now becoming apparent that mammalian Toll receptors are very similar to those found in *Drosophila* and show remarkable specificity for different ligands (*see* Table 1).

2.2. Toll-Like Receptors

Among the most characterized of these are TLR2, which is responsible for the recognition of peptidoglycan or lipopeptide from Gram-positive bacteria *(3)*, and TLR4, which recognizes lipopolysaccharide from Gram-negative bacteria *(4)*. Studies with both of these receptors have shown that they activate the NF-κB pathway, which regulates cytokine expression through the adaptor molecule MyD88. Activation of the NF-κB leads to the initiation of the adaptive immune response by production of inflammatory cytokines such as interleukin (IL)-1, IL-6, chemokines, IL-8, tumor necrosis factor (TNF)-α, and IL-12. Eight other TLRs have been identified with TLR-9 recently being identified as responsible for mediating the host cellular response to bacterial DNA—consisting of an unmethylated pair of nucleotides, CpG, plus their flanking regions *(4,5)*.

TLR9 appears to interact with and detect these unmethylated "CpG motifs." These CpG motifs are around 20 times more common in bacterial than mammalian DNA, therefore, the likelihood is that this receptor will only be activated by bacterial, viral, or retroviral DNA. TLR9 deficient (TLR9$^{-/-}$) mice do not show any response to CpG DNA and the in vivo CpG-mediated T-helper type-1 immune response was also abolished in these animals *(2)*. Studies with immobilized CpGs suggest that the sequences must be internalized to stimulate cells *(6)*; this implies that the TLR9 receptor is an intracellular receptor, rather than a cell-surface protein. The suggested uptake and activation via

Table 1
Toll-Like Receptors (TLRs) and Their Ligands

Name	Organ/cellular distribution (mRNA/protein)	Ligand/function
TLR1	Leukocytes	Associates with and regulates TLR2 response
TLR2	Monocytes, granulocytes	Interacts with peptidoglycan and lipoproteins from Gram-positive bacteria
TLR3	Dendritic cells	Interacts with dsRNA, induces production of type I interferons
TLR4	Monocytes	Interacts with microbial lipoproteins, CD14-dependent response to LPS
TLR5	Leukocytes, prostate, ovary, liver, lung	Interacts with microbial lipoproteins
TLR6	Leukocytes, ovary, lung	Interacts with microbial lipoproteins, associates with and regulates TLR2 response
TLR7	Spleen, placenta, lung	Interacts with Imiquimod, homology to TLR8
TLR8	Leukocytes, lung	Interacts with Imiquimod,
TLR9	Leukocytes	Receptor for CpG bacterial DNA

mRNA, messenger RNA.

TLR9 is as follows: bacterial CpG-DNA (from lysed bacterial cells) or mimicking CpG-oligodeoxynucleotide (ODN) binds first to an unidentified cell-surface DNA-binding protein. This binding is sequence independent and does not bring about activation but does induce endocytosis of the DNA. DNA can also be internalized by pinocytosis, although less efficiently. Upon endosomal maturation/acidification, any CpG motifs present in the DNA become sequence-specifically engaged by TLR9 *(7)*. Activated TLR9 recruits the adaptor protein MyD88 (also important in signaling via TLR2 and TLR4), followed by IRAK and TRAF6 triggering a signaling cascade that leads to activation of NF-κB.

3. ORIGIN OF CpG IMMUNOTHERAPY RESEARCH

The area of DNA vaccines and CpG DNA is widely considered to be a relatively new area, but perhaps it is just our understanding that is a recent development. It is more than 100 yr since William Coley initiated his research in immunotherapy following the discovery of a cancer patient who had failed all standard treatment options but who had complete recovery after two attacks of erysipelas, a severe infection caused by *Streptococcus pyogenes*. Subsequently, using a culture from Robert Koch, Coley succeeded in inducing tumor regression in a patient and published his first paper on the new method in 1893 *(8)*. Nearly 900 patients with advanced malignancy were treated over the next 43 yr with what became known as "Coley Toxins." Greater than 40% of these patients achieved sustained clinical remissions, a rate that has not been surpassed even by modern chemotherapy. In recent years, it has been suggested that specific bacterial DNA sequences, or CpG DNA, may have contributed to the therapeutic activity of Coley's extracts.

3.1. Stimulatory Sequences

The therapeutic effects of bacterial DNA toward tumors were first reported by Tokunaga *(5,9)*. Six base self-complementary palindromic sequences in the bacterial DNA were subsequently identified, which appeared to be responsible for these immune stimulatory effects *(10)*. Active palindromes were found to include AACGTT, AGCGCT, ATCGAT, CGATCG, CGTACG, CGCGCG, GCGCGC, and TCGCGA, all of which contain at least one CpG dinucleotide. These bacterial DNA fragments were found to activate NK cells and induce interferon (IFN) production, whereas vertebrate DNA does not. In vertebrate genomes, CpG dinucleotides are suppressed and are present at approx 25% of the frequency that would be predicted if base utilization was random. Additionally, CpGs are generally methylated in vertebrate DNA, but not in bacterial or viral DNA. These factors are thought to contribute to the ability of CpG DNA to serve as a PAMP indicating the host is under attack from a pathogen. As a result, the presence of bacterial DNA or mimicking synthetic oligodeoxynucleotides may directly activate cells of the innate immune system and particularly dendritic cells, NK cells, and macrophages.

Many applications for the use of CpG DNA are currently being investigated, these include cancer immunotherapy similar to that first suggested by Coley, as a vaccine adjuvant owing to its effects on T-cell responses, and as a treatment from autoimmune diseases. However, this chapter addresses the effects of CpG DNA as a generic broad-spectrum therapy against infectious diseases.

3.2. The Effects of Sequence and Species

Bacterial DNA from a range of species has been investigated for its immunostimulatory effects with DNA from *Escherichia coli* being found to be among the most effective whereas DNA from *C. perfringens* was found to be the least effective at stimulating the immune system *(11)*. This is thought to reflect differences in the content of CpG motifs and the presence of potentially inhibitory DNA sequences in these different DNAs. More recently, it has been shown that synthetic DNA fragments (ODN) which are rich in CpG motifs are able to stimulate the innate immune system *(12)*. Such oligonucleotides are more effective than crude bacterial DNA in stimulating such responses and have the advantage that their makeup can be modified to precisely tailor the nature of the host response. It has been shown that although all CpG motifs appear to require the expression of TLR9, different synthetic sequences activate different immune cell types to different degrees, and sequences that elicit a response in rodents do not necessarily stimulate the same response in primates because of evolutionary divergence in their TLR9 sequences. As a consequence, it may be necessary to modify the sequences used depending on the animal being investigated. For example, we have shown that although the CpG 1826 is highly stimulatory for mouse lymphocytes, it is essentially nonstimulatory for human and chimpanzee B cells *(13)*. We have identified that the optimal "mouse CpG-S motif" is GACGTT, whereas the preferred "human CpG-S motif" is GTCGTT, however, this sequence is also highly stimulatory for mouse cells. This suggests that murine lymphocytes have a broader ability to bind CpG motifs than human cells.

3.3. The Effects of Backbone Chemistry

The backbone of the synthetic DNA has also been found to alter the immuno-stimulatory effects of CpGs. The phosphorothioate (PS) backbone confers both nuclease resistance and improved cellular uptake on the CpGs *(14)*. Pisetsky and Reich *(15)* have determined that both base sequence and backbone chemistry influence immune activation and that this may raise the possibility of the design of agents with specific patterns of immune modulation. Additionally, Yu et al. *(16)* have determined that in PS ODNs the immunostimulatory activity is significantly reduced when the 5'-end of the oligo is not accessible rather than the 3'-end, suggesting that the 5'-end plays a critical role in immunostimulatory activity.

3.4. CpG Classes

Currently, two classes of CpG ODN have been published on the basis of their structure and immunostimulatory properties. The first ODN class, CpG-A ODNs have a structure with PS guanine-rich sequences called "polyG motifs" on the 5'- and 3'-ends and a palindromic phosphodiester core containing one or more CpG motifs *(17–19)*. CpG-A ODNs have been found to induce the highest production of IFN-α and marked NK cell activation, but relatively low levels of B cell activation. In contrast, CpG-B ODNs have a fully PS-modified backbone and induce only modest levels of IFN-α, much weaker NK-cell activation, but excellent B-cell activation *(17,20)*. Both CpG-A and CpG-B have been shown to have protective effects against challenges with viral, bacterial, or protozoal pathogens *(12,21–23)*.

4. IMMUNE ACTIVATION BY CpG DNA

The stimulatory effects of bacterial DNA was first demonstrated by Shimada *(24)* and Yamamoto *(25)* who found that it could enhance NK-cell activity. It was then demonstrated by Messina et al. *(26)* that such DNA could also stimulate B cells. It was in the mid-1990s that we discovered the immunostimulatory activity of bacterial DNA is dependent on an unmethylated CpG dinucleotide in particular sequence context *(27)*. The optimal sequence for murine immune activation was identified as $R_1R_2CGY_1Y_2$ where R_1 is a purine (preferably G), R_2 is a purine or T, and Y_1 and Y_2 are pyrimidines. Klinman et al. *(28)* subsequently demonstrated that these sequences also induced upregulation of a wide variety of cytokines.

4.1. Macrophages

Murine macrophages have been shown to be rapidly activated by CpG ODN via NFκB to secrete IL-12 and TNF-α *(29)*. The IL-12 is then able to induce IFN-γ from NK cells, which leads to the further stimulation of macrophages. In vitro CpG DNA treatment of murine macrophages has been shown to induce a biphasic TNF-α response to subsequent lipopolysaccharide challenge *(6)*. This study also revealed that the prolonged exposure of macrophages to CpGs resulted in the upregulation of IL-10, which acts in an autocrine manner to inhibit TNF-α production. This suggests that although the initial effects of CpGs are well-characterized, there is less known about prolonged exposure that may result in complex autocrine and paracrine feedback mechanisms.

CpG DNA has also been shown to stimulate the upregulation of expression of messenger RNA encoding the chemokines macrophage inflammatory protein (MIP)-1α, MIP-1β, MIP-2, regulated upon activation normal T-cell expressed and secreted (RANTES), monocyte chemoattractant protein (MCP)-1, and interferon α-inducible protein (IP)-10. Increases in these chemokines are found both at the site of injection and also at the local draining lymph nodes within 6 h of administration. These chemokines are known to play a vital role in the migration and stimulation of inflammatory cells that contribute to the development of CpG induced immune responses *(30)*.

4.2. Monocytes

The effects of CpGs on monocytic cells have not been extensively studied, but in contrast with mice, purified human monocytes do not express TLR9. However, CpG treatment of human peripheral blood mononuclear cells (PBMC) or whole blood secondarily activates the monocytes to produce IL-6 and TNF-α *(31)*. Microglial cells and astrocytes, both of which are closely related to monocytes, are also activated by CpG-B ODN in mice *(32)*. However, despite monocyte activation and increase in cytokine production within mixed populations of cells, highly purified human monocytes do not respond to CpG stimulation *(33)*, consistent with the lack of TLR9 expression in these cells.

4.3. Dendritic Cells

In humans, CD123+ (plasmacytoid) dendritic cells and B cells have been found to express the TLR9 receptor *(34–36)*. The PDC have been shown to produce high levels of type I IFN and Th1-promoting cytokines and chemokines, which in turn, leads to the rapid activation of many other cell types including NK cells, macrophages, and other types of dendritic cells. CpGs have also been found to induce the maturation of immature dendritic cells, transiently increase antigen processing and also increase the half-life of peptide-class II major histocompatibility complexes that leads to the sustained presentation of antigen *(37)*.

4.4. NK Cells

CpG DNA has been reported to promote NK-cell function both directly and indirectly in mice. The DNA has been shown to act indirectly by the activation of monocytes and macrophages to produce IL-12, TNF-α, and IFN; these cytokines then induce IFN-γ production by NK cells, which enhances their cytotoxicity *(38)*. However, in humans synthetic CpGs have been shown to induce NK cells to produce IFN-γ with an increased CD69 expression and an increased cytotoxicity. Interestingly, the response of human NK cells was found to be sequence dependent with the sequence GACGATCGTC found to be the most potent inducer of IFN-γ production from NK cells *(39)*.

4.5. Complement

There is little information available regarding the effects of synthetic oligonucleotides on the complement system. The components of the complement system would seem to be likely candidates to interact with the DNA, especially if it is administered intravenously. Henry et al. *(40)* demonstrated that systemic CpG administration can cause massive complement activation leading to haemodynamic collapse in primates; however, the concentrations used were excessively high and these effects have not been observed in other models. A wide range of proteins, bacteria, viruses, and fungi can activate complement; this may be of importance particularly if the DNA is complexed, for example, in liposomes. The activation of complement would be expected to severely limit the half-life of DNA in blood, and this may have a detrimental effect on this type of therapy.

5. PROTECTION AGAINST INTRACELLULAR INFECTION

As described earlier, synthetic oligodeoxynucleotides have been shown to mimic the effects of bacterial DNA and induce lymphocytes and macrophages to secrete polyreactive antibodies and cytokines including IFN-γ, IL-6, IL-12, IL-18, and TNF-α. The rapid induction of these effectors of the innate immune system is known to be critical in controlling the early spread of intracellular pathogens. The finding that Toll receptors are so functionally well-conserved and that immune recognition of unmethylated CpG motifs occurs in a similar way in the most diverse of species has suggested the hypothesis that pathogen recognition may confer a selective advantage on the host. In recent years, a range of challenge organisms, bacterial, viral, and protozoan have been used to assess the efficacy of synthetic CpG DNA as a generic medical countermeasure (*see* Table 2).

Many of the agents of particular relevance to BW weapon defense are intracellular pathogens, with few specific vaccines or chemotherapies available. The possible development of immunostimulation by CpG DNA as an effective single therapy against a broad range of these diseases would be of invaluable use.

5.1. Francisella tularensis

Francisella tularensis is the causative agent of tularemia in humans and in other animals *(41)*. Although this disease is endemic in various areas (e.g., North America, Northern Europe) where it is most commonly transmitted by ticks, the organism is infectious by the aerosol route and is therefore considered to be of high importance in the development of therapies for BW defense (*see* Chapter 20). Four subspecies of *F. tularensis* have been identified: subsp. *tularensis* (type A) strains are highly virulent in man, with a very low infectious dose; subsp. *holarctica* (type B), of which there are three biovars: I, II and *japonica*, subsp. *mediaasiatica,* which are of moderate virulence; and subsp. *novicida,* which are nonpathogenic in immunocompetent humans. To date, no work has been reported on the protective effects of CpG ODN against challenge with *F. tularensis* subsp. *tularensis*. Rather, more work has been carried out with the live vaccine strain (LVS) of *F. tularensis*, this is an attenuated subsp. *holarctica* strain in humans, however, it is fully virulent in mice and is a useful model of the disease. Elkins et al. *(12)* demonstrated that both bacterial DNA and synthetic ODNs protect against lethal challenge with *F. tularensis* LVS (and also *Listeria monocytogenes*) (*see* Fig. 1). Human placental DNA, methylated CpG DNA, and GpC DNA were administered in the same way and no protective effects were observed, this confirms the specific recognition of bacterial CpG sequences and the subsequent induction of a protective immune response.

Table 2
Protection Achieved by Administration of CpG-ODN

Organism	CpG ODN	Immune response	Protection achieved	Ref.
Francisella tularensis LVS	CpG-B GCTAGACGTTAGCGT	IFN-γ IL-12, TNF-α	100% to 10^3 intraperitoneally	12,22
Burkholderia mallei	CpG-A (2216) CpG-B (2006)	No details available	30% to 60 LD_{50} intraperitoneally	21
Ebola virus	No details available	No details available	Partial to 10^2–10^3 LD_{50}	43
Bacillus anthracis	No details available	No details available	Partial to 10^2–10^3 LD_{50}	43
Listeria monocytogenes	CpG-B TCTCCCAGCGTGCGCCAT	IFN-γ IL-12	approx 2 log reduction (liver)	12,22
Plasmodium yoelii	CpG-B (1826) TCCATGACGTTCCTGACGTT	IFN-γ IL-12	100% to 50 sporozoites intravenously	23
Mycobacterium avium	TCCATGACGTTCCTGACGT	No details available	0.9 log reduction (spleen)	45,48
Leishmania major	TCCATGACGTTCCTGATGCT	IFN-γ, IL-12 NO	100% to 2×10^5 parasites	44
Polymicrobial sepsis	TTCATGACGTTCCTGATGCT	↑ activated neutrophils	↑ survival, ↓ counts	49
Herpes simplex virus type 2	No details available	No details available	Local protection	46

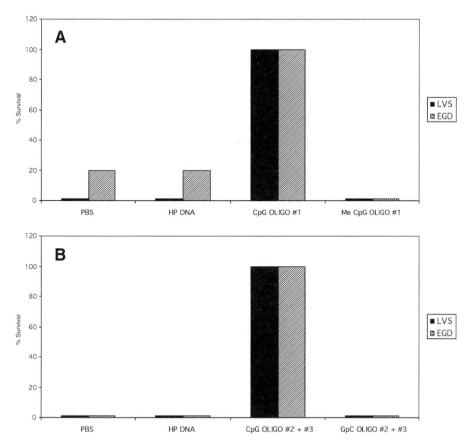

Fig. 1. Oligonucleotide DNA protects mice from lethal *F. tularensis* LVS or *L. monocytogenes* (strain EGD) infection. Groups of five BALB/cByJ were treated with (**A**) PBS, 20 µg HP DNA, oligo #1 (CpG oligo #1, TCT CCC AGC GTG CGC CAT) or Me-#1 (Me-CpG oligo#1, as oligo #1 but with methylated C's at positions 9, 13, and 15); or (**B**) 50 µg of HP DNA, 50 µg of an equal mixture of oligos #2 and #3 (CpG oligo #2, GCT AGA CGT TAG CGT +#3, TCA ACG TTG A), or 50 µg of an equal mixture of oligos #2' and #3' (GpC oligo #2' + #3') on day 0. Mice were challenged with 10^3 LVS (filled bars) or 2×10^5 *L. monocytogenes* strain EGD (hatched bars) intraperitoneally on day 3; actual priming and challenge doses were confirmed by plate count at the time of inoculation. Mice were observed for morbidity and mortality through day 30. Time to death of those mice that died ranged from day 4 to day 8. These experiments are representative of five total experiments (**A**) and three total experiments (**B**) of similar design. (Taken from ref. *12*. Copyright 1999. The American Association of Immunologists, Inc.)

This work suggested that the protection achieved was highly dependent on lymphocytes—particularly B cells as well as on the production of IFN-γ suggested earlier. Optimal protection was achieved 2–3 d after pretreatment with bacterial (and synthetic) DNA and persisted for up to 2 wk (*see* Fig. 2). In addition, it was found that mice that survived an otherwise lethal challenge with *F. tularensis* LVS went on to develop pathogen specific secondary immunity. This work has suggested that although in the first instance CpGs activate the innate immune system, subsequent exposure to pathogens results in the development of immune memory.

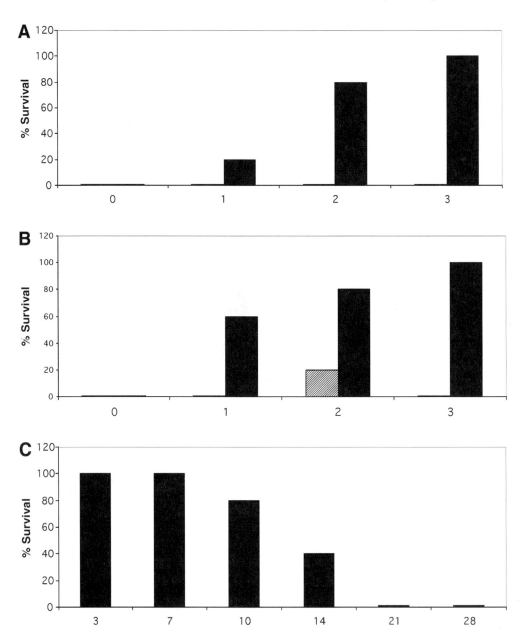

Fig. 2. Time-course of oligonucleotide-induced protection of mice from lethal *F. tularensis* LVS infection. Groups of five BALB/cByJ mice were treated with 20 µg of oligo #1 (CpG oligo, filled bars), 20 µg of Me-CpG oligo #1 (Me Oligo, hatched bars), or PBS (not shown) 0–28 d before challenge with 10^3 or 10^4 LVS intraperitoneally; within an experiment, the day of DNA inoculation was varied and challenge performed on all groups on the same day. Mice were observed for morbidity and mortality through day 30. Time to death of those mice that died, including all PBS-treated mice, ranged from day 4 to day 7. In **A, B,** and **C,** experiments are representative of three total experiments of similar design. (Taken from ref. *12*. Copyright 1999. The American Association of Immunologists, Inc.)

Klinman et al. *(42)* have shown that the protective effects of CpGs to challenge with both *L. monocytogenes* and *F. tularensis* can be extended dramatically by repeatedly administering two to four times per month. In this case, protection was shown to be associated with an increase in the number of spleen cells that could be triggered by subsequent pathogen exposure to secrete IFN-γ and IL-6. In all experiments, the animals were found to remain healthy and suffer no ill effects either macro- or microscopically upon tissue examination, suggesting that repeated administration of CpGs may provide a safe means of conferring long-term protection against a range of infectious pathogens.

5.2. Other Potential BW Agents

Klinman et al. *(43)* also demonstrated that 10–50 µg of CpG ODN administered by numerous of routes partially protected mice from a 10^2–10^3 LD_{50} systemic challenge of both Ebola virus or *Bacillus anthracis*, both agents of high importance.

Protective effects to another BW agent *Burkholderia mallei*, (the causative agent of Glanders) has recently been demonstrated *(21)*. In this study, CpG DNA was administered intraperitoneally 2 d before intraperitoneal or aerosol challenge with virulent *B. mallei*. At a challenge dose, which resulted in the deaths of all control mice by day 2 (60 LD_{50} intraperitoneally), 30% of CpG DNA treated mice were surviving 3 wk postchallenge. In aerosol challenge experiments (14–20 LD_{50}), all control animals were dead by day 6, whereas 20–50% of CpG treated animals survived to 3 wk postchallenge. However, sterile immunity was not achieved in animals which had been dosed with CpG DNA.

5.3. Other Organisms

Krieg et al. *(22)* demonstrated that the administration of synthetic ODN containing CpG motifs in vivo resulted in an increase in serum IL-12 which lasted for at least 8 d, and an increase in IFN-γ, which returned to baseline within 48 h. The production of these Th1-like cytokines induced protection against lethal challenge with *Listeria monocytogenes* in susceptible BALB/c mice. It was shown that protection was achieved within 48 h of pretreatment with CpGs and persisted for at least 2 wk, it was also suggested that this protection was dependent on IFN-γ secretion.

Zimmerman et al. *(44)* demonstrated the protective effects of CpG DNA against lethal challenge with the intracellular pathogen *Leishmania major*. In this study animals were treated up to 20 d after challenge with CpG ODN and curative effects were observed. These results reveal the potential for their use as a postexposure therapy. However, many of the BW agents of interest are highly virulent organisms where the disease process is much shorter than this, so it would seem likely that the immunostimulation achieved by postexposure therapy would only be effective if given immediately postchallenge.

5.4. Delivery Routes

Some studies have suggested that delivery of CpG ODN to the mucosal surface where challenge occurs gives greater levels of protection than systemically delivered ODN. In the case of *Mycobacterium tuberculosis* infection, a single intranasal administration of CpG ODN, but not an intraperitoneal administration, protected against an

M. tuberculosis aerosol challenge 6 wk later *(45)*. This is supported by the observation that transmucosal (intravaginal) delivery of CpG ODN gives superior levels of protection compared to intramuscular ODN delivery against lethal challenge with herpes simplex virus type 2 by the vaginal route *(46)*. In this study, animals treated 24 h before challenge showed minimal vaginal pathology and very low viral counts, mice treated shortly after infection were also protected, but those treated 24 and 72 h postchallenge were not.

These data suggest that the most appropriate delivery route for CpG ODN in protection against inhaled BW agents might be directly to the lung mucosae. This route of administration has the potential added advantage of being less invasive than conventional routes of administration, and would potentially reduce any systemic side effects.

6. CLINICAL TRIALS AND PROSPECTS FOR THE FUTURE

Currently, no generic therapies are licensed for human use against BW agents. However, one CpG-B ODN (CpG 7909, Coley Pharmaceutical Group) is currently in human clinical trials for enhancing the potency of vaccines against infectious disease, and for improving immunotherapy of cancer and allergy. Based on information gathered in over 250 human subjects who have received CpG 7909, this oligonucleotide appears to be well-tolerated in humans at immune stimulatory doses *(47)*. These data suggest that serious adverse effects are likely to be uncommon in further trials with different CpG ODN and that the prospects are good for development as a generic therapy against BW agents.

7. THE USE OF CpG AS A NONSPECIFIC IMMUNOMODULATOR

The data presented here describe the possible use of CpG ODN as an immunostimulatory therapy against both bacterial and viral agents. Although data demonstrating protection against agents of particular relevance to BW countermeasure research are relatively scarce, the data currently available are largely encouraging. When combined with the published data showing protection to challenge with a range of other intracellular pathogens they suggest that the possibility of using this technology against BW agents is a very good prospect for the future. Although much of the data demonstrate protection levels at around 10-fold, this could significantly reduce casualties in the event of an immediate biological release. As the development of new CpG ODN, improved formulations, and delivery systems progresses, it seems likely that the protective effects so far observed will be improved, and this will quickly lead to licensing applications for this use.

If the data generated in this area continue to improve and protection is demonstrated to more agents of relevance, the CpG ODN would be of invaluable use in the event of the deliberate release of an unknown agent, and could significantly reduce casualties and mortality.

REFERENCES

1. Medzhitov, R., Preston-Hurlburt, P., Janeway, C. A. Jr. (1997) A human homologue of the *Drosophila* Toll protein signals activation of adaptive immunity. *Nature* **388,** 394–397.
2. Hemmi, H., Takeuchi, O., Kawai, T., et al. (2000) A toll-like receptor recognizes bacterial DNA. *Nature* **408,** 740–745.

3. Brightbill, H. D., Libraty, D. H., Krutzik, S. R., et al. (1999) Host defence mechanisms triggered by microbial lipoproteins through toll-like receptors. *Science* **285,** 732–736.

4. Poltorak, A., He, X. L., Smirnova, I., et al. (1998) Defective LPS signalling in C3H/HeJ and C57BL/10ScCr mice: Mutations in Tlr4 gene. *Science* **282,** 2085–2088.

5. Tokunaga, T., Yamamoto, H., Shimada, S., et al. (1984) Antitumor activity of deoxyribonucleic acid fraction from *Mycobacterium bovis* BCG. I. Isolation, physicochemical characterization, and antitumor activity. *J. Natl. Cancer Inst.* **72,** 955–962.

6. Krieg, A. M. (2000) The role of CpG motifs in innate immunity. *Curr. Opin. Immunol.* **12,** 35–43.

7. Wagner, H. (2001) Toll meets bacterial CpG-DNA. *Immunity* **14,** 499–502.

8. Wiemann, B. and Starnes, C. O. (1994) Coley's toxins, tumor necrosis factor and cancer research: a historical perspective. *Pharmacol. Ther.* **64,** 529–564.

9. Tokunaga, T., Yamamoto, S., and Namba, K. (1988) A synthetic single-stranded DNA, poly(dG,dC), induces interferon-α/β and -γ, augments natural killer activity, and suppresses tumor growth. *Jpn. J. Cancer Res.* **79,** 682–686.

10. Kuramoto, E., Yano, O., Kimura, Y., et al. (1992) Oligonucleotide sequences required for natural killer cell activation. *Jpn. J. Cancer Res.* **83,** 1128–1131.

11. Neujahr, D. C., Reich, C. F., and Pisetsky, D. S. (1999) Immunostimulatory properties of genomic DNA from different bacterial species. *Immunobiology* **200,** 106–119.

12. Elkins, K. L., Rhinehart-Jones, T. R., Stibitz, S., Conover, J. S., and Klinman, D. M. (1999) Bacterial DNA containing CpG motifs stimulates lymphocyte-dependent protection of mice against lethal infection with intracellular bacteria. *J. Immunol.* **162,** 2291–2298.

13. Krieg, A. M. (1999) Mechanisms and applications of immune stimulatory CpG oligodeoxynucleotides. *Biochim. Biophy. Acta* **1489,** 107–116.

14. Zhao, Q., Matson, S., Herrara, C. J., Fisher, E., Yu, H., Waggoner, A., and Krieg, A. M. (1993) Comparison of cellular binding and uptake of antisense phosphodiester, phosphorothioate, and mixed phosphorothioate and methylphosphonate oligonucleotides. *Antisense Res. Dev.* **3,** 53–56.

15. Pisetsky, D. S. and Reich, C. F. (1998) The influence of base sequence on the immunological properties of defined oligonucleotides. *Immunopharmacology* **40,** 199–208.

16. Yu, D., Zhao, Q., Kandimalla, E. R., and Agrawal, S. (2000) Accessible 5'-end of CpG containing phosphorothioate oligodeoxynucleotides is essential for immunostimulatory activity. *Bioorg. Med. Chem. Lett.* **10,** 2585–2588.

17. Ballas, Z. K., Rasmussen, W. L., and Krieg, A. M. (1996) Induction of NK activity in murine and human cells by CpG motifs in oligodeoxynucleotides and bacterial DNA. *J. Immunol.* **157,** 1840–1845.

18. Krug, A., Rothenfusser, S., Hornung, V., et al. (2001) Identification of CpG oligonucleotide sequences with high induction of IFN-alpha/beta in plasmacytoid dendritic cells. *Eur. J. Immunol.* **31,** 2154–2163.

19. Krieg, A. M. (2002) CpG motifs in bacterial DNA and their immune effects. *Annu. Rev. Immunol.* **20,** 709–760.

20. Boggs, R. T., McGraw, K., Condon, T., et al. (1997) Characterisation and modulation of immune stimulation by modified oligoncleotides. *Antisense Nucleic Acid Drug Dev.* **7,** 461–471.

21. Waag, D., Heppner, D. G., and Krieg, A. M. (2002) The protective efficacy of CpG oligonucleotides against Glanders. 102nd General Meeting, American Society for Microbiology.

22. Krieg, A. M., Love-Homan, L., YI, A.-K., and Harty, J. T. (1998) CpG DNA induces sustained IL-12 expression in vivo and resistance to *Listeria* monocytogenes challenge. *J. Immunol.* **161,** 2428–2434.

23. Gramzinski, R. A., Doolan, D. L., Sedegah, M., Davis, H. L., Kreig, A. M., and Hoffman, S. L. (2001) Interleukin-12 and gamma interferon dependent protection against malaria conferred by CpG oligodeoxynucleotide in mice. *Infect. Immun.* **69,** 1643–1649.

24. Shimada, S., Yano, O., and Tokunaga, T. (1986) In vivo augmentation of natural killer cell activity with a deoxyribonucleic acid fraction of BCG. *Jpn. J. Cancer Res.* **77,** 808–816.

25. Yamamoto, S., Yamamoto, T., Shimada, T., et al. (1992) DNA from bacteria, but not vertebrates, induces interferons, activates natural killer cells and inhibits tumor growth. *Microb. Immunol.* **36,** 983.

26. Messina, J. P., Gilkeson, G. S., and Pisetsky, D. S. (1991) Simulation of in vitro murine lymphocyte proliferation by bacterial DNA. *J. Immunol.* **147,** 1759–1764.

27. Krieg, A. M., Yi, A. K., Matson, S., et al. (1995) CpG motifs in bacterial DNA trigger direct B cell activation. *Nature* **374,** 546–549.

28. Klinman, D. M., Yi, A. K., Beaucage, S. L., Conover, J., and Krieg, A. M. (1996) CpG motifs present in bacterial DNA rapidly induce lymphocytes to secrete interleukin 6, interleukin 12 and interferon gamma. *Proc. Natl. Acad. Sci. USA* **93,** 2879–2883.

29. Chu, R. S., Askew, D., Noss, E. H., Tobian, A., Krieg, A. M., and Harding, C. V. (1999) CpG oligodeoxynucleotides down-regulate macrophage class II antigen processing. *J. Immunol.* **163,** 1188–1194.

30. Takeshita, S., Takeshita, F. Haddad, D. E., Ishii, K. J., and Klinman, D. M. (2000) CpG oligodeoxynucleotides induce murine macrophages to up-regulate chemokine mRNA expression. *Cell. Immunol.* **206,** 101–106.

31. Hartmann, G. and Krieg, A. M. (1999) CpG DNA and LPS induce distinct patterns of activation in human monocytes. *Gene Ther.* **6,** 893–903.

32. Schluesener, H. J., Seid, K., Deininger, M., and Schwab, J. (2001) Transient in vivo activation of rat brain macrophages/microglial cells and astrocytes by immunostimulatory multiple CpG oligonucleotides. *J. Neuroimmunol.* **113,** 89–94.

33. Bauer, M., Heeg, K., Wagner, H., and Lipford, G. B. (1999) DNA activates human immune cells through a CpG sequence-dependent manner. *Immunology* **97,** 699–705.

34. Krug, A., Towarowski, A., Britsch, S., et al. (2001) Toll-like receptor expression reveals CpG DNA as a unique microbial stimulus for plasmacytoid dendritic cells which synergises with CD40 ligand to induce high amounts of IL-12. *Eur. J. Immunol.* **31,** 3026–3037.

35. Kadowaki, N., Ho, S., Antonenko, S., et al. (2001) Sunsets of human dendritic cell precursors express different toll-like receptors and respond to microbial antigens. *J. Exp. Med.* **194,** 863–870.

36. Hornung, V., Rothenfusser, S., Britsch, S., et al. (2002) Quantitative expression of toll-like receptor 1-10 mRNA in cellular subsets of human peripheral blood mononuclear cells and sensitivity to CpG oligodeoxynucleotides. *J. Immunol.* **168,** 4531–4537.

37. Askew, D., Chu, R. S., Krieg, A. M., and Harding, C. V. (2000) CpG DNA induces maturation of dendritic cells with distinct effects on nascent and recycling MHC-II antigen-processing mechanisms. *J. Immunol.* **165,** 6889–6895.

38. Tokunaga, T., Yano, O., Kuramoto, E., et al. Synthetic oligonucleotides with particular base sequences from the cDNA encoding proteins of *Mycobacterium bovis* BCG induce interferons and activate natural killer cells. *Microbiol. Immunol.* **36,** 55.

39. Iho, S., Yamamoto, T., Takahashi, T., and Yamamoto, S. (1999) Oligonucleotides containing palindrome sequences with internal 5'-CpG-3' act directly on human NK and activated T cells to induce IFN-gamma production in vitro. *J. Immunol.* **163,** 3642–3652.

40. Henry, S. P., Giclas, P. C., Leeds, J., et al. (1997) Activation of the alternative pathway of complement by a phosphorothioate oligonucleotide: potential mechanism of action. *J. Pharmacol. Exp. Ther.* **281,** 810–816.

41. Ellis, J., Oyston, P. C. F., Green, M., and Titball, R. W. (2002) *Francisella tularensis.* *Clin. Micro. Rev.,* in press.

42. Klinman, D. M., Conover, J., and Coban, C. (1999) Repeated administration of synthetic oligodeoxynucleotides expressing CpG motifs provides long-term protection against bacterial infection. *Infect. Immun.* **67,** 5658–5663.

43. Klinman, D. M., Verthelyi, D., Takeshita, F., and Ishii, K. J. (1999) Immune recognition of foreign DNA: a cure for bioterrorism? *Immunity* **11,** 123–129.
44. Zimmermann, S., Egeter, O., Hausmann, S., et al. (1998) Cutting edge: CpG oligodeoxynucleotides trigger protective and curative Th1 responses in lethal murine leishmaniasis. *J. Immunol.* **160,** 3627–3630.
45. Vogels, M. T. and van der Meer, J. W. (1992) Use of immune modulators in non-specific therapy of bacterial infections. *Antimicrob. Agents Chemother.* **36,** 1–5.
46. Sajic, D., Ashkar, A. A., Patrick, A. J., et al. (2002) Transmucosal delivery of CpG ODN applied to the genital mucosa protects mice against intravaginal HSV-2 infection. 9th Conference on Retroviruses and Opportunistic Infections.
47. Krieg, A. M., et al. Clinical trial information. www.coleypharma.com
48. Jiang, W., Quinn, A., and Frothingham, R. (2002) Balb/c mice treated with CpG oligodeoxynucleotide controlled *Mycobacterium avium* infection. 102nd General Meeting, American Society for Microbiology.
49. Weighardt, H., Feterowski, C., Veit, M., Rump, M., Wagner, H., and Holzmann, B. (2000) Increased resistance against acute polymicrobial sepsis in mice challenged with immunostimulatory CpG oligodeoxynucleotides is related to an enhanced innate effector cell response. *J. Immunol.* **165,** 4537–4543.

15

Decontamination

Robert J. Hawley and Joseph P. Kozlovac

1. DECONTAMINATION

Decontamination is defined as disinfection or sterilization of toxin- or agent-contaminated articles to make them safe for use or disposal. Disinfection is the selective elimination of certain undesirable microorganisms to prevent their transmission whereas sterilization is the complete destruction of microbial life *(1–3)*. The operational definition of sterilization is a carefully monitored process that will assure that the probability of an item being contaminated by a microbe to be equal to or less than one in a million (10^{-6}) *(4,5)*.

The preferred methods of environmental decontamination are determined only after a careful analysis of the risks involved—risks to both personnel responding to a situation and the environment. An evaluation of the situation is accomplished by employing risk-management procedures with guidelines for conducting a risk assessment *(6–10)*. Risk assessment is a method for reducing all hazards to the minimal acceptable level and is an expression of potential loss in terms of hazard severity, accident probability, and exposure to the hazard. Risk management is the systematic application of policies, practices, and resources to the assessment and control of risk affecting human health, human safety, and the environment. The severity of the hazard must be considered by assessing the expected consequence, which is defined as the degree of injury or occupational illness that could occur from the hazard. The probability of an accident or illness occurring after a given exposure to the hazard must also be determined. Finally, and most importantly, what level of environmental risk will the affected individuals or community accept? The answer to this question will most likely dictate the degree of aggressiveness of a decontamination process. The approach to a decontamination process must be based on many issues *(11,12)*. They include health risks with consideration of regulatory requirements, public perception (e.g., the acceptance of the process by the public), environmental concerns, scientific data showing the efficacy of the process, political influence, the time involved for the process, and economic impact. Consideration must also be given to any potential collateral damage caused by the decontamination process. Finally, the public accepts that the process provided the outcome sought. These issues will hopefully contribute information to establish a rational and reasonable approach to the decontamination process. Without a doubt, the most important consideration is involvement and education of the public so that people may voluntarily accept some level of risk.

From: *Infectious Diseases: Biological Weapons Defense: Infectious Diseases and Counterterrorism*
Edited by: L. E. Lindler, F. J. Lebeda, and G. W. Korch © Humana Press Inc., Totowa, NJ

How do you gain public confidence for acceptance that an area or building is decontaminated, and that the area or building is "clean" enough for them to re-enter and return to normalcy? Historically, decontamination strategies have been ultraconservative with sterilization as the goal rather than disinfection or decontamination, as earlier defined, which would have been more than adequate. Unfortunately, this conservative approach is often driven by fear and politics rather than good science.

The criteria for decontamination are strongly influenced by public concerns—the public may demand zero risk, that is, zero living organisms after the decontamination process. However, the result of a decontamination procedure is influenced by both the sampling and assay (determination of efficacy) procedures. What must be realized is that many microorganisms that could potentially be used in a biological warfare or terrorism scenario may be naturally present in certain communities or areas of the country. Examples include *Bacillus anthracis*, the causative agent of anthrax that is indigenous to many farming areas *(13,14)*, such as in Louisiana, Mississippi, Illinois, California, Missouri, Iowa, and the Dakotas. *Yersinia pestis* is the causative agent of human and animal plague and is found in many rural areas of the western United States *(15,16)*. *Francisella tularensis,* originally isolated in Tulare County, CA, although it is enzootic in all areas of the continental United States, is the causative agent of rabbit fever and tularemia in humans *(17,18)*, and *Clostridium botulinum*, commonly found in soil, has a potent toxin that can cause botulism in humans as a result of improper food processing *(19)*. As these microorganisms (or their toxic metabolic products) may be present in the community and their documented involvement in incidents are sporadic and rather uncommon, the requirements for zero concentration of the agent (e.g., absence of the agent) after a decontamination process and zero risk is not necessary (*see* also, refs. *11* and *12*). Therefore, an assessment of exposure to the hazard considers the number of persons exposed and the duration or frequency of the exposure. A risk assessment will provide guidance for choosing the appropriate decontaminant, protection of responding personnel, and the subsequent management of those individuals that may be potentially exposed to an environmental contaminant. A risk assessment is never complete because the process is a constant review of implemented procedures, policies, and plans—a risk assessment of a situation is actually a snapshot of the scenario at a given time.

Environmental decontamination procedures can be discussed from two approaches, surface decontamination and area (space) decontamination. For surface decontamination, the effectiveness of a decontaminant depends on decontaminant concentration, concentration of the agent, type of agent, time of contact, and the environmental conditions *(20–23)*. There are a number general groups of decontaminants such as alcohols, halogens, quaternary ammonium compounds, phenolics, and glutaraldehyde. These decontaminants are used primarily for nonporous surfaces. Many of these decontaminants are only active against certain groups of microorganisms, whereas inactive against others *(24)*. Although some of the halogen-containing decontaminants are corrosive, they can be chemically modified to an environmentally acceptable form. The activity of chlorine-containing disinfectants, such as sodium hypochlorite solutions, can be neutralized with sodium thiosulfate *(24)*. The range of etiologic agents inactivated by various decontamination techniques is extensively documented *(3,23,24,26–31)* and is represented in Table 1.

Table 1
Decontamination Agents for Etiologic Agents

Etiologic agent(s)	Decontamination agent(s)	Reference(s)
Bacillus subtilis spores	Sodium hypochlorite	Rutala and Weber *(3)*
Various vegetative bacteria, bacterial spores, viruses, and protozoa	Sodium hypochlorite, ozone, chlorine dioxide, ultraviolet light	Weavers and Wickramanayake *(22)*
B. subtilis spores	Peracetic acid, sodium hypochlorite, hydrogen peroxide, formaldehyde	Alasri et al. *(23)*
Staphylococcus aureus, *B. subtilis* spores	Sodium hypochlorite, dichloroiso-cyanurate sodium	Bloomfield and Uso *(25)*
Various vegetative bacteria, bacterial spores, viruses, fungi, and protozoa	Aldehydes, peroxygens, phenols, halogen-releasing agents, vapor-phase sterilants, quaternary ammonium, compounds, alcohols	McDonnell and Russell *(26)*
Various vegetative bacteria, *Bacillus* spores, *Giardia*, *Cryptosporidium*	Gaseous sterilizing agents: Ethylene oxide, propylene oxide, formaldehyde, β-Propiolactone, hydrogen peroxide, ozone, chlorine dioxide, peracetic acid, and plasma gases	Joslyn *(27)*
S. albus	Propylene glycol vapor	Puck, Robertson, and Lemon *(28)*
Bacterial spores (*Clostridium* and *Bacillus* species)	Phenols, cresols, alcohols, quaternary ammonium compounds, aldehydes, chlorine-releasing agents, peroxygens, ethylene oxide, β-Propiolactone, ozone	Russell *(29)*
B. subtilis spores	Formaldehyde vapor	Songer et al. *(30)*

2. SURFACE DECONTAMINATION

The efficacy of decontaminating inanimate surfaces with liquid household bleach is under investigation at the US Army Medical Research Institute of Infectious Diseases (USAMRIID) *(32,33)*. Undiluted liquid household bleach inactivated 99.8% of the spore population (a 5 $\log_{10}$ reduction in viability) of *B. anthracis* after 1 min of contact time. Similarly, after 1 min of contact, an *Escherichia coli* population was completely inactivated (a 6 $\log_{10}$ reduction in viability). *E. coli* was used as a Gram-negative model in these experiments to simulate *Y. pestis* and other Gram-negative bacteria that are more fastidious in their growth requirements and are more dangerous to handle. Further experiments were conducted to determine the efficacy of 0.26% sodium hypochlorite (a 1:20 dilution of liquid household bleach, 2625 parts per million free, available chlorine in unbuffered water). Results showed a 100% inactivation of the spore population (a 5 $\log_{10}$ reduction in viability) of *B. anthracis* after 15 min of contact time to 0.26% sodium hypochlorite. Using 0.5% sodium hypochlorite (a 1:9.5 dilution of liquid household bleach, about 5500 parts per million free, available chlorine in unbuffered water), a greater than 90% inactivation of the spore population (up to a 3 $\log_{10}$

reduction in viability) of *B. anthracis* after 5 min of contact time was observed. Experiments in progress continue to refine the contact time data for inactivating *B. anthracis* spores and to determine the influence of extraneous organic material on inactivation kinetics.

Although sodium hypochlorite (NaOCl) is a useful broad-spectrum surface disinfectant *(34,35)*, it may not always be the best choice of disinfectant. In fact, in certain situations the use of bleach as a disinfectant could create a more hazardous byproduct. For instance, using NaOCl solutions to inactivate aflatoxin B_1 would be inappropriate as it may lead to the formation of aflatoxin B_1-2,3,-dichloride, which is a potent carcinogen and mutagen. In this situation, sodium hypochlorite alone is not the recommended method of inactivation and if used, should be diluted to 1–1.5% NaOCl followed by the addition of acetone (5% v/v final concentration) to ensure elimination of the carcinogen hazard *(36)*. Caution is emphasized during the addition of acetone to the strong sodium hypochlorite solution because of the potential for a violent haloform reaction. The detoxification of T-2 mycotoxins is another case when a NaOCl solution used alone would be inappropriate and inadequate for the task. Sodium hypochlorite (2.5%) alone will not inactivate T-2 mycotoxins even after a 30-min exposure. However, when combined with 0.25 *N* sodium hydroxide, the mixture will completely inactivate T-2 mycotoxins *(37)*. Therefore, it is critical when performing a risk assessment that the mechanism of inactivation be well-understood before deciding which surface disinfectant will be used to inactivate the agent (microbe or toxin) of interest.

Federal and commercial programs have begun to identify, evaluate, and demonstrate practical approaches to decontaminate surface materials in response to the growing concern of domestic biological terrorism *(38)*. The purpose of exploring new technologies and systems is to develop a response plan to address decontamination of a building that has been contaminated with a biological agent. Because many of these technologies involve proprietary information, only a brief description is provided here.

1. Diligen II (DII) is a system that uses ozone and moisture, generated from ultraviolet lamps operating at a 254-nm wavelength, producing highly oxidative gaseous species. In this system, microorganism deactivation occurs at a rate 30–50 greater than if ozone was solely used. At the end of the decontamination process, the gaseous species produced are destabilized and recombine to form oxygen and water. Carbon dioxide is the byproduct of any reaction with microorganisms.
2. Reactive Nanoparticle technology (Nantek, Inc., Manhattan, KS) uses reactive nanoparticles of halogenated metal oxides that are effective against both chemical and biological agents (including Gram-positive and Gram-negative bacteria, toxins, and a bacteriophage—the latter a simulant of a human virus).
3. L-Gel (Lawrence Livermore Laboratory, Livermore, CA) is a gelled decontamination material. The gel is designed to adhere to the undersides of horizontal surfaces and vertical spaces and is sprayed onto the surfaces to be decontaminated. The gel interacts with and damages the cell membrane of the biological agent by oxidizing the organic lipid layers.
4. A broad-spectrum antimicrobial nanoemulsion developed by the University of Michigan Center for Biological Nanotechnology is reported to be a nonirritant, nontoxic, and safe for the environment. The nanoemulsion is reported to have a shelf-life of 2 yr. Although it does not require any special storage, it must be kept from freezing and drying. Its action against *B. anthracis* spores involves initiating partial germination of spores to weaken the spore wall, followed by spore disruption and disintegration. This process begins within 30 min with complete inactivation of spores in 2–3 h.

5. An aqueous foam (Sandia National Laboratories, Albuquerque, NM) is reported to neutralize chemical warfare agents, such as soman, persistent nerve agent, and mustard. It also neutralizes biological warfare agents, such as *B. anthracis*. The mechanism of neutralization has been reported to involve enzyme technology and agent-binding protein chemistry.

6. Activated solution of hypochlorite, developed by the Naval Biological Laboratory during 1967 and 1968, is reported to be effective against *B. subtilis* var. *globigii*, a simulant for *B. anthracis* (anthrax). The general formula, by weight percent, is calcium hypochlorite (0.5), sodium dihydrogen phosphate (0.5), Triton X-100 (0.05), and water (98.95).

7. GD-5 decontaminant solution (Odenwald Werke Rittersbach, GmbH of Elztal-Rittersbach, Germany) is a mixture of aminoalcholates and a nonionic surfactant. Its mechanism of action is based on the nucleophilic substitution of chemical warfare agents. It was shown to have limited activity (decrease of about 10–100 spores during test decontamination procedures) against *B. subtilis* var. *globigii*, the simulant for *B. anthracis* (anthrax).

A decontamination procedure for nonporous surfaces using sodium hypochlorite was adopted for the metal mail sorting slots at the Boca Raton Post Office, FL, on October 15, 2001. This was a collaborative effort of the US Environmental Protection Agency (EPA) and the USAMRIID. Published decontamination procedures *(3,33,39)* document the efficacy of sodium hypochlorite against *B. anthracis* (anthrax) and *B. subtilis* spores. This decontamination procedure could also be applied to other work surfaces, computer equipment, file cabinets, vinyl floors, and painted walls and ceilings.

The EPA regulates the use of materials or solutions for decontamination or disinfection. That is, only those products registered by the EPA may be used for a particular application. However, nonregistered products may be used only after the EPA grants them an emergency exemption.

3. DEMONSTRATION OF DECONTAMINATION OPERATIONS

Individuals tasked to decontaminate such areas should wear personal protective equipment (PPE) for the purpose of protecting them from a potential splash during the decontaminating process. PPE should include a Tyvek® coverall to protect their street clothes, shoe covers to protect their shoes, a minimum of a N95 half-face disposable respirator to protect against nuisance dusts, eye protection (wraparound goggles or full-face shield), and two pairs of surgical (latex or nitrile) gloves. For the Boca Raton facility, EPA personnel wore a full-face respirator with combination filters, a Tyvek coverall and hood, rubber boots, and two pairs of nitrile gloves. PPE should be appropriate for both the biological agent and the decontaminating agent. Decontamination personnel applied a 0.5% sodium hypochlorite (a 1:10 dilution of liquid household bleach [5.25%], about 5500 parts per million [ppm] free, available chlorine in unbuffered water) solution to affected nonporous surfaces for a minimum contact time of 5 min. After this time, the decontaminated areas were wiped twice with a water-moistened cloth or sponge to remove any residual bleach.

Samples were obtained after the decontamination process to validate its efficacy. Upon completion of the decontamination procedure, clean-up materials (bleach, moistened cloths, and sponges) were disposed of using the normal household waste stream. The absence of organisms as compared to previous sampling data results indicated the adequacy of a 5-min contact time. At the point of exit from the decontaminated area, personnel removed their PPE in reverse order of donning, removing the outer pair of surgical gloves, Tyvek coverall, respirator, and rubber boots. The last item removed were the second pair of nitrile gloves. Personnel immediately washed their hands with soap and warm water for at least 30 s.

Two procedures may be recommended for decontaminating porous surfaces (carpeting and cloth-covered furniture). Individuals tasked to decontaminate porous surface areas should wear PPE as described in one of the earlier situations. Their procedures upon exit from the decontaminated area should also follow those described previously.

If it is determined that the materials are dispensable, then carpeted and cloth-covered areas or materials identified as contaminated or potentially contaminated could be decontaminated in place by application of 0.5% sodium hypochlorite solution. Treated materials would then be removed and disposed of appropriately and the materials replaced as required. Carpeted and/or cloth-covered areas or materials identified as not contaminated could be vacuumed with a high-efficiency particulate air (HEPA)-filtered vacuum to minimize airborne allergenic particulates and help provide for better indoor air quality.

For nondispensable items, an alternative method for decontaminating porous surfaces is a vacuum process to remove the microbial burden. Individuals tasked to decontaminate porous surface areas should wear PPE as previously described. Carpeted and/or cloth-covered areas or materials could be treated with a steam extractor type of vacuum unit (such as a Stanley Steemer®, Electrolux Carpet Machine, Rug Doctor®, or equivalent) equipped with a HEPA filter to filter the exhaust air. The steam applied to the carpet is then vacuumed into a reservoir containing 0.25% sodium hypochlorite solution. The extracted fluid containing carpet debris, dust, and environmental contaminants (allergens, mold spores, and so on) is treated with sodium hypochlorite to effect decontamination of any living organisms and microbial spores. The treated extracted fluid can be safely discarded into the sanitary sewer system.

4. AREA OR SPACE DECONTAMINATION

The second approach to decontamination is area or space decontamination, that is, decontamination of material within enclosed spaces. This can be accomplished by using various gases *(40)*. Ethylene oxide (epoxyethane, ETO) is a flammable and explosive gas, and is classified as both a mutagen and a carcinogen. The microbicidal activity of ETO is caused by alkylation of sulfhydryl, amino, carboxy, phenolic, and hydroxyl groups in the spore or vegetative cell. The primary mechanism of its bactericidal and sporicidal activity is reaction of ETO with nucleic acids. ETO is used because of its ability to inactivate most bacteria, molds, yeasts, and viruses, but its use is limited because of the many dangers mentioned. The use of ETO requires a EPA air permit under certain circumstances because of air quality emission standards. Propylene oxide (epoxy propane) hydrolyzes in the presence of moisture to form nontoxic propylene glycol. Propylene glycol vapor *(29)* is odorless, tasteless, and nonirritating to the respiratory mucosa. The microbicidal mode of action of propylene oxide has been shown to be the alkylation of DNA guanines, resulting in single-strand breaks. β-propiolactone (BPL) is approx 4000 times more active than ETO and 25 times more effective than formaldehyde. The microbiological activity of BPL is caused by alkylation of DNA. However, there is limited use of this decontaminant because BPL lacks the ability to penetrate material and is carcinogenic in mice. Formaldehyde is more widely recognized as a fumigant for buildings and rooms *(31,41–43)*, and equipment *(44)* and is the most commonly recommended decontaminant for an area. Formaldehyde gas is capable of killing microorganisms and detoxifying *C. botulinum* toxin. The microbicidal activity of formaldehyde is to denature proteins. Ammonium bicarbonate can be used to neutralize formaldehyde gas. Although formaldehyde vapor is explosive at concentrations between 7.0 and 73.0% by volume in air, these concentrations should not be reached if standard decontamination procedures (using 0.3–0.6 g/ft^3 of paraformaldehyde in the presence of 60–90% relative humidity with a minimum contact time of 6 h) *(31)* are used. Although widely used and recommended as a surface and area sterilant, formaldehyde is a safety hazard because it is a carcinogen. In addition, it is a powerful reducing agent, has limited penetrating ability, and is potentially explosive. Environmental release of formaldehyde is also highly regulated.

Because of the difficulties encountered with some of the decontaminants described above, technologies are emerging that may provide alternative sterilants. One alternative is the powerful oxidant chlorine dioxide (CD), a greenish-yellow gas, which is an effective sterilant even at a concentration range between 10–20 mg/L *(45,46)*. The EPA under the Federal Insecticide, Fungicide, and Rodenticide Act registered CD as a sterilizing agent in 1988. CD is noncarcinogenic, nonflammable, is not an ozone-depleting chemical, and no serious human toxicities are associated with the acute or chronic ingestion of CD. However, CD is considered a mucous membrane irritant and inhalation of excessive amounts can result in pulmonary edema. The threshold limit value time-weighted average (period of safe exposure during 8 h) for CD is 0.1 parts per million *(47)*, which is also the reported odor threshold. After an area is treated, CD can be converted to sodium sulfate using sodium thiosulfate. Because of the selective reactivity of CD, materials such as titanium, stainless steel, silicone rubber, ceramics, polyvinyl chloride, and polyethylene are unaffected by exposure to the gas. However, uncoated copper and aluminum are highly affected. In addition, certain formulations of polycarbonates and polyurethanes develop a marked change in color and tensile properties. The effect on decontamination of a computer central processing unit (CPU) was recently reported *(48)*. An IBM 330-p100 CPU was exposed to five successive CD processes. The CPU hard drive was configured with typical files and diagnostic software (PC doctor). Each exposure was 10 mg/L for 30 min. There was no effect after the first two exposures. However, after the third exposure fan noise was detected and after the fifth exposure the Windows Operating System would not execute. In contrast to chlorine or chlorine-containing solutions, CD is not influenced by the presence of organic materials and is unaffected by pH variations between 6 and 10. CD reacts with carbohydrates by oxidizing the primary hydroxyl groups to aldehydes and then to carboxylic acids. Oxidation occurs at the double bond with lipids. The effect on peptides and proteins is mainly oxidation, substitution, and addition reactions. The lethal activity of CD on spores is dependent on hydration of the spores for optimal activity—a relative humidity of 50% or higher is optimal for sterilization. A CD test system was shown to inactivate paper strip biological indicators containing 10^6 *B. subtilis* var. *niger* spores after 60 min of exposure to CD. CD has been used extensively for water purification and disinfection in the United States and Europe and in the food industry to disinfect fruits and vegetables and to bleach fats and fatty oils. CD has also been used in scrubbing systems to remove or control odors associated with sulfur compounds and fish- and meat-processing plants.

As a result of anthrax (*B. anthracis* spores) contamination of the Hart Senate Office Building (an enclosed area, although not air-tight) in Washington, DC, the EPA Environmental Response Team fumigated affected areas with CD on December 1, 2001. Additional fumigation was done on the air-handling system on December 30, 2001. Selected areas were again fumigated in January 2002. During each of these three occasions, the sporicidal efficacy of the CD decontamination technology was challenged. Collateral damage was not minimal, as many office furniture items (such as couches), office filing cabinets, carpet flooring, and computer equipment were removed after CD decontamination and subsequently destroyed by incineration.

Another alternative, ozone, is not a new sterilant. It was used to sterilize the water supply of Lille, France, in 1899. It has potential as a sterilant for medical devices and, in fact, is used in many healthcare facilities because it is highly oxidizing. The gas is compatible with titanium, stainless steel, silicone rubber, ceramics, polyvinyl chloride, and polyurethane. A recent report *(49)* discussed the efficacy of ozone in the presence of water as a decontaminating strategy for decontaminating facilities involved in a terrorist attack. Collateral damage and residual chemical hazards associated with the use of ozone in a cleanup operation would be minimal.

A relatively new alternative sterilization system is based on the vapor phase of hydrogen peroxide *(50)*. The system provides a rapid, low-temperature technique that because of its low toxicity *(51)*, eliminates much of the potential public health hazard associated with decontaminants such as formaldehyde and ethylene oxide. In the cold sterilization process, 35% liquid hydrogen peroxide (300,000 ppm) is vaporized to yield 700–1200 ppm. The hydroxyl radical, a strong oxidant, is believed to have microbicidal activity through attack on membrane lipids, DNA, and other essential cell components. The hydrogen peroxide vapor is unstable and degrades to the nontoxic residues of water vapor and oxygen. Any enclosure that can be sealed, such as small rooms or an enclosed cabinet (up to 7500 ft^3), can be sterilized with existing portable equipment. More recently, a high-capacity system has been used to decontaminate areas up to 200,000 ft^3. These high-capacity systems were used successfully to decontaminate mail facilities contaminated with *B. anthracis* spores. The process is effective at temperatures ranging from 4 to 80°C. The vapor phase hydrogen peroxide sterilization system appears to be safe and is effective against a variety of microorganisms. Historically, aqueous phase hydrogen peroxide has been used as a surface disinfectant in various food service and dairy industries. A 3% solution of hydrogen peroxide has been frequently used as an antiseptic for minor cuts and abrasions, as a mouthwash (diluted), and as a disinfectant of hospital fabrics *(52)*. However, because aqueous phase hydrogen peroxide has limited efficacy against the more resistant bacterial spores, its use as a sterilant has not been widely investigated. A few investigators *(53,54)* demonstrated that vaporized hydrogen peroxide (VHP®) was an effective sporicide at fairly low concentrations (0.5 to < 10.0 mg/L) over a wide range of temperatures (4–80°C). The process usually involves a dehumidification step, an area conditioning (VHP injection and concentration) phase, a sterilization phase, and finally, an aeration phase. The phases will vary in the amount of time they take to be completed and will vary dependent upon the area being decontaminated. A critical factor in performing a successful decontamination is humidity. An area to be decontaminated should be conditioned to have a relative humidity not greater than 30%. This step ensures that the air can contain enough hydrogen peroxide to successfully sterilize the area. If a low relative humidity is not achieved, then condensation will occur because hydrogen peroxide interacts with water vapor *(55)*. Upon successful dehumidification, vapor phase hydrogen peroxide is continuously injected into the area during the room conditioning and sterilization phase. Even when near saturation levels have been achieved during the conditioning phase, hydrogen peroxide must continuously be added during the sterilization phase albeit at a lower injection rate to replace the hydrogen peroxide that has decomposed to oxygen and water *(56)*. An aeration or ventilation cycle is begun when the sterilization cycle is complete. This cycle may be accomplished using the hydrogen peroxide generator or the building ventilation system.

VHP is an attractive option for use as a sterilization methodology for numerous reasons:

1. It is an environmentally friendly process because through a catalytic process VHP breaks down into oxygen and water. There is no need for neutralization procedures or periods of aeration as required for other gas sterilants, such as formaldehyde or ethylene oxide that may have "toxic" residues.
2. Chemical compatibility and corrosion of materials does not seem to be an issue even though hydrogen peroxide is a powerful oxidizer because only very low levels of VHP are used during the sterilization process. VHP has been tested to determine if the sterilant could be used safely with various types of scientific and business equipment including computers, microscopes, camera lens, various types of film and recording media, telephones, electric drills, and pipet aids. The equipment that was sterilized suffered no apparent ill effects and continued to be operated successfully even after several exposures *(57)*.
3. VHP is effective at low temperatures and can be used to decontaminate items and equipment unable to withstand the higher temperatures used in steam sterilization and dry heat sterilization processes.

Although VHP is a promising new technology, it is not appropriate for all decontamination applications. Some of the limitations of VHP include:

1. Some materials absorb hydrogen peroxide such as cellulose products (which are highly absorbent) and make sterilization difficult to achieve. Cellulosic materials also release the vapor slowly, increasing the aeration time needed to achieve a level of 1 ppm and thus creating a potential occupational exposure hazard *(56)*. Materials such as polyethylene, PVC, polyester, and polypropylene composites were noted to have limited permeability to VHP *(54)*.
2. VHP will not sterilize standing liquids, will condense into standing liquids, and will no longer be able to perform as an effective sporicide.
3. There are a few materials that are not compatible with VHP such as nylon, which becomes brittle after repeated exposure *(58)* and various neoprene gaskets. Some types of paints such as epoxy paint on metal surfaces, will also bubble and peel after repeated exposure and, at least in one case, an epoxy, monolithic floor has pitted after repeated exposures (Kozlovac, personal communication). Other materials such as copper and nickel alloys could be affected and should be considered before using this decontamination technology because they cause hydrogen peroxide to catalytically decompose. In addition, materials containing organic dyes and organic sulfides react with hydrogen peroxide *(59)*.

4.1. The National Cancer Institute at Frederick Experience With VHP

During the construction of a human immunodeficiency virus Research Facility, a room was specified for decontaminating equipment that could not be readily decontaminated in place. Although formaldehyde was originally going to be the decontaminating agent of choice, safety personnel at the Frederick campus were evaluating and validating a VHP generator for space decontamination. When finally constructed, the decontamination room would employ a VHP generator. This generator, the STERIS 1000 VHP Biodecontamination System, had been purchased earlier by the National Cancer Institute (NCI)-Frederick. The room, which is about 400 ft^3, was designed to be easily sealable. The room supply and exhaust system is sealed by leak-proof dampers equipped with Viton® gaskets (the original gasket material was replaced after repeated exposures because of degradation caused by incompatibility with VHP). The decontamination room is also equipped with a large stainless steel fan that aids in circulation of VHP to all areas of the room during the decontamination phase of the operation. The walls are coated with epoxy paint and the floor is of poured epoxy. The entryway is a conventional, epoxy-painted steel door that is sealed with plastic and pressure-sensitive tape during a decontamination cycle. During this cycle, the VHP generator is connected to ports outside the room and the unit can be monitored directly by the operator. The generator is able to maintain a slight negative pressure throughout the operation to ensure that the disinfectant does not escape to surrounding laboratory areas. When the decontamination process is completed, the supply and exhaust system dampers are opened to aid in the aeration of the space. The decontamination room employing VHP has been used repeatedly to successfully decontaminate many types of equipment over the past several years. The only negative impacts upon the room after repeated exposures to VHP is the replacement of the original supply and exhaust damper gaskets, peeling of epoxy-based paint on metal surfaces, and slight pitting of the poured epoxy floor.

Another alternative decontamination process, gas plasma sterilization *(60)* uses radio frequency energy and hydrogen peroxide vapor to create a low-temperature hydrogen peroxide gas plasma to achieve relatively rapid sterilization. Radio waves break apart the hydrogen peroxide vapor into reactive species (hydroperoxy, hydroxyl free radicals, water, and oxygen), which form a gas plasma that interacts with membranes, enzymes, or nucleic acids to disrupt and kill microorganisms. The advantage of this process is that the process temperature does not exceed 40°C. However, the efficacy of this process remains questionable.

A process that is being explored, especially for decontaminating mail, is radiation sterilization or cold sterilization by electron-beam (E-beam) technology or γ-irradiation. Radiation sterilization is known as a cold process because sterilization can be achieved at room temperature. This technology has been used to sterilize thermally unstable materials used in the biomedical field and food processing industry. This technology is not new to the field of sterilization. Johnson and Johnson introduced the first commercial application using E-beam technology to the industry in 1956. Because of the unreliability of the available equipment, further investigations into commercial application of this technology were not considered *(61)*. However, in the 1960s, there emerged γ-irradiator technology, which did not have reliability issues. Because of improved reliability in electron accelerators and other control components, the medical device industry and the US Postal Service are re-evaluating sterilization by E-beam technology.

Regardless of the method used, the primary means of inactivating organisms is to disrupt DNA chains by secondary energetic species (e.g., free radicals, electrons).

When matter absorbs high-energy radiation, molecules and atoms that were in a stable state become excited or charged; this process is defined as ionization *(62)*. The typical dose required for sterilization of bacterial spores is reported as 2.5 megarads although the dose required to inactivate vegetative bacteria is much less (0.25 megarad) (J.T. Moore, personal communication). A brief discussion on the advantages and disadvantages of E-beam technology and γ-irradiation facilities as it relates to processing bulk, unscreened mail is presented below. This issue is currently being vigorously debated among health physicists and radiation safety professionals within the United States.

4.2. E-Beam Irradiation Facilities

Two factors: voltage and the available amperage determine the capacity of an E-beam facility. Typical medical device sterilization uses high-energy electrons, usually 10 million electron volts (10 MeV). This type of E-beam facility has a capacity comparable to a multimillion curie [60]cobalt facility. Electron penetration into a product directly correlates to the energy of the electron and the density of the material to be sterilized. This is the main disadvantage of E-beam technology. Even 10 MeV units will have a only a short effective range, which may require mail to be removed from mail bags to be placed in trays or boxes for processing. With double-sided irradiation, an E-beam system was able to penetrate up to 35 in. of material with a bulk density of 0.10 g/cm^3 *(61)*. However, in a bulk mail operation, material would most likely need to be transferred from larger containers such as mail bags into smaller boxes and trays before sterilization. This creates the possibility of contaminating the handling area and the individuals performing the repacking operation. A major advantage of E-beam irradiation over γ-irradiation is the decreased exposure time, which is measured in minutes rather than hours. Although E-beam sterilization and γ-irradiation will have similar effects on materials because of the decreased exposure time, less oxidative damage will occur with E-beam sterilization, as free radicals will interact for only a short period of time in and around the material to be sterilized. Another advantage of E-beam is that if an exothermic or explosive reaction occurs due to irradiation of vulnerable materials (accidentally or intentionally), only the E-beam facility would be damaged or destroyed, which would not release radiation or cause radiological contamination problems.

4.3. γ-Irradiation Facilities

One of the advantages of γ-irradiation is that a γ-ray (source examples include cobalt-60 and cesium-137) has considerably more penetrating power than an electron. The reason for this is that γ-rays do not have electron mass. One disadvantage for using γ-irradiation instead of E-beam irradiation is that it has a considerably longer processing time. The parameter that will control the exposure time required to sterilize, is the bulk density and irradiation dose. Typical batch processing in medical sterilization requires from 3 to 12 h depending on the batch *(63)*. One of the main disadvantages, especially when irradiating unscreened mail containing unknown materials, is the possibility that a vulnerable material, upon exposure to a high radioactive field, could become explosive or initiate an exothermic reaction. Such an adverse reaction could damage the source transfer mechanism of the irradiator or, in a worst-case scenario, cause a breach in the source capsules. This would cause a major radiation contamination problem throughout the facility.

The effectiveness of each decontamination (or sterilization) process can be determined by monitoring the biological activity of spore preparations *(35,38,42,43,64)* usually consisting of a combination of *B. atropheus* (10^6) and *Geobacillus stearmotherophilus* (10^5). To determine the adequacy of different methods of decontamination or sterilization, a variety of different uncombined spore preparations can be used. These include *B. pumilus*, *B. atropheus*, *G. stearothermophilus,* which are commercially available, and *B. globigii*, and *B. subtilis globigii.* Spore preparations are prepared as dried preparations on filter paper (spore strips), stainless steel coupons, or aluminum foil, or as a combined unit consisting of a paper carrier of the spores and a vial of growth medium containing a pH indicator system. After the decontamination, the dried preparations, and a control preparation not exposed to the decontamination process, are placed in tryptic soy broth and incubated at an appropriate time and temperature to determine spore viability. For the combined unit, the vial of growth medium is ruptured and the paper carrier of the spores is released into the released growth medium. Preparations used as a control and those subjected to the decontamination process are incubated as described earlier.

In summary, decontamination is the disinfection or sterilization of agent-contaminated articles to make them safe for use or disposal. The emphasis is on making the article safe, whether accomplished by selectively eliminating certain undesirable microorganisms to prevent their transmission or completely destroying microbial life. The method(s) of decontamination should be determined only after a careful analysis of the risks involved to both personnel and the environment. Although there are many different technologies available for decontamination, each will have advantages and disadvantage when considering the material(s) being decontaminated. Without a doubt, the chosen method of decontamination will be strongly influenced by concerns of the public. Although the public may demand zero risk, this goal may not be logical, rational, practical, or even achievable. To minimize any confusion or misperception, it is imperative that the public be educated and actively involved in the decision-making process to convince them to voluntarily accept some level of risk. To gain public confidence so it will accept the finding that an area or building is completely decontaminated is not insurmountable. Through their active and cooperative involvement, the public should be successfully convinced by authorities that an area or building is "clean" enough for them to re-enter and return to the normal activities of life.

ACKNOWLEDGMENTS

The authors gratefully acknowledge Ms. Katheryn F. Kenyon, Dr. Peter B. Jahrling, Dr. Patricia L. Worsham, LTC George W. Korch, Evelyn Hawley, and Tammy Kozlovac, for their gracious contributions and critical review of the manuscript. This project has been funded in part with Federal funds from the National Cancer Institute, National Institutes of Health, under contract No. N01-CO-12400.

DISCLAIMER STATEMENT

The content of this publication does not necessarily reflect the views or policies of the Department of Health and Human Services, nor does mention of trade names, commercial products, or organizations imply endorsement by the US Government.

REFERENCES

1. Block, S. (2001a) Definition of terms, in, *Disinfection, Sterilization, and Preservation,* 5th ed. (Block S, ed.), Lippincott, Williams & Wilkins, Phialdelphia, PA, pp. 19–28.
2. Kortepeter, M. (2001a) Decontamination, in *USAMRIID's Medical Management of Biological Casualties Handbook* (Kortepeter, M., Christopher, G. W., Cieslak, T. J., et al., eds.), U.S. Army Medical Research Institute of Infectious Diseases, Fort Detrick, pp. 161–165.
3. Rutala, W. and Weber, D. (1997) Uses of inorganic hypochlorite (bleach) in health care facilities. *Clin. Microbiol. Rev.* **10,** 597–610.
4. Favero, M. S. and Bond, W. W. (2001) Chemical disinfection of medical and surgical materials, in *Disinfection, Sterilization, and Preservation,* 5th ed. (Block, S., ed.), Lippincott, Williams & Wilkins, Philadelphia, PA, pp. 881–917 .
5. Favero, M. (2002) Issues in laboratory decontamination strategies: large areas, new pathogens, and prions. *Managing Risk in Animal Care and Use,* 7th National Symposium on Biosafety, Atlanta, GA, January 30.
6. Army Regulation 385-10. (2000) Abatement program, in *The Army Safety Program*, Headquarters, Department of the Army, Washington, DC, pp. 12–14.
7. Fleming, D. O. (2000) Risk assessment of biological hazards, in *Biological Safety Principles and Practice*, 3rd ed. (Fleming, D. O. and Hunt, D. L., eds.), ASM, Washington, DC, pp. 57–64.
8. Hammer, W. (1989) Appraising plant safety, in *Occupational Safety Management and Engineering,* 4th ed. (Hammer, W., ed.), Springer-Verlag, Englewood Cliffs, NJ, pp. 227–246.
9. Sidell, F. R., Patrick, W. C., III, and Dashiell, T.R. (1998) On-scene procedures, in *Jane's Chem-Bio Handbook* (Sidell, F. R., Patrick, W. C., III, Dashiell, T. R., eds.), Jane's Information Group, Alexandria, VA, pp. 9–13.
10. Tempest Publishing. (1998b) Scene assessment and control, in *First Responder Chem-Bio Handbook – A Practical Manual for First Responders,* Version 1.5 (Tempest Publishing, ed.), Tempest Publishing, Alexandria, VA, pp. A-1-2-A-1-7.
11. Alexander, L. (1998) Decontaminating civilian facilities: biological agents and toxins. Institute for Defense Analyses (IDA Paper P-3365), Alexandria, VA. U.S. Dept. Commerce, Natl. Techn. Inform. Ser. (UG447D2961998), January.
12. Raber, E., Jin, A., Noonan, K., McGuire, R., and Kirvel, R. D. (2001) Decontamination issues for chemical and biological warfare agents: how clean is clean enough? *In. J. Env. Health Res.* **11,** 128–148.
13. Stein, C. D. and Van Ness, G. B. (1955) A ten year survey of anthrax in livestock with special reference to outbreaks in 1954. *Vet. Med.* **50,** 579–588.
14. Kiel, J. L., Parker, J. E., Alls, J. L., et al. (2000) Rapid recovery and identification of anthrax bacteria from the environment. *Ann. NY Acad. Sci.* **916,** 240–252.
15. Swearengen, J. R. and Worsham, P. L. (2000) Plague, in *Emerging Diseases of Animals,* Chapter 13 (Brown, C. and Bolin, C., eds.), ASM Press, Washington, DC, pp. 259–279.
16. Inglesby, T. V., Dennis, D. T., Henderson, D. A., et al. (2000) Plague as a biological weapon. Medical and public health management. *J. Am. Med. A* **283,** 2281–2290.
17. McCoy, G. W. and Chapin, C. W. (1912) *Bacterium tularense*, the cause of a plague-like disease of rodents. *Pub. Health. Bull.* **53,** 17–23.
18. Jellison, W. L. and Parker, R. R. (1945) Rodents, rabbits and tularemia in North America: some zoological and epidemiological considerations. *Am. J. Trop. Med.* **25,** 349–362.
19. Hatheway, C. L. (1990) Toxigenic Clostridia. *Clin. Microbiol. Rev.* **3(1),** 66–98.
20. Jones, L. A., Hoffman, R. K., and Phillips, C. R. (1968) Sporocidal activity of sodium hypochlorite at subzero temperatures. *Appl. Microbiol.* **16,** 787–791.
21. Malloch, R. A. and Stoker, M. G. P. (1952) Studies on the susceptibility of *Rickettsia burnetii* to chemical disinfectants, and on techniques for detecting small numbers of viable organisms. *J. Hyg.* **50,** 502–514.

22. Scott, G. H. and Williams, J. (1990) Susceptibility of *Coxiella burnetii* to chemical disinfectants. *Ann. NY Acad. Sci.* **590,** 291–296.

23. Weavers, L. K. and Wickramanayake, G. B. (2001) Kinetics of the inactivation of microorganisms, in *Disinfection, Sterilization, and Preservation,* 5th ed. (Block, S., ed.), Lippincott, Williams & Wilkins, Philadelphia, PA, pp. 65–78.

24. Alasri, A., Valverde, M., Roques, C., and Michel, G. (1992) Sporicidal properties of peracetic acid and hydrogen peroxide, alone and in combination, in comparison with chlorine and formaldehyde for ultrafiltration membrane disinfection. *Can. J. Microbiol.* **39,** 52–60.

25. Vesley, D., Lauer, J. L., and Hawley, R. J. (2000) Decontamination, sterilization, disinfection, and antisepsis, in *Biological Safety Principles and Practice,* 3rd ed. (Fleming, D. O. and Hunt, D. L., eds.), ASM, Washington, DC, p. 387.

26. Bloomfield, S. F. and Uso, E. E. (1985) The antibacterial properties of sodium hypochlorite and sodium dichloroisocyanurate as hospital disinfectants. *J. Hosp. Infect.* **6,** 20–30.

27. McDonnell, G. and Russell, A. D. (1999) Antiseptics and disinfectants: activity, action, and resistance. *Clin. Microbiol. Rev.* **12,** 142–179.

28. Joslyn, L. J. (2001) Gaseous chemical sterilization, in *Disinfection, Sterilization, and Preservation,* 5th ed. (Block, S., ed.), Lippincott, Williams & Wilkins, Philadelphia, PA, pp. 337–359.

29. Puck, T. T., Robertson, O. H., and Lemon, H. M. (1943) The bactericidal action of propylene glycol vapor on microorganisms suspended in air. II. The influence of various factors on the activity of the vapor. *J. Exp. Med.* **78,** 387–406.

30. Russell, A. D. (1990) Bacterial spores and chemical sporicidal agents. *Clin. Microbiol. Rev.* **3,** 99–119.

31. Songer, J. R., Braymen, D. T., Mathis, R. G., and Monroe, J. W. (1972) The practical use of formaldehyde vapor for disinfection. *Health Lab. Sci.* **9,** 46–55.

32. Hawley, R. J. and Eitzen, E. E. Protection against biological warfare agents, in *Disinfection, Sterilization, and Preservation,* 5th ed. (Block, S., ed.), Lippincott, Williams & Wilkins, Philadelphia, PA, pp. 1161–1167.

33. Hawley, R. J. and Eitzen, E. E. (2001) Biological weapons—a primer for microbiologists. *Ann. Rev. Microbiol.* **55,** 235–253.

34. Babb, J. R., Bradley, C. R., and Ayliffe, G. A. Y. (1980) Sporicidal activity of glutaraldehydes and hypochlorites and other factors influencing their selection for the treatment of medical equipment. *J. Hosp. Infect.* **1,** 63–75.

35. Sagripanti, J.-L., and Bonifacino, A. (1996) Comparative sporicidal effect of liquid chemical germicides on three medical devices contaminated with spores of *Bacillus subtilis.* *Am. J. Infec. Control.* **24(5),** 364–371.

36. Castegnaro, M., Friesen, M., Michelon, J., and Walker, A. (1981) Problems related to the use of sodium hypochlorite in the detoxification of aflatoxin B1. *Am. Ind. Hyg. Assoc. J.* **42,** 398–401.

37. Morin, R. and Kozlovac, J. (2000) Biological toxins, in *Biological Safety Principles and Practice,* 3rd ed. (Fleming, D. O. and Hunt, D. L., eds.), ASM, Washington, DC, pp. 261–272.

38. O'Conner, L. E. (2001) A comparison of decontamination technologies for biological agent on selected commercial surface materials. Aberdeen Proving Ground, MD: U.S. Army Soldier and Biological Chemical Command.

39. National Antimicrobial Information Network Fact Sheet. http://ace.orst.edu/info/nain/, Corvallis OR: Oregon State University, 2001.

40. Joslyn, L. J. (2001) Gaseous chemical sterilization, in *Disinfection, Sterilization, and Preservation,* 5th ed. (Block, S., ed.), Lippincott, Williams & Wilkins, Philadelphia, PA, pp. 338–340.

41. Taylor, L. A., Barbeito, M. S., and Gremillion, G. G. (1969) Paraformaldehyde for surface sterilization and detoxification. *Appl. Microbiol.* **17(4),** 614–618.

42. Abraham, G., LeBlanc Smith, P. M., and Nguyen, S. (1997) The effectiveness of gaseous formaldehyde decontamination assessed by biological monitoring. *J. Am. Biol. Safety Assoc.* **2(1)**, 30–38.
43. Cheney, J. E. and Collins, C. H. (1995) Formaldehyde disinfection in laboratories: limitations and hazards. *Br. J. Biomed. Sci.* **52**, 195–201.
44. Rayburn, S. R. (1990) Design and use of biological safety cabinets, in *The Foundations of Laboratory Safety: A Guide for the Biomedical Laboratory* (Rayburn, S. R., ed.), Springer-Verlag, New York, pp. 89–101.
45. Kowalski, J. B. (1998) Sterilization of medical devices, pharmaceutical components, and barrier isolation systems with gaseous chlorine dioxide, in *Sterilization of Medical Products*, vol. VII. (Morrissey, R. F. and Kowalski, J. B., eds.), Polysciences Publications, Champlain, NY, pp. 313–323.
46. Knapp, J. E. and Battisti, D. L. (2001) Chlorine dioxide, in *Disinfection, Sterilization, and Preservation,* 5th ed. (Block, S., ed.), Lippincott, Williams & Wilkins, Philadelphia, PA, pp. 215–227.
47. ACGIH. (2001) Chlorine dioxide. chemical substances, in *Threshold Limit Values for Chemical Substances and Physical Agents and Biological Exposure Indices*, American Conference of Governmental Industrial Hygenists (ACGIH), Cincinnati, OH, p. 21.
48. Morrissey, R., Kowalski, J., and Battisti, D. (2002) J&J Experience with Technologies Under Consideration for Remediation of Anthrax-Contaminated Sites/Items, Presented at an Environmental Protection Agency *Meeting on Anthrax Remediation Issues*, Washington, DC, January 10.
49. Currier, R. P., Torraco, D. J., Cross, J. B., Wagner, G. L., Gladden, P. D., and Vandenberg, L. A. (2001) Deactivation of clumped and dirty spores of *Bacillus globigii. Ozone Sci. Eng.* **23**, 285–294.
50. Block, S. (ed.) (2001) Peroxygen Compounds, in *Disinfection, Sterilization, and Preservation,* 5th ed. Lippincott, Williams & Wilkins, Philadelphia, PA, pp. 185–204.
51. ACGIH. (2001) Hydrogen peroxide. chemical substances in *Threshold Limit Values for Chemical Substances and Physical Agents and Biological Exposure Indices*, American Conference of Governmental Industrial Hygenists (ACGIH), Cincinnati, OH, p. 68
52. Neely, A. and Maley, M. (1999) The 1999 Lindberg Award: 3% hydrogen peroxide for the gram-positive disinfection of fabrics. *J. Burn Care Rehabil.* 471–477.
53. More, F. and Perkinson, R. (1979) Cold gas sterilization using H_2O_2. U.S. Patent 4,169,123.
54. Joslyn, L. J. (2001) Gaseous chemical sterilization, in *Disinfection, Sterilization, and Preservation,* 5th ed. (Block, S., ed.), Lippincott, Williams & Wilkins, Philadelphia, PA, p. 344.
55. Jahnke, M. and Lauth, G. (1997) Biodecontamination of a large volume filling room with hydrogen peroxide. *Pharm. Eng.* **17(4)**, 3–12.
56. Jones, R., Drake, J., and Eagleson, D. (1993) Using hydrogen peroxide vapor to decontaminate biological safety cabinets. *Acumen* **1(1)**, 1–3.
57. Heckert, R., Best, M., Jordan, L., Dulac, G., Eddington, D., and Sterritt, W. (1997) Efficacy of vaporized hydrogen peroxide against exotic animal viruses. *Appl. Environ. Microbiol.* **63(10)**, 3916–3918.
58. Rickloff, J. and Graham, G. (1989) Vapor phase hydrogen peroxide sterilization. *J. Healthcare Mat. Manag.* **7(5)**, 45–48.
59. Widmer, A. and Frei, R. (1999) Decontamination, disinfection and sterilization, in *Manual of Clinical Microbiology*, 7th ed. (Murray, P., Baron, E., Pfaller, M., et al., eds.), ASM Press, Washington, DC, pp. 138–164.
60. Joslyn, L. J. (2001) Gaseous chemical sterilization, in *Disinfection, Sterilization, and Preservation,* 5th ed. (Block, S., ed.), Lippincott, Williams & Wilkins, Philadelphia, PA, pp. 345, 346.

61. Calhoun, L., Allen, J., Shaffer, H., Sullivan, G., and Williams, C. (1997) Electron-beam systems for medical device sterilization. *Med. Plastics Biomat. Mag.* 26.
62. Hansen, J. M. and Shaffer, H. L. (2001) Sterilization and preservation by radiation sterilization, in *Disinfection, Sterilization, and Preservation,* 5th ed. (Block, S., ed.), Lippincott, Williams & Wilkins, Philadelphia, PA, pp. 731.
63. Hansen, J. M. and Shaffer, H. L. (2001) Sterilization and preservation by radiation sterilization, in *Disinfection, Sterilization, and Preservation,* 5th ed. (Block, S., ed.), Lippincott, Williams & Wilkins, Philadelphia, PA, p. 740.
64. Raven Biological Laboratories. (2002) Regarding changes to taxonomy of *Bacillus* organisms. Technical notice rev$_2$. Tuesday, Aug., 20, 2002: Kansas City, MO.

PART III

EMERGING THREATS AND FUTURE PREPARATION

16

Definition and Overview of Emerging Threats

Luther E. Lindler, Eileen Choffnes, and George W. Korch

1. INTRODUCTION

The risks posed by bioterrorism and the proliferation of biological weapons capabilities have increased concern about how the rapid advances in genetic engineering and biotechnology could enable the production of biological weapons with unique and unpredictable characteristics. The nature of the biotechnology problem—indeed the nature of the biological research enterprise—is vastly different from that of theoretical and applied nuclear physics in the late 1930s. Evolving biotechnology presents an inextricably linked combination of opportunity and danger and that distinction turns on projected consequences and attributed intentions at the level of fundamental research. Matthew Meselson gave a stark warning of the potential dangers posed by the destructive applications of biotechnology at the annual meeting of the National Academy of Sciences in May 2000.

> "Every major technology—metallurgy, explosives, internal combustion, aviation, electronics, nuclear energy—has been intensively exploited, not only for peaceful purposes but also for hostile ones. Must this also happen with biotechnology, certain to be a dominant technology of the coming century? During the century just begun, as our ability to modify fundamental life processes continues its rapid advance, we will be able not only to devise additional ways to destroy life but will also be able to manipulate it—including the processes of cognition, development, reproduction, and inheritance. A world in which these capabilities are widely employed for hostile purposes would be a world in which the very nature of conflict has radically changed. There in could lie unprecedented opportunities for violence, coercion, repression, or subjugation."

As noted earlier, biotechnology can be used for destructive purposes, but it also holds vast promise for countering bioterrrorism threats. For example, genomic sequence analysis of pathogens can lead to the design of more effective vaccines and antibiotics. Biotechnology may also be used for large-scale production of therapeutics to counter biological agents.

The "dual" nature of biotechnology is evident in recent scientific publications. For example, an Australian research group attempted to sterilize mice by immunizing them against an important reproductive protein (discussed in detail in Subheading 3.3.). To do so, this protein was inserted into the poxvirus genome to produce the antigen in the mice. A gene for interleukin (IL)-4 was also inserted into this poxvirus vector, because

From: *Infectious Diseases: Biological Weapons Defense: Infectious Diseases and Counterterrorism*
Edited by: L. E. Lindler, F. J. Lebeda, and G. W. Korch © Humana Press Inc., Totowa, NJ

IL-4 is known to enhance antibody formation. Although the original intent was simply to sterilize the mice, the researchers found that the engineered poxvirus construct was more virulent. The construct resulted in the death of genetically resistant, vaccine-protected, and wildtype mice. This example illustrates the current potential, through biotechnology, to enhance the potency of disease-causing agents.

Because the fundamental knowledge from which these dangers emerge is common-place around the world and the potential benefits of biotechnology for medicine and defense are too great, efforts to prohibit or reverse such research and investigations may be futile, at best. However, the potential adverse impacts associated with the ex-ploitation of these technological advances over the next 5–15 yr cannot be ignored. History has demonstrated that research in biology conducted without any military ap-plication in mind may still contribute to the production of biological weapons. In this context, the next generation of biological warfare (BW) agents may mimic physiologi-cally active compounds and disregulate fundamental life processes including repro-duction, apoptosis, cognition, and enhancement or suppression of the immune response. Microbes used for bioremediation purposes may also be modified to target strategic materials and infrastructures.

Dr. Anna Johnson-Winegar, Deputy Assistant to the Secretary of Defense for Chemi-cal and Biological Defense has made the following remarks.

> "[Although] gene-based weaponry is not currently a credible threat, the sophisticated methods which we now have to probe the human genome, . . . , introduce the possibility that these techniques may be used to create weapons. Viruses may be developed that can be genetically targeted to a particular nationality or race based on certain genetic charac-teristics. Biological weapons may be created that are tailored to produce symptoms weeks after exposure but are contagious much earlier, allowing the agent to spread for extended periods prior to medical experts becoming aware that an epidemic has started. Biological agents may be used to produce debilitating but not fatal diseases, requiring the use of tremendous resources for palliative care. The strain on the medical resources and psycho-logical strength of a society could potentially be crippling."

The current military Biodefense Research Program (BDRP) focuses on agents listed on the Department of Defense (DOD) validated threat list. With the birth of recombi-nant DNA technology in the early 1970s, the possibility that new agents might be con-structed for offensive purposes became a reality. Military planners in the BDRP program office began to seriously consider this possibility in the early to middle 1990s. Their concerns were borne out with the defection of one of the leaders in the former Soviet Union offensive bioweapons programs. Ken Alibeck described a significant project within this program specifically aimed at the use of recombinant technologies to modify classic agents as well as develop new agents with unique pathogenic proper-ties. This program was referred to as "bonfire" in his book about covert former Soviet Union bioweapons development *(3)*. The bonfire project attempted to make relatively simple (by today's standards) modifications of agents such as the incorporation of an-tibiotic resistance genes in classic bacterial agents. Russian bioweaponeers were also purported to have modified classic agents such as *Yersinia pestis* such that they pro-duced dramatically different pathologies compared with the unaltered pathogen. Inter-estingly, some hints of these activities were published in the open literature although many have not been independently confirmed.

The weapons alluded to in the previous paragraph all began as one of the classic agents considered for use in BW. However, the possibility exists for development of chimeras that do not exist in nature through the use of recombinant technologies. The study and development of agents isolated from nature that are yet to be discovered is also a possibility that must be considered in planning for future threats. Possible examples of both of these potential agents will be discussed later. However, it should be pointed out that the intent of this chapter is not to specifically discuss the weaponization of these agents but more to address the fact that these bioweapons are a distinct set of unconventional agents that require unconventional countermeasures to deter their possible development and use.

From what was aforementioned, it is clear that emerging threats can be divided into two groups. The first are ones that began with a classic platform or agent, this is the weaponization of disease agents. The second group would be comprised of agents that do not exist in nature and are produced by man. It should be pointed out that the definitions of these two groups may, in some cases, be arbitrary because classic agents may produce new or mixed pathologies after modification. In this instance, the question is when does the agent cease to be the classic agent such that it should be considered a new agent? The purpose of this chapter is to introduce the reader to these current and future possibilities as well as give examples of modified agents that appear in the open literature.

1.1. Definition of a Validated Threat That Has Been Modified

Agents in this category are ones that fall into the classic agents but have been modified to circumvent normal countermeasures or therapies. Some in the community refer to these as "improved agents." Examples of these will be discussed in Subheading 2. and include agents made antibiotic resistant or vaccine resistant.

1.2. Definition of Potential Threats That Could Be Developed

These agents are ones that may include a modified classic agent that now produces new and unique pathology. Modified agents could be created by recombinant technologies. These agents include generation after next organisms or toxins that are manmade to target specific biological systems. Agents in this category might also include ones that have newly emerged and are amenable to weaponization or that encode some properties necessary for pathogenesis but lack others that are critical to cause disease. These may be referred to as "advanced" agents by some in the community. Possible examples of these are presented in Subheading 3. It is important to note that these agents can be created outside natural evolutionary pressures.

2. EXAMPLES OF MODIFIED VALIDATED THREATS

2.1. Recombinant Anthrax

In 1997, the DOD medical community was alerted to just how serious a threat genetic modification was to their planned anthrax vaccination program for military personnel. A small group of Russian scientists at the State Research Center for Applied Microbiology in Oblensk published a paper in the journal *Vaccine,* which demonstrated that the addition of a single gene to a strain of *Bacillus anthracis* could cause disease in vaccinated animals *(21)*. This research center was one that Alibeck had mentioned in his book as specializing in constructing recombinant threat agents *(3)*. These researchers added a cereolysin gene from *Bacillus cereus* to a fully virulent *B. anthracis* strain. The cereolysin *AB* genes encode a functional hemolysin. Hamsters immunized with live *B. anthracis* harboring only pOX1 encoding the anthrax toxin and not pOX2 encoding the capsule displayed an immune index of 140 when challenged with the unmodified (cereolysin negative) recombinant. In contrast, hamsters immunized with the same strain and challenged with the recombinant cereolysin-producing strain were not protected (immune index approx 1). Thus, mice could be well-protected by live immunization with a crippled strain of *B. anthracis* but were not protected when challenged with the cereolysin producing recombinant organism. This "vaccine breakthrough" could be overcome if the cereolysin gene was included in the live *B. anthracis* vaccine strain used to immunize the animals. These results brought into question the utility of vaccination of the entire military population and weather simple genetic modification might circumvent that program. It should be noted that these results have not been independently confirmed at this time.

2.2. Antibiotic Resistance

The classic bacterial biothreat agents are generally susceptible to most antibiotics used to treat the infections *(5,9,11,24,26)*. However, multidrug resistance has been reported for *Y. pestis* but is confined to the island of Madagascar *(13,15)*. Doxycycline is one of the primary antibiotics recommended for treatment of infections caused most of the high-risk bacterial threat agents (US Army Medical Research Institute if Infectious Diseases Medical Management of Biological Casualties Handbook, http:// www.usamriid.army.mil/education/bluebook.html). The Russian offensive program is purported to have invested in the generation of recombinant organisms that were resistant to the common therapies such as antibiotic treatment *(3)*. This is consistent with the desire to produce offensive biological weapons for which there was no current cure *(3)*. The idea that they were producing antibiotic-resistant BW agents is supported by several publications in the open literature. Gorelov et al. generated a multidrug resistant vaccine strain of *Brucella abortus (14)*. This strain was resistant to doxycycline, streptomycin, ampicillin, and rifampicin. The drug-resistant strain was generated by spontaneous selection for rifampicin resistance and by transformation with a "hybrid" plasmid. The researchers went on to demonstrate that the vaccine strain retained the ability to immunize animals against brucellosis. This latter point was important because recombinant strains of pathogenic organisms can be altered in terms of biological properties in some instances. In relation to recombinant antibiotic resistant *B. anthracis*, Pomerantsev and Staritsyn *(22)* studied the stability of a tetracycline resistance plasmid pCET in vegetative cells and in spores. These studies included conditions for stable maintenance, complete loss and integration of the plasmid into the chromosome of *B. anthracis*. Experiments to test stability of the added phenotype would be necessary for the development of antibiotic resistant *B. anthracis* strains as a BW agent, which is consistent with Alibeck's assertion that the former Soviet Union offensive BW program developed strains of the organism that were resistant to five different antibiotics *(3)*. Generation of multiply antibiotic-resistant strains of *Pseudomonas mallei* (*Burkholderia mallei*) and *P. pseudomallei* (*B. pseudomallei*), which cause glanders and melioidosis, respectively, have also been described in the open literature *(1,2,25)*.

These papers describe genetic manipulation by transformation and conjugation as well as the effect of plasmid maintenance has on virulence of the organism. Taken together, these papers as well as others described in Subheading 2. of this chapter, demonstrate the emphasis that the former Soviet Union BW offensive program placed on alteration of antibiotic resistance of the agents under development.

2.3. Recombinant Francisella tularensis

In 1993, Borzenkov et al. published experiments describing the construction of an attenuated strain of *Francisella tularensis* harboring a construct expressing the human β-endorphin gene *(6)*. The production of the recombinant bioactive peptide was reported to cause dose-dependent effects consistent with endorphin expression in mice infected with the recombinant strain. This is the first report of a bioactive peptide being delivered by a threat agent and having a physiological effect in animals. The following year, the same group reported construction of recombinant strains of *Yersinia, Francisella,* and *Brucella* producing human endorphin *(7)*. Although not specifically reported for obvious reasons, these recombinant organisms might be expected to produce altered pathology following infection that might confound treatment of the disease. For example, the animal might demonstrate signs of the bacterial infection but also signs of an overdose of a drug such as an opiate. Although these effects are theoretically possible, it is unknown what real effects recombinant organisms of this type might have.

3. POTENTIAL THREATS

3.1. Organisms That Develop in Nature That Might Be Weaponized

Many traits must be considered when BW agents are developed. These concepts are briefly discussed in Chapter 3. Accordingly, it is conceivable that a pathogen could emerge in the future through natural selection that meets the criteria for weaponization, and therefore, might become a threat agent. There have been numerous new diseases in recent history any of which could potentially be characterized for weaponization. The most recent example of a newly emerged disease was the Sudden Acute Respiratory Syndrome (SARS) epidemic *(27)*. The virus that causes SARS might be considered as a BW agent because it was highly infectious, communicable and caused mortality. Besides being an example of a natural emerging threat, SARS is also an example of how we might recognize, respond, and limit damage because of a bioterrorist attack. Accordingly, planners for future bioterrorist attacks could use the public health and research community response to the SARS epidemic to gain insight into how to possibly reduce the impact of agent release.

3.2. Low Virulence or Nonpathogenic Organisms That Could Be Genetically Modified

A more theoretical group of organisms that might be developed into BW agents in the laboratory are ones that are of low pathogenicity but that encode some factors associated with virulence. The addition of specific genes could then result in the creation of a more virulent organism. This process can be thought of as the laboratory equivalent of what occurs in nature. The process from nonpathogen to pathogen is believed to be primarily driven by lateral gene transfer events *(20)*. The resulting pathogen depends on the traits that are added to the ancestral bacteria. The study of evolution of pathogens in this manner has been greatly supported and accelerated by genomic sequencing efforts and comparisons between completed genomes. One specific example of the close relationship between nonpathogenic and highly pathogenic members of a genus can be see in the comparison of *Y. pestis* and *Yersinia pseudotuberculosis*. These two organisms are highly related at the whole genome level yet cause vastly different diseases *(8)*. A detailed description of the differences between *Y. pestis* and *Y. pseudotuberculosis* can be found in Chapter 22. The emergence of a new pathogenic organism is thought to be through "genetic sampling" such that new combinations of genetic materials coalesce and allow an organism to occupy a new niche in nature. Theoretically, this might be possible to duplicate in the laboratory using recombinant techniques and, therefore, must be considered in future preparations to counter bioterrorism and BW threats.

3.3. The Mousepox That Roared

A relatively recent publication by Jackson et al. *(16)* had important implications in the field of genetically engineered or emerging threats. These researchers demonstrated that a modified mousepox virus, ectromelia (ECTV) could: a) cause lethal infections in normally genetically resistant mice; and b) cause lethal infections in mice previously immunized against infection with ECTV. The genetic modification included in this strain of ECTV was the inclusion of the gene encoding the normal cytokine IL-4 into the genome of the virus. These experiments were performed under the auspices of enhancing the immune response to other recombinant antigens carried on the virus. The creation of the supermousepox and the possibility that similar experiments could be done with smallpox had obvious implications on further development of an already formidable bioweapon. These implications were noted in prominent scientific journals and reignited discussions about the open nature of publication of scientific results and implications such publications have for national security *(4,12,19)*.

4. COUNTERMEASURES: WHAT CAN WE DO TO PREPARE?

4.1. Genome Sequencing and Database Development

Possibly one of the greatest difficulties will be the identification of the new agent that is causing the disease. This was seen more than 20 yr ago when the agent of Legionnaire's disease could not be isolated. Of course the first step is the isolation of the agent but then soon follows the identification needed to help provide proper therapy for infected patients. The recent emergence of SARS is a good example of how rapid sequencing capability can provide useful information during an infectious disease epidemic. Two different groups were able to grow and isolate the virus from infected tissue culture cells at about the same time *(10,17)*. These studies used electron microscopic examination, random polymerase chain reaction sequencing, and immunoreactivity to identify the agent as a coronavirus. Two weeks later, the complete genome sequence of the SARS virus was reported by two independent groups *(18,23)*. Knowledge of the complete genome sequence allowed the exact identification of the virus as well as the determination of the phylogeny that gave rise to this new strain. The fact that SARS has a relatively small genome of approx 27 kb facilitated the rapid sequencing, assembly, and molecular characterization of this newly emerged virus. Of course, this would be more difficult with larger bacterial genomes that are megabases in size. However, complete sequence information may not be necessary to determine the identity of the organism involved in the outbreak at least sufficiently enough to allow proper treatment.

The databases used to analyze the genome sequences obtained in the earlier SARS example were standard databases such as GenBank. Development of more sophisticated databases that concentrate on virulence factors, pathogen genetic traits, and other characteristics associated with pathogenicity may be needed. Well-annotated and developed datasets of this type will be useful for research purposes such as genomic sequencing projects and the identification of potential virulence properties. Genome sequencing projects and use of databases of this type may be useful in the identification of low-virulence or nonpathogenic organisms that might be genetically modified (*see* Subheading 3.2.). A virulence factor database of this type would also be useful for the characterization of novel agents postevent as well.

4.2. Genotyping

The development of a large genotyping database for the primary threat agents would allow us to identify newly emerging strains of these organisms. The success of such a project would depend greatly on international cooperation because most of the diseases caused by the primary agents are not prevalent in the United States. Not only would such a genetic fingerprint database help identify new strains of these organisms, but it would also support attribution efforts in the event of a bioterrorist attack. Accordingly, a genotype database capability is absolutely critical for monitoring and countering emerging threats. More information can be found about genotyping BW pathogens in Chapter 21.

4.3. Detailed Study of Emerged Pathogens

The investigation of how new pathogens arise in nature could lend insight into how an aggressor might modify an organism to use as a new threat. The more details that are learned about pathogenesis of various infectious diseases will greatly enhance our ability to identify and respond to the use of a novel agent. Primarily, the more we know about the "pathosphere" will enhance our ability to detect traits of pathogens and characterize these new organisms. Investment in monitoring organisms circulating in animals will also support our ability to avoid "tactical surprise" because many diseases such as SARS and influenza arise in the human population through close contact with domestic animals. In fact, emerging infectious disease surveillance is a natural partner in the fight against bioterrorism. Many programs within this discipline have been harnessed for this purpose (*see* Chapter 17 for more details).

4.4. Investment in Research on Nonspecific Immunity

In the event that a genetically modified agent were to be used, it is likely that we would not have on-hand a specific vaccine or therapeutic. Therefore, it is likely that we will be forced to rely on nontraditional measures for treatment of infected individuals. These treatments could come in the form of cytosine and guanosine (*see* Chapter 14) or the use of specific immunomodulators. Research in this area could be critical for countering an attack with a previously unknown threat agent.

5. CONCLUSIONS

The number of scenarios that an ill-intended group might invent is almost limitless certainly to the point that all possibilities could not be programmed in any reasonable manner. Even with good intelligence, we cannot be assured that a covert group will not develop novel agents. For this reason, our best defense is one of developing knowledge in key areas that will be useful should an event occur. This chapter attempts to address some of these key areas including genomic sequencing, informatics, forensic genotyping, emerging disease monitoring, and research. Linking all of these elements together to form a national shield against the use of modified or novel agents is our best and only viable defense.

ACKNOWLEDGMENTS

We thank Ted Plasse for reviewing the manuscript and making helpful suggestions.

DISCLAIMER

This chapter is the opinion of the authors and does not represent the view of the Department of Defense or of the Department of the Army.

REFERENCES

1. Abaev, I. V., Akimova, L. A., Shitov, V. T., Volozhantsev, N. V., and Svetoch, E. A. (1992) Transformation of pathogenic pseudomonas by plasmid DNA. *Mol. Gen. Mikrobiol. Virusol.* 17–20.
2. Abaev, I. V., Astashkin, E. I., Pachkunov, D. M., Stagis, N. I., Shitov, V. T., and Svetoch, E. A. (1995) *Pseudomonas mallei* and *Pseudomonas pseudomallei*: introduction and maintenance of natural and recombinant plasmid replicons. Mol. Gen. Mikrobiol. Virusol. 28–36.
3. Alibeck, K. and Handleman, S. (1999) *Biohazard.* Random House, New York.
4. Atlas, R. M. (2002) Public health. National security and the biological research community. *Science* **298,** 753, 754.
5. Bodur, H., Balaban, N., Aksaray, S., Yetener, V., Akinci, E., Colpan, A., and Erbay, A. (2003) Biotypes and antimicrobial susceptibilities of *Brucella* isolates. *Scand. J. Infect. Dis.* **35,** 337, 338.
6. Borzenkov, V. M., Pomerantsev, A. P., and Ashmarin, I. P. (1993) The additive synthesis of a regulatory peptide in vivo: the administration of a vaccinal *Francisella tularensis* strain that produces beta-endorphin. *Biull. Eksp. Biol. Med.* **116,** 151–153.
7. Borzenkov, V. M., Pomerantsev, A. P., Pomerantseva, O. M., and Ashmarin, I. P. (1994) Study of nonpathogenic strains of *Francisella, Brucella* and *Yersinia* as producers of recombinant beta-endorphin. *Biull. Eksp. Biol. Med.* **117,** 612–615.
8. Brubaker, R. R. (1991) Factors promoting acute and chronic diseases caused by yersiniae. *Clin. Microbiol. Rev.* **4,** 309–324.
9. Coker, P. R., Smith, K. L., and Hugh-Jones, M. E. (2002) Antimicrobial susceptibilities of diverse *Bacillus anthracis* isolates. *Antimicrob. Agents Chemother.* **46,** 3843–3845.
10. Drosten, C., Gunther, S., Preiser, W., et al. (2003) Identification of a novel coronavirus in patients with severe acute respiratory syndrome. *N. Engl. J. Med.* **348,** 1967–1976.
11. Esel, D., Doganay, M., and Sumerkan, B. (2003) Antimicrobial susceptibilities of 40 isolates of *Bacillus anthracis* isolated in Turkey. *Int. J. Antimicrob. Agents* 22, 70–72.
12. Finkel, E. (2001) Australia. Engineered mouse virus spurs bioweapon fears. *Science* **291,** 585.
13. Galimand, M., Guiyoule, A., Gerbaud, G., et al. (1997) Multidrug resistance in *Yersinia pestis* mediated by a transferable plasmid. *N. Engl. J. Med.* **337,** 677–680.

14. Gorelov, V. N., Gubina, E. A., Grekova, N. A., and Skavronskaia, A. G. (1991) The possibility of creating a vaccinal strain of *Brucella abortus* 19-BA with multiple antibiotic resistance. *Zh. Mikrobiol. Epidemiol. Immunobiol.* 2–4.

15. Guiyoule, A., Gerbaud, G., Buchrieser, C., et al. (2001) Transferable plasmid-mediated resistance to streptomycin in a clinical isolate of *Yersinia pestis. Emerg. Infect. Dis.* **7,** 43–48.

16. Jackson, R. J., Ramsay, A. J., Christensen, C. D., Beaton, S., Hall, D. F., and Ramshaw, I. A. (2001) Expression of mouse interleukin-4 by a recombinant ectromelia virus suppresses cytolytic lymphocyte responses and overcomes genetic resistance to mousepox. *J. Virol.* **75,** 1205–1210.

17. Ksiazek, T. G., Erdman, D., Goldsmith, C. S., et al. (2003) A novel coronavirus associated with severe acute respiratory syndrome. *N. Engl. J. Med.* **348,** 1953–1966.

18. Marra, M. A., Jones, S. J., Astell, C. R., et al. (2003) The Genome sequence of the SARS-associated coronavirus. *Science* **300,** 1399–1404.

19. Mullbacher, A. and Lobigs, M. (2001) Creation of killer poxvirus could have been predicted. *J. Virol.* **75,** 8353–8355.

20. Ochman, H., Lawrance, J. G., and Groisman, E. A. (2000) Lateral gene transfer and the nature of bacterial innovation. *Nature* **405,** 299–304.

21. Pomerantsev, A. P., Staritsin, N. A., Mockov Yu, V., and Marinin, L. I. (1997) Expression of cereolysine AB genes in *Bacillus anthracis* vaccine strain ensures protection against experimental hemolytic anthrax infection. *Vaccine* **15,** 1846–1850.

22. Pomerantsev, A. P. and Staritsyn, N. A. (1996) Behavior of heterologous recombinant plasmid pCET in cells of *Bacillus anthracis. Genetika* **32,** 500–509.

23. Rota, P. A., Oberste, M. S., Monroe, S. S., et al. (2003) Characterization of a novel coronavirus associated with severe acute respiratory syndrome. *Science* **300,** 1394–1399.

24. Smith, M. D., Vinh, D. X., Nguyen, T. T., Wain, J., Thung, D., and White, N. J. (1995) In vitro antimicrobial susceptibilities of strains of *Yersinia pestis. Antimicrob. Agents Chemother.* **39,** 2153, 2154.

25. Verevkin, V. V., Volozhantsev, N. V., Miakinina, V. P., and Svetoch, E. A. (1997) Effect of TRA-system of plasmids RP4 and R68.45 on *Pseudomonas mallei* virulence. *Vestn. Ross. Akad. Med. Nauk.* 37–40.

26. Wong, J. D., Barash, J. R., Sandfort, R. F., and Janda, J. M. (2000) Susceptibilities of *Yersinia pestis* strains to 12 antimicrobial agents. *Antimicrob. Agents Chemother.* **44,** 1995, 1996.

27. Ziebuhr, J. (2003) SARS—unprecedented global response to a newly emerging disease. *Int. J. Med. Microbiol.* **293,** 229–231.

17

Department of Defense Global Emerging Infections System Programs in Biodefense

Julie A. Pavlin and Patrick W. Kelley

1. THE DEPARTMENT OF DEFENSE GLOBAL EMERGING INFECTIONS SYSTEM

One of the great fallacies of the mid-20th century was that infectious diseases were nearing elimination. In the face of those prognostications, more than 25 new infectious diseases were recognized for the first time between 1975 and 2000. These new scourges included HIV, Ebola, Legionnaire's Disease, Hantavirus pulmonary syndrome, deadly new strains of influenza, and new forms of drug-resistant bacteria and malaria. Rather than nearing extinction as a broad class of human suffering, infectious diseases remain the leading cause of death worldwide. The ability of microbes to adapt to new pressures, including antibiotic usage coupled with changes in society, technology, and the environment make it likely that the microbial threat will remain a threat to humanity, and even suggests the possibility of regional and global epidemics comparable to the worst in history.

Although naturally occurring microbial threats remain a perennial threat, the politics of international relations and terrorism result in the additional threat of the use of weaponized biological agents. The fall of the Soviet Union and the position of the United States as the sole global superpower, coupled with the growing sophistication of various state and nonstate sponsored adversaries, have contributed to a situation of increased risk of biological warfare (BW). In current circumstances, a glut of underemployed bioweaponeers combined with advances in the science of microbiology may empower otherwise weak adversaries to asymmetrically wage BW.

Infectious diseases are more than an issue of individual health. There has been an increasing appreciation of their effects on international trade, the stability of families, institutions, and societies, and military readiness. Under this broader context, the control of infectious diseases is increasingly seen as a fundamental element of national security. Such considerations in the early 1990s prompted groups such as the National Academy of Sciences, the Centers for Disease Control and Prevention (CDC), and the World Health Organization (WHO) to develop plans for addressing and mitigating the threat of emerging and re-emerging infectious diseases. The Department of Defense (DOD) figured heavily in the recommended actions from these deliberative bodies because of its wide spectrum of domestic and international assets for

From: *Infectious Diseases: Biological Weapons Defense: Infectious Diseases and Counterterrorism*
Edited by: L. E. Lindler, F. J. Lebeda, and G. W. Korch © Humana Press Inc., Totowa, NJ

infectious disease surveillance, research, and control. These recommendations in June 1996 led to Presidential Decision Directive NSTC-7 on Emerging Infections. This directive formally expanded the mission of the DOD to support global surveillance, training, research, and response to emerging infectious disease threats.

The DOD Global Emerging Infections System (DOD-GEIS) is the centrally coordinated DOD response to the Presidential Decision Directive. Using Army, Navy, and Air Force preventive medicine and infectious disease personnel plus unique DOD assets such as the overseas medical research units in Egypt, Kenya, Peru, Thailand, and Indonesia and the availability of a global military health care network, DOD-GEIS has developed sophisticated programs to enhance surveillance for new and re-emerging infections; develop and integrate relevant military public health systems; improve prevention and control strategies; and leverage international and DOD public health infrastructure through the facilitation of training, networking, and capacity building.

DOD-GEIS surveillance has a primary focus on traditional military threats such as influenza and other respiratory diseases, drug-resistant malaria, and drug-resistant enteric organisms. However, the emergence of new or unfamiliar diseases to include agents of bioterrorism and BW is clearly of concern. These represent a particular challenge because available laboratory diagnostic methods may be nonexistent, very limited, or insensitive.

1.1. GEIS and Biodefense

Detecting new and reemerging infections, to include bioterrorism, not only requires laboratory capabilities but also prompt recognition of an aberration in community health. Delays in recognition can lead to considerable morbidity and mortality even when a specific preventive or therapeutic modality is available. Many of the disease emergences over the last 25 yr have been characterized by delayed recognition or diagnosis. For example, the appearance of West Nile encephalitis in New York City in 1999 was manifest as weeks of human and animal morbidity before the problem was recognized as an old disease in a new location.

Whether the goal is to detect a new syndrome such as AIDS or Hantavirus pulmonary syndrome or the insidious initial manifestations of a deliberate attack with a biological agent, the recognition across a population of unusual syndromes or a change in the frequency of common syndromes or symptom patterns may be an important harbinger. This is different from the traditional clinical and laboratory approach to public health surveillance that tends to focus on tracking well-defined diseases of public health significance. A complementary epidemiologic approach has been embraced by DOD-GEIS as key to maintaining a comprehensive, alert public health system. The concept of epidemiologists playing a central role in the detection of biological attacks and other emerging infections is not a new one. In 1952, Alexander Langmuir, the founder of CDC's Epidemic Intelligence Service noted:

> "The detection and control of saboteurs are the responsibilities of the FBI, but the recognition of epidemics caused by sabotage is peculiarly an epidemiologic function .... Therefore any plan of defense against biological warfare sabotage requires trained epidemiologists, alert to all possibilities, and available for call at a moment's notice anywhere in the country." *(1)*

The expectation is that early detection of emerging infections, to include deliberate biological attacks, will require a system of innovative techniques to detect a wide range of possible scenarios across a dispersed population. These may range from isolated cases, such as the anthrax letter attacks of Fall 2001, through small-scale events such as an attack against a group of people in a building or at a gathering, to a more extensive attack against one or more population centers. The mobility of modern society presents added challenges because cases from a common point infection may disperse across a community or even the globe. Case clusters would initially be undetectable at the level of clinicians or individual health care facilities but would require consolidation over larger catchment areas. Even more insideous, low-impact attacks may indicate "experiments" or failed attempts for a larger impact by a determined adversary. Thus, the goal is not only early detection of large and small outbreaks but also the rapid epidemiologic assessment of the situation so as to optimally deploy limited response assets and to empower civil leaders with credible information for risk communication to an anxious population. The DOD, as a result of having a singular global medical informatics backbone, is in a unique position to pioneer innovative approaches to community-based, near real-time detection of changes in health indicators. DOD-GEIS has made adaptation of these unique assets a feature of response to the President's call for enhanced public health surveillance, systems research, and integration.

2. USING SURVEILLANCE TO IMPROVE BIODEFENSE

2.1. Need for Improved Disease Surveillance

The advent of relatively focal biological attacks in the United States in 2001 emphasized what has long been suspected—that the public health infrastructure had deteriorated over time and the medical system was not prepared for this contingency (2–4). We need to plan and be prepared to prevent illness and death that may result from a biological terrorist attack. Similar to any emerging infection, early detection is key to controlling the spread of an outbreak. Detection and control of a disease outbreak depends on a strong and flexible public health systems at local, state, and federal levels (5).

One of the primary goals of public health is to prevent disease in a community. Therefore, one must have knowledge of existing disease rates, risk factors for these diseases, and the effectiveness of preventive measures. The first step in gaining this knowledge is a working surveillance system that rapidly allows the public health practitioner to know the health status of the community. Indeed, public health surveillance is a core element of public health practice. Unfortunately, most infectious disease surveillance systems are passive and rely on practitioners voluntarily reporting to the public health system (6). Not only do reports often take weeks to months to receive, but gross underreporting is usually the norm. A recent review of reportable disease reporting in the US military revealed the Army centrally reported 45% of hospitalized reportable disease cases when compared to International Classification of Diseases, 9th Revision (ICD9) discharge diagnoses during the period January–June 2001 (7).The Navy and Air Force each reported 18% of these cases over the same time period (8,9). Additionally, most are based on laboratory results that, although improving the specificity of the report, increases the lag time between the onset of illness and the report being sent. In the previous review, of those diseases that were reported by the Army, 45% were reported within 1 wk of hospital discharge and 76% were reported within 1 mo *(7)*. For bioterrorism, if the notification of something unusual occurring reaches the health department quickly, then the investigation, treatment, prophylaxis, and preventive measures can be started that much sooner. In many instances, early response can allow significant improvements in morbidity, mortality, and decrease costs *(10)*. Therefore, we must improve our public health surveillance systems to allow rapid acquisition of important disease incidence information.

2.1.1. Historical Disease Outbreaks

Recent disease outbreaks in the United States demonstrate characteristics that serve as important lessons in developing surveillance systems. The outbreak of Legionnaires' Disease in Pennsylvania in 1976 shows how an unknown pathogen acquired via respiratory exposure from a common source can present *(11)*. This outbreak mimics a bioterrorist attack with an aerosolized agent. The situation was complicated by a population that dispersed after exposure, so cases appeared throughout the state. This can also happen with a bioterrorist attack and can confuse the investigation. In 2001, the index case of anthrax in Florida had recently traveled to North Carolina, which made the investigation and search for the source of infection that much more difficult. With the wide range of potential incubation periods inherent in agents that could be used for bioterrorism, similar scenarios should be anticipated. Surveillance systems that can rapidly compare diseases seen throughout the state or even the country are necessary.

Other lessons learned from recent disease outbreaks in the United States include the impact of zoonotic illnesses. With hantavirus infections in the southwestern United States, rodents brought the virus into homes as their populations expanded as a result of fluctuations in environmental conditions *(12)*. In 1999, West Nile virus was first identified as an autochthonous disease in New York City *(13)*. This event had features one would anticipate from a bioterrorist event, but most experts have determined this to have been a natural, accidental introduction. Human cases were preceded by deaths in wild and zoo-kept birds, although the significance of the association was not realized at first. Both of these outbreaks demonstrate the need to keep in mind both the ability of various vectors to transmit potential bioterrorist-induced disease and the impact of a new disease on other species.

2.1.2. Need for Early Recognition of Disease Outbreaks

Developers of surveillance systems must determine their priorities based on their objectives. Because surveillance can be used for many purposes, the reason for the surveillance is of the utmost importance in determining which qualities are essential. For surveillance systems that monitor long-term trends in disease rates or evaluate the effectiveness of a public health program, accuracy is needed more than timeliness. However, to rapidly detect and respond to a nascent disease outbreak, quickly acquiring disease incidence data and analyzing it is of crucial concern. Although accuracy is not unimportant to disease outbreak investigations, the initial notification of a potential outbreak can be based on less accurate data, as long as it allows more in-depth investigation after the alert. In fact, the entire purpose of disease outbreak surveillance is notification that a more thorough and accurate investigation needs to be performed.

This may be as simple as a phone call to a local clinic inquiring as to the status of patients or as comprehensive as door-to-door documentation of illness.

The early recognition that something unusual is happening in a community can improve the public health response, even before the entire investigation is completed. If evidence is sufficient that a disease of high morbidity or mortality is present, the initial presentation of that disease outbreak can suggest the initial or continuing means of exposure. For example, the disease may present in a way that suggests person-to-person spread. If this is the case, then certain preventive measures such as closing of schools, altering public gatherings, and so on, can be instituted even before the specific etiologic agent is identified. This was done during the influenza pandemic in 1918, before they knew the cause of the epidemic. Even with diseases of lower virulence, measures can be taken to decrease the potential spread of an illness, such as recommendations to confine new ill recruits to the hospital to decrease transmission in crowded barracks situations. Should the surveillance data suggest other transmission routes, such as water- or vector-borne, then early measures can target water distribution systems or integrated pest management operations.

Another important element that surveillance can provide is to identify whether the epidemic curve generates secondary cases, which would be expected with only a limited number of bioterrorist agents (e.g., plague or smallpox), or the kinetics yield a discrete "peak" more consistent with a nonpropagated outbreak.

Information rapidly obtained from a disease surveillance system can also assist in providing information to decision makers. Although not of the highest accuracy, initial information obtained by surveillance systems can include geographic information on disease occurrence, disease virulence, and general signs and symptoms of the illness. This information can then be used to determine at-risk populations and to inform people what symptoms they should look for, what they should do (stay home, seek medical attention) and what areas seem to be most affected. In addition, this basic information can help public officials best allocate limited resources. For example, if it is recommended that antibiotics be used for treatment, certain stockpiles of medication can be directed to the areas most impacted. Personnel resources can be similarly allocated.

Whereas early response based on nonspecific information can be very helpful, the best use of early recognition of a potential disease outbreak is the indication to conduct an investigation to find more accurate information. In particular, a specific microbiological diagnosis will be most helpful in instituting preventive measures. Often in clinical settings, especially with diseases of low severity, diagnostic specimens are not taken. If the disease is not severe, it is common practice to treat patients empirically and save time and money on laboratory tests that probably will not affect the outcome of the patient's illness, as the patient often recovers before the laboratory diagnosis is obtained. However, the first cases in a disease outbreak, if investigated, can provide crucial information to prevent or limit the spread of the outbreaks through proper treatment and prophylactic protocols. For example, the index case of anthrax in Florida had meningeal symptoms that prompted the physician to take cerebrospinal fluid for culture and Gram stain *(14)*. The use of diagnostic tests allowed a more rapid recognition of the cause of the disease and assisted with recognition of future cases and the institution of preventive measures. In this case, the disease presentation and severity contributed to the taking of diagnostic specimens. In other disease outbreaks caused by pathogens such as Norwalk or influenza viruses, although there are appropriate preventive or treatment measures available, the lack of severity of the disease may result in few diagnostic tests performed. The result of this omission is that the outbreak can continue and future patients will not receive the most appropriate care as they could have with knowledge of the disease-causing agent. Nor will the most effective preventive measures be enacted at the earliest possible opportunity. Early indication of unusual disease patterns can allow health departments to request appropriate diagnostic tests on current and future patients in order to obtain the correct diagnosis quickly and improve the ability to prevent and treat future cases.

An additional way that surveillance systems can assist public health is in the ability to provide important demographic information that can assist in the outbreak investigation. If surveillance systems are linked to patient identifiers, then the investigators can rapidly perform chart reviews, determine geographic locations of high case density, and even contact the patient to determine current health status, risk factors, or to obtain diagnostic specimens. Although privacy concerns are paramount and must adhere to local law, it is in the course of proper public health practice that these investigations are carried out to protect the health of a community.

2.2. Ways to Improve Surveillance

For rapid detection of a bioterrorist attack or any disease outbreak, the speed of data acquisition and analysis must be improved to be of use in mitigation efforts. This can be done in various of ways, including instituting new data collection methods, using previously collected health data in new ways, and using nontraditional sources of data to track the health of a community. A summary of potential data sources is outlined in Table 1. A combination of many types of data sources may provide the most sensitive system.

2.2.1. Institution of a New Surveillance System

The most useful data can usually be obtained from surveillance systems that are designed specifically for the purpose intended. If tracking infectious disease incidence for bioterrorism detection is the purpose, then the surveillance system can be designed to capture information that can assist in this detection. Some of the data elements that might be of use are included in Table 2.

The most accurate information is obtained through active surveillance systems that continually query patients, providers, or other personnel on new potential cases. Although of great use in detecting unusual disease trends, these systems are often labor intensive and not well-accepted by those having to provide the information. One way to improve the acceptability is to give feedback to the provider or other person contributing the information to let them know how their work is assisting in disease detection, and also allow them to tailor their treatment regimens with the knowledge of surrounding disease trends. For the most rapid disease information transfer, the system should be automated and the data entered and reported electronically.

Many of these new data source systems have been tried in various of situations. Some have been used in event-driven scenarios—that is, for a limited time period around an event of high public exposure and, thus, higher than usual potential threat of

Table 1
Potential Sources of Data for Infectious Disease Surveillance

Typical health surveillance	Reportable diseases
	Laboratory-based surveillance
	Specific disease surveillance (e.g. influenza)
Existing health data not normally used for surveillance	Billing data with diagnostics for inpatients and outpatients
	Prescription and over-the-counter pharmacy sales
	Laboratory test ordering and results
	Radiology test ordering and results
	Intensive care unit admissions
	Emergency room utilization
	Medical advice call-in lines
	Internet hits for medical information
	911 calls or ambulance run information
	Data from medical examiner
Nonhealth data sources	School and work absenteeism
	Road and transit usage
	Entertainment venues usage
	Weather data
	Vector data

Table 2
Example of Ideal Data Fields for Disease Outbreak Investigations

Age
Gender
Onset of illness
Symptoms
Vital signs
Work/school/day care and home locations of patient
Recent travel
Potential exposures through day care or restaurants
Any ill contacts
Attended any recent large public events
Occupation
Underlying illnesses
Medications used or prescribed
Lab tests ordered and results

bioterrorism *(15)*. They have also been used on an ongoing basis in some localities with varying amounts of participation and automation. Although the experience to date has been that these systems have the potential to provide very useful and timely information, they have had varying degrees of acceptance and utility. The greatest detriment has been the need for additional work for the healthcare provider to enter the information. A decrease in data entry resulting from providers' lack of time is often realized when the data is needed the most (e.g., during an outbreak situation). An additional problem for those used only during or after an event is the lack of pre-existing data for comparison. Surveillance systems need to provide more than a snapshot in time to be useful. In fact, the definition of surveillance includes the criteria of "ongoing" *(16)*. Public health surveillance must demonstrate change or lack of change in disease rates over time. Therefore, if a surveillance system is only used for a 2- to 3-wk time period, it will be very difficult to determine abnormal patterns of disease incidence because the baseline rate is not established.

2.2.2. Use of Previously Existing Health Data for New Surveillance Methods

There are many sources of health data that exist for reasons other than public health surveillance. Many of these serve a logistic or financial purpose. Some examples are outpatient and inpatient diagnostic coding for insurance claims purposes, tallies of hospital admissions or emergency room visits for personnel allocation, or records of pharmacy prescriptions for legal documentation. With the increasing use of an electronic medical record, other information such as laboratory test ordering and results, radiology orders and results, and even vital signs can be retrieved from electronic databases. Although many of these sources were not created for a public health surveillance purpose, the amount of information available that can be useful for tracking disease trends is absolutely astounding.

Because these sources of data were not intended for surveillance, some aspects of their collection, format or content may not be ideal for monitoring disease trends. First, and most important, the data may not be collected in a timely fashion, or it may be difficult to retrieve soon after collection. An example of this is insurance claims data for billing purposes that may take weeks to be processed. Second, the data may not be in an ideal or even electronic format, making useful retrieval difficult. Third, information may not be available that would make it ideal for a surveillance system. For example, if a system is designed to track diarrheal illnesses, certain information such as recent travel or eating history would be beneficial but is unlikely to be available on an electronic database. However, although not ideal, the data can still be useful for public health purposes.

Finally, issues with privacy may complicate access to data. The privacy issues are both personal and commercial. To access personal medical information, stringent privacy protection elements must be in place. Even without specific identifying information such as name or social security number, demographic information such as date of birth, gender, race, address, or even zip code can be used in aggregate to identify someone. Therefore, care must be taken to ensure that the data are held securely, and any information released for use by various public health personnel must have appropriate anonymity algorithms in place to ensure that identity is not gleaned from basic demographic information. Access to information by law enforcement agencies for leads or clues in a bioterrorist attack may also need to be considered.

The other concern is the sensitivity regarding commercial privacy. Many sources of data are held by for-profit hospitals, clinics, pharmacies, and other contracting agencies. Access to the data might be hindered by the desire of these organizations to keep the data private to protect their profits and methods from competitors. These are legitimate concerns and may necessitate strict legal agreements between data sources and recipients.

2.2.3. Use of Nontraditional Sources of Data for Detection of Disease Outbreaks

In addition to previously collected health-related data, there are other sources of information that might prove useful for early warning of a disease outbreak. As people become ill, they demonstrate certain behaviors that may be measurable. These could include changes in road or public transit use, a decrease in the use of entertainment venues such as restaurants and movie theaters, or an increase in school or work absenteeism. There is also information such as weather conditions or changes in vector populations that may prove useful in predicting conditions that foster disease outbreaks *(17,18)*. However, many of these sources of data are not yet proven to be of use in disease outbreak prediction or detection; indeed most have not yet even been captured for that purpose. Because there are less privacy concerns resulting from no medical information being included, these sources may be easier to obtain and may be worth investigating further.

2.3. Examples of New Surveillance Systems

Several new surveillance systems using various data resources are being developed by states, cities, academic institutions, private companies, and federal institutions including the DOD. Many of these have demonstrated remarkable utility in monitoring the health status of communities. A sample of some of these systems are outlined here.

2.3.1. New York City Diarrheal Diseases Surveillance

New York City has three complementary systems to monitor for outbreaks of diarrheal illness. They include sales of over-the-counter antidiarrheal medications, the number of stool samples submitted for testing, and the incidence of gastroenteritis in nursing home populations *(19,20)*. The first two are examples of nontraditional health indicator surveillance methods, whereas the third represents a form of specific health surveillance initiated for a specific purpose. Through monitoring of sales of over-the-counter drugs, the New York City Department of Environmental Protection has been able to detect anomalies in sales data that could herald a gastrointestinal outbreak *(20)*. Similarly, in retrospect, one of the first changes recorded during a Cryptosporidium outbreak in Minnesota was the increase in over-the-counter antidiarrheal medication sales *(21)*. The monitoring of laboratory test ordering such as stool sample submissions as opposed to laboratory test results allows a much more rapid notification of a potential change in disease incidence. These systems trade specificity for sensitivity but quickly recommend investigations to determine what disease agent is causing illness.

2.3.2. New York City 911 Disease Surveillance

In 1998, the New York City Department of Health began monitoring chief complaints for 911 calls in the city *(22)*. The calls are coded with a diagnosis from a specific list. They chose to monitor those potentially indicative of an influenza outbreak such as "difficulty breathing" or "sick." Review of data previous to 1998 revealed a temporal association between a rise in calls for these complaints and annual influenza outbreaks. Since its inception, the system has detected influenza outbreaks earlier than any other traditional influenza surveillance system in New York City and provides information on long-term historical cycles of respiratory disease *(22)*.

2.3.3. University of Pittsburgh Emergency Room Surveillance

The University of Pittsburgh has developed a surveillance system using routinely generated outpatient data from emergency rooms for real-time outbreak and disease surveillance (RODS). This system utilizes ICD9 codes generated by the triage nurse at the time of presentation to the emergency room and by the clinician who sees and diagnoses the patient. Using sophisticated algorithms, RODS is able to detect changes in the number of patients presenting with certain types of symptoms and diseases, taking into account such confounders as day of the week, time of day, season, and other variables *(23,24)*.

2.3.4. Harvard University Outpatient Surveillance

A similar system has been developed by the Harvard University Medical School, the Massachusetts Department of Public Health, and the CDC using data from the Harvard Vanguard Medical Associates, a large group practice located in eastern Massachusetts *(25)*. They used ICD9 codes generated at 14 health clinics that provide ambulatory care including scheduled appointments and same day and urgent care visits in greater Boston. In one study looking at lower respiratory diagnoses, they demonstrated daily and seasonal variation, as well as differences by age groups and gender. With census tract information, they were able to track changes in disease occurrence geographically.

2.3.5. Web-Based Surveillance System

A consortium of private companies have developed the computerized surveillance and response tool Lightweight Epidemiology Advanced Detection and Emergency Response System (LEADERS) *(26,27)*. This system includes not just surveillance tools but the ability to track response assets geographically and share them among various emergency response and medical groups via an application service provider. Another element is a rapid diagnostic module using polymerase chain reaction techniques *(26)*. The surveillance module contains the ability to design a computerized information sheet requesting specific information for disease monitoring in emergency rooms. This information is entered via the website and then shared among participating medical facilities. Statistical analysis can be performed with this data for detection of abnormal levels of illness *(27)*. LEADERS also has the ability to pull various information from a computerized medical record and analyze it to detect variations indicative of a disease outbreak.

2.3.6. New Mexico's Emergency Room Surveillance

Researchers at the Sandia National Laboratory, Los Alamos National Laboratory, University of New Mexico, and the New Mexico Department of Health have developed a surveillance method using newly gathered data to detect changes in disease patterns in emergency room visits in New Mexico *(28)*. The system, the Rapid Syndrome Validation Project (RSVP), uses handheld computers with touch screens for the provider to enter basic demographic and diagnostic data on their patients. Its added features include a direct reporting link to the health department for patients with sufficiently suspicious disease patterns and immediate feedback to the practitioner on information of disease patterns being seen in the area.

2.3.7. DOD-GEIS Outpatient Surveillance System

The GEIS has also developed a surveillance system using outpatient (both emergency room and outpatient clinics) data generated at military treatment facilities (MTFs). The Electronic Surveillance System for the Early Notification of Community-based Epidemics (ESSENCE) uses ICD9 diagnostic codes generated by the healthcare provider near the time of patient visit to track various potential infectious disease patterns. The ICD9 codes are divided into seven syndrome groups most likely to represent infectious disease presentations. Outpatient data from all MTFs are received from a central server and processed to demonstrate changes in visits for the various syndrome groups. As with most of the other surveillance systems, the data can be displayed demographically by age and gender and geographically by zip code. Provision of this information on a secure website allows sharing of the data with appropriate public health personnel.

2.4. The Ability of ESSENCE to Detect Outbreaks

ESSENCE has detected many fluctuations in diseases since the pilot project was first instituted for the national capital area in 1999. These include expected yearly influenza epidemics as well as other random disease outbreaks. After September 11, 2001, the system was expanded to include coverage of all MTFs that contribute outpatient data into this electronic system. This includes all but the most forward deployed military forces, including installations in Asia and Europe.

2.4.1. Detection of Annual Influenza Outbreaks

Influenza outbreaks occur during the winter season in most of the temperate world, including the United States. Each year's influenza epidemic has different characteristics including the timing and length of peak activity, and the severity of the outbreak. However, there is always a yearly increase in people presenting for influenza-like illness (fever and cough or sore throat), pneumonia-related deaths, and isolation of influenza viruses from laboratory samples. Using ESSENCE to follow visits that have been coded by the provider as any kind of respiratory ailment, we can follow respiratory illness year round and detect within 2–3 d when any outbreaks begin, including the yearly influenza epidemics.

The data collected by ESSENCE can be compared to data from more traditional surveillance systems, such as that collected by the CDC. Figure 1 shows both surveillance systems for influenza season 1999–2000 using sentinel physicians who report the percent of patients who meet the case definition of influenza-like illness (ILI). To make a direct comparison, we have figured the ESSENCE data in a similar format as the CDC data by calculating the percent of visits on a weekly basis for a respiratory illness. The average percent of patients with a respiratory complaint is higher than that seen with the CDC surveillance. This is expected, because they do not have to meet the same stringent ILI case definition. The codes included in the respiratory syndrome group are listed in Table 3, which are less restrictive, as a patient only has to be diagnosed with one of these to be included. Regardless, the similarity of the epidemic curve is striking, and ESSENCE detects the influenza outbreak as well as more traditional data sources. The benefit of ESSENCE is that the data are received in 1–3 d and do not require additional work by the provider, whereas the CDC data are not available for public consumption for a longer period of time. It also requires the sentinel physicians to perform additional work to create this dataset.

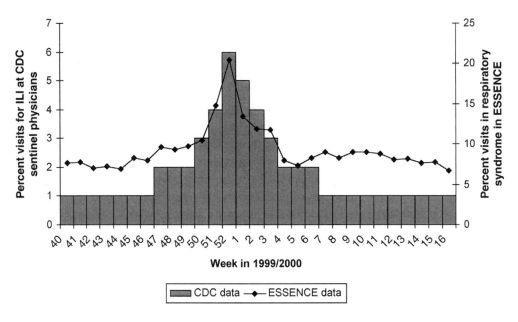

Fig. 1. Comparison of ESSENCE data in the national capital area and national CDC influenza data for 1999–2000.

Table 3
ICD9 Codes Included in the Respiratory Syndrome Group

ICD9 code	Description
003.22	Pneumonia, salmonella
020.3	Plague, primary pneumonic
020.4	Plague, secondary pneumonic
020.5	Plague, pneumonic NOS
021.2	Tularemia, pulmonary
022.1	Anthrax, pulmonary
031.0	Disease, pulmonary d/t mycobacteria
031.8	Disease, mycobacterial NEC
031.9	Disease, mycobacterial NOS
032.0	Diphtheria, faucial
032.1	Diphtheria, nasopharyngeal
032..2	Diphtheria, anterior nasal
032.3	Diphtheria, laryngeal
032.89	Diphtheria NEC
032.9	Diphtheria NOS
033.0	Whooping cough, Bordetella pertussis
033.1	Whooping cough, Bordetella parapertussis
033.8	Whooping cough NEC
033.9	Whooping cough NOS
034.0	Sore throat, streptococcal
052.1	Varicella pneumonitis

(continued)

Table 3 (continued)

ICD9 code	Description
055.1	Pneumonia, postmeasles
055.2	Otitis media, postmeasles
073.0	Ornithosis w/pneumonia
079.0	Infection, adenovirus
079.1	Infection, ECHO virus
079.2	Infection, Coxsackie virus
079.3	Infection, rhinovirus
079.6	Infection, respiratory syncytial virus
079.82	SARS associated coronavirus
079.88	Infection, chlamydial NEC
079.89	Infection, viral NEC
079.98	Infection, chlamydial NOS
079.99	Infection, viral NOS
381.00	OM, acute nonsuppurative NOS
381.01	OM, acute serous
381.03	OM, acute sanguinous
381.04	OM, acute allergic serous
381.4	OM, chronic nonsuppurative NOS
381.50	Salpingitis, Eustachian NOS
381.51	Salpingitis, acute Eustachian
382.00	OM, acute suppurative NOS
382.01	OM, acute suppurative w/drum rupture
382.02	OM, acute suppurative in disease CE
382.4	Otitis supprative NOS
382.9	Otitis media NOS
460	Nasopharyngitis, acute
461.0	Sinusitis, acute maxillary
461.1	Sinusitis, acute frontal
461.2	Sinusitis, acute ethmoidal
461.3	Sinusitis, acute sphenoidal
461.8	Sinusitis, acute NEC
461.9	Sinusitis, acute NOS
462	Pharyngitis, acute
463	Tonsillitis, acute
464.00	Laryngitis, acute, w/o obstruction
464.01	Laryngitis, acute w/ obstruction
464.10	Tracheitis, acute, w/o obstruction
464.20	Laryngotracheitis, acute w/o obstruction
464.21	laryngotracheitis, acute w/ obstruction
464.30	Epiglottitis, acute w/o obstruction
464.31	Epiglottitis, acute w/ obstruction
464.4	Croup
464.50	Supraglottis, unspecified w/o obstruction
464.51	Supraglottis, unspecified w/ obstruction
465.0	Laryngopharyngitis, acute

(continued)

Table 3 (continued)

ICD9 code	Description
465.8	Acute URI of other multiple sites
465.9	Acute URI of unspecified site
466.0	Bronchitis, acute
466.1	Bronchiolitis, acute
466.11	Bronchiolitis, acute, d/t RSV
466.19	Bronchio acute d/t infectious organism
478.9	Disease, upper respiratory NEC/NOS
480.0	Pneumonia, adenovirus
480.1	Pneumonia d/t respiratory syncytial virus
480.2	Pneumonia d/t parainfluenza virus
480.3	Pneumonia d/t SARS
480.8	Pneumonia d/t virus NEC
480.9	Pneumonia d/t virus NOS
481	Pneumonia d/t pneumococca virus
482.0	Pneumonia d/t Klebsiella pneumoniae
482.1	Pneumonia d/y Pseudomonas
482.2	Pneumonia d/t Hemophilus influenzae
482.30	Pneumonia d/t Streptococcus NOS
482.31	Pneumonia d/t Streptococcus Group A
482.32	Pneumonia d/t Streptococcus Group B
482.39	Pneumonia d/t Streptococcus NEC
482.40	Pneunonia d/t Staphylococus NOS
482.41	Pneumonia d/t Staphylococcus aureus
482.49	Pneumonia d/t Staphylococcus NEC
482.81	Pneumonia d/t anaerobes
482.82	Pneumonia d/t Escherichia coli
482.83	Pneumonia d/t gram-negative NEC
482.84	Pneumonia d/t Legionnaires' disease
482.89	Pneumonia, bacterial NEC
482.9	Pneumonia, bacterial NOS
483.0	Pneumonia d/t Mycoplasma pneumoniae
483.1	Pneumonia d/t Chlamydia
483.8	Pneumonia D/T organism NEC
484.1	Pneumonia in cytomegalic inclusion disease
484.3	Pneumonia in whooping cough
484.5	Pneumonia in anthrax
484.6	Pneumonia in aspergillosis
484.7	Pneumonia in systemic mycoses
484.8	Pneumonia in other infectious disease CE
485	Bronchopneumonia, organism NOS
486	Pneumonia, organism NOS
487.0	Influenza w/pneumonia
487.1	Influenza w/respiratory manifestation NEC
487.8	Influenza w/manifestation NEC
490	Bronchitis NOS

(continued)

Table 3 (continued)

ICD9 code	Description
494.1	Bronchiectasis with acute exacerbation
511.0	Pleurisy w/o effusion or TB
511.1	Pleurisy, w/bacterial effusion, not TB
511.8	Pleurisy, effusion NED, not TB
511.9	Effusion, pleural NOS
513.0	Abscess, lung
513.1	Abscess, mediastinum
514	Congestion/hypostasis, pulmonary
5517.3	Acute chest syndrome
518.0	Collapse, pulmonary
518.4	Edema, acute lung NOS
518.81	Failure, acute respiratory
518.82	Insufficiency, pulmonary NEC
518.84	Respiratory failure, acute & chronic
519.2	Mediastinitis
519.3	Disease, mediastinum NEC
769	Syndrome, respiratory distress
782.5	Cyanosis
784.1	Pain, throat
786.00	Abnormality, respiratory NOS
786.05	Shortness of breath
786.06	Tachypnea
786.07	Wheezing
786.09	Abnormality, respiratory NEC
786.1	Stridor
786.2	Cough
786.3	Hemoptysis
786.52	Painful respiration
786.7	Abnormal chest sounds
786.9	Symptons involving respiratory system/chest NEC

NOS, not otherwise specified; NEC, not elsewhere classified; d/t, due to; w/, with; w/o, without; OM, otitis media; CE, classified elsewhere; URI, upper respiratory infection; RSV, respiratory syncytial virus; SARS, severe acute respiratory syndrome; TB, tuberculosis.

2.4.2. Detection of Multiple Gastrointestinal Outbreaks Nationwide

In January 2002, the ESSENCE system detected spikes in the gastrointestinal ICD9 syndrome code group at the Marine Corps Recruit Depot in San Diego, CA, Fort Monmouth, NJ, Aberdeen Proving Ground, MD, and Fort Leonard Wood, MO (*see* Fig. 2). Because of the near-simultaneous occurrence of these outbreaks, investigations were undertaken to determine the potential source and cause and also to ensure that nothing else suspicious occurred that could be considered a warning of a bioterrorist attack. The largest outbreak occurred in San Diego, and a medical records review was conducted to ascertain the characteristics of the outbreak.

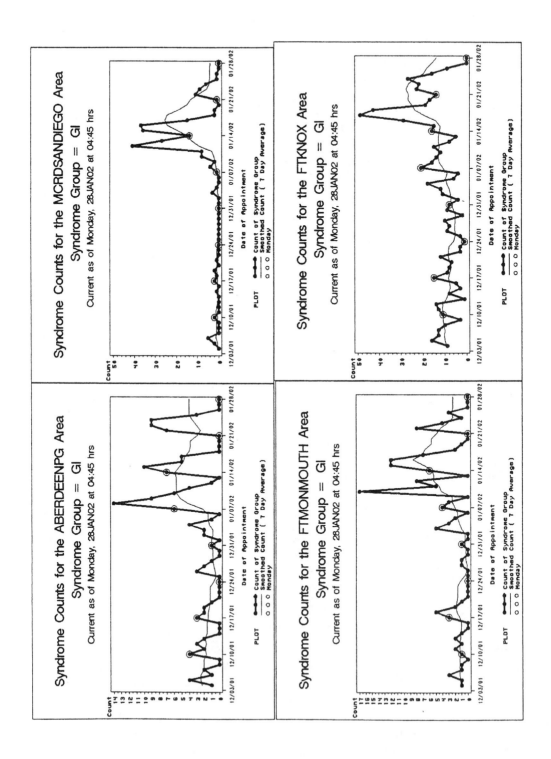

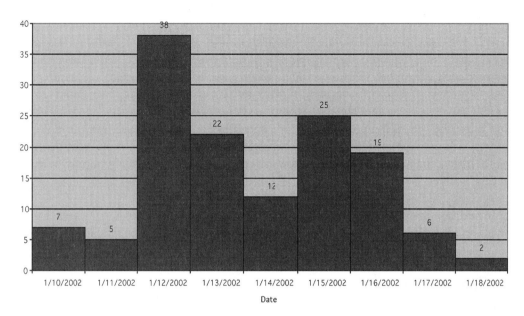

Fig. 3. Epidemic curve of individual cases at MCRD, San Diego, CA.

On investigation, the earliest record of gastrointestinal illness occurred in a Marine who worked in the dining facility. He was ill for 3 d before being evaluated and removed from working with food. Within 2 d of the onset of his illness, illness began to occur in many different trainee companies. The epidemic curve representing unique individuals as recorded by ESSENCE is shown in Fig. 3. It is possible that after initial spread via food, spread continued person-to-person in the barracks environment. Diagnostic studies of stool specimens revealed Norwalk-like viruses that are known to spread not only by water and food but also airborne between people.

Investigations at Fort Leonard Wood and Aberdeen Proving Ground also revealed an afebrile illness of acute onset and short duration characterized by vomiting and diarrhea. No stool samples were available for analysis, but the clinical picture points to a Norwalk-like virus as well. Preventive medicine personnel were notified and told to be on a heightened alert for more gastroenteritis cases at these and other installations. The ability of ESSENCE to demonstrate outbreaks in disparate locations and to compare the results of investigations can assist in detecting bioterrorist attacks.

2.5. Evaluation of New Surveillance Systems

The CDC has issued recommendations on the evaluation of surveillance systems *(4)*. Surveillance systems should be periodically evaluated to ensure they are efficient and effective. As these new health indicator surveillance systems are still mostly unproven, special emphasis should be placed on their evaluation and subsequent improvement. Information on what aspects made the system more efficient or useful should be made available to others who are developing similar systems.

Fig. 2. *(opposite page)* Example of ESSENCE data detecting multiple simultaneous GI outbreaks at Aberdeen Proving Ground, MD, Fort Monmouth, NJ, Fort Knox, KY, and Marine Corps Recruit Depot in San Diego, CA.

The attributes of simplicity, flexibility, data quality, acceptability, sensitivity, predictive value positive, representativeness, timeliness, and stability should be assessed during an evaluation *(4)*. Some attributes will be more important to some surveillance systems than for others. Early warning systems for infectious disease outbreaks will rank timeliness first, with acceptability, flexibility, sensitivity, and representativeness coming closely thereafter. The data quality and predictive value positive, although still important, will be less important than for a specific reportable disease. If a surveillance system is somewhat inaccurate, but is consistently inaccurate then it can still be quite useful in detecting fluctuations in disease incidence. Additionally, the grouping of cases into larger syndromes done in many of these surveillance systems represents larger categories that compensate for minor variations in diagnoses.

In addition to the traditional attributes to consider, new surveillance systems based on automated data sources will have other concerns. These include standard user interface, data format and coding, compatible hardware and software, quality assurance, and strict adherence to security and confidentiality *(5)*.

At the end of a surveillance system evaluation, recommendations should be made to improve the system. However, efforts to improve some attributes may detract from others. After accounting for elements that cannot be changed (e.g., security restrictions that may impede timeliness, but cannot be removed), those elements that are most important should be identified and given highest priority for improvement.

Although the pressure is often apparent to rapidly start using data for surveillance before first evaluating its usefulness, we must continue to prove the effectiveness and sensitivity of data sources before establishing them as reliable public health information. Care must be taken to ensure that the data being utilized has meaning in the public health community and that the output being generated is derived from appropriate information. With the great amount of data available for analysis, it may be tempting to try to use as much as possible to find an answer. Each data source must be able to stand alone as a useful tool, although it may be more useful in combination with other sources.

In addition, the issue of false-positives must be considered. The surveillance systems should be set at an alert level that is as sensitive as possible without overburdening the responders. In many cases, the "false"-positive may not actually be "false," it may just be a small outbreak of little consequence that has low morbidity and no mortality and rapidly resolves without revealing a source. Evaluation of these incidents may prove difficult, but attempts should be made to ascertain the true false-positive rate.

2.6. The Future of Health Indicator Surveillance Systems

As previously described, there are many initiatives to develop surveillance systems using traditional and nontraditional data sources. Probably the best system will use a combination of many data sources to achieve the highest sensitivity and specificity—a system of systems. The need for extreme timeliness will drive the creation of new, time-sensitive surveillance.

2.6.1. Integration of Military and Civilian Systems

To have the most sensitive surveillance system, information from as many segments of society as possible is important. This is termed the representativeness of a system— if it concentrates on only one geographic, ethnic, or socioeconomic section of a population, then it cannot accurately represent the status of the entire community. Similarly,

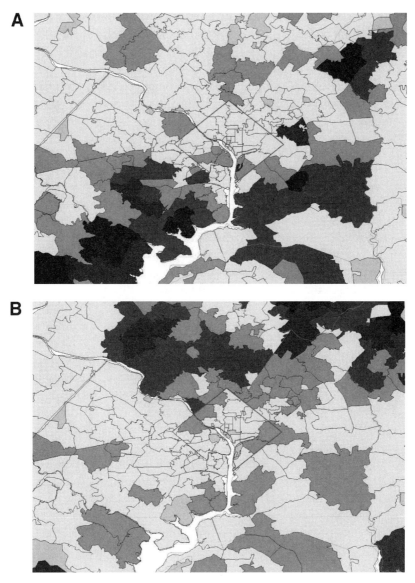

Fig. 4. **(A)** Density of outpatient visits for defined syndromes captured by ESSENCE at MTFs in the national capital region. **(B)** Same map for data captured from a civilian HMO.

if a surveillance system only takes information from military beneficiaries, it will miss important other elements, both geographically and socioeconomically, in tracking disease rates.

Current ESSENCE surveillance information includes data from active duty, retirees, and family members, and thus, has a good representative slice regarding gender and age range. However, there are geographic areas that are not as well-represented if only military data are available. As Fig. 4 demonstrates, the density of use of MTFs by military beneficiaries in the national capital area varies across the region. Integration of civilian health data from local hospitals, health maintenance organizations, and regional billing centers is being collected through collaboration with civilian academic institutions. We find that the civilian data complement the military data very well by providing information on geographic areas that are not as well-represented in the military catchment (Fig. 4). In addition to the outpatient data, other civilian sources, such as over-the-counter pharmacy sales, school absenteeism, and veterinary information (e.g., wildlife die-off, veterinary clinic chains) is being added to the surveillance system. Again, a system of systems is the most sensitive way to detect variations in disease rates, and these systems must include collaborations between many organizations and institutions.

2.6.2. Nationwide Integration and Access

The CDC is developing the National Electronic Disease Surveillance System (NEDSS) to improve the management of and enhance currently existing surveillance systems *(5)*. This will allow public health professionals to more rapidly detect and respond to outbreaks of infectious diseases, whether from natural sources or bioterrorism. It will use standard data formats to electronically link many different surveillance systems. In addition, it will provide a communications infrastructure to allow rapid communication between different public health sectors and provide agreements on data access, sharing and confidentiality *(5)*. Recent funding by the Department of Health and Human Services will assist in providing funds to local and state health departments to assist in this integration. This type of system will greatly improve the current state of surveillance, with many current systems running on different platforms, including many paper-based systems. In particular, there are large government suppliers of health data, such as Medicare and Medicaid, that already have health-related databases that should be made available through a national plan. All state, local, and military health departments should assist in building a national network of information.

Although a national system is needed, the information must still be viewed and interpreted locally. The ownership of surveillance systems must be kept with the local users, who will be the ones to respond. However, the data should be available and shared across jurisdictions to give state and national epidemiologists the tools to evaluate a composite view of health status and to monitor for spread of infectious disease outbreaks.

3. LABORATORY SURVEILLANCE AND CAPABILITIES TO IMPROVE BIODEFENSE

3.1. Laboratory-Based Surveillance

Traditional surveillance systems rely heavily on laboratory reporting to track infectious disease trends. Because laboratory diagnoses provide the most specific information in a infectious disease surveillance system, they are essential for accurate monitoring. Although lab-based surveillance is not yet very timely, it is still of critical importance, especially in the evaluation of specific preventive measures. In bioterrorism defense, laboratory surveillance allows the public health community to track the spread of certain types of disease agents and, therefore, understand what pathogens are circulating in a given area. In bioterrorism detection, new or unusual strains can potentially be a strong indicator that an intentional attack has occurred *(29)*. The strain of Salmonella causing illness in The Dalles, OR, in 1984 was one of the principal clues in determining that the outbreak was intentional *(30)*. With emphasis on cutting costs in healthcare, many patients are treated empirically without the benefit of microbiological diagnoses, especially when the illness is not severe or when the test result may arrive too late to benefit the patient *(31)*. However, with recent increasing threats of bioterrorism in the United States, the need for laboratory-based surveillance is greater than ever.

3.1.1. DOD Laboratory-Based Global Influenza Surveillance

The DOD-GEIS has sponsored the Air Force influenza surveillance program since 1997. This program was initiated in 1976 under the title Project Gargle. Since then, the influenza surveillance program has used sentinel sites worldwide to isolate, identify, and study circulating influenza viruses *(32)*. It is a part of the WHO global surveillance network and supplies isolates and reports to the CDC, WHO, and the Vaccines and Related Biological Products Advisory Committee.

Influenza is a highly contagious virus and has the potential to undergo major antigenic shift, which could expose much of the population to a virus to which they have no underlying immunity. Infection with influenza virus can incapacitate the victim, and it can be a lethal infection, especially in the very young and very old. If antigenic shift results in an especially virulent form, as apparently occurred in 1918, a disease with high mortality in all age groups may occur. For these reasons, the DOD strives to protect its servicemembers against this disease. This is done not only through annual vaccination programs, but also through the Air Force's active surveillance program to monitor isolates throughout the world and anticipate any changes that may require new vaccines or other preventive measures.

The influenza surveillance program is an example of a highly successful system to monitor changes in microbiological flora nationally and internationally to effect appropriate preventive measures. Strengthening of systems such as this, especially those that monitor diseases that could be used as or engineered into a lethal bioweapon, is essential for biodefense.

3.1.2. The Naval Health Research Center's Respiratory Disease Laboratory

In addition to the Air Force influenza program, the Naval Health Research Center (NHRC) in San Diego, CA surveys bacterial and viral respiratory pathogens at military installations in the United States *(34)*. Population-based surveillance for febrile respiratory pathogens at basic training centers includes testing for influenza, parainfluenza, respiratory syncytial virus, and adenovirus. As major military installations, especially those that house recruits, could be bioterrorist targets, an active surveillance system that is confirmed by laboratory testing is crucial to monitor the health of these populations, follow changes in circulating pathogens, and evaluate preventive measures. NHRC also conducts surveillance on common bacterial causes of respiratory illness, in particular, *Streptococcus pyogenes* and *S. pneumoniae*, both of which can cause severe disease, especially in crowded recruit populations. Most importantly, with both the Air Force and NHRC surveillance systems, data are available for public health interpretation via websites.

3.1.3. Antibiotic Resistance Surveillance

The growing natural resistance of many bacteria to commonly used antibiotics is an additional reason to improve laboratory based surveillance. Tracking the incidence of antibiotic resistant bacteria and monitoring changes over large geographic areas can greatly assist in addressing and mitigating this growing concern. The possibility of engineering disease agents to be antibiotic-resistant is already described, and laboratories must retain the capability to rapidly determine antibiotic sensitivity *(33)*. Electronic laboratory files can provide a large amount of information and can be linked to pharmacy data to monitor the use of antibiotics, as well as resistance patterns *(34)*. Recent studies have demonstrated that electronic laboratory reporting greatly increased the number, completeness, and timeliness of reports received *(35)*. The DOD-GEIS is working with military and commercial laboratories to improve surveillance of antibiotic resistance patterns *(36)*.

3.2. Laboratory Response to Bioterrorism

The public health and hospital laboratories will remain key players in biodefense. Even if detected quickly, only through rapid and accurate diagnosis will a bioterrorist attack be mitigated to the greatest extent possible. It is essential that all laboratories are trained to suspect and recognize potential biological terrorism agents, and furthermore, that the laboratory knows the appropriate reference chain for any suspicious or unusual pathogens. To assist in this endeavor, the Association of Public Health Laboratories with the CDC has developed a network of civilian laboratories designated as the Laboratory Response Network (LRN) *(37)*.

The LRN is a pyramidal structure in which the lowest (Level A) of four levels of laboratories provides initial evaluation and sample referrals to increasingly more sophisticated laboratories. Each level has different responsibilities in the detection, confirmation, and typing of specimens and different requirements to save suspected or known bioterrorism agent isolates *(37,38)*. The network is evolving rapidly as the plans and procedures are developed and distributed. An understanding of the LRN and collaboration with clinical laboratories to quickly mobilize available resources will greatly increase the ability to recognize a bioterrorism attack and implement appropriate curative and postexposure disease prevention measures. Additional information about the LRN, including lab protocols, is available through the CDC website (http://www.bt.cdc.gov).

3.2.1. The Virtual Public Health Laboratory Directory

Advances in laboratory technology in recent years has fostered the question of how to provide these new techniques at every laboratory level. However, many of these new tests are performed on an *ad hoc* basis, may be unlicensed, and require specific expertise to run them. A system designed to optimize the delivery of advanced technology cannot rely on the physical presence of these capabilities at every level. However, an inventory of available resources that is updated and provides contact information and instructions on how to obtain reference testing can easily be made available through a Web-based system *(39)*. For this reason, the DOD-GEIS is developing a virtual public health lab directory to accomplish this mission.

Within the DOD alone, there are numerous medical laboratories located throughout the world that have a wide range of testing capabilities. Some are research laboratories, whereas others are hospital-based. Within the research community, there are a large number of specialized tests that could be available, but there is no established DOD system to define or facilitate coordination or communication. Most hospital clinicians may have no idea that a DOD laboratory can provide a specific test, let alone how to contact them or send it. Several of these assays are not performed under the regulatory controls necessary for clinical laboratory certification, nor do they represent devices licensed by the Food and Drug Administration because of their research status. Along with improvements in the Web-based linkages, attention needs to be placed on validation of these procedures. In addition, the CDC and state and university laboratories can provide assistance in specialized areas, and may be easier to use as a result of proximity. However, there are no formal support agreements between DOD and state laboratories. During a time of crisis, lack of an established plan can result in confusion and wasted time.

In light of these issues, it was decided at a Military Public Health Laboratory Symposium held in 1999 that the DOD medical system must become aware of the availability and accessibility of specialized laboratory testing worldwide *(40)*. In addition, lines of communication must be opened within the DOD and with civilian partners to ensure the most prudent use of resources. The first step in addressing these concerns will be the release of the DOD virtual public health lab directory, a joint collaborative effort between the DOD-GEIS and the Armed Forces Institute of Pathology. In addition, efforts to archive and store clinical specimens of interest from those with known or potential infectious disease etiologies for future study is also being undertaken.

4. CONCLUSION

The US military has been involved with developing defenses against biological warfare for many decades. These efforts have featured research into vaccines, therapeutics, diagnostics, and various other countermeasures. Most of the doctrine developed has been based on battlefield scenarios in which deployed forces are arrayed against a defined enemy. However, the specter of biological terrorism on the homeland perpetrated by a unique set of actors with nontraditional agendas raises many new challenges to old defensive assumptions. One of these is the greatly increased challenge of defining, recognizing, and responding to an unexpected threat before its full consequences are felt. It is clear that with the homeland as a potential target, some of the approaches to threat mitigation that are appropriate to a fielded military force are less practical to communities of civilians or garrison military structures. An important ally in this threat to internal national security is the public health community and a key function of the public health community is the ongoing assessment of community health through surveillance. DOD-GEIS has assumed a pioneering role in creating new public health systems to meet this unprecedented challenge. Many of the innovations made possible by the military's unique global medical information systems are equally beneficial detecting naturally occurring and deliberate outbreaks of infectious diseases. However, it is only through partnering with civilian public health agencies that it will be possible to apply these techniques on the scale necessary to build a truly national civil biodefense infrastructure needed for early detection and effective management of these threats. In numerous readiness exercises, the need for crisp and accurate information has been seen as central to effective crisis management. Public health surveillance is thus a foundation stone in any comprehensive system for biodefense.

REFERENCES

1. Langmuir, A. D. and Andrews, J. M. (1952) Biological warfare defense: the Epidemic Intelligence Service of the Communicable Disease Center. *Am. J. Public Health* **42,** 235–238.
2. O'Toole, T. (2001) Emerging illness and bioterrorism: implications for public health. *J. Urban Health* **78,** 396–402.
3. Inglesby, T. V., Grossman, R., and O'Toole, T. (2001) A plague on your city: observations from TOPOFF. *Clin. Infect. Dis.* **32,** 435, 436.
4. Khan, A. S. and Ashford, D. A. (2001) Ready or not - preparedness for bioterrorism. *N. Engl. J. Med.* **345,** 287–289.
5. Centers for Disease Control and Prevention. (2001) Updated guidelines for evaluating public health surveillance systems: recommendations from the guidelines working group. *MMWR* **50,** 1–30.
6. Thacker, S. B. and Berkelman, R. L. (1998) Public health surveillance in the United States. *Epidemiol. Rev.* **10,** 164–190.
7. Army Medical Surveillance Activity. (2001) Completeness and timeliness of reporting of hospitalized notifiable cases, US Army, January 1995–June 2001. *MSMR* **7,** 12–15.
8. Army Medical Surveillance Activity. (2001) Completeness and timeliness of reporting of hospitalized notifiable cases, US Navy, January 1998–June 2001. *MSMR* **7,** 16–19.
9. Army Medical Surveillance Activity. (2001) Completeness and timeliness of reporting of hospitalized notifiable cases, US Air Force, January 1998–June 2001. *MSMR* **7,** 20–23.
10. Kaufmann, A., Meltzer, M., and Schmid, G. (1997) The economic impact of a bioterrorist attack: are prevention and postattack intervention programs justifiable? *Emerg. Infect. Dis.* **3,** 83–94.
11. Fraser, D. W., Tsai, T. R., Orenstien, W. et al. (1977) Legionnaires' disease: description of an epidemic of pneumonia. *N. Engl. J. Med.* **297,** 1189–1197.
12. Centers for Disease Control and Prevention. (1993) Outbreak of Hantavirus infection—Southwestern United States, 1993. *MMWR* **42,** 495, 496.
13. Fine, A. and Layton, M. (2001) Lessons from the West Nile viral encephalitis outbreak in New York City, 1999: implications for bioterrorism preparedness. *Clin. Infect. Dis.* **32,** 277–282.
14. Centers for Disease Control and Prevention. (2001) Update: investigation of anthrax associated with intentional exposure and interim public health guidelines, October, 2001. *MMWR* **50,** 889–893.
15. Khan, A. S., Morse, S., and Lillibridge, S. (2000) Public-health preparedness for biological terrorism in the USA. *Lancet* **356,** 1179–1182.
16. Thacker, S. B. (2000) Historical development, in *Principles and Practice of Public Health Surveillance*, 2nd ed. (Teutsch, S. M. and Churchill, R. E., eds.), Oxford University Press, New York.
17. Thomson, M., Connor, S., O'Neill, K., and Meert, J. -P. (2000) Environmental information for prediction of epidemics. *Parasitol. Today* **16,** 137, 138.
18. Dowell, S. F. (2001) Seasonal variation in host susceptibility and cycles of certain infectious diseases. *Emerg. Infect. Dis.* **7,** 369–374.
19. Miller, J. R. and Mikol, Y. (1999) Surveillance for diarrheal disease in New York City. *J. Urban Health* **76,** 388–390.
20. Mikol, Y., Miller, J., and Ashendorff, A. (2000) Diarrheal disease surveillance programs: New York City's experience. International Conference on Emerging Infectious Diseases. Centers for Disease Control and Prevention, Atlanta, GA.
21. Proctor, M. E., Blair, K. A., and Davis, J. P. (1998) Surveillance data for waterborne illness detection: an assessment following a massive waterborne outbreak of Cryptosporidium infection. *Epidemiol. Infect.* **120,** 43–54.

22. Pavlin, J. A., Kelley, P. W., Mostashari, F., et al. (2002) Innovative surveillance methods for monitoring dangerous pathogens, in *Institute of Medicine (US). Biological Threats and Terrorism: Assessing the Science and Response Capabilities.* National Academy of Sciences, Washington, DC, pp. 185-196.

23. Connolly, C. (2002) Bush promotes plans to fight bioterrorism. *The Washington Post* (Feb 6) **Sect A,** 3.

24. Espino, J. U., Tsui, F. -C., and Wagner, M. Realtime outbreak detection system (RODS). Available from http://www.health.pitt.edu/rods/rods.htm. Accessed on 11 Feb 2002.

25. Lazarus, R., Kleinman, K. P., Dashevsky, I., DeMaria, A., and Platt, R. (2001) Using automated medical records for rapid identification of illness syndromes (syndromic surveillance): the example of lower respiratory infection. *BMC Public Health* **1,** 9.

26. Idaho Technology. Idaho technology inc. Detection and identification of bio-warfare agents. Available from http://www.army-technology.com/contractors/nbc/idaho. Accessed on 2/11/2002.

27. Schafer, K. LEADERS (Lightweight Epidemiology Advanced Detection & Emergency Response System). Available from http://www.tricare.osd.mil/conferences/2001/agenda.cfm. Accessed on 2/12/2002.

28. New Mexico Department of Health. Rapid Syndrome Validation Project (RSVP) Project Description. Available from http://epi.health.state.nm.us/rsvpdesc/default.asp. Accessed on 2/11/2002.

29. Pavlin, J. A. (1999) Epidemiology of bioterrorism. *Emerg. Infect. Dis.* **5,** 528–530.

30. Torok, T. J., Tauxe, R. V., Wise, R. P., et al. (1997) A large community outbreak of salmonellosis caused by intentional contamination of restaurant salad bars. *JAMA* **278,** 389–395.

31. Skeels, M. R. (2000) Laboratories and disease surveillance. *Mil. Med.* **165(Suppl. 2),** 16–19.

32. Canas, L. C., Lohman, K., Pavlin, J. A., et al. (2000) The Department of Defense laboratory-based global influenza surveillance system. *Mil. Med.* **165(Suppl. 2),** 52–56.

33. Alibek, K. and Handelman, S. (1999) *Biohazard: The Chilling True Story of the Largest Covert Biological Weapons Program in the World: Told from the Inside by the Man Who Ran It.* Random House.

34. O'Brien, T. F., Eskildsen, M. A., and Stelling, J M. (2000) The complex processes of antimicrobial resistance and the information needed to manage them. *Mil. Med.* **165(Suppl. 2),** 12–15.

35. Effler, P., Ching-Lee, M., Bogard, A., Ieong, M.-C., Nekomoto, T., and Jernigan, D. (1999) Statewide system of electronic notifiable disease reporting from clinical laboratories. Comparing automated reporting with conventional methods. *JAMA* **282,** 1845–1850.

36. Davis, S. R. (2000) The state of antibiotic resistance surveillance: an overview of existing activities and new strategies. *Mil. Med.* **165(Suppl. 2),** 35–39.

37. Gilchrist, M. J. R. (2000) A national laboratory network for bioterrorism: evolution from a prototype network of laboratories performing routine surveillance. *Mil. Med.* **165(Suppl. 2),** 28–31.

38. Centers for Disease Control and Prevention. (2000) Biological and chemical terrorism: Strategic plan for preparedness and response. *MMWR* **49(RR-4),** 1–14.

39. Asher, M. S. (2000) A civilian-military virtual public health laboratory network. *Mil. Med.* **165(Suppl. 2),** 1–4.

40. Bolton, J. C. and Gaydos, J. C. (2000) Workshop group B: a Department of Defense (DOD) directory of public health laboratory services for infectious agents and public health laboratory system. *Mil. Med.* **165(Suppl. 2),** 66–69.

18

Information Resources and Database Development for Defense Against Biological Weapons

Frank J. Lebeda, Murray Wolinsky, and Elliot J. Lefkowitz

Men are most apt to believe what they least understand. *-Montaigne*

The concern for man and his destiny must always be the chief interest of all technical effort. *-Albert Einstein*

1. INTRODUCTION

The events in the United States on September 11, 2001, the subsequent dissemination of anthrax through the mail, and the existence of biological weapons programs in other nations have raised the public's concern about the detection and medical management of biological agents, whether on the battlefield or in a civilian environment. This concern is heightened by advances in molecular biology, and the ease of information flow via the Internet (http://www.usamriid.army.mil/education/index.html).

Potential biological weapons include a large variety of microorganisms as well as toxins from microbes, plants, and animals that produce disease or death in humans, livestock, or crops *(1–3)*. The use of these biological threat agents by states, terrorists, or nonstate-sponsored criminals differs in scope and intent. Biological warfare (BW) is associated with state-supported military programs, although bioterrorism is usually considered to be conducted by lone individuals or small groups against civilians or property to create fear, lower public trust of their government, and to generate publicity for their causes (http://www.fema.gov/hazards/terrorism/). Biocrimes have been associated with vengeance, extortion, and murder. Social and economic disruptions in the civilian sector are also expected to occur. Assessment of these threat agents is a function of the capability and the intent of the users and the vulnerability of their targets.

Preparing for and responding to a terrorist threat from the use of harmful biological organisms and their products begins with the collection, analysis, and dissemination of information regarding the potential threat. This chapter reviews the availability, use, and development of databases that can support current biodefense initiatives in basic and applied research. These initiatives include the development of environmental detectors, diagnostic reagents, animal models, new vaccines, and antimicrobial drugs. Our discussion begins with a general summary of publicly available biological databases and follows with a discussion of existing database efforts that have a specific

From: *Infectious Diseases: Biological Weapons Defense: Infectious Diseases and Counterterrorism*
Edited by: L. E. Lindler, F. J. Lebeda, and G. W. Korch © Humana Press Inc., Totowa, NJ

biodefense focus. We then provide an overview of some of the technical aspects of database development and conclude with a discussion of some of the analytical techniques that depend on or utilize these research databases.

2. BIOLOGICAL DATABASES

The first publicly available database of biological sequence information was published in 1965 by Margaret O. Dayhoff *(4)*. This Atlas of Protein Sequence and Structure was only available as a printed copy and contained the sequences of approx 50 proteins. Establishment of a database of nucleic acid sequences began in 1979 through the efforts of Walter Goad at the US Department of Energy's Los Alamos National Laboratory (LANL) *(5)* and separately in the early 1980s at the European Molecular Biology Laboratories (EMBL). In 1982 the database established at LANL received funding from the National Institute of Health (NIH) and was christened GenBank. The first official release of the GenBank database contained the sequences of approx 600 DNA and RNA molecules *(6)*. Today, the successor of the original Dayhoff protein sequence database, the Protein Information Resource (PIR-PSD) *(7)* contains more than 280,000 protein sequences, whereas GenBank contains more than 17 million sequence records. This explosive growth in sequence information has primarily occurred as a result of the genomic sequencing efforts initiated as a part of the human genome project. Genomic sequencing projects span the phyla of all biological kingdoms, including Bacteria, Archaebacteria, Plants, and Animals. These projects generate information in the form of raw sequences that today comprise large percentages of the available protein and nucleic acid sequence databases. In addition to sequence data, experiments that are designed to investigate large-scale gene expression (microarrays) and protein composition (mass spectrometry analysis) generate huge datasets that comprise a massive information source for the biological scientist. The field of bioinformatics has the challenge of providing for the storage, retrieval, analysis, and display of this information in a manner that allows the research scientist, whether from a basic or clinical research background, to ask and answer questions of relevance to their work. This is no less true for research into biological weapons defense, where, as can be seen throughout the many organism-specific chapters of this book, the generation and analysis of genomic information is a key resource for further investigations *(8–10)*.

2.1. Sequence Databases

Bioinformatic databases essentially began with the collection of protein and nucleic acid primary sequence data. Today, available databases have expanded to include a large variety of "specialty" databases that concentrate on specific subsets of sequences and may provide "value-added" information in the form of more extensive annotation and/or analytical information. In addition, databases that collect nonsequence information such as the results of structural determination studies, gene expression data, or clinical information are also available. However, given that so much of our current scientific research efforts are focused on providing a more complete understanding of biological processes by understanding their underlying genetic basis, having a readily available comprehensive database of genomic sequence information from various model organisms is critical to providing a solid foundation on which biological research depends. Indeed, the raison-d'être of the Human Genome Project proceeds from this goal *(11)*. The primary repositories of existing sequence information come from the three organizations that comprise the International Nucleotide Sequence Database Collaboration. These three sites are GenBank, maintained at the National Center for Biotechnology Information (NCBI) *(12)*; EMBL, at the European Molecular Biology Laboratory *(13)*; and the DNA DataBank of Japan (DDBJ) *(14)*. Because all sequence information submitted to any one of these entities is shared with the others on a daily basis, any researcher only needs to query one of these to get the most up-to-date set of available sequences. Using GenBank as an example, access to their sequence database for searching and downloading sequence records is available through the Entrez web interface (http://www.ncbi.nih.gov/Entrez/). GenBank is essentially a repository of nucleotide sequences. But NCBI also provides access to several protein sequence databases. These include the Swiss-Prot *(13)*, PIR *(7)*, and PDB *(15,16)* databases, as well as sequences translated directly from GenBank nucleotide sequence records where the sequence annotation identifies coding sequence features. Although at the present time, essentially all sequences in the protein databases are derived from, or at least represented in GenBank, many of the other protein-specific databases contain additional information in the form of descriptive annotations that add value to the sequence records themselves.

2.1.1. Sequence Annotation

Sequence annotation is a critical step in taking raw biological sequence information and providing meaningful descriptive information to aid subsequent research. Annotation is the process whereby biological features present in any nucleotide or protein sequence are delineated and mapped to their primary sequence location. In essence, an inference is made as to the function of a particular primary sequence or sequence structure. Features such as open reading frames, eukaryotic gene structures, regulatory elements, and functional sequence motifs are among the many types of pieces of information identified during the annotation process. GenBank maintains an extensive guide for researchers to follow in the annotation process (http://www.ncbi.nih.gov/ Sitemap/samplerecord.html and http://www.ncbi.nlm.nih.gov/projects/collab/FT/ index.html). This guide provides a common vocabulary that can be used in the understanding of the functional significance of any particular sequence but also allows for searching and retrieval of particular sequence subsets based on the annotation record. This common vocabulary is then useful for both human-directed and computer-automated searches. Generally, GenBank leaves the process and extent of sequence annotation up to the individual sequence submitter. Therefore, the annotation provided with any particular sequence in comparison to that provided with another may vary extensively. One of the goals of some of the publicly available protein databases such as PIR and Swiss-Prot is to provide more extensive and more accurate descriptive information for each protein record. This annotative information may be initially derived from the sequence record provided by the sequence submitter, but it is then extended during the annotation process employed by the database curators. More recently, NCBI has established the Reference Sequence (RefSeq) database project (http://www.ncbi.nih.gov/ RefSeq/index.html). RefSeq attempts to provide reference sequences for genomes, genes, messenger RNAs, proteins, and RNA sequences that can be used, in NCBI terminology, as "a stable reference for gene characterization, mutation analysis, expression studies, and polymorphism discovery." RefSeq should also provide a more highly curated and annotated set of sequence records to the research community.

In addition to the sequences themselves and their annotation records, sequence databases provide various of other types of biological information that may be linked to sequence records as appropriate. As an example, each sequence in GenBank has links to appropriate references in the PubMed literature database from which the sequence record may have been derived. NCBI also provides a Web-based taxonomy browser (http://www.ncbi.nlm.nih.gov/Taxonomy/taxonomyhome.html.index.cgi) for access to taxonomically specified sets of sequence records as well as information concerning the taxonomic classification of the organism from which any particular sequence was derived. The sequence records also provide, as available, links to information on chromosomal location and genomic mapping data, higher order structural information (PDB), mutational analysis and genetic disorders online Mendelian (OMIM), homologs in other species (Homologene), single nucleotide polymorphisms, and expressed sequence tags and possible alternative splicing events (Unigene). Links to appropriate records in these other databases are provided by the NCBI Entrez search interface. Links to other relevant resources are provided by Entrez "LinkOut" capabilities (http://www.ncbi. nih.gov/entrez/linkout/doc/linkoutoverview.html). In addition to advances in large-scale sequencing technologies, advances in our ability to analyze gene and protein expression on a large scale have increased the number and breadth of sequence-associated biological databases. The recent establishment of gene expression databases at Stanford (http://genome-www.stanford.edu/microarray/) *(17)* and NCBI (http://www.ncbi.nlm.nih.gov/geo/) *(18)*, among others *(19)*, represent recent examples of this trend.

2.2. Genomic Databases

The GenBank sequence database includes complete genomic sequences (or chromosomal sequences) from "finished" genomic sequencing projects, as well as large "contigs" (or contiguous assemblies of individual sequences) that are fully assembled and accurate but may be derived from ongoing sequencing projects. Although the term "finished" may have different meanings dependent on the particular research lab and sequencing project that is underway, in general, it refers to completion of a particular sequencing milestone for which the determination of all sequence information is complete to some specified degree of accuracy. Given the large number of ongoing sequencing projects that have generated significant, but not yet finished, sequence, and given that government-funded sequencing projects must release this sequence information at regular intervals, NCBI has established specialized Web pages that make unfinished sequence information from ongoing genomic sequencing projects available for use by other researchers (http://www.ncbi.nih.gov/Genomes/). In addition, this site also provides a separate genomics database where more direct access to complete genomes from any organism can be found. Several public sites also provide various visualization and analytical tools that makes the process of mining of these large genomic sequence databases for specific information accessible to any researcher—even those inexperienced in using data mining and sequence searching tools. In addition to a genome browser available at the NCBI website, EMBL and the Sanger Institute provide a genome browser at their Ensembl site, http://www.ensembl.org/ *(20),* and the University of California, Santa Cruz, provides a genome browser as well at http://genome.ucsc.edu/ *(21).*

Organismal biology at the sequence level provides vast opportunities for scientific discovery. Better understanding of the genetic basis of human disease, as well as better understanding of infectious diseases and host–parasite interactions are key goals in these initiatives. Accessing databases and analysis tools similar to those described above is critical in making use of the vast amounts of data generated by these projects. Whether one is interested in the genetic basis of diabetes, the infectious process utilized by microorganisms involved in sexually transmitted disease, or, as for the present volume, organisms that might be used as weapons of bioterrorism, an effective research program must have ready access to the relevant genetic data. These data not only include the pertinent sequence data but also the corresponding annotation record along with appropriate analytical and visualization tools that can process the data. Although all of these resources are available from NCBI, EMBL, DDBJ, and others, these institutions serve all of the biological sciences and, therefore, do not try and provide more specialized databases directed at specific research problems. Therefore the user community and funding agencies have recognized the usefulness of developing specialized, model organism databases that provide gene and genomic information of particular interest to a specific community of researchers. One example of these specialized databases is the Los Alamos Sexually Transmitted Disease database (STDgen; http://www.stdgen.lanl.gov/) of genomic information derived from microorganisms responsible for, or associated with, sexually transmitted diseases. The complete genomic sequences of organisms such as chlamydia, mycoplasma, treponema, papillomaviruses, and herpesviruses are included in this database. Another model organism database is the Poxvirus Bioinformatics Resource Center (http://www.poxvirus.org), which provides a database of genomic information from various poxvirus strains and species, emphasizing variola virus, the causative agent of smallpox. This bioinformatics resource is funded by the US NIH and the US Defense Advanced Research Projects Agency (DARPA) to specifically address the potential use of poxviruses, either naturally occurring or engineered, as agents of bioterrorism. It provides an information resource to support research into the development of environmental detectors, diagnostic reagents, antiviral drugs, and new vaccines. A more general resource directed at microbial genomes is available from The Institute for Genomic Research (TIGR). TIGR provides the comprehensive microbial resource (http://www.tigr.org/tigr-scripts/CMR2/CMRHomePage.spl), which collects complete genomic sequences from all publicly available sources of both prokaryotic and archaebacterial microbial species *(22)*. There are many other databases and websites directed at providing specialized subsets of sequence information. There are also quite a few organism-specific databases such as those for *Plasmodium falciparum (23)*, *saccharomyces (24)*, *Caenorhabditis elegans (25)*, and *Drosophila (26)*. An important aspect to these databases is that in addition to providing appropriate subsets of gene and genome sequences, they also attempt to provide a more comprehensive annotation for the available sequence records. The curation effort required to more fully annotate gene and genome sequence records can be extensive, but the "value-added" knowledge obtained through such efforts is critical in providing a useful database resource as an aid in furthering traditional laboratory-based efforts at answering scientific problems. These resources also provide a substantial number of analytical tools that can be utilized to mine the sequence data and help answer questions regarding the biology—especially the comparative biology—of these organisms. An excellent resource for information on available biological databases is the Database Issue of Nucleic Acids Research that is published in January of each year *(27)*.

2.3. Gene Databases

Many of the efforts directed at providing sequence-based model organism resources have utilized an organism-, or disease-based perspective. Another useful perspective would be to develop a database that organizes information around gene or protein function. Several databases and corresponding search and analysis tools exist that categorize proteins according to function. These include the Clusters of Orthologous Groups database at NCBI (http://www.ncbi.nih.gov/COG/) *(28)* and the iProClass Protein Classification Database at PIR (http://pir.georgetown.edu/iproclass/) *(7)*. These databases provide the means to make functional inferences for new or unclassified proteins on the basis of shared primary sequence domains with proteins of known function. They also frequently include descriptive records providing substantial annotation for each protein and functional domain as well as links to other sources of information. The Gene Ontology Consortium effort (http://www.geneontology.org/) *(29)* is designed to help establish a common vocabulary to support all annotation and organizational projects. Use of a common vocabulary can aid efforts to classify, organize, cluster, search for, and understand the structures and functions of genes and other biological entities.

The utility of organizing information around function rather than source can also be extended to more specialized databases to study biological processes at a more general level such as microbial pathogenicity. For research directed at providing a defense against the use of microorganisms as agents of bioterrorism, a better understanding of the processes involved in pathogenesis, including the microbial genes collectively known as virulence factors, would certainly be important. A virulence factor database of genes involved in pathogenicity would include microbial toxins, antibiotic resistance genes, metalloproteases, adhesins, invasins, hemolysins, and so on (*see* ref. *30* for a review). Such a database would be useful in studying common mechanisms of virulence and help to delineate common "themes" utilized by microorganisms to cause disease. A virulence factor database would also be critical in detecting organisms engineered to be more potent bioterrorist threats. Only by knowing the composition, organization, and function of the genes that comprise naturally occurring organisms can we hope to be able to detect unnatural or altered organisms with new combinations of genetic elements. Efforts to develop such a virulence factor database are currently in progress through a joint effort of the Walter Reed Army Institute for Research (WRAIR), the US Army Medical Research Institute of Infectious Diseases (USAMRIID), the University of Alabama at Birmingham, and the LANL.

3. BIODEFENSE DATABASES

In the previous section, we provided a general overview of biological databases, focusing on databases that store sequence-derived information. In any research with an emphasis on biodefense, it will be important to not only access biological sequence information but also access information relevant to all aspects of a potential biological warfare attack including surveillance, environmental, diagnostic, epidemiological, and other biomedical information. Here, we focus on databases that have more specific relevance to the biodefense community.

It is assumed that reducing the threats posed by biological agents can be aided by developing databases that are designed to assist in selecting the appropriate responses that will guard against disease contagion and lethality *(31)*. These responses obviously depend on the rapid and accurate identification of disease outbreaks but also depend on knowledge of many other factors the details of which remain to be defined and established.

For example, vaccination records of those individuals who are at risk could be used to determine those who are currently immunized to a given threat or epidemic. Antibiotic resistance data could also prove to be crucial to initiating efficacious responses to bacterial disease outbreaks. These databases will certainly need to assimilate the large amount of molecular genomic data from threat microbes that have been or will be collected and published and make the information available in a cogent form to government and academic laboratories and to state and municipal public health systems. The mere existence of such databases may also help deter the intentional use of bioagents if they are perceived to mitigate their threat capabilities *(32)*.

3.1. The User Community

Database development and design goals depend on the questions being asked. However, before these questions can be properly addressed the user community needs to be accurately identified and asked about the types of information they need. This feedback process may not be an easy task for building biodefense-related databases because the users may not know what kinds of questions to ask at the early stages of development. For example, most current life-scientists are neither computer nor database experts and may not be willing to learn to use complex interfaces or query languages. Some of these users may simply want to browse and explore websites rather than to become experts in the use of more complicated information retrieval systems. Therefore, database developers will be challenged to build user-friendly query interfaces and to provide visualization tools to view the retrieved information in a meaningful way (*see* Subheadings 4. and 5.). It is anticipated that any biodefense database project will only partially satisfy the user community needs at any moment and that change, expansion, and continuous improvement will characterize this dynamic information resource.

It is clear from the outset that the "customers" will be defined as a diverse group of individuals who represent a broad spectrum of communities: first responders, scientists from various fields of expertise, policy analysts who help formulate threat assessments and response policies, and senior decision makers. The first responder communities will of course differ for chemical and biological events. For example, fire, police, and emergency medical teams will be present at the site of a chemical attack at a time close to the time at which the attack was initiated. Whereas emergency room nurses and physicians in walk-in hospital facilities will be involved hours, days, or weeks following a biological incident at facilities that may be fairly distant from the attack site. It is also evident that, given the wide range of interests and areas of expertise of these potential users, an interconnected network of several databases needs to be considered and that specific databases will need to be tailored for a particular group's interest.

To decide what a system of databases should contain, the potential uses must be predefined. For biodefense "preparedness," a standard set of descriptive terms usually includes surveillance, detection, diagnosis, response, and training. Besides providing collections of information, these databases and their associated sites on the Web will provide guidelines, standards, training, and educational material. Such a system should also foster interaction and coordination among government, academia, and industry. The following subheadings provide examples of databases and information resources from military and nonmilitary government organizations and academic sites that focus on these preparedness issues along with issues and concerns for securing computer environments.

3.2. Department of Defense Databases Related to Biodefense

3.2.1. Medical Information Systems

The DOD maintains several centrally managed Military Health System (MHS) clinical information technology systems. The Composite Health Care System (CHCS) is the DOD's integrated medical information database. It provides automated medical information system support to all military treatment facilities (MTFs) for active and retired military personnel and their families. More than 8 million CHCS records for MHS beneficiaries exist worldwide in more than 700 DOD hospitals and clinics. Among its many features in maintaining administrative data for patients and outpatients, the CHCS is interfaced to 40 other clinical and administrative systems. The future Composite Health Care System II (CHCS II) is a clinical information system that will generate and maintain a comprehensive, lifelong, computer-based patient record for each beneficiary. CHCS II will support various of programs to help the MHS determine disease prevalence, management and outcomes. Finally, the Preventive Health Care Application (PHCA) is currently being installed and tested. PHCA is a computerized health maintenance system that assists health care providers at 56 MTFs to help deliver and track clinical preventative services (http://tricare.osd.mil/immunization/militaryimmunization.html).

3.2.2. Army Medical Information and Surveillance Systems

The central epidemiological resource for the Army is the Army Medical Surveillance Activity (AMSA; http://amsa.army.mil/AMSA/amsa_ns_home.htm), which is a part of the US Army Center for Health Promotion and Preventive Medicine. AMSA operates the Defense Medical Surveillance System (DMSS), which contains a database of recent and archival data on diseases and medical events (e.g., hospitalizations, ambulatory visits, reportable diseases, HIV tests, acute respiratory diseases, and health-risk appraisals). The Medical Surveillance Monthly Report (MSMR) is a Web-accessible AMSA publication that is patterned after the CDC's Morbidity and Mortality Weekly Report. The MSMR disseminates the medical surveillance information from the DMSS database to provide summaries for notifiable diseases, trends of illnesses of special surveillance interest; field reports of disease outbreaks and case occurrences. Through DMSS, AMSA provides the sole link between the DOD Serum Repository and other databases to combine statistics from the Army and the other services. Currently, the serum repository is the world's largest, containing nearly 26 million frozen serum specimens, and is used for medical surveillance, diagnoses, and epidemiological studies.

3.2.3. Immunization Tracking

Presently, each service uses its own immunization tracking system to record vaccination data for active duty personnel (http://www.vaccines.army.mil/default.aspx?cnt=resource/ITS). These systems include the Air Force Complete Immunization Tracking Application (AF-CITA), the Army Medical Occupational Data System (MODS), and the Navy/Marines/Coastguard Shipboard Automated Medical System (SAMS; https://imcenter.med.navy.mil/its/default.asp). Each system is capable of transmitting immunization data about uniformed service members to the Defense Enrollment Eligibility Reporting System (DEERS), which is a centralized database for providing, among other services, medical readiness data (http://www.dmdc.osd.mil/deers/). Personnel with appropriate access can query this data repository for status reports on their military unit via the Immunization Compliance Reporting System website. Presently, more than 16 million immunization records are stored by AMSA from DEERS. The new DEERS, scheduled to begin in 2003, will consolidate medical information from more than 120 different databases (http://www.af.mil/news/Apr2002/n20020429_0682.asp). The service-specific systems will be replaced with a single DOD immunization tracking system when the CHCS II and the Theater Medical Information Program (http://www.tricore.osd.mil/peo/tmip/applications.htm) become active.

3.2.4. Telemedicine

The Telemedicine Project at the Walter Reed Army Medical Center (http://telemedicine.wramc.amedd.army.mil/Index.htm) provides worldwide support of deployed military units and humanitarian missions. This project is integrated with medical information databases and is linked to the National Library of Medicine and the DOD CHCS. Telemedicine consultations rely on computerized consult sheets that were developed using database management software and represent a multimedia medical record that includes traditional text information (histories, physical exams, lab results, radiological interpretations, etc.) along with high resolution digitally compressed images (e.g., X-rays) used in preventive medicine, infectious disease, and other disciplines. This approach is based on a computerized two-way audio communication and image transfer linked with satellite video teleconferencing, allowing data transmission between deployed military medical units and supporting military hospitals.

3.2.5. Syndromic Surveillance

Presently, no US agency is charged with providing medical care to domestic mass causalities as a result of deliberate or natural disasters *(33)*. Before September 11, 2001, public health officials primarily kept track of information such as childhood immunizations, HIV/AIDS cases, and other more prevalent communicable diseases. After September 11, priorities in some of the larger cities were changed to focus on early warnings of chemical or biological weapons usage. These changes involve, for example, detecting higher-than-normal frequencies of ambulance runs, absences from work or school, sales of over-the-counter flu medications, and numerous of other nontraditional indicators. To have this nation's massive public health system evolve from a decentralized set of local data collection organizations into a national sentinel network of syndromic surveillance is a far-reaching goal that has just begun to develop *(34)*.

The DOD agency at the forefront of these novel surveillance efforts is the DARPA, the military's central research and development organization. DARPA manages and directs projects where the cost–benefit ratio is high but where the potential benefits could provide dramatic advances in technology. An important example of this extremely high-risk, high-payoff approach is DARPA's sponsorship of the ARPANET, the forerunner of the Internet *(35)*.

In the realm of early warning of diseases, a DARPA Information System Office study demonstrated the feasibility of identifying an abnormal health event following an intentional exposure by analyzing nontraditional measures of infection days prior to detection by more traditional methods. The study mined diverse databases containing retail consumer and healthcare-related purchases looking for purchase patterns that could be indicative of disease outbreaks. More recently, DARPA has sponsored the development of the Enhanced Consequence Management Planning And Support System (ENCOMPASS) for syndromic surveillance (http://www.darpa.mil/dso/trans/pdf/encompass.pdf). ENCOMPASS exploits Web-accessible and local software tools to dynamically act on data from different sources. This system consists of two integrated components. The incident command management system is involved with the activities of the Incident Commander, first responders, and various emergency centers. The DARPA Syndromic Surveillance System (D-S^3) is designed to detect sudden changes in occurrence of a predetermined set of patients' signs/symptoms (e.g., fever) and to advise epidemiologists of possible exposures to a biological agent. Although no disease outbreak has been reported by a syndromic surveillance approach *(33)*, the potential for setting an early alarm supports the time and cost required for this type of effort. The fact that there are other biosurveillance systems being independently developed in the commercial sector also raises compatibility issues for future interconnections among these diverse systems *(34)*.

3.2.6. Biosensors and Medical Countermeasures

Other DARPA-sponsored research program areas that are related to surveillance include detection and genomic sequencing. One of DARPA's programs is Biological Warfare Agent Detection, which involves biosensor technologies and tissue-based biosensors. Through its Information Awareness Office, DARPA has sought to develop a biosurveillance system that will be integrated with biosensor technologies for the early detection of intentional exposures of military and civilian populations to biological agents. Biosensor approaches under development include upconverting phosphors, antibodies, and mass spectrometry. Analyzed data from these approaches will be integrated with data contained in heterogeneous databases to distinguish between naturally occurring and abnormal disease outbreaks; to identify the responsible pathogens, to find the points of release, and to notify the relevant response agencies.

A DARPA program involved with medical countermeasures is Pathogen Genomic Sequencing, whose goal is to identify potential molecular targets in these organisms for use in detection, diagnosis, and therapy. Bioinformatic and database tools are to be developed to study the dynamic pathways involved in pathogenesis and to compare them to related nonvirulent strains. At the time of this writing, the *P. falciparum* Genome Database (http://www.tigr.org/tdb/edb2/pfa1/htmls/) is still an ongoing project. The TIGR and the Malaria Program of the Naval Medical Research Center, The Sanger Centre, and Stanford University are each responsible for analyzing specific chromosomes of this organism. DARPA also funds genome sequencing projects for *Bacillus cereus,* which produces a lethal toxin along with diarrheal and emetic enterotoxins, and for *B. thuringiensis israelensis*, both of which are related to *B. anthracis*. DARPA is also funding genome sequencing for *Brucella suis* (brucellosis) and *Coxiella burnetii* (Q fever). Complementing these DARPA-sponsored efforts are several other completed or ongoing genome sequencing projects that are being funded by other government agencies and public organizations (*see* Table 1 and http://www. genomesonline.org).

3.2.7. DOD-Related Biomedical Databases

The TriAgency (Lawrence Livermore National Laboratory, LANL, USAMRIID) ChemBio NonProliferation Portal is part of the Chemical and Biological National Security Program in Threat Reduction. This site includes case studies of biological agent outbreaks, epidemiological studies, software tools, and genomics databases. After September 11, access to this portal has been restricted and public access is under review pending analysis of the overall security of government information systems.

In the course of drug discovery research that has been conducted at several federal and academic laboratories, the Army has acquired a chemical inventory of more than 350,000 samples that reside at the US Army Medical Research and Material Command Repository, located at the WRAIR (http://www.tatrc.org). The inventory includes compounds that have been screened to counteract malaria and Leishmania (WRAIR); antivesicants and AChE reactivators (US Army Medical Research Institute of Chemical Defense); antivirals (USAMRIID); *Cryptosporidia* (US Department of Agriculture); retroviruses, staphylococcus, enterococcus, and streptococcus (The Ohio State University); babesiosis (CDC); and mycobacteria, toxoplasma, and fungi (National Institute of Allergies and Infectious Diseases). To cope with tracking each compound and retaining links to experimental data, a novel laboratory management system was developed, the Chemical Information System. Several features are incorporated in this system to handle this large number of compounds. Biological data from experimental test systems are captured and converted to appropriate formats. These biological data are integrated together with a compound's chemical properties, geometry (shape), and molecular connectivity. Its pharmacaphore interactions are stored as nonparametric,-binary fingerprints that are based on atomic positions, binding affinities, and geometry. Compounds are compared and grouped by using Tanimoto, Taversky, and other metrics to calculate Euclidian distances to identify nearest chemical neighbors that share toxicity or other relevant properties and can be used in structure–activity relationship studies.

The Chemical Biological Defense Information Analysis Center (CBIAC) (http://www.cbiac.apgea.army.mil/) is a DOD Information Analysis Center under contract to the Office of the Secretary of Defense and administratively managed by the Defense Technical Information Center (DTIC). The CBIAC is a focal point for DOD Chemical and Biological Defense scientific and technical information. It provides services to DOD organizations, other government groups, and their approved contractors. Access to the following databases are limited to authorized users: CBIAC Bibliographic Database, Chemical Defense Materials Database, and the DTIC Databases. The CBIAC includes BW defense technology information concerning warning and identification, domestic preparedness, individual and collective protection, medical effects and treatment, environmental fate and effects, and decontamination.

Table 1
DOD Involvement With Ongoing or Completed Genome Projects

Organisms	Diseases	Sequencing institutions	Database/Data analysis sites	Funding organizations
Plasmodium falciparum	Malaria	Sanger Center, Stanford, TIGR, NMRC	Sanger Centre[a] PFDB: TIGR[b] PlasmoDB[c]	Wellcome Trust, ONR, NIAID, Burroughs Wellcome Fund
Bacillus anthracis Ames strain	Anthrax	TIGR[d]	TIGR	ONR, DOE, NIAID, Porton Down (DERA)
Bacillus cereus	Food poisoning	Integrated Genomics, Inc.	Integrated Genomics, Inc.	DARPA
Bacillus thuringiensis israelensis	Microbial insecticide	Integrated Genomics, Inc.	Integrated Genomics, Inc.	DARPA
Brucella suis	Brucellosis	TIGR	TIGR	DARPA, NIAID
Burkholderia mallei (ATCC 23344)	Glanders	USAMRIID, TIGR	TIGR	DARPA, NIAID
Coxiella burnetii	Q fever	TIGR	TIGR	DARPA, NIAID
Francisella tularensis Schu 4	Tularemia	Univ of Uppsala WRAIR MDS	MDS Univ of Uppsala[e]	USAMRMC, UKMOD, MDS, DARPA
Rickettsia typhi	Typhus	Baylor College of Medicine, University of Texas Medical Branch	Baylor College of Medicine, University of Texas Medical Branch	DARPA, NIAID
Clostridium perfringens	Gas gangrene	TIGR	TIGR	DARPA, NIAID
Poxviruses	Smallpox	St. Louis Univ., Univ. Alabama Birmingham, Univ. Victoria	Poxvirus Bioinformatics Resource Center[f]	DARPA, NIAID

(Adapted from Genomes On-Line Database [GOLD™] at http://www.genomesonline.org and citations under References.)

[a]http://www.sanger.ac.uk/Projects/P_falciparum/blast_server.shtml
[b]http://www.tigr.org/tdb/edb2/pfa1/htmls/
[c]http://www.plasmodb.org/
[d]http://www.tigr.org/
[e]http://artedi.ebc.uu.se/Projects/Francisella/
[f]http://www.poxvirus.org/

3.2.8. DOD and Distributed Computer Resources

Large-scale computational chemistry in drug discovery programs involving consortia among commercial and academic partners has begun to use edge-distributed computing technology, which involves having many PCs working during idle moments on small tasks in parallel across the Internet. Each PC runs an Internet screensaver application (agent). In 1997, the first large distributed-net project used thousands of independent, general purpose personal computers for cryptographic problems. Later, the SETI@home project in 1999 demonstrated the successful application of distributed computing in analyzing data collected from radiotelescopes in searching for nonrandom signals from extraterrestrial sources.

In a study related to biodefense against anthrax, the To Have Information and Knowledge (THINK) software project developed at Oxford University was sponsored by the government of the United Kingdom and corporate sponsors. The approach used for their Anthrax Research Project involved screensaver software distributed on a worldwide system of approx 1 million personal computers to quantitatively analyze and evaluate the results *(36–38)*. Within 1 mo, more than 35 billion known and predicted low-molecular-weight structures were tested with a flexible docking program for their ability to dock to the anthrax lethal factor. The most favorable structures have been made available to the US DOD and to the United Kingdom (http://www.grid.org) .

Also within this category of distributed systems exists LEGION, an object-oriented metasystem software project that is sponsored in part by DARPA, the DOD High Performance Computing Modernization Program, and other US government agencies (http://legion.virginia.edu/index.html). This collection of software services is designed to connect millions of hosts and trillions of objects that are linked via high-speed connections to create the illusion of a single virtual computer for the user. CENTURION, the LEGION software testbed, contains applications for computational chemistry projects germane to biodefense applications (http://legion.virginia.edu/centurion/Applications.html). These include the CHARMM suite of programs for protein dynamics calculations *(39)*; COMPLIB, which compares DNA sequences; the DARPA-supported Assisted Model Building with Energy Refinement (AMBER) program package *(40)*; and the GAUSSIAN98 program suite for semiempirical and *ab initio* molecular orbital (http://www.gaussian.com/index.htm).

3.3. DOD Database Security Issues for Nonclassified Data

Beyond the functional objectives in developing a new Web-accessible database (e.g., Web-hosting, data storage needs, cost estimates, hyperlinks to other databases, helpdesk capabilities, back-up procedures, etc.) decisions need to be made on issues such as user accessibility, and requirements for coordinating and administering public key certificates (http://iase.disa.mil/) for secure, encrypted access. For an open-ended database in which the general public can view the information, there is no legal requirement concerning the information on the site and it is not regulated under the Electronic Communications Privacy Act (http://personalinfomediary.com/ECPA1986_text.htm). Typically, the data are read-only so the information cannot be changed at the website by the casual user. If there is any sensitive, yet nonclassified information, a protected section can be created to limit the user base. Access in this case would be restricted with user registration and password protection. Limited access could include only those end users who are government and civilian contractor personnel. The Content Management Control Authority would administer the information and determine which documents or data can be uploaded and stored as they are developed. The institute or managing facility would be responsible for maintaining and storing the information and managing passwords. If the material in the database involves information derived from DOD personnel medical records, the entire system is considered a MHS, and as such, the hardware, software applications, and networks would undergo an extensive certification and accreditation process prior to deployment.

3.4. Future Directions

A distributed set of relevant but heterogeneous databases exist within academia and government that need to be efficaciously accessed and exploited for their roles in defending against naturally occurring or intentional biothreats. Different actions and solutions are being considered. It is envisioned that overall database integration will prove to be too costly to implement (http://img.cs.man.ac.uk) *(41)* and that no single (unique) database schema could be efficiently used, but having a single, consistent user interface would be extremely desirable. A common language will be needed to query multiple sources, and several metasearch engines will need to be built that can pose queries based on different models of data storage and access. A standard, common representation of all database content (e.g., in XML format) will also be needed. In this way, new, specialized databases could readily be added to the existing set.

From a pragmatic view, maximizing the quality of information sharing among government agencies requires information-gathering standards that assess quantity, accuracy, verifiability, and reliability. Various obstacles can inhibit sharing of data not the least of which is interagency cooperation (http://www.brook.edu/dybdocroot/fp/projects/homeland/homeland.htm).

Future large-scale databases will be represented by multimedia, virtually centralized repositories of information. New technologies will have to be developed to design, populate, and use such databases. Large-scale databases will probably be distributed, continuously updated in near-real-time, and provide automatic and semiautomated analyses that can be examined by machines and humans. New methods will be required to answer complex, less-than-specific queries. Detection of subtle changes in a population's health status will need to be quickly and correctly identified so that the execution of appropriate procedures (evacuation, quarantines, treatments) can be quickly initiated. Cost-effective adaptable schema must be created to accommodate future growth and new types of information. Perhaps of greatest concern is that of maintaining and protecting individual privacy.

4. DATABASE FUNDAMENTALS

In this section, we take the perspective of a researcher who has decided that he or she needs to develop a new Web-accessible database and attempt to sketch the considerations involved in developing, maintaining, and making available a useful database. Gibas and Jambeck provide a somewhat longer treatment in the present spirit *(42)*. We try to complement their treatment as much as possible.

We begin by providing a quick overview of the types of efforts needed to provide a Web-connected database. We then discuss how data travel between the database and the user and the software architecture needed to accomplish this task securely. Then we use a (currently) hypothetical database on β-helix proteins to attempt to illuminate database and site design considerations. Finally, we provide some guesses about future directions of database technology.

4.1. Building a Secure Web-Accessible Relational Database

Much of the effort in developing a high-quality database is dedicated to tasks other than that of designing, building, populating, and maintaining the database proper. Although these tasks remain demanding, relational databases—overwhelmingly the most common favorite—have been around for decades: relational database management systems are mature and the issues are generally well-understood.

Most of the complexity—and flux—is currently located in providing access to these databases. Browser-based interfaces provide the most popular current paradigm for database interaction regardless of whether the database is located on the user's machine, a local area network (LAN), or the Internet. Browsers provide remote access, a familiar interface for various users, and a desirable level of platform independence. However, one must now deal with a complex array of rapidly evolving choices of technologies, including Web (and application) servers, security, page design and scripting, and use of Web-based program applets or servlets. Moreover, visual (graphical) means of interrogating databases and expressing search results are common, and enabling such visual access—particularly interactively through a Web browser—may require relatively complex coding. Further, many current biological databases also provide analytical features that again may require complex coding. So, even relatively simple databases demand various skills ranging from the highly analytical to the artistic.

Generally, a team of individuals is required to design, implement and maintain a worthwhile data resource (*see* Table 2). Many of the skills shown are equally relevant for e-business applications *(43)*, thereby exacerbating the well-known scarcity of bioinformatically qualified individuals. Of course, some of these skills or needs may not be required in any particular application, particularly if the database is intended as a private resource. We touch on most of the required skills here. However, it is good to realize that much of the following discussion may be expected to possess a relatively short "shelf-life" as technologies mature.

4.1.1. (Secure) Connectivity

Data must potentially travel a long and complex path from the database to a user (*see* Fig. 1). This fact has at least two implications: first, the database provider must furnish and maintain all the hardware and software resources necessary to reach the network; and second, the indirect nature of this connection magnifies security risks *(44)*.

The architecture shown in Fig. 1 is only one of many possible. The Web server and the data server reside on two distinct machines. The data server is located on a LAN together with the databases themselves and developer resources. The Web server is sited in a "demilitarized zone" between internal and external firewalls. Depending on one's host institution, all or part of this (or other) architecture may be dictated to the data resource provider—and firewalls (and possibly the Web server) may be provided.

Table 2
**Roles and Responsibilities of Team Members Involved in Developing
a Web-Accessible Database**

Role	Typical responsibilities
Systems administrator	Provides for the physical well-being of the machines and the network, and provides for system backups.
Website administrator	Maintains the Web server and the application server, and is responsible for website security.
Site designer	Designs and creates specifications for the overall structure and feel (Graphical User Interface) of the website.
Page designer	Implements the website through Html coding and scripting.
Data architect	Creates the database schema.
Database administrator	Maintains the database server and provides for database backup.
Annotators	Responsible for the information content of the database.
Curators	Provide scientific quality control of the database information.
Developers	Responsible for development of java servlets, applets, visualization tools, and analytical tools.

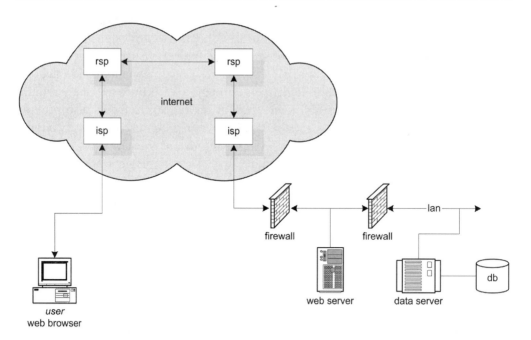

Fig. 1. The data path between the database and user.

Once the data leaves the host institution, it embarks on its path through the Internet; this takes it across two Internet service providers (ISPs)—one at each end—and a series of regional service providers (RSPs). The data then makes its way through a LAN (not shown) to eventually arrive at the user's desktop.

The numerous and complex physical hardware and network interconnections required to move data from the database are accompanied by even more complicated

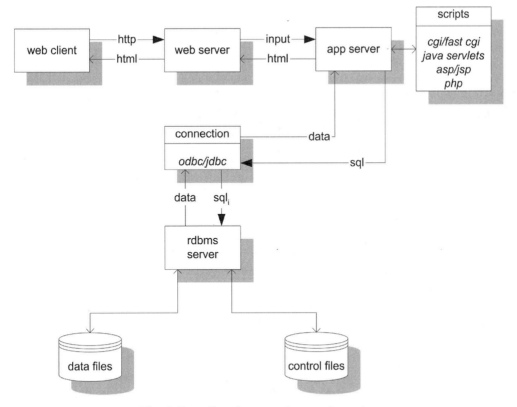

Fig. 2. Data flow from a software viewpoint.

software interconnections. Figure 2 shows a generic version of several relatively popular software configurations. Much of the complexity in developing contemporary biodatabases is at this level, rather than in the more traditional area of database design and maintenance.

The user accesses the data in the database through a Web browser. This browser sends HTTP requests to a Web server and receives information back in the form of HTML pages. In turn, the Web server communicates with a so-called application server, which may be an integrated component of the Web server itself, or a separate piece of software. In the oldest but still very popular architecture, the application server communicates with other programs—including the database server—with scripts written in Perl *(45)*. Java servlets *(46)*, Microsoft Active Server Pages (ASPs) and other technologies, such as those based on the PHP hypertext processor *(47)* or the Python-based Zope product, are also utlized. It is also possible and common to combine these technologies—Java servlets and Perl scripts frequently coexist.

Through any of these mechanisms, the application server communicates with the database server through a database *connection*. The connection can be either a software connection to a specific database (e.g., Oracle or Sybase), or it can be a more general type of connection such as that provided by Open Database Connectivity or the Java equivalent *(48)* that insulates the rest of the system from the underlying database. The application server communicates with the generic connection using a standard (vendor-neutral) dialect of Structure Query Language (SQL) and the generic connection then translates, if necessary, to the specific dialect of SQL spoken by the relational database management system being used. In theory—and in practice—the existence of generic connection components allows a great deal of freedom to choose an underlying database engine and removes a great deal of the risk inherent in making such a choice.

4.2. Types of Databases

Relational databases are the overwhelmingly dominant type of database technology employed today. Both older and newer technologies exist; however, for a combination of reasons including feature adequacy, technological maturity, efficiency, widespread standardization, and perhaps inertia, relational databases appear to possess advantages over both their predecessors and their would-be successors. Of the older architectures, perhaps only the so-called "flat-file databases"—that is, collections of files containing data in some private format—are still used, particularly for those databases intended solely for a researcher's private use. These databases are used for convenience and often represent a developmental stage in the transition of an informatics system to a more conventional database architecture. The Sequence Retrieval System *(49)* represents a flat file indexing system still in widespread use by numerous bioscientists. There are a host of newer (many of which are no longer "new") architectures, including object relational and object-oriented databases and knowledge bases *(50,51)* (e.g., Prolog, which allows one to store "rules" as well as "facts"). The need to store new types of data, including images and audio, and more complex structured data, as well as inherent limitations of the relational database model will lead to the gradual supplanting of relational databases by more powerful architectures; however, relational databases will remain the main game for some time to come. There is one current development that might invalidate this statement: relational database systems are currently being paired with mechanisms to improve data exchange. By far the most widespread mechanisms of data exchange are based on eXtendable Markup Language (XML). XML can be used for data storage as well as for data exchange and, indeed, XML-based databases are now making an appearance *(51–53)*. Because XML-based database architectures mature and approach relational architectures in access speed, security, and administrative features, they may be expected to challenge the hegemony of relational database systems.

4.2.1. The Relational Model

There are a huge number of introductions to the relational database model and its query language SQL. Gibas and Jambeck provide a good short introduction *(42)*. The book by Joe Celko *(54)* is also a good introduction. Here, we provide only a quick taste in the context of a hypothetical example. Consider a database that contains information about β-helices, a particular protein structural motif that is associated with cell invasion and attachment, which is disproportionately represented in pathogens, both viral and bacterial. For each identified β-helix, one might be interested in sequence information: both DNA sequences for a coding gene and the actual amino acid sequence; the structure itself, either as experimentally observed or computationally predicted; and also any references in the literature that may be available. Additionally, one would obviously be interested in properties of the encoding gene, especially any functional properties that may be known, and one would also like to know something about the organism in which the gene was found, especially whether it is a pathogen.

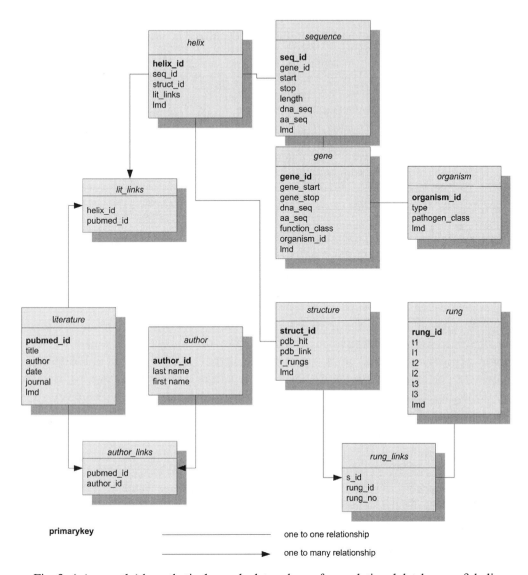

Fig. 3. A (currently) hypothetical sample data schema for a relational database on β-helices.

Relational databases organize this information in linked tables as shown in Fig. 3. The diagram in Fig. 3 is an example of a database schema and represents the organization of the database. Each table consists of rows and columns, just as in a spreadsheet. The rows (or records) contain the actual data about each β-helix or affiliated object. The columns or fields describe the type of information. In a pure relational database, each field is a simple datatype such as those shown in Table 3.

The key point here is that complex, or nested, datatypes are not allowed in a pure relational database. So, for example, lists or sets, have to be "simulated" using the table structure. This requires that tables be linked together using specific fields, called keys. In the hypothetical β-helix database, at least three examples of this requirement are presented. Specifically, each β-helix may be referenced by several publications in the

Table 3
Data Types Supported by the Pure Relational Database Model

Data type	Description
int	Integer (whole number)
float, real	Computer approximation of a real number
char, text	Character-string data
date	Year, month, day
blob	Binary large object—an uninterpreted type which may be used to store information such as image data

literature (hence, the *lit_links* table), each reference may have several authors (hence, the *author_links* table), and the β-helix itself is composed of a series of rungs (hence, the *rung_links* table). The rung_links table provides an additional field because the order of the rungs is important (unlike, presumably the order of references).

There is a well-established set of relational database design principles. These principles are typically phrased in terms of rules for data *normalization* which provide for construction of a well-ordered data schema—the set of database tables and other structures that hold the information *(55)*. In addition, there is a large amount of literature on the nature of database transactions, much of which is critical for databases used for financial transactions but of less relevance to biological databases, which are generally "read-only" for the vast majority of users.

The primary points we wish to make concerning relational databases include the following.

- Designing a database is a skilled activity and requires an understanding of the data, of the expected queries, and of the limitations/features of the relational architecture.
- Querying the data directly requires an understanding of the table structure.
- Adding fields to tables within databases is easy, but more substantial alterations can be costly.

We also note that it is generally necessary to associate data with a curator name or identifier and a "last-modified-date" (shown in Fig. 3 as the fields *lmd* in various tables). Finally, we note that the use of so-called "comment" fields frequently leads to abuse— "parsing" comment fields to extract information not specifically allowed for in the table structure is a depressingly common activity.

4.2.2. Choosing a Relational Database Management Systems

There are a large number of database systems in common use. Oracle is the market leader. Microsoft's SQL Server is a popular choice on Windows platforms. Microsoft Access is an easy-to-use "starter" system, adequate for learning and for small databases. The bioinformatics community has embraced the free database management systems MySQL and PostgresSQL, both of which are available for Windows and Unix systems and both of which have excellent performance and numerous features. Many of these systems are integrated with Web servers, application servers, and other software. This is particularly true for recent releases of Oracle. As stated earlier, transaction control is not generally critical for most bioinformatic databases, and our primary recommendation for choosing a database management system is that whichever system has the most local institutional support is probably the right pick.

4.3. Providing User Access to the Database

Once the database is in place and appropriate security measures have been instituted, the issue of how users interact with the database must be confronted. As stated earlier, the most common "front-end" for databases is now the Web browser. Therefore, biological databases are generally accessed as part of a website. This website will generally provide numerous services to users. The site may provide "raw" access to the database in which the user enters a SQL query and receives the query results as a served HTML page. Raw SQL access requires the user to know the table structure, so the site should provide access to this table structure, as well as any other necessary explanatory material.

However, entering SQL queries directly is not a task that should be imposed on most users—including sophisticated ones. Rather, one should provide "canned" queries where the user can build a query by choosing from drop-down lists or entering specific terms.

In addition, many Web-enabled biological databases show the results of particularly interesting analyses that were performed using the underlying database. Furthermore, it is generally necessary to provide alternate interfaces to curators or data entry specialists who are given permission to modify the underlying database (as opposed to general users who cannot).

A site map such as that shown in Fig. 4 is fairly common. Designing the website requires as much attention as designing the underlying database. The primary usability criterion for websites is that pages should download quickly. Most surveys indicate that download speed is at least three times as important as appearance.

Sites have an information architecture and should be designed for easy navigation. At all times, the user should know where they are in the architecture (or hierarchy) and which options are available to them. The visual appearance of the site should facilitate navigation and provide a uniform experience, especially for sites containing a large number of heterogeneous pages.

Also note that issues of configuration and version control must be managed. Specifically, one often has to manage four sites in parallel—release and development versions for both public (read-only) and privileged (read-write) users. Frequently, the development versions of the site are hosted on different hardware from the release versions.

5. DATA ANALYSIS AND VISUALIZATION

5.1. Analysis

As indicated earlier, databases of biological sequence information contain not only the sequences themselves, but also an annotation record that provides descriptive information concerning the structure and function of the sequenced molecules. Frequently, an even more thorough analysis of the sequence information may be warranted. The analytical tools to be used may be provided by a website setup to run various analytical programs (sequence similarity searching with Basic Local Alignment Search Tool [BLAST] is a frequently available), or may be provided by sequence analysis software packages or stand-alone analysis tools. The results of different analyses can

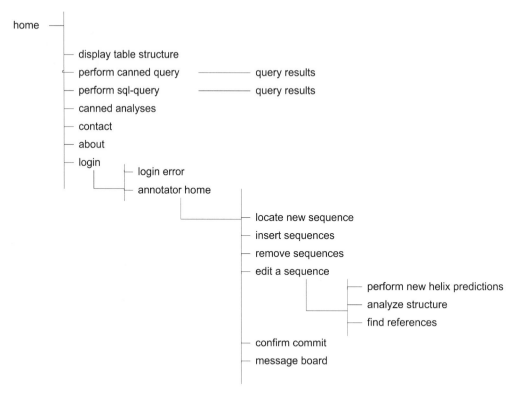

Fig. 4. Beginnings of a website map.

then be provided either as static information derived from the analytical work already performed by the curator or as dynamic information that has been generated as the result of a specific request by a researcher utilizing a website. As an example, the Poxvirus Bioinformatics Resource Center provides numerous analytical tools that are accessible from Web-based forms allowing for network access to analysis tools that, in general, will be run on poxvirus sequences made available from the Resource Center's integrated database. Examples include BLAST (http://www.poxvirus.org/search.asp), textual and graphical ortholog gene comparisons (http://www.poxvirus.org/orthologs.asp), and gene sequence search interfaces (http://www.poxvirus.org/gene_search.asp). Similar sets of Web-based analysis tools designed to integrate closely with existing information stored in a sequence database are available at many of the organism-specific sites mentioned in Subheading 2.

Pattern identification and comparison might be considered to be one of the hallmark goals of any bioinformatic work. Whether we are trying to map out the gene structure of an organism, identify unique pathogenicity islands in a microbial genome, or compare the similarity between the gene sets of two different microbial strains, we are in effect using pattern matching algorithms to satisfy all of these goals. Visualization tools (*see* Figs. 5–7) that generate graphical summaries of database information that has been subjected to pattern matching searches have the potential to greatly enhance our ability to discern important, characteristic patterns in the data.

5.1.1. Detection of Newly Emerging or Engineered Threats

The annotation and analysis procedures utilized by any basic sequencing and analysis pipeline along with the database and Web application developed to support these procedures can be used for the rapid identification of unknown or possibly genetically engineered biological threats. Whereas the detection of anticipated biological threats such as anthrax will usually proceed on the basis of scripted laboratory procedures using common protocols for immunological, polymerase chain reaction, or hybridization probe-based techniques; the detection and identification of unanticipated threats, such as unexpected zoonoses, or natural or engineered recombinants may require a more generic approach. One means of dealing with this problem is through development of a rapid identification process that combines random, shotgun sequencing of isolated genomic nucleic acid from the unknown organism, with a sequence assembly and annotation engine. The assembly and annotation engine would be used to assemble the shotgun sequences into larger sequence contigs and then sequence similarities would be detected by automated database searching schemes utilizing both large-scale (GenBank) and curated model organism or gene pathogen databases. Information from these analyses would then be used to assemble a genetic map of the organism that should allow for the identification of its basic genetic background (the parental organism or vector) along with the detection of any unusual or unexpected genetic information such as virulence factors or regulatory regions. One would be looking for unique combinations of genes present in a unique genomic context. Because of the nature of a shotgun sequencing approach, this map will not be complete; however, generally, it need not be. There should be sufficient information to identify important differences from known organisms, and the rough genetic map generated can be refined as necessary using directed, "finishing" sequencing schemes to fill in gaps.

5.2. VISUALIZATION

Databases provide vast repositories for storage and retrieval of information. This information is useless unless desired subsets of this information can be packaged in a form that is meaningful to the individuals who would like to utilize this information. Generating reports in tabular form is a common method for preparing summaries of database information, but frequently, tabular data are not the best means to identify important patterns in many types of data. In addition, the underlying relational structure of most databases is best hidden from users or camouflaged by providing canned or alternate access that does not require knowledge of the table structure. Graphical tools provide particularly effective means of interacting with databases. Interaction can be dynamic—not precanned—and allows complex sets of data to be represented simultaneously and graphically. Creating graphical representations of information can be as simple as importing the data into a spreadsheet program such as Microsoft Excel or SigmaPlot and using the built-in graphing tools to generate figures. Alternatively, more elaborate programs can be developed that allow user interaction from webpages to create customized graphic illustrations. Currently, three technologies are available for providing such access in a largely browser- and platform-independent fashion. The oldest of these technologies is that supplied by Java applets. Macromedia's Flash plug-in has been considerably enhanced recently and the Flash plug-in is actually installed

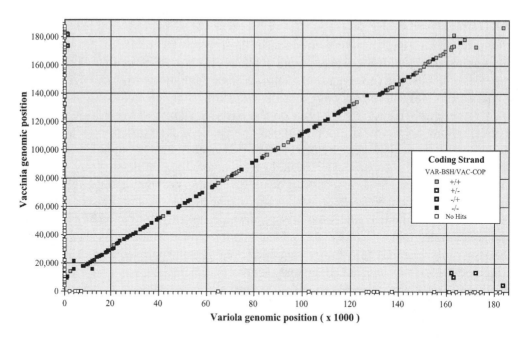

Fig. 5. Conserved ortholog comparison between *Variola major* virus strain Bangladesh, and *Vaccinia* virus strain Copenhagen generated by the Java-based application at http://www.poxvirus.org/pairs_comp.asp.

in more browsers than is the Java plug-in. The most recent technology is an XML-derivative termed Simple Vector Graphics, which is rapidly becoming available on most platforms.

The Poxvirus Bioinformatics Resource Center website provides a tool for creating a comparison plot of conserved gene order between any two poxvirus genomes (http://www.poxvirus.org/pairs_comp.asp). This Web-based application gets its input from a user-submitted html form, downloads the desired data from the poxvirus database, and then uses a Java-based applet to generate a figure that is displayed on the user's screen. Figure 5 shows an example of such a Java-based synteny plot. These types of Web-based graphical tools are being seen much more frequently and are becoming much more sophisticated. Some of the most elaborate visualization tools currently available are those for displaying human genome project data. The Ensembl browser of the EMBL European Bioinformatics Institute and the Sanger Institute (http://www.ensembl.org/) provides access to current assemblies of the human, mouse, and *Drosophila* genomic databases.

Figure 6 shows an advanced graphical interface to a sequence database developed at LANL by Karla Atkins. This tool is used as a front-end to numerous sequence databases and provides interactive and dynamic access to the data.

Fig. 6. *(opposite page)* Dynamic interactive visualization using Java. *Bacillus anthracis* virulence plasmid pX01 showing open reading frames and other genomic features. (Figure provided by K. Atkins, Los Alamos National Laboratory.)

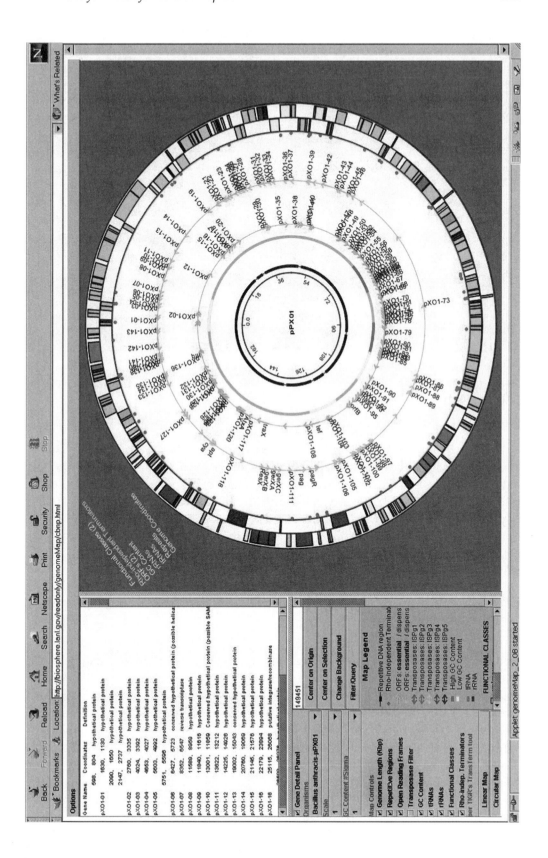

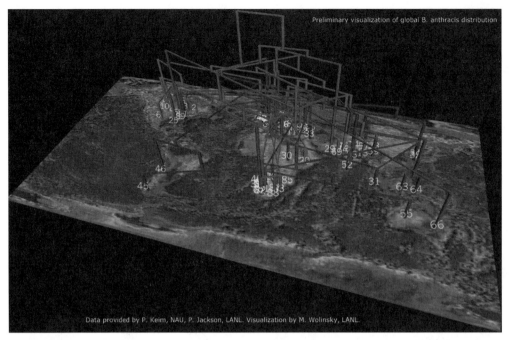

Fig. 7. Dynamic interactive visualization using VRML. These data can be rotated and zoomed interactively in a browser. Both phylogenetic and geographical data can be displayed simultaneously.

Databases intended to support biothreat reduction will also be increasingly used in conjunction with other data. In the biothreat reduction area, combining biological data with geographic data will be particularly important. A preliminary visualization capability, also developed at LANL, which uses Virtual Reality Markup Language technology (now being replaced with an XML-based version—X3D), allows interactive access to both phylogenetic data and geographical data for pathogens. A visualization of this data for *Bacillus anthracis* using data supplied by Paul Jackson (LANL) and Paul Keim (Northern Arizona University) is shown in Fig. 7.

6. SUMMARY

Protecting military and civilian populations from the use of biological weapons involves preparation and research at multiple levels. These needs include the development of environmental detectors, diagnostic reagents, animal models, antimicrobial drugs, and new, more effective vaccines. All of these areas need to be able to deal with pathogens on the current lists of microbial agents thought to be potential offensive threats, as well as recognize novel and/or engineered pathogens not yet recognized as threat agents. The availability of bioinformatic databases and analytical resources provides an information backbone that supports all research, both basic and applied, into providing a defense against the use of biological weapons. This research support ranges from the development and refinement of biological signatures for detection and diagnosis; to the recognition of unique patterns of engineered genes arising from sophisticated development of offensive weapons; to providing a better understanding of the relationship between expression of particular genes and the ability of any pathogen to cause disease. The amount of information generated by genomic, proteomic, expression array, and other modern, high-throughput biological techniques is huge. Combined with information generated by public health and clinical endeavors, this represents an extensive resource for biodefense research and response. It is the job and responsibility of the bioinformaticist to take these resources and restructure them so that the biodefense researcher and responder can be fully aware and make the best use of all of this critical information.

ACKNOWLEDGMENTS

The authors express their thanks for the information so generously provided to them by Drs. Kevin Anderson, Alison Deckhut, Eric Eisenstadt, Edward Eitzen, Maria Y. Giovanni, George Korch, Gerry Myers, Piush Patel, W. Graham Richards, and Bruno Sobral. The work described herein was funded in part by NIAID/DARPA grant (U01-AI48706) to EJL, and USAMRIID Research Plan ET-00-04 to FJL. The mention of a company or a commercial product does not constitute an endorsement. The views expressed in this chapter are those of the authors and are not necessarily endorsed by Department of Defense or by the Department of Energy.

REFERENCES

1. Drell, S. D., Sofaer, A. D., and Wilson, G. D. (1999) Hoover Institution on War Revolution and Peace. *The New Terror: Facing the Threat of Biological and Chemical Weapons.* Hoover Institution Press, Stanford, CA.
2. DaSilva, E. J. (1999) Biological warfare, bioterroism, biodefense and the biological and toxin weapons convention. *Elec. J. Biotechnol.* **2.**
3. Lederberg, J. (1999) *Biological Weapons: Limiting the Threat.* MIT Press, Cambridge, MA.
4. Dayhoff, M. O and National Biomedical Research Foundation. (1965) *Atlas of Protein Sequence and Structure*, 1st ed. National Biomedical Research Foundation, Sliver Spring, MD.
5. Kanehisa, M. I. (1982) Los Alamos sequence analysis package for nucleic acids and proteins. *Nucleic Acids Res.* **10,** 183–196.
6. Burks, C., Fickett, J. W., Goad, W. B., et al. (1985) The GenBank nucleic acid sequence database. *Comp. Appl. Biosci.* **1,** 225–233.
7. Wu, C. H., Huang, H., Arminski, L., et al. (2002) The Protein Information Resource: an integrated public resource of functional annotation of proteins. *Nucleic Acids Res.* **30,** 35–37.
8. Mount, D. W. (2001) *Bioinformatics: Sequence and Genome Analysis.* Cold Spring Harbor Laboratory Press, Cold Spring Harbor, NY.
9. Setubal, J. C. and Meidanis, J. (1997) *Introduction to Computational Molecular Biology.* PWS, Boston, MA.
10. Kelle, A., Dando, M., Nixdorff, K., and North Atlantic Treaty Organization, Scientific Affairs Division (2001) *The Role of Biotechnology in Countering BTW Agents.* Kluwer Academic Publishers, Boston, MA.
11. Collins, F. S., Patrinos, A., Jordan, E., Chakravarti, A,. Gesteland, R., and Walters, L. (1998) New goals for the U.S. Human Genome Project: 1998–2003. *Science* **282,** 682–689.
12. Wheeler, D. L., Church, D. M., Lash, A. E., et al. (2001) Database resources of the National Center for Biotechnology Information. *Nucleic Acids Res.* **29,** 11–16.
13. Stoesser, G., Baker, W., van den Broek, A., et al. (2002) The EMBL nucleotide sequence database. *Nucleic Acids Res.* **30,** 21–26.
14. Tateno, Y., Imanishi, T., Miyazaki, S., et al. (2002) DNA Data Bank of Japan (DDBJ) for genome scale research in life science. *Nucleic Acids Res.* **30,** 27–30.

15. Berman, H. M., Westbrook, J., Feng, Z., et al. (2000) The protein data bank. *Nucleic Acids Res.* **28**, 235–242.
16. Westbrook, J., Feng, Z., Jain, S., et al. (2002) The Protein Data Bank: unifying the archive. *Nucleic Acids Res.* **30**, 245–248.
17. Sherlock, G., Hernandez-Boussard, T., Kasarskis, A., et al. (2001) The Stanford Microarray Database. *Nucleic Acids Res.* **29**, 152–155.
18. Edgar, R., Domrachev, M., and Lash, A. E. (2002) Gene Expression Omnibus: NCBI gene expression and hybridization array data repository. *Nucleic Acids Res.* **30**, 207–210.
19. Gardiner-Garden, M. and Littlejohn, T. G. (2001) A comparison of microarray databases. *Brief Bioinform.* **2**, 143–158.
20. Hubbard, T., Barker, D., Birney, E., et al. (2002) The Ensembl genome database project. *Nucleic Acids Res.* **30**, 38–41.
21. Kent, W. J., Sugnet, C. W., Furey, T. S., et al. (2002) The human genome browser at UCSC. *Genome Res.* **12**, 996–1006.
22. Peterson, J. D., Umayam, L. A., Dickinson, T., Hickey, E. K., and White, O. (2001) The comprehensive microbial resource. *Nucleic Acids Res.* **29**, 123–125.
23. Collaboration TPGD (2001) PlasmoDB: An integrative database of the *Plasmodium falciparum* genome. Tools for accessing and analyzing finished and unfinished sequence data. The Plasmodium Genome Database Collaborative. *Nucleic Acids Res.* **29**, 66–69.
24. Ball, C. A., Jin, H., Sherlock, G., et al. (2001) Saccharomyces Genome Database provides tools to survey gene expression and functional analysis data. *Nucleic Acids Res.* **29**, 80, 81.
25. Stein, L., Sternberg, P., Durbin, R., Thierry-Mieg, J., and Spieth, J. (2001) WormBase: network access to the genome and biology of *Caenorhabditis elegans*. *Nucleic Acids Res.* **29**, 82–6.
26. Consortium TF. (2002) The FlyBase database of the *Drosophila* genome projects and community literature. *Nucleic Acids Res.* **30**, 106–108.
27. Baxevanis, A. D. (2002) The molecular biology database collection: 2002 update. *Nucleic Acids Res.* **30**, 1–12.
28. Tatusov, R. L., Natale, D. A., Garkavtsev, I. V., et al. (2001) The COG database: new developments in phylogenetic classification of proteins from complete genomes. *Nucleic Acids Res.* **29**, 22–28.
29. Consortium GO. (2001) Creating the gene ontology resource: design and implementation. *Genome Res.* **11**, 1425–1433.
30. Finlay, B. B. and Falkow, S. (1997) Common themes in microbial pathogenicity revisited. *Microbiol. Mol. Biol. Rev.* **61**, 136–169.
31. Myers, G. (2000) Bioinformatics support for the CBNP at Los Alamos National Laboratory. Proceedings of the chemical and biological nonproliferation program. *CBIAC* 101, 102.
32. Lebeda, F. J. (1997) Deterrence of biological and chemical warfare: a review of policy options. *Mil. Med.* **162**, 156–161.
33. Okie, S. (2002) U.S. health care system grapples with new role. *The Washington Post* A3.
34. Bunk, S. (2002) Early warning. *Scientist* **16**, 14, 15.
35. Glowniak, J. (1998) History, structure, and function of the Internet. *Semin. Nucl. Med.* **28**, 135–144.
36. Davies, E. K., Glick, M., Harrison, K. N., and Richards, W. G. (2002) Pattern recognition and massively distributed computing. *J. Comput. Chem.* **23**, 1544–1550.
37. Glick, M., Grant, G. H., and Richards, W. G. (2002) Pinpointing anthrax-toxin inhibitors. *Nat. Biotechnol.* **20**, 118, 119.
38. Glick, M., Robinson, D. D., Grant, G. H., and Richards, W. G. (2002) Identification of ligand binding sites on proteins using a multi-scale approach. *J. Am. Chem. Soc.* **124**, 2337–2344.
39. Brooks, B. R., Bruccoleri, R. E., Olafson, B. D., States, D. J., Swaminathan, S., and Karplus, M. (1983) CHARMM: a program for macromolecular energy, minimization, and dynamics calculations. *J. Comp. Chem.* **4**, 187–217.

40. Pearlman, D. A., Case, D. A., Caldwell, J. W., et al. (1995) AMBER, a package of computer programs for applying molecular mechanics, normal mode analysis, molecular dynamics and free energy calculations to simulate the structural and energetic properties of molecules. *Comp. Phys. Commun.* **91,** 1–44.

41. Baker, P. G., Brass, A., Bechhofer, S., Goble, C., Paton, N., and Stevens, R. (1998) *TAMBIS: Transparent Access to Multiple Bioinformatics Information Sources.* Proc. 6th Int. Conf. on Intelligent Systems for Molecular Biology, (Glasgow, J., et al., eds.), AAAI, New York, pp. 25–34.

42. Gibas, C. and Jambeck, P. (2001) Developing Bioinformatics Computer Skills. 1st ed. O'Reilly, Cambridge, MA. (*See especially* chapters 13 and 14.)

43. Graff, J. (2001) *Cryptography and E-Commerce: A Wiley Tech Brief.* John Wiley, New York.

44. Stein, L. D. (1998) *Web Security: A Step-By-Step Reference Guide.* Addison-Wesley, Reading, MA.

45. Tisdall, J. D. (2001) *Beginning Perl for Bioinformatics,* 1st ed. O'Reilly, Beijing.

46. Brogden, W. B. (2002) *SOAP Programming with Java.* Sybex, San Francisco, CA.

47. Ullman, L. E. (2001) *PHP for the World Wide Web.* Peachpit Press, Berkely, CA.

48. Speegle, G. D. (2002) *JDBC: Practical Guide for Java Programmers.* MK/Morgan Kaufmann, San Francisco, CA.

49. Etzold, T., Ulyanov, A., and Argos, P. (1996) SRS: information retrieval system for molecular biology data banks. *Meth. Enzymol.* **266,** 114–128.

50. Brown, P. G. (2001) *Object-Relational Database Development: A Plumber's Guide.* Prentice Hall, Upper Saddle River, NJ.

51. Chaudhri, A. B. and Zicari, R. (2001) *Succeeding with Object Databases: A Practical Look at Today's Implementations with Java and XML.* Wiley, New York.

52. Rubin, D. L., Shafa, F., Oliver, D. E., Hewett, M., and Altman, R. B. (2002) Representing genetic sequence data for pharmacogenomics: an evolutionary approach using ontological and relational models. *Bioinformatics* **18(Suppl. 1),** S207–215.

53. Wang, L., Riethoven, J. J., and Robinson, A. (2002) XEMBL: distributing EMBL data in XML format. *Bioinformatics* **18,** 1147, 1148.

54. Celko, J. (1995) *Instant SQL Programming.* Wrox Press, Birmingham, UK.

55. Dutka, A. F. and Hanson, H. H. (1989) *Fundamentals of Data Normalization.* Addison-Wesley, Reading, MA.

19

Genomic Efforts With Biodefense Pathogens

Rekha Seshadri, Timothy D. Read, William C. Nierman, and Ian T. Paulsen

1. INTRODUCTION

Events following the attacks on New York City and Washington, DC on September 11, 2001, have served to underscore the need for extensive research on biological warfare (BW) and other agents in order to aid the initiative to fight terrorism worldwide. During the Cold War era, the former USSR covertly developed, tested, and stockpiled immense amounts of biological weapons in an effort to build the largest and most advanced biological warfare program in the world. The knowledge developed in these laboratories and manufacturing sites has since undoubtedly spread to other regimes and terrorist organizations. Research on these agents of bioterrorism concern is of highest priority to enhance diagnostic, preventative, and therapeutic measures. Pathogens that may be potentially adapted for biological warfare include those causing smallpox (*Variola*), anthrax (*Bacillus anthracis*), plague (*Yersinia pestis*), tularemia (*Francisella tularensis*), brucellosis (*Brucella abortus, B. melitensis, B. suis, B. canis*), Q fever (*Coxiella burnetii*), botulism (*Clostridium botulinum*), glanders (*Burkholderia mallei*), and enterotoxin B producing *Staphylococcus* spp. All of these agents constitute considerable threat to military personnel and civilians alike in the dreaded event of a bioterrorist affront.

Whole-scale genome sequencing of various of potential BW agents are underway at The Sanger Center, The Institute for Genomic Research (TIGR), and other institutions. This chapter highlights some of the prominent features of the individual genomes of organisms being sequenced by TIGR. The information characteristically gleaned from whole genome analysis includes novel gene sequences, coding capacity, metabolic and transport capabilities, virulence determinants, and so on. For BW pathogens, the expectation is that genome sequence will aid in the development of better vaccines, detection assays, and therapeutics and pave the way toward a comprehensive understanding of their fundamental biological processes. Detection of genetically engineered variants that may have been enhanced in their pathogenicity by introduction of nonindigenous genes would also be possible. State-of-the art techniques and equipment have allowed rapid and efficient sequencing of entire genomes. A brief description of the procedure follows.

From: *Infectious Diseases: Biological Weapons Defense: Infectious Diseases and Counterterrorism*
Edited by: L. E. Lindler, F. J. Lebeda, and G. W. Korch © Humana Press Inc., Totowa, NJ

2. DETERMINING WHOLE-GENOME SEQUENCES AT TIGR

TIGR has pioneered a random shotgun genome-sequencing strategy that was first used to sequence and assemble the 1.83-Mb genome of *Haemophilus influenzae* Rd *(1)* in 1995 and has since been used successfully in the completion of more than 60 other microbial genomes to date (a list of completed genomes can be found at http:// www.tigr.org/tdb/mdb/mdbcomplete.html). Currently, this method involves the construction of random small (2.0 kb) and medium (10 kb) insert plasmid libraries from genomic DNAs, sequencing both ends of randomly selected clones from these libraries to provide approx eightfold sequence coverage of the genome and assembly of random sequence fragments using TIGR assembler programs. The sequences from medium-insert clones provide "scaffolding" for linking assemblies and contigs during genome closure. Any remaining gaps are resolved by polymerase chain reaction (PCR), direct genome-walking, and primer-walking of the library templates. Overall accuracy of the inferred genome structure and all repeat sequences are confirmed by PCR and walking repetitive elements. Subsequent annotation of the genome involves use of various computing software developed to optimize identification of open reading frames (ORFs) and intergenic regions, and to facilitate other analyses. ORFs are identified using TIGR gene-finding "GLIMMER" *(2,3)* software and these ORFs are then searched against an internal nonredundant amino acid database (nraa) comprised of all proteins made up of GenBank, Protein Information Resource (PIR), and SWISS-PROT. The search algorithm is BLAST-Extend-Repraze, which performs a basic local alignment search tool (BLAST) against the nraa *(4)*, identifies potential frameshifts or point mutations, and maximally extends regions of similarity across frameshifts. All proteins are additionally searched against two sets of hidden Markov models (HMMs; constructed from multiple alignments of proteins sharing the same function or belonging to the same family): Pfam HMMs *(5)* and TIGRFAMS *(6)*. Results of all these searches are used by the preliminary annotation tool, "auto-Annotate," which assigns common name, gene symbol, Enzyme Commission number and TIGR role category and rapidly generates a preliminary gene list. This initial automated annotation is followed by a manual curation of each gene assignment. In addition, sequences are analyzed for the presence of transfer RNAs (tRNAs), ribosomal RNAs (rRNAs), codon usage, nucleotide biases, ribosome binding sites, insertion elements, terminator regions, frameshifts, repeat regions, paralogous gene families, signal sequences, membrane spanning regions, predicted cell localization, and structural or functional motifs.

TIGR provides the academic research community complete access to genomic sequence and results of sequence analysis through the TIGR Microbial Database on the World Wide Web (www.tigr.org/tdb/tdb.html). Initial release of the sequence data is in the form of contigs assembled at threefold sequence coverage, with monthly updates thereafter, until completion of the genome. The assemblies are searchable through the TIGR BLAST Search Engine for Unfinished Microbial Genomes (www.tigr.org/cgi-bin/BlastSearch/blast) and the assemblies can be downloaded through the ftp server. At the completion of sequencing and analysis phases, the database will provide the complete DNA sequence and the translation of all ORFs on an ftp site, gene identifications and alignments, and a searchable list of all the genes and their metabolic role categories. The Comprehensive Microbial Resource (CMR; http://www.tigr.org/tigr-scripts/CMR2/ CMRHomePage.spl) allows cross-genome analyses for all the completed bacterial genomes or any sub-set of genomes; analysis includes GC plots, comparison of clusters of orthologous groups of proteins, computer-generated two-dimensional gel models, recent duplications, and so on *(7)*. It also allows retrieval of data based on user-specified parameters such as role assignments, membrane topology, molecular weight, p*I*, and so on. Databases such as the CMR and other initiatives help further our understanding of microbial physiology and evolution using genome-sequence derived information.

3. SEQUENCE ANALYSIS OF BIODEFENSE AGENTS AT TIGR

The interaction between host and pathogen may be envisioned as a battle where attacks and counteroffensives are mounted and clever tactics have been devised by both microbe and host over the years. Each pathogen has evolved a unique parasitic "strategy" that allows it to counter host defenses and establish infection. Therefore, in addition to their BW potential, the select agents serve as important paradigms for bacterial pathogenesis and further our understanding of host–pathogen interactions and adaptations. Sequencing projects for *Bacillus anthracis, Clostridium perfringens, Coxiella burnetii, Brucella suis,* and *Burkholderia mallei* are at different stages of completion at TIGR, and an overview of the current status of the respective projects as well as general genome features are presented.

The information gained from the sequencing projects of BW pathogens will be essential for the development of countermeasures against the BW threat in terms of identifying vaccine candidates and therapeutic and diagnostic reagents. The genome sequence will also enable production of DNA microarrays to analyze gene expression during the infectious process, and identify host specificity factors that account for differences in pathogenicity of intraspecific strains. Microarray analysis also has the potential for identifying strains that have been genetically manipulated to function as BW agents, either by comparative genome hybridiazation studies or by confirming altered gene expression profiles.

3.1. B. anthracis

Anthrax, caused by *B. anthracis*, is primarily a zoonosis that causes cutaneous, inhalation, or gastrointestinal infections in humans with consequences that are frequently fatal *(8)*. This nonmotile, Gram-positive, facultatively anerobic bacillus is an ideal candidate for BW because of the ease of dissemination and production of highly resilient spores capable of surviving under adverse physical and chemical circumstances, including heat, ionizing radiation, and pressure *(9,10)*. Spores enter via skin abrasions, orally, or by inhalation and initially target macrophages, followed by development of systemic disease. Little is known regarding the initial intracellular phase of infection or how subsequent escape from the macrophage occurs, leading to bacteremia. The pathogenic process in humans is poorly understood; patients succumb to various of symptoms including toxin-triggered shock, septicemia, meningitis, and respiratory failure *(11)*. The key virulence genes are located on two large plasmids: pX01 (181 kb) and pX02 (96 kb). The tripartite exotoxin composed of subunits designated lethal factor, protective antigen (PA), and edema factor is found in a pathogenicity island located on pX01 *(12,13)*. A poly-D-glutamic acid capsule located on pX02 is also a major virulence component *(14,15)*. The principal antigen in the vaccines used currently by the

US and UK militaries is the cellular-binding toxin component PA. These vaccines, although offering basic protection from infection, suffer several problems with administration such as requirement of too many initial and booster doses and lack of cross-protection *(16)*. Sequencing of the *B. anthracis* genome offers prospects for a better understanding of mechanisms mediating persistence, host interaction, pathogenesis, survival, replication, germination, and other phenomena. The design of safer and more efficacious vaccines is also much anticipated.

3.1.1. General Features of the B. anthracis Genome

Sequencing of a *B. anthracis* Ames Δ (pXO1-, pXO2-) genome received from collaborators at the Defence Science and Technology Laboratory in Porton Down, UK, has been completed *(16a)*. The 5.23-Mb chromosome has an average G+C content of 35.4% and has been preliminarily determined to encode approx 5750 genes that have an average gene length of approx 710 nucleotides. Biological roles have been assigned to approx 38.7% of the predicted genes; approx 29.3 % are similar to hypothetical genes in other organisms (full-length database matches to conceptual translations in other species, these are referred to as "conserved hypothetical" proteins), approx 11.4% match genes of unknown function (database match is to a group of proteins that are members of a defined family, but whose function is unknown) and approx 20.6% represent unique or "hypothetical" genes (with no significant similarity to other sequenced genes), accounting for a coding capacity of approx 84.8%. Ninety-six tRNA genes have been identified. The ORFs with assigned function are classified into functional role categories that allow reconstruction of various metabolic pathways and transporter profiles. A graph representing the distribution of ORFs in each of these functional role categories is shown (*see* Fig. 1). Examination of the gene list suggests the presence of some previously unidentified chromosomally encoded virulence determinants such as enterotoxins, secreted metalloproteases, and other mediators of host–pathogen interactions. An interesting feature of the *B. anthracis* genome is the number of potentially important proteins encoded, for which corresponding phenotypes have not been demonstrated. These functions include hemolysis, motility, and resistance to the antibiotics penicillin and tetracycline.

In addition to the "index" Ames strain, TIGR sequenced the "Florida" isolate of the Ames strain from a victim of the anthrax attack in Fall 2001 to draft (averge 8X sequence coverage). Using a statistical method to aggregate sequence quality scores, 60 novel polymorphisms between the previously indistinguishable isolates were determined computationally and subsequently confirmed by resequencing. The majority of differences were found on the pXO1 and pXO2 plasmids. However, the "Florida" Ames plasmids were compared to reference plasmid sequences from Pasteur and Sterne strains *(17,18)*, which are more distantly related, whereas the chromosomes that were compared belonged to the same strain (Ames). The 11 single nucleotide polymorphisms on the chromosome included nonsynonymous mutations in important conserved genes for ABC transporters, sporulation regulator *spo0A,* and starvation response gene *relA*. The "Florida" pXO1 plasmid had two large DNA inversions compared to the previously sequenced Sterne strain, one of which consisted of the entire 44.8-kb pathogenicity island *(19)*. Screening the polymorphisms in various of *B. anthracis* strains showed that the "Florida" isolate was from the same lineage as strains distributed through the

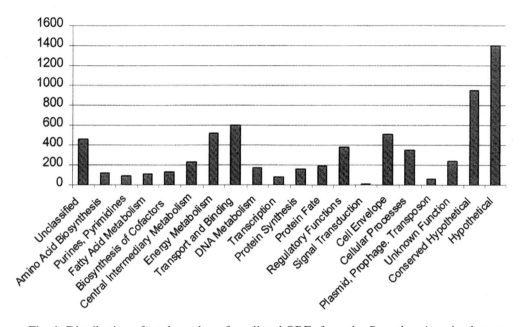

Fig. 1. Distribution of total number of predicted ORFs from the *B. anthracis* main chromosome sequence into different functional role categories.

US Army Medical Research Institute of Infectious Disease in Fort Detrick, MD, and was clearly differentiated from the only other natural strain with the same Variable Number of Tandem Repeat pattern *(20)*. This work also announced the value of comparative genome sequencing for microbial forensic studies and has been summarized in a recent report *(21)*.

3.2. C. burnetii

C. burnetii is the etiological agent of "Q-fever," an acute "influenza-like" illness with a characteristic debilitating, periorbital headache, and cyclic fever *(22)*. Instances of chronic disease manifest as endocarditis and hepatitis, and patients have poor prognosis for recovery *(23)*. Domestic livestock are the primary reservoir, but the host range encompasses arthropods, birds, rodents, and other wild vertebrates *(22,24)*. Infection arises primarily via aerosol transmission and constitutes a serious threat for military personnel and civilians alike. Taxonomically placed amidst the γ-Proteobacteria, closest to *Legionella* spp., this "rickettsia" (historical description) is an obligately intracellular, Gram-negative parasite that resides within the unique replicative niche of the phagolysosome of its eukaryotic host (professional and nonprofessional phagocytes) *(25)*. *C. burnetii* is highly adapted to thrive in this discouraging compartment where low pH, hydrolytic enzymes, and other likely stresses such as oxygen and nitrogen radicals are the norm *(26)*. In addition, the organism has evolved a novel nonsporulating developmental strategy to survive extracellularly for extended periods of time *(27)*. Resistance to heat, desiccation, pressure (up to 35,000 psi in French press), and osmotic and oxidative stress has been demonstrated *(28)*. Therefore, all of these characteristics bestow eligibility to *C. burnetii* as a potential BW agent. Difficulty in cultivation and paucity of available genetic tools to study the organism make the genome sequence information extremely valuable to investigators. The elucidation of mechanisms contributing to extracellular persistence, high infectivity, intracellular trafficking and survival, morphological differentiation, and other aspects of its pathogenic mode are of primary importance.

3.2.1. General Features of the C. burnetii Genome

The genome of the Nine Mile, Phase I (RSA493) strain has been completely sequenced and assembled at TIGR *(28a)*. This tick-isolate was originally identified in Missoula, MT, in 1937 and is highly virulent, with multiple incidents of lab infections reported. The 1.99-Mb circular chromosome possesses an average G+C content of 42.6%. Initial automated annotation suggests the chromosome encodes approx 2527 ORFs with an average gene length of 722 bp. Manual curation of the individual gene assignments was yet to be performed as of January 1, 2002. The coding capacity is approximately 89%, which does not suggest extensive gene loss as seen in the case of other Rickettsial species; *R. prowazekii* and *R. conorii* have coding capacities of 76 and 81%, respectively *(29)*. Approximately 43% (1089) of the predicted ORFs were given a functional assignment, whereas 10.9% (275) were conserved hypothetical, *viz.*, similar to hypothetical proteins from other bacteria. A large proportion, 38.9% or 982, were hypothetical, that is, not similar to any other sequences deposited in GenBank to date, and 7.2% matched genes of unknown function. A graph representing the distribution of ORFs in each functional role category is shown *(see* Fig. 2). About 42 genes encoding transfer RNAs corresponding to the different iso-acceptor tRNA species have been identified. Only a single operon encoding rRNAs is seen as suspected previously *(30)*, and presumably, partly accounts for the slow replication time (6–12 h). Examining gene duplications or expansion of certain gene families may provide information regarding recent lifestyle changes such as adaptation to life in a phagolysosome. Comparison with other obligate intracellular organisms reveals some unexpected features in the *C. burnetii* genome, such as an abundance of transporters and a prominent number of transposases *(20)* and IS elements relative to the *C. trachomatis* and *R. prowazekii* genomes. Unsurprisingly, there is very little evidence for recent lateral gene transfer events as evinced by unusual nucleotide composition and comparison to other sequenced genomes. A chi-square analysis of trinucleotide composition across the entire genome is often performed to detect regions of atypical composition as previously demonstrated *(31)*. An initial survey of metabolic enzymes confirms previously suspected limitations in biosynthetic capabilities such as amino acid biosynthesis. A moderate number of virulence-associated genes with potential roles in invasion and colonization have been identified.

3.3. B. suis

Brucella spp. belong to the α-2 subclass of Proteobacteria, and are small, nonmotile, Gram-negative, zoonotic pathogens with broad host range and worldwide distribution *(32,33)*. Infection occurs via inhalation, consumption of contaminated foodstuffs, or by direct contact with an infected animal *(34)*. Resultant abortion and infertility in cattle leads to large economic losses *(32)*. In humans, a debilitating acute disease termed "undulant fever" occurs, with diverse pathological manifestations including malaise and myalgia. In some instances, chronic brucellosis characterized by endocarditis,

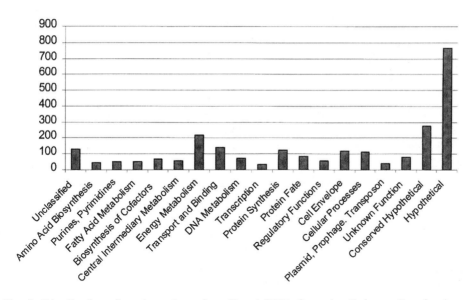

Fig. 2. Distribution of total number of predicted ORFs from the *C. burnetii* main chromosome sequence within different functional role categories.

arthritis, meningitis, and other osteoarticular and neurological complications occurs *(35)*. Patients respond to large doses of antibiotics such as tetracycline, gentamicin, and streptomycin administered over an extended period of time; untreated disease is often fatal *(36,37)*. There are no human brucellosis vaccines presently; vaccines for military use are under development *(38)*. The organism is a facultatively intracellular coccobacillus that enters the host through mucosal surfaces and replicates within specialized vacuoles in professional and nonprofessional phagocytic cells, causing minimal cytopathogenic effects. Localization of *B. suis* and *B. melitensis* within the rough endoplasmic reticulum (RER), followed by large-scale proliferation, has been demonstrated *(39,40)*. Genome analysis of this organism will help reveal putative virulence strategies, identify potential vaccine candidates, and aid in developing protocols to distinguish *B. suis* biovars. Comparative analysis of the *B. suis* genome and the recently published *B. melitensis* genome *(41)* and the *B. abortus* genome (currently being sequenced by the US Department of Agriculture (USDA) and University of Minnesota) may reveal factors determining host specificity and pathogenic strategies and help in studying divergence between Brucella species.

3.3.1. General Features of the B. suis Genome

The genome of the swine isolate, *B. suis* 1330 has been completely sequenced and is comprised of two circular chromosomes of 2,109,237 bp (chromosome 1) and 1,208,734 bp (chromosome 2) that have average G + C contents of 57.2 and 57.3%, respectively *(41a)*. Chromosome 1, encoding 2149 ORFs with an average gene length of 851 nucleotides, possesses a coding capacity of 86.8%; chromosome 2, encoding 1202 ORFs with an average gene length of 892 nucleotides, has a coding capacity of 88.8%. Of the total number of ORFs, 2132 (approx 63.6%) have a predicted function, 563 (approx 16.8%) are conserved hypothetical, 494 (approx 14.7%) are unique, and

162 (approx 4.9%) match genes of unknown function (*see* Fig. 3). Fifty-five tRNAs with specificity for all 20 amino acids and three rRNA operons have been identified.

Chromosome 2 possesses "plasmid-like" replication genes as well as a cluster of conjugation-associated genes, supporting the hypothesis that the small chromosome may have been originally acquired as a megaplasmid that was subsequently stabilized, perhaps to confer selective advantage in the recently colonized animal host. Multiple regions of potential, recent lateral gene transfer events are suggested by anomalous DNA composition. A modest number of "typical" putative virulence determinants such as adhesins, invasins are apparent, no toxins are present, and a large putative (approx 50 kb) pathogenicity island have been identified. Comparisons between the *B. suis* genome and other α-Proteobacterial genomes, viz., *Agrobacterium tumefaciens*, *Mesorhizobium loti*, and *Sinorhizobium* spp. have confirmed the close relationship and particularly in the case of *M. loti,* have identified extensive regions of synteny (conserved gene order). Fairly comprehensive metabolic capabilities and some additional functions normally associated with soil-dwelling bacteria have been revealed. The recently published sequence of *Brucella melitensis* provides an overview of basic physiological and metabolic properties and general features of that genome. Comparison of the *B. suis* genome with that of *B. melitensis* revealed extensive similarity and gene synteny. A large proportion (greater than 90%) of *B. suis* and *B. melitensis* genes share 98–100% identity at the nucleotide level. Based on the whole genome nucleotide alignments, a finite number of *B. suis* and *B. melitensis* genes were identified that are completely absent in the other genome. Most of these differences appear to be caused by phage-related integration events. A detailed comparative analysis with *B. melitensis, B. abortus,* and other closely related bacteria will provide important insight into the evolution and acquisition of virulence factors and development of host-specific adaptations.

3.4. B. mallei

B. mallei, the etiological agent of glanders, is an obligate parasite associated with solipeds (horses, mules, and donkeys). Humans in direct contact with infected animals are at highest risk of acquiring disease *(42)* with frequently fatal consequences. The organism is a nonmotile, obligately aerobic, Gram-negative bacillus, a member of the β-subgroup of the proteobacteria, and is closely related to *Burkholderia pseudomallei*, the causative agent of melioidosis *(43)*. Symptoms of acute glanders following a 1- to 14-d incubation period include fever, malaise, delirium, and pains of the joints, muscles, and so on *(42,44)*. Disease may progress to coma or death within 10–36 d if untreated with antibiotics such as sulfadazine *(44)*. Occasionally, chronic disease may occur. No licensed vaccines are currently available.

Few reports describing virulence factors, pathogenesis, or genetic analysis of *B. mallei* exist because of its eradication from most developed countries for more than 50 yr. Capsular polysaccharide is the only identified virulence determinant thus far. Because little is known about the basic mechanisms of *B. mallei* pathogenesis, the availability of the complete annotated genome sequence of this organism is much anticipated and will hopefully aid in the development of much-needed vaccines, therapeutics, and effective diagnostics.

The Sanger Centre has been funded to sequence the genome of *B. pseudomallei*, the causative agent of melidosis, which is closely related to *B. mallei (43)*. *B. pseudomallei*

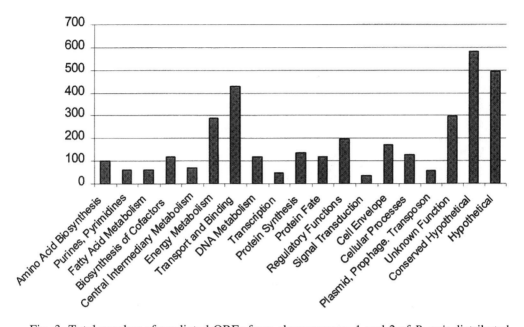

Fig. 3. Total number of predicted ORFs from chromosomes 1 and 2 of *B. suis* distributed into different functional role categories.

and *B. mallei* share morphological, biochemical, and antigenic characteristics, and their disease manifestations are similar; however, some notable phenotypic differences do exist and the diseases are epidemiologically and geographically distinct. The Sanger Centre is currently sequencing the approx 6-Mb genome of strain K96243, a clinical isolate from Thailand, consisting of two chromosomes of approx 3.5 and 2.5 Mb each. The Sanger Centre has generated greater than 10-fold sequence coverage of this genome, representing essentially the entire genome in assemblies (http://www.sanger.ac.uk/Projects/B_pseudomallei/).

3.4.1. General Features of B. mallei Genome

TIGR has completed the shotgun sequencing phase of the 5.9-Mb genome of *B. mallei* ATCC 23344 and conducted preliminary analyses of the ORFs as of January 1, 2002. A total of 81,354 random reads from both ends of plasmid clones were assembled into 270 contigs and nine groups. The genome was compared to the *B. pseudomallei* K96243 shotgun sequence from The Sanger Centre. Preliminary studies indicate that many *B. mallei* and *B. pseudomallei* genes are 99–100% identical at the nucleotide level. However, there appear to be significant differences in gene content and order between the two species. The automated annotation protocol has identified approx 4978 ORFs, of which approx 55% have be assigned biological function, approx 9% match genes of unknown function, approx 20% (999) are conserved hypothetical, and nearly 16% are novel genes (*see* Fig. 4). Predicted ORFs with significant similarity to invasin proteins from other pathogenic bacteria as well as some toxins are evident. A notable number of alternate sigma factors and components of types I, II, and III, secretion systems may also be present.

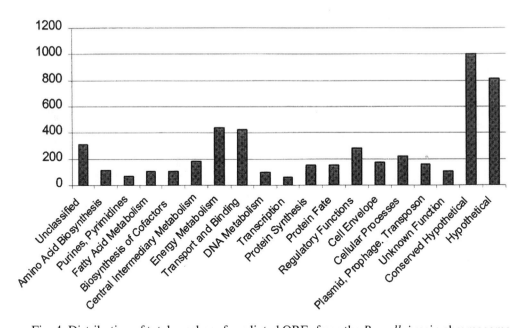

Fig. 4. Distribution of total number of predicted ORFs from the *B. mallei* main chromosome sequence within different functional role categories.

3.5. Clostridium perfringens

C. perfringens is a ubiquitous, saprophytic bacterium, found at high levels in the large intestine, on the skin, and in soil and freshwater sediments *(45)*. *C. perfringens* can cause a wide spectrum of diseases in humans and animals. In people, *C. perfringens* is the cause of gas gangrene (myonecrosis), enteritis necroticans, food poisoning, and nonfood-borne enterotoxemic infections. *C. perfringens* can grow at an extremely rapid rate; generation times as short as 10 min have been reported at optimum growth temperatures. This rapid growth rate is considered a major factor in the organism's ability to spread rapidly to healthy tissues in a gangrene infection. As a species, *C. perfringens* is one of the most prolific producers of toxins; 13 different plasmid-encoded toxins have been identified so far. Many deadly human bacterial pathogens are included in the genus *Clostridium*, including *C. perfringens*, *C. botulinum*, *C. tetani*, *C. difficile*, and many others. The genus *Clostridium* contains anaerobic, spore-forming, rod-shaped, bacteria that do not respire sulfur compounds. *C. perfringens* is most closely related to the nonpathogenic bacterium *C. butyricum.*

Clinical cases of gangrene are treated by surgical debridement of dead tissue and administration of large doses of antibiotics. There is no effective vaccine against *C. perfringens* gangrene infections in humans at the present time. However, vaccination with a C-terminal domain fragment of α-toxin-protected mice against challenge with virulent *C. perfringens* in a gangrene model *(46)*, suggesting a strategy that may be used in the future. If left untreated, the disease is always fatal because of severe toxin-induced shock following bacteremia.

The production of a heat-resistant spore is considered to be a major factor in *C. perfringens'* ability to cause disease. *C. perfringens* spores are ubiquitous in the environment and are considered to be the main source of contamination in traumatic and postsurgical wounds. The heat-resistant spore has been the vehicle most often cited in theoretical and actual uses of *C. perfringens* as a BW agent. Spore development is not as well-understood in the clostridia as it is in *Bacillus* species; the genome sequence of *C. perfringens* will allow researchers to identify key components of the sporulation process by genomic comparison to other sporulating bacteria. Toxin production has historically been the main focus of studies of *C. perfringens* gangrene infections; however, the recent discovery that *C. perfringens* can persist inside macrophages by escaping the phagosome under aerobic conditions *(47)* opens up surprising new aspects of its pathogenic potential.

3.5.1. General Features of the C. perfringens Genome

The genome of the *C. perfringens* type strain ATCC 13124 (NCTC 8237) is currently being sequenced, and as of January 1, 2002, random sequencing was complete and closure of this genome is commencing. This strain is a type A human gangrene isolate that has been shown to exhibit the highest level of virulence in animal models *(48)*, produces large amounts of all of the gangrene-associated toxins, sporulates *(49)*, and has been the standard strain used for antimicrobial sensitivity testing for many years. Additionally, TIGR has undertaken sequencing of plasmids from other strains: 6234 LI (beta toxin, type C), JGS1721 (epsilon toxin, type D), and JGS1987 (iota toxin, type E). The toxin-encoding plasmids have an estimated average size of 100 kb. *C. perfringens* has a circular chromosome of approx 3.6 Mb with an overall G + C content of approx 28.5%. About 3798 ORFs have been predicted preliminarily with an average gene length of 752 nucleotides. The percent coding capacity is currently estimated at 79.3%, with approx 51% of ORFs having assigned function, approx 12% conserved hypothetical, approx 11% unknown gene function, and approx 26% representing unique ORFs (*see* Fig. 5). Numerous of striking virulence genes such as phospholipases, hyaluronidases, hemolysins, and other toxins (some previously characterized) are immediately apparent. Factors mediating attachment to host cells and other aspects of the infectious process may also be predicted from the genome sequence.

C. perfringens strain 13 complete genome sequence was recently reported by Shimizu et al *(50)*. In contrast to the ATCC strain being sequenced at TIGR, this strain has a significantly smaller genome size of 3.03 Mb and encodes only 2660 protein coding regions and 10 rRNA operons. The overall G + C content is about the same (28.6%). Some phenotypic differences that characterize strain 13 include extremely poor sporulation and only moderate virulence in animal gangrene models relative to other strains. Genome sequence analysis has revealed interesting aspects of its metabolism such as presence of saccharolytic enzymes, absence of enzymes of the tricarboxylic acid cycle, respiratory chain, and many amino acid biosynthetic pathways. More than 20 putative virulence factors such as enterotoxins, fibronectin-binding proteins, other adhesins and hemolysins, and so on were newly identified as well.

Sequencing projects of two other clostridia, *C. acetobutylicum* (http://www.cric.com/sequence_center/bacterial_genomes/) and *C. tetani* (http://www.ncbi.nlm.nih.gov/htbin-post/Taxonomy/wgetorg?name=Clostridium+teta-ni), are near completion, whereas sequencing projects for *C. difficile* (http://www.sanger.ac.uk/Projects/C_difficile/), *C. botulinum* (http://www.sanger.ac.uk/ Projects/C_botulinum/), and *Clostridium* species BC1 (http://www.ncbi.nlm.nih.gov/ htbin-post/Taxonomy/

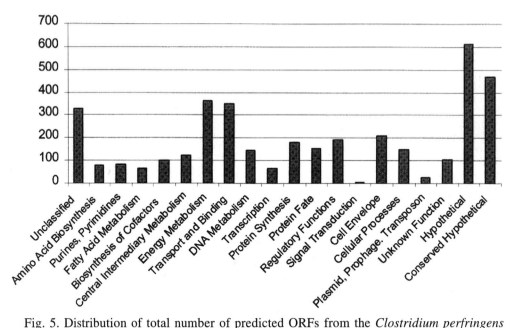

Fig. 5. Distribution of total number of predicted ORFs from the *Clostridium perfringens* main chromosome sequence into different functional role categories.

wgetorg?name=Clostridium+BC1) are in earlier stages. The availability of these sequences will permit comparative genomic analyses of *C. perfringens* strain ATCC 13124 with strain 13, and with these different species and provide powerful insight into the evolution of these strains as well as the species as a whole.

4. POSTGENOMIC STUDIES AND CONCLUSIONS

Sequencing projects of the BW pathogens are at different stages of completion and the process of "mining" these data for meaningful information has only just begun. A major rate-limiting step in our pursuit of a comprehensive understanding of microbes and their genomes is the limitations of available methods to assign function to the numerous "hypothetical" ORFs encountered in every genome. It is apparent that generation of sequence data has functional characterization of genes *(51)*. The accuracy of bioinformatic annotation of a genome is also unclear; there has been little reported in terms of systematic experimentation to confirm functional assignments of genes on a genome-wide scale.

Various of postgenomic approaches to investigate gene function have been developed, including global gene expression (microarrays), global protein analysis (proteomics, mass spectrometry, protein-linking experiments), global mutagenesis, protein overexpression screens, "in-silico studies," comparative genomics, three-dimensional structural predictions, biochemical pathways, gene expression hierarchy, and so on. All of these approaches have been enabled or facilitated by the availability of complete genome sequences. A long-term goal is to use these myriad strategies to design effective vaccines and develop therapeutics and diagnostic measures for each of these BW agents. Such methods have already been demonstrated in other bacterial pathogens with rewarding results. Particularly noteworthy is the study identifying novel vaccine candidates against *Neisseria meningitidis* serogroup B strains *(52)*. The approach involved identifying 570 candidate surface-exposed or exported antigens from the genome sequence, expressing these genes (350 ORFs were successfully expressed) in *Escherichia coli,* and development of immune-sera against purified protein. These were further tested for suitability in conferring protection against heterologous Meningococcus B strains by using enzyme-linked immunsorbent assay and fluorescence activated cell sorting (FACS) techniques. Several vaccine candidates were identified from the genome using this method, which are currently undergoing clinical trials.

Global transposon mutagenesis is a highly prolific and successful strategy used to identify central effectors of virulence in pathogenic models. In particular, the "signature-tagged mutagenesis" technique *(53)*, which allows rapid screening of large mutant pools (each mutant is "labeled" with a unique DNA "signature-tag") by selecting for loss of function (e.g., attenuation in an animal model). This strategy has been employed with widespread success in numerous bacterial and a fungal pathogen and has led to the identification of many novel virulence factors in those paradigms *(54,55)*. Complete genome sequences facilitate large-scale mutagenesis projects as seen in the case of the study to determine the minimal number of genes essential for cellular life of *Mycoplasma* spp. *(56)*. Numerous genes nonessential for growth in in vitro conditions were identified by large-scale transposon mutagenesis. The study suggested that only 265–330 *M. genitalium* genes were essential for growth and may represent the minimal genome required for life.

The production of microarrays to perform whole genome expression analysis under various in vitro and in vivo conditions or to identify intraspecies divergence has also become highly practicable in recent times. One approach consists of PCR amplifying ORFs identified from genome sequencing, spotting these in a high-density array on glass slides (or chips or other templates), followed by hybridization with fluorescently labeled cDNA prepared from total RNA procured from the organism cultivated under test or control conditions. Specialized imaging and analysis software allow quantification of signal intensities from fluorescing spots and calculate mRNA levels in the cell corresponding to each ORF. For example, the complete set of 4290 *E. coli* ORFs were amplified and RNA expression patterns of cultures in exponential or transitional stages of growth in rich and minimal media were analyzed to further our understanding of *E. coli* physiology *(57)*. A microarray approach has also been used to monitor alterations in mRNA expression of *M. tuberculosis* following isoniazid treatment *(58)*.

It is anticipated that microarray expression analysis of the biodefense pathogens will provide insights into mechanisms of molecular pathogenesis. Microarrays have been used successfully in strain comparisons, a notable example being the study of *H. pylori* genetic diversity within the ecological niche of the gastrointestinal tract of a single host. Differences in the genetic composition among single-colony isolates obtained from the same source patient were examined and found to be highly polymorphic *(59)*. Another example of comparative genome hybridizations to study strain diversity is a *Vibrio cholerae* study. A *V. cholerae* O1 El Tor strain microarray comprised of 3632 ORFs (representing 93.5% of the genome) was constructed to compare the gene content of El Tor isolates obtained from different epidemic instances worldwide. Although strain isolates are highly similar, many unique genes were identified that may have contributed to the relative success of certain strains over others in causing pandemics of cholera. They concluded that these genes (located on a "pandemic island") might represent an increased adaptation to the human host resulting in more efficient and persistent infections *(60)*. A technique designated "TraSH" (transposon site hybridization) combines high-density insertional mutagenesis with microarray hybridization for mapping pools of mutants, and allows functional characterization of the complete complement of genes required for growth under different conditions. TraSH was used to identify genes required for growth of *M. bovis* BCG on minimal but not rich medium. Genes of both previously known and unknown function were identified in this study *(61)*.

Comparative genome analysis of closely related strains can yield useful information regarding physiological and other differences. It is anticipated that in the relatively near future, there will be partial or complete sequences of multiple strains of various pathogens, including BW agents. Examining variance in gene content will help understand subtle nuances of bacterial adaptations in response to specific host conditions, as well as other aspects of species divergence. A comparison of the genome sequence of enterohaemorrhagic *E. coli* O157:H7 with nonpathogenic *E. coli* K12 revealed candidate genes contributing to virulence, differences in metabolic capacities, and so on, and evidence of extensive gene transfer, all contributing to an unexpectedly high level of diversity between the two strains *(62)*.

Advances in structural and functional genomics as well as computational biology have allowed investigators to gain insights into fundamental biological processes such as physiology, genetics, evolution and other aspects of microbial lifestyles and adaptations. We are optimistic that genome analysis of the BW agents and comparison to other pathogenic (and nonpathogenic) organisms will help in identification of the wide range of effectors contributing to virulence, host-specificity, resistance ,and other phenotypes, and these can subsequently be used to rapidly develop efficacious prophylactic and remedial measures.

REFERENCES

1. Fleischmann, R. D., Adams, M. D., White, O., et al. (1995) Whole-genome random sequencing and assembly of *Haemophilus influenzae* Rd. *Science* **269,** 496–512.
2. Salzberg, S. L., Delcher, A. L., Kasif, S., and White, O. (1998) Microbial gene identification using interpolated Markov models. *Nucleic Acids Res.* **26,** 544–548.
3. Delcher, A. L., Harmon, D., Kasif, S., White, O., and Salzberg, S. L. (1999) Improved microbial gene identification with GLIMMER. *Nucleic Acids Res.* **27,** 4636–4641.
4. Altschul, S. F., Gish, W., Miller, W., Myers, E. W., and Lipman, D. J. (1990) Basic local alignment search tool. *J. Mol. Biol.* **215,** 403–410.
5. Bateman, A., Birney, E., Durbin, R., Eddy, S. R., Howe, K. L., and Sonnhammer, E. L. (2000) The Pfam protein families database. *Nucleic Acids Res.* **28,** 263–266.
6. Haft, D. H., Loftus, B. J., Richardson, D. L., et al. (2001) TIGRFAMs: a protein family resource for the functional identification of proteins. *Nucleic Acids Res.* **29,** 41–43.
7. Peterson, J. D., Umayam, L. A., Dickinson, T., Hickey, E. K., and White, O. (2001) The comprehensive microbial resource. *Nucleic Acids Res.* **29,** 123–125.
8. Dixon, T. C., Meselson, M., Guillemin, J., and Hanna, P. C. (1999) Anthrax. *N. Engl. J. Med.* **341,** 815–826.

9. Manchee, R. J., Broster, M. G., Anderson, I. S., Henstridge, R. M., and Melling, J. (1983) Decontamination of *Bacillus anthracis* on Gruinard Island? *Nature* **303**, 239, 240.

10. Mock, M. and Fouet, A. (2001) Anthrax. *Annu. Rev. Microbiol.* **55**, 647–71.

11. Hanna, P. C. and Ireland, J. A. (1999) Understanding *Bacillus anthracis* pathogenesis. *Trends Microbiol.* **7**, 180–182.

12. Mikesell, P., Ivins, B. E., Ristroph, J. D., and Dreier, T. M. (1983) Evidence for plasmid-mediated toxin production in *Bacillus anthracis. Infect. Immun.* **39**, 371–376.

13. Pezard, C,. Berche, P., and Mock, M. (1991) Contribution of individual toxin components to virulence of *Bacillus anthracis. Infect. Immun.* **59**, 3472–3477.

14. Green, B. D., Battisti, L., Koehler, T. M., Thorne, C. B., and Ivins, B. E. (1985) Demonstration of a capsule plasmid in *Bacillus anthracis. Infect. Immun.* **49**, 291–297.

15. Uchida, I., Sekizaki, T., Hashimoto, K., and Terakado, N. (1985) Association of the encapsulation of *Bacillus anthracis* with a 60 megadalton plasmid. *J. Gen. Microbiol.* **131(Pt. 2)**, 363–367.

16. Little, S. F. and Knudson, G. B. (1986) Comparative efficacy of *Bacillus anthracis* live spore vaccine and protective antigen vaccine against anthrax in the guinea pig. *Infect. Immun.* **52**, 509–512.

16a. Read, T. D., et al. (2003) The genome sequence of *Bacillus anthracis* AMES and comparison to closely related bacteria. *Nature* **423(6935)**, 81–86.

17. Okinaka, R., Cloud, K., Hampton, O., et al. (1999) Sequence, assembly and analysis of pX01 and pX02. *J. Appl. Microbiol.* **87**, 261, 262.

18. Okinaka, R. T., Cloud, K., Hampton, O., et al. (1999) Sequence and organization of pXO1, the large *Bacillus anthracis* plasmid harboring the anthrax toxin genes. *J. Bacteriol.* **181**, 6509–6515.

19. Thorne, C. B. (1993) Bacillus anthracis, in Bacillus subtilis *and Other Gram-Positive Bacteria.* American Society for Microbiology, Washington, DC, pp. 113–124.

20. Keim, P., Price, L. B., Klevytska, A. M., et al. (2000) Multiple-locus variable-number tandem repeat analysis reveals genetic relationships within *Bacillus anthracis. J. Bacteriol.* **182**, 2928–2936.

21. Read, T. D., Salzberg, S. L., Pop, M., et al. (2002) Comparative genome sequencing for discovery of novel polymorphisms in *Bacillus anthracis. Science* **9**, 9.

22. Baca, O. G. and Paretsky, D. (1983) Q fever and *Coxiella burnetii*: a model for host-parasite interactions. *Microbiol. Rev.* **47**, 127–149.

23. Broqui, P., Dupont, H. T., Drancourt, M., et al. (1993) Chronic Q fever. *Arch. Int. Med.* **153**, 642–648.

24. Babudieri, C. (1959) Q fever: a zoonosis. *Adv. Vet. Sci.* **5**, 81–84.

25. Weisburg, W. G., Dobson, M. E., Samuel, J. E., et al. (1989) Phylogenetic diversity of the *Rickettsiae. J. Bacteriol.* **171**, 4202–4206.

26. Reiner, N. E. (1994) Altered cell signaling and mononuclear phagocyte deactivation during intracellular infection. *Immunol. Today* **15**, 374–381.

27. Wiebe, M. E., Burton, P. R., and Shankel, D. M. (1972) Isolation and characterization of two cell types of *Coxiella burnetii* phase I. *J. Bacteriol.* **110**, 368–377.

28. Williams, J. C., Johnston, M. R., Peacock, M. G., Thomas, L. A., Stewart, S., and Portis, J. L. (1984) Monoclonal antibodies distinguish phase variants of *Coxiella burnetii. Infect. Immun.* **43**, 421–428.

28a. Seshadri, R., et al. (2003) Complete genome sequence of the Q-fever pathogen C*oxiella burnetii. Proc. Natl. Acad. Sci. USA* **100(9)**, 5455–5460.

29. Ogata, H., Audic, S., Renesto-Audiffren, P., et al. (2001) Mechanisms of evolution in *Rickettsia conorii* and *R. prowazekii. Science* **293**, 2093–2098.

30. Afseth, G., Mo, Y. Y., and Mallavia, L. P. (1995) Characterization of the 23S and 5S rRNA genes of *Coxiella burnetii* and identification of an intervening sequence within the 23S rRNA gene. *J. Bacteriol.* **177**, 2946–2949.

31. Tettelin, H., Saunders, N. J., Heidelberg, J., et al. (2000) Complete genome sequence of *Neisseria meningitidis* serogroup B strain MC58. *Science* **287,** 1809–1815.
32. Nicoletti, P. (1980) The epidemiology of bovine brucellosis. *Adv. Vet. Sci. Comp. Med.* **24,** 69–98.
33. Roux, J. (1979) [Epidemiology and prevention of *brucellosis*]. *Bull. World Health Org.* **57,** 179–194.
34. Young, E. J. (1988) Brucellosis: a model zoonosis in developing countries. *APMIS* **Suppl. 3,** 17–20.
35. Young, E. J. (1995) An overview of human brucellosis. *Clin. Infect. Dis.* **21,** 283–289; quiz 290.
36. Hall, W. H. (1990) Modern chemotherapy for brucellosis in humans. *Rev. Infect. Dis.* **12,** 1060–1099.
37. Young, E. J. (1983) Human brucellosis. *Rev. Infect. Dis.* **5,** 821–842.
38. Hoover, D. L., Crawford, R. M., Van De Verg, L. L., et al. (1999) Protection of mice against brucellosis by vaccination with *Brucella melitensis* WR201(16MDeltapurEK). *Infect. Immun.* **67,** 5877–5884.
39. Detilleux, P. G., Deyoe, B. L., and Cheville, N. F. (1990) Penetration and intracellular growth of *Brucella abortus* in nonphagocytic cells in vitro. *Infect. Immun.* **58,** 2320–2328.
40. Detilleux, P. G., Deyoe, B. L., and Cheville, N. F. (1990) Entry and intracellular localization of *Brucella* spp. in Vero cells: fluorescence and electron microscopy. *Vet. Pathol.* **27,** 317–328.
41. DelVecchio, V. G., Kapatral, V., Redkar, R. J., et al. (2002) The genome sequence of the facultative intracellular pathogen *Brucella melitensis*. *Proc. Natl. Acad. Sci. USA* **99,** 443–448.
41a. Paulsen, I. T., et al. (2002) The *Brucella suis* genome reveals fundamental similarities between animal and plant pathogens and symbiants. *Proc. Natl. Acad. Sci. USA* **99(20),** 13,148–13,153.
42. McGilvray, C. D. (1944) The transmission of glanders from horse to man. *Can. J. Public Health* **35,** 268–275.
43. Stanton, A. T. and Fletcher, W. (1925) Melidosis and its relation to glanders. *J. Hyg.* **23,** 347–363.
44. Neubauer, H., Meyer, H., and Finke, E. J. (1997) Human glanders. *Revue Internationale Des Services De Sante Des Forces Armees* **70,** 258–265.
45. Rood, J. I. and Cole, S. T. (1991) Molecular genetics and pathogenesis of *Clostridium perfringens*. *Microbiol. Rev.* **55,** 621–648.
46. Williamson, E. D. and Titball, R. W. (1993) A genetically engineered vaccine against the alpha-toxin of *Clostridium perfringens* protects mice against experimental gas gangrene. *Vaccine* **11,** 1253–1258.
47. O'Brien, D. K. and Melville, S. B. (2000) The anaerobic pathogen *Clostridium perfringens* can escape the phagosome of macrophages under aerobic conditions. *Cell. Microbiol.* **2,** 505–519.
48. Stevens, D. L., Tweten, R. K., Awad, M. M., Rood, J. I., and Bryant, A. E. (1997) Clostridial gas gangrene: evidence that alpha and theta toxins differentially modulate the immune response and induce acute tissue necrosis. *J. Infect. Dis.* **176,** 189–195.
49. Netherwood, T., Chanter, N., and Mumford, J. A. (1996) Improved isolation of *Clostridium perfringens* from foal faeces. *Res. Vet. Sci.* **61,** 147–151.
50. Shimizu, T., Ohtani, K., Hirakawa, H., et al. (2002) Complete genome sequence of *Clostridium perfringens*, an anaerobic flesh-eater. *Proc. Natl. Acad. Sci. USA* **99,** 996–1001.
51. Nelson, K. E., Paulsen, I. T., Heidelberg, J. F., and Fraser, C. M. (2000) Status of genome projects for nonpathogenic bacteria and archaea. *Nat. Biotechnol.* **18,** 1049–1054.

52. Pizza, M., Scarlato, V., Masignani, V., et al. (2000) Identification of vaccine candidates against serogroup B meningococcus by whole-genome sequencing. *Science* **287,** 1816–1820.

53. Hensel, M., Shea, J. E., Gleeson, C., Jones, M. D., Dalton, E., and Holden, D. W. (1995) Simultaneous identification of bacterial virulence genes by negative selection. *Science* **269,** 400–403.

54. Hong, P. C., Tsolis, R. M., and Ficht, T. A. (2000) Identification of genes required for chronic persistence of *Brucella abortus* in mice. *Infect. Immun.* **68,** 4102–4107.

55. Tsolis, R. M., Townsend, S. M., Miao, E. A., et al. (1999) Identification of a putative *Salmonella enterica* serotype typhimurium host range factor with homology to IpaH and YopM by signature-tagged mutagenesis. *Infect. Immun.* **67,** 6385–6393.

56. Hutchison, C. A., Peterson, S. N., Gill, S. R., et al. (1999) Global transposon mutagenesis and a minimal Mycoplasma genome. *Science* **286,** 2165–2169.

57. Wei, Y., Lee, J. M., Richmond, C., Blattner, F. R., Rafalski, J. A., and LaRossa, R. A. (2001) High-density microarray-mediated gene expression profiling of *Escherichia coli. J. Bacteriol.* **183,** 545–556.

58. Wilson, M., DeRisi, J., Kristensen, H. H., et al. (1999) Exploring drug-induced alterations in gene expression in *Mycobacterium tuberculosis* by microarray hybridization. *Proc. Natl. Acad. Sci. USA* **96,** 12,833–12,838.

59. Israel, D. A., Salama, N., Krishna, U., et al. (2001) *Helicobacter pylori* genetic diversity within the gastric niche of a single human host. *Proc. Natl. Acad. Sci. USA* **98,** 14,625–14,630.

60. Dziejman, M., Balon, E., Boyd, D., Fraser, C. M., Heidelberg, J. F., and Mekalanos, J. J. (2002) Comparative genomic analysis of *Vibrio cholerae*: genes that correlate with cholera endemic and pandemic disease. *Proc. Natl. Acad. Sci. USA* **99,** 1556–1561.

61. Sassetti, C. M., Boyd, D. H., and Rubin, E. J. (2001) Comprehensive identification of conditionally essential genes in mycobacteria. *Proc. Natl. Acad. Sci. USA* **98,** 12,712–12,717.

62. Perna, N. T., Plunkett, G., 3rd, Burland, V., et al. (2001) Genome sequence of enterohaemorrhagic *Escherichia coli* O157:H7. *Nature* **409,** 529–533.

20

Genomics for Biodefense

Exploiting the Francisella tularensis *Genome Sequence*

Siv G. E. Andersson, Mats Forsman, Petra C. F. Oyston, and Richard W. Titball

1. INTRODUCTION

Francisella tularensis is the aetiological agent of tularemia, a plague-like disease of rodents capable of being transmitted to man. Tularemia is a zoonosis, found in a wide range of animals such as rabbits, hares, rodents, and beavers *(1)*. Transmission occurs usually through the bite of an insect, such as a tick, biting fly, or mosquito *(2–5)* but can also be through ingestion of infected foodstuffs *(3)* and drinking water *(6)*, or through inhalation of the bacterium *(7)*. In humans, the most common presentation is ulceroglandular tularemia, a disease typified by flu-like symptoms, normally with a low mortality rate *(8)*. An ulcer forms at the site of infection, which can persist for several months. Other forms of tularemia, such as typhoidal, gastrointestinal, and pneumonic tularemia, are more serious diseases and may have mortality rates up to 60%, depending on the type of strain causing infection *(7)*. *F. tularensis* subspecies *tularensis* is one of the most infectious pathogens known, with an infectious dose of less than 10 colony-forming units (CFU) in humans *(9,10)*.

F. tularensis subspecies *tularensis* has been an organism of concern in the defense against biological attack since the large state-funded biological weapons programs of the 1950s, when the United States first evaluated the organism as a biological weapon, and it was subsequently incorporated into weapons by the USSR (reviewed in ref. *11*). Now that the emphasis has shifted toward defending against biological terrorism, the same features of this organism that attracted the attention of the superpowers decades ago are still pertinent: a highly infectious organism inducing a potentially fatal disease, with no widely available licensed vaccine *(12)*. In the bioterrorism context, pneumonic tularemia is of greatest concern, compared to naturally occurring infections that normally present as ulceroglandular tularemia.

1.1. Phylogenetic Context of F. tularensis

Phylogenetic studies based on 16S rRNA sequences (*see* Fig. 1) have indicated that *F. tularensis* and *Francisella philomiragia* are members of a separate family, the *Francisellaceae (13)*. The *Francisellaceae* are closely related to members of

From: *Infectious Diseases: Biological Weapons Defense: Infectious Diseases and Counterterrorism*
Edited by: L. E. Lindler, F. J. Lebeda, and G. W. Korch © Humana Press Inc., Totowa, NJ

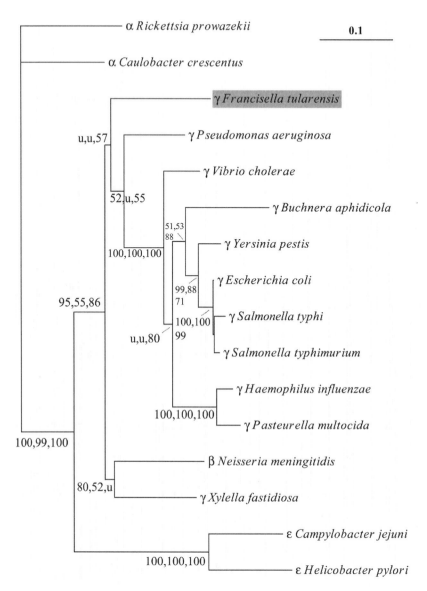

Fig. 1. The position of *F. tularensis* in a 16S rRNA minimum evolution tree. Bootstrap values are presented for the minimum evolution (based on 500 replicates), parsimony (500 replicates), and maximum likelihood (100 replicates) methods in that order. Alignments are collected from the Ribosomal Database Project (http://rdp.cme.msu.edu/html/) *(16)*. Parameter values used in minimum evolution and maximum likelihood are calculated with Modeltest *(17)*. Phylogenetic analysis are made with PAUP *(18)*. Abbreviations: α, β, γ, and ε: alpha-, beta-, gamma- and epsilon-proteo bacterium respectively; u, unresolved node in the used method. (From ref. *13* with permission.)

the γ-subclass of *Proteobacteria* including *Wolbachia persica*, the *Dermatocor andersoni* symbiont, and *Ornithodorous moubata* symbiont B, a group of arthropod parasites and symbionts *(13–15)*. The γ-proteobacteria contains many bacteria for which complete genome sequencing data is available, such as *Escherichia coli, Salmo-*

Table 1
Subspecies of *F. tularensis*

Subspecies	Other name	Location	Severity of disease in humans
tularensis	type A	N. America	Severe, 30% fatality rates
holarctica	type B	N. America and Europe	Moderate
mediasiatica		Central Asia	Moderate
novicida		N. America, Europe, and Australia	Mild

nella enterica var Typhi, *S. enterica* var Typhimurium, *Haemophilus influenzae,* and *Helicobacter pylori.* This should provide a wealth of information for comparative analyses, helping to identify unique as well as shared features of the *F. tularensis* genome sequence.

1.1.1. Biotypes of F. tularensis

Numerous of biotypes or subspecies of *F. tularensis* have been proposed. Originally, the species was divided into two biotypes (A and B) on the basis of virulence, ecological characteristics, and citrulline ureidase activity. Subsequently, biotype A was reclassified as subspecies *tularensis,* whereas biotype B has been designated subspecies *holarctica* (reviewed in ref. *19*). More recently, it has been suggested that *F. tularensis* should be divided into four subspecies; *F. tularensis* subsp. *tularensis, holarctica, mediasiatica,* and *novicida* (*see* Table 1; ref. *20*). These four subspecies display a very close phylogenetic relationship, despite showing marked variations in their virulence for mammals and originating from different regions in the Northern Hemisphere (*see* Table 1).

The most virulent of these isolates belong to subspecies *tularensis,* and before the introduction of effective antibiotic treatment, human infections caused by such strains resulted in a mortality rate of up to 30% *(21,22)*. This highly virulent subspecies is found predominantly in the United States and Canada. The European isolates belong primarily to the subspecies *holarctica,* and although such isolates may cause severe disease and are highly infectious, they rarely result in human mortality. Japanese strains are presently also included in the subspecies *holarctica,* whereas those from Central Asia constitute a separate subspecies, *F. tularensis* subsp. *mediasiatica (20)*.

Although *F. tularensis,* subsp. *tularensis* was formerly believed to be confined to the Northern America, recent studies have reported the occurrence of this subspecies in Europe as well *(23)*. Vice versa, *F. tularensis,* subsp. *holarctica* is mainly found in Europe but has also been identified in North America. Studies of *F. tularensis* have shown that contamination with the organisms may persist for more than a year in water *(24,25)*. Moreover, recent data suggest that *F. tularensis* may also be able to survive in protozoa for long periods of time *(26,27)*.

2. WHY SEQUENCE THE *F. tularensis* GENOME?

F. tularensis is a facultative intracellular pathogen *(28)*; however, in contrast to many other intracellular pathogens, only a few virulence factors and genes required for infection and survival in vivo have been identified *(29–33)*. Thus, very little is currently known about *F. tularensis* at the molecular level, why it is so infectious, and how it causes disease. Also, although there is a live-attenuated vaccine (strain LVS; ref. *10*), the basis of attenuation and how it induces a protective immune response are not known, and the vaccine is not fully licensed. One of the problems in analyzing the contribution of a specific gene to virulence is that producing defined isogenic mutants in *F. tularensis* has yet to be achieved, although methods have been described for producing mutants in *F. novicida (34)*. Transposon mutagenesis has been employed successfully and has been used to identify some genes involved in macrophage survival and growth.

The many microbial genome projects have provided lists of potential genes involved in pathogenicity, virulence, adhesion, colonization of host cells, immune response evasion, and antibiotic resistance. By sequencing the genome of *F. tularensis* and searching for genes with similarities to previously described virulence systems in other organisms, some clues may be obtained about the source of virulence and these systems may then be selected as targets for transposon mutagenesis and further experimental characterization. Likewise, strain-specific sequence variation related to differences in virulence phenotypes may be used for the development of new detection methods based on, for example, DNA microarrays. Genome sequence information may also be useful for the construction of a rationally attenuated vaccine and/or for the identification of vaccine candidates, as previously described for *Neisseria meningitidis (35)*.

For all of these reasons, a project to sequence the genome of a virulent strain of *F. tularensis*, strain SchuS4, was initiated by a consortium of European and US laboratories (see http://artedi.ebc.uu.se/Projects/Francisella/). The results of this project are discussed in Section 3. A second project to sequence the genome of the LVS strain (derived from a virulent *F. tularensis* subspecies *holarctica* strain) has recently commenced in the United States; comparison of the two genomes will eventually yield many insights into *Francisella* physiology, virulence, and antigenicity.

3. PRELIMINARY ANALYSIS OF THE *F. tularensis* STRAIN SCHUS4 GENOME

When the *F. tularensis* SchuS4 genome project was initiated, only 34 gene sequences from *F. tularensis* had been deposited with GenBank. Confirmation that the assembled *F. tularensis* contigs was of high quality was obtained by searching the *F. tularensis* contigs with the *Francisella* gene sequences already contained in GenBank *(36)*. We have identified 25 of the 34 known *Francisella* sequences in our dataset. The remaining 9 sequences that were not found in our dataset are encoded on two cryptic plasmids, pOM1 *(37)* and pNFL10 *(38)*. This was to be expected because these plasmids have been found in strain LVS and in *F. novicida,* respectively, but not in *F. tularensis,* subsp. *tularensis.*

3.1. Genome Size and Base Composition of the **F. tularensis** Genome

Preliminary results from the strain SchuS4 genome sequencing project suggest a total genome size of 1.8 Mbp, which is in good agreement with previous estimates of 1.8–2.0 Mb *(36)*. The G + C content of the genome is approx 34 %, which is also in good agreement with previous estimates of 30–36%. The analysis has identified about 1800 open reading frames (ORFs) with an average G + C content of 33.8%. The relatively high A + T content is particularly striking at sites where nucleotide substitutions have no effect on amino acid usage, such as in noncoding regions and at third codon positions. Thus, *F. tularensis* genes have a significant codon bias with only 23.3% of the third nucleotide being G or C, as compared to a G + C content of 43.9 and 34% at first and second codon positions, respectively. The striking pattern in codon usage in *F. tularensis* genes will be very useful for training programs to automatically identify ORFs as genes in the *F. tularensis* genome.

3.2. Metabolic Features

To get an overview of the information contained in the genome of *F. tularensis*, we searched for similarities to other previously identified genes and sorted all sequences with significant similarity into their different functional categories (*see* Fig. 2). Because *F. tularensis* is a member of the γ-proteobacteria, it is of particular interest to compare the fraction of genes in the different categories of *F. tularensis* to those of other members of this subdivision, such as for example *E. coli*. As expected from their different genome sizes, 1.8 vs 4.7 Mb, respectively, the total number of predicted genes is lower in *F. tularensis* than in *E. coli*. The difference is particularly striking in categories such as biosynthesis, regulation, and transport, whereas the relative fraction of genes coding for information processes, such as replication, transcription, and translation is more similar in the two species.

Metabolic reconstructions of particularly interesting pathways have identified genes that may be used to construct live-attenuated vaccine strains of *F. tularensis*. These include genes involved in purine and aromatic amino acid biosynthesis *(36)* as well as other gene products involved in central intermediary metabolism *(39)*. We have also identified at least 17 of the 37 *E. coli* genes that are necessary for lipopolysaccharide (LPS) biosynthesis in our dataset (L. Lindler, unpublished observations). Of the 20 LPS biosynthetic genes not found in our searches, 9 may be specific to *E. coli* synthesis. LPS biosynthesis is important because it is related to pathogenesis of *F. tularensis (40)*.

4. STRAIN IDENTIFICATION AND TYPING METHODS

The identification of *F. tularensis* and differentiation of its subspecies has traditionally been accomplished by growth characteristics and biochemical analysis *(20)*. Besides being time-consuming and tedious, cultivation renders a high risk of laboratory-acquired infection. In view of these problems, diagnosis of tularemia has relied mainly on serology. However, antibodies are usually not detected before the second week of disease *(41)*. Moreover, *F. tularensis* is a fastidious bacterium and isolation direct from the environment of the bacterium is hampered because other bacteria may be favored on most media used for growth of *F. tularensis (42)*.

The genus *Francisella* is antigenically coherent and the subspecies are almost indistinguishable by serological methods, although the LPS of *F. tularensis,* subsp. *novicida* discriminates the subspecies *(43)*. Despite a dramatic difference in virulence between the subspecies, *F. tularensis* appears to be a genetically homogenous species. Thus, in a bioterrorism scenario there is a need to develop rapid screening methods for identification of species and high resolution typing methods, which permit the differentiation of the four subspecies of *F. tularensis* and the identification of individual strains.

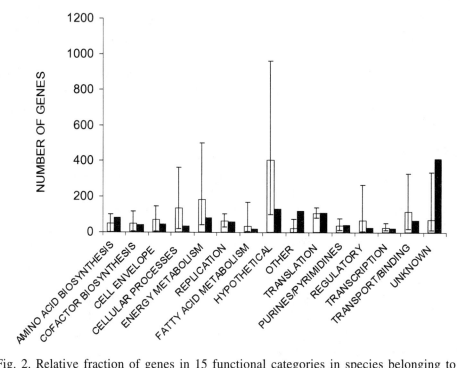

Fig. 2. Relative fraction of genes in 15 functional categories in species belonging to 20 members of the γ-proteobacteria for which complete genome sequence data is available (open bars). Error bars indicating the lowest and highest numbers of genes in each category. The number of *F. tularensis* genes in the 15 functional categories are shown as solid bars. Other, genes with similarities to genes with previously identified gene functions that are not related to any of the other defined categories; hypothetical, genes with similarities to genes in the public databases with no assigned function; unknown, genes with no hits to sequences in the public databases. (Reproduced from ref. *39* with the kind permission of Blackwell Scientific Limited.)

4.1. Pregenomic Molecular Methods for the Identification of F. tularensis

The first reported molecular identification of *F. tularensis* was based on differences in 16S rRNA sequences *(44)*. RNA-hybridization was used on spleen tissues and wound specimens as diagnostic measures *(44,45)*. Subsequently, on the basis of *Francisella*-specific 16S rRNA sequence signatures, polymerase chain reaction (PCR)-based methods have been developed allowing identification of *Francisella* strains at the genus level and differentiation at the species level *(46)*. Another molecular target is a gene encoding a 17-kDa lipoprotein from *F. tularensis* strain LVS *(47)*. This gene is conserved in *F. tularensis* and *F. philomiragia* isolates *(48)*. PCR targeting this gene has been applied for sensitive and specific detection of *F. tularensis* in blood from infected animals *(49)*. PCR-based identification of the 17-kDa lipoprotein gene and the *Francisella* 16S rRNA sequence has been applied and found sensitive for detection of *F. tularensis* DNA in wound specimens from tularemia patients *(50,51)*. PCR amplification of the rRNA gene cluster combined with endonuclease digestion has been used for typing of *Francisella* strains. This strategy enabled differentiation at the species level but not at the subspecies level *(52)*.

Repetitive extragenic palindromic sequence (REP)-PCR has been applied to identify strains of *F. tularensis,* subsp. *novicida,* but patterns from *F. tularensis,* subsp. *holarctica* and *F. tularensis,* subsp. *tularensis* strains were found to be similar *(53).* Recent studies have evaluated the use of PCR based on the use of various arbitrary primers as well as of primers specific to REP and enterobacterial repetitive intragenic consensus sequences *(54,55).* It was concluded that the methods were useful for rapid and a technically simple strategy for discrimination of subspecies but not individual strains. A 30-bp sequence heterogeneity among the genomes of various *F. tularensis* strains was found by use of PCR and arbitrary priming; by targeting this genomic region a PCR was developed that distinguished the two clinically most important subspecies *tularensis* and *holarctica (51).* Pregenomic molecular identification methods for *F. tularensis* are summarized in Table 2.

4.2. Postgenomic Molecular Methods for the Identification of F. tularensis

The genome-sequencing project of *F. tularensis* strain ShuS4 generated a well-defined genomic library, which has been used to create a whole genome DNA microarray. To identify discriminatory deletion regions, a set of strains belonging to the various subspecies has been investigated by the microarray to discover regions of difference that are useful for classification and identification *(56).*

The whole genome microarray analysis of *F. tularensis* subspecies divided the *F. tularensis* strains into four major genetic groups: *F. tularensis,* subsp. *tularensis,* *F. tularensis,* subsp. *holoarctica,* and *F. tularensis* strains originating from Japan (*holoarctica*). The single representative of *F. tularensis,* subsp. *novicida* showed a unique hybridization pattern. Interestingly, the relatively low virulent *F. tularensis,* subsp. *mediasiatica* strains, which have only been isolated in the Central Asian Republics of the former USSR, clustered with the highly virulent *F. tularensis,* subsp. *tularensis* strains isolated in North America (*see* Fig. 3).

One region of chromosomal difference identified by microarray analysis was demonstrated to be variable in size. Interestingly, each subspecies was unique in this region. Alignment of this region and comparison to the *F. tularensis,* subsp. *tularensis* Shu4 sequence revealed a deletion of 389 bp in *F. tularensis,* subsp. *tularensis* strains from Japan. Likewise, a 598 bp deletion in the *F. tularensis,* subsp. *holarctica* strains, a 68 bp deletion in *F. tularensis* subsp. *mediasiatica* strains and two large deletions in the *F. tularensis,* subsp. *novicida* strains were identified. Thus, all four suggested subspecies of *F. tularensis* could be discriminated by one specific PCR utilizing one single primer pair flanking this region *(56).* In addition, this specific PCR also distinguished strains originating from Japan.

Bacterial genomes frequently contain hypervariable short-sequence repeats arranged in tandem, and this has been proven an attractive target for high-resolution bacterial strain typing *(57).* The detection of different copy number of repeats in different strains provides a high level of discriminatory power in bacterial strain typing. This kind of repeat, variable-number tandem repeats (VNTRs), was also found in the SchuS4 genome and have been evaluated for strain typing of *F. tularensis.* By use of two highly variable loci, it was possible to identify strains of the same subspecies and the method fulfilled the criteria for routine typing of individual isolates *(55).* Another study *(58)* employed multiple-locus variable number of repeat analysis (MLVA) for typing of

Table 2
Pregenomic Molecular Identification Methods
for *F. tularensis*

Methods	Target	References
Hybridization		
Dot-blot	16S rRNA	*44,45*
PCR		
Specific	16S rDNA, 17-kDa gene	*46,49–51*
	30-bp heterogenity	
Quantitative	16S rDNA, 17-kDa gene	*95–97*
Ribotyping	16S –23S rDNA	*52*
REP	DNA-fingerprint	*51,53,54*
ERIC	DNA-fingerprint	*51,54*
RAPD	DNA-fingerprint	*51,54*
PCR-EIA	17-kDa gene	*96*

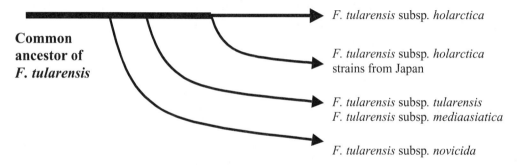

Common ancestor of *F. tularensis*

F. tularensis subsp. *holarctica*

F. tularensis subsp. *holarctica* strains from Japan

F. tularensis subsp. *tularensis*
F. tularensis subsp. *mediaasiatica*

F. tularensis subsp. *novicida*

Fig. 3. Schematic depiction of proposed evolutionary pathway within *F. tularensis* as inferred from microarray hybridizations. The scheme is based on the presence or absence of deleted regions detected by microarray hybridizations. Note that the distances between certain branches may not correspond to actual phylogenetic differences calculated by other methods.

individual isolates of *F. tularensis*. Six VNTR loci, including the two loci used by Johansson and his colleagues *(55)*, were identified and used to resolve 56 isolates into 39 unique types. Although subspecies classification seems to be possible with MLVA, this approach might be most powerful for discrimination of individual strains. Further analyses of the genome sequence have identified several additional MLVA loci. This will enable even higher resolution for the identification of individual strains and, hence, facilitate the tracing of the outbreak source, which will be pertinent in distinguishing unusual outbreaks from bioterrorism.

Analyses of the genome sequence data have suggested several other potential typing strategies, which are being explored. An obvious approach that has been facilitated with the availability of the genome sequence is primer design for multi-locus sequence typing. Other examples include insertion sequence (IS)-element-based typing methods and methods targeting potentially variable genomic regions adjacent to inverted and forward repeat sequences in the genome.

5. DEVELOPMENT OF VACCINES AND ANTIMICROBIALS

5.1. Live-Attenuated Vaccines

A live-attenuated strain of *F. tularensis* (strain LVS) derived from the type B strain was originally isolated in the former USSR and has been used extensively in humans during the 20th century. Several human trials with this vaccine were reported in the 1960s, which indicated that immunization with this vaccine yielded good protection against inhalation challenge with 2000 CFU of *F. tularensis* strain SchuS4 *(59–61)*. The effectiveness of this vaccine has also been confirmed by a retrospective study in laboratory workers where the incidence of typhoidal tularemia fell from 5.7 to 0.27 cases per 100 workers after a vaccination program was introduced *(62)*. This vaccine also offered some protection against the ulceroglandular form of the disease. The LVS vaccine has previously been granted Investigational New Drug status by the Food and Drug Administration (FDA) but, to date, the full licensing of the vaccine has not been granted. The basis of attenuation of the LVS strain is not known, and for reasons which are not known, this strain is attenuated in the murine model of disease only when given by the intradermal route *(63)*.

An alternative approach to the development of an effective and licensable tularemia vaccine exploits the finding that in principle, any attenuated mutant can be used as vaccine. Based on the knowledge of the methodologies that have previously been applied to other bacterial pathogens to devise defined attenuated mutants and on the availability of the partial genome sequence of *F. tularensis*, it should be possible to develop a rationally attenuated vaccine also for *F. tularensis*, strain SchuS4.

5.1.1. The Shikimate Pathway

Genes that encode enzymes in the shikimate pathway have previously been targeted in bacteria such as *S. enterica* var Typhimurium, *Salmonella enterica* var Typhi, *Shigella flexneri*, *Pasturella multocid,* and *Aeromonas salmonicida* to construct attenuated mutants that are highly effective live vaccines *(64–71)*. The shikimate pathway is required both for the biosynthesis of aromatic amino acids as well as for the generation of *para*-aminobenzoic acid (pABA), 2,3 dihydroxybenzoic acid (DHB), ubiquinone, menaquinone, and enterochelin *(72)*. At least in the case of *S. enterica* var Typhimurium, attenuation is thought to be caused by the inability of the bacterium to generate pABA and/or DHB, neither of which are freely available in the host-cell cytoplasm *(73)*. Although shikimate pathway mutants (or so-called aro mutants) are often highly effective vaccines, some pathogens such as *Rickettsia prowazekii* appear to lack all of the necessary genes in this pathway *(74)*. In other pathogens such as *Yersinia pestis*, inactivation of the *aroA* gene did not result in significant attenuation of the bacterium *(75)*.

The finding that *F. tularensis* strain SchuS4 is able to grow in the media lacking aromatic amino acids indicates that a pathway for the biosynthesis of these amino acids is functional in the bacterium *(36)*. Using existing knowledge about the shikimate pathway in other bacteria, the genes that could potentially encode enzymes in this pathway (*see* Fig. 4) have been identified from the *F. tularensis* strain SchuS4 partial genome sequence *(36,39)*. This analysis supports the hypothesis that this pathway is functional, at least for the generation of aromatic amino acids, although some differences have been noted on comparison with the pathway in *E. coli*. For reasons that are not clear, but might relate to differential regulation of this pathway, there is redundancy of

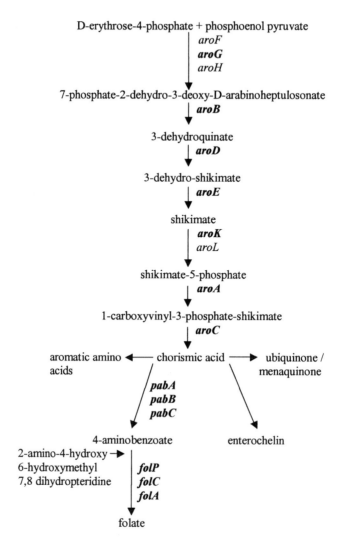

Fig. 4. Aromatic amino acid biosynthesis pathway as identified in *E. coli.* Chorismic acid, which is the product of the shikimate biosynthesis pathway, serves as the starting point for the biosynthesis of aromatic amino acids, *p*-aminobenoic acid, and folic acid, enterochelin, and ubiquinone, and menaquinone. The attenuation of virulent bacteria is thought to be a result of their inability to synthesize in *p*-aminobenoic acid, folic acid or enterochelin. Genes that encode enzymes required for the conversion of each of the intermediates in the pathway are shown italicized. Shown in bold are genes in *F. tularensis,* which appear to encode homologs of these enzymes that have been identified in other bacteria. (Reproduced from ref. *36* with the kind permission of Mary Ann Liebert, Inc.)

phospho-2-dehydro-3-deoxyheptonate aldolase (AroF, AroG, or AroH) and shikimate kinase enzymes (AroK and AroL) in *E. coli.* In *F. tularensis* SchuS4, only a single gene encoding each of these enzymes has been identified *(36,39).* Notwithstanding, these differences in all of the enzymes necessary for the biosynthesis of chorismate and aromatic amino acids are apparently encoded by *F. tularensis.* However, this does not in itself indicate that mutations within genes in this pathway would result in attenuation, because as noted earlier in *S. enterica* var Typhimurium, it is the inability to produce terminal products such as pABA or DHB that is growth-limiting in vivo. To date, we have been able to identify all of the necessary genes in the pABA pathway apart from *pabC*. However, we have also noted that PabC proteins from other bacteria show only a low level of sequence similarity, suggesting that the unambiguous identification of this gene in *F. tularensis* might be difficult *(36)*.

5.1.2. The Purine Biosynthetic Pathway

An alternative biosynthetic pathway, which has been disrupted in *Brucella melitensis (76)*, *Mycobacterium tuberculosis (77)*, *Y. pestis (78)*, *Bacillus anthracis (79)* *Salmonella enterica* var Dublin*,* or *S. enterica* var Typhimurium *(80)* to yield attenuated mutants, is required for the biosynthesis of purines. However, the precise effects of mutations in this pathway on the degree of attenuation are difficult to predict. The virulence features of *Yersinia pestis (78)*, *B. anthracis (79)*, and *Salmonella (80)* are most reduced by mutations that act after the production of inosine 5'-monophosphate (IMP) in the purine biosynthetic pathway. In contrast, in *B. melitensis (76)* and *M. tuberculosis (77)* virulence is markedly attenuated by mutations that act before the production of IMP. In part, this might reflect the relative functions of the purine biosynthetic and salvage pathways.

In the partial genome sequence of *F. tularensis* strain SchuS4, we have identified all of the genes that could encode proteins necessary for the *de novo* synthesis of purine nucleotides (ref. *36*; *see* Fig. 5). We have also identified genes that potentially encode proteins required for the salvage of adenine, adenosine, deoxyadenosine, or hypoxanthine in *E. coli (81)*. However, to date we have not been able to identify genes putatively coding for guanosine kinase (*gsk*) or guanine phosphoribosyltransferase (*gpt*), which are required for the growth of *E. coli* when guanine or xanthine precursors are provided to mutants in the *de novo* pathway. Overall, our findings suggest that part of the purine salvage pathway is functional in *F. tularensis* strain SchuS4 *(36)*.

5.1.3. The Construction of Defined Attenuated Mutants

Although we have identified two pathways that might be interrupted to yield a defined attenuated mutant of *F. tularensis*, to date the construction of mutants has proven to be difficult. Methodologies that have been used to generate allelic replacement mutants of *F. novicida (34)* have not yet been successfully used with *F. tularensis*. The lack of such a genetic system is clearly a major hurdle to be overcome in the near future if an improved live vaccine is to be devised.

5.1.4 Subunit Vaccines

It has long been a goal to identify subunits derived from *F. tularensis* that induce a protective immune response. Immunization of mice with LPS from *F. tularensis* does show some potential for protection against low virulence strains *(82,83)* and might be exploited as one component of a subunit vaccine, especially if in complex with a polypeptide derived from *F. tularensis*. Previous workers have identified numerous cell surface proteins that appear to be recognized by T cells from individuals immunized with the LVS vaccine. Some of these polypeptides have been evaluated as protective subunits in a murine disease model, with disappointing results *(82,84,85)*.

Recently, numerous of workers have demonstrated the feasibility of identifying proteins that induce a protective immune response from the genome sequence of the pathogen of interest *(35,86–89)*. This *in silico* approach to the identification of vaccines has

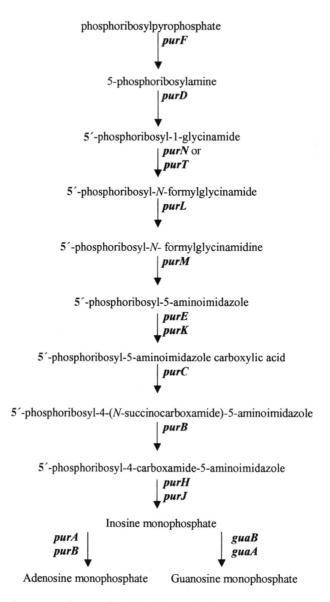

Fig. 5. The *de novo* pathway of purine biosynthesis as previously identified in *E. coli* and identified in *F. tularensis* by genomic sequencing and homology searches. Gene designations are as reported for *E. coli* loci. Genes that encode enzymes required for the conversion of each of the intermediates in the pathway are shown italicized. Shown in bold are genes in *F. tularensis,* which appear to encode homologs of these enzymes that have been identified in other bacteria. (Reproduced from ref. *36* with the kind permission of Mary Ann Liebert, Inc.)

been termed reverse vaccinology *(89).* Candidate vaccine proteins are identified based on the assumption that vaccine antigens will be exposed on the cell surface and by using algorithms that predict their likely cellular location. Proteins destined for the cell surface are likely to possess signal sequences and are also likely to lack motifs for anchoring in the inner membrane of the bacterial cell *(86).* When these criteria are applied to all of the predicted proteins encoded within the bacterial genome, a subset of candidate proteins are selected for testing in a suitable animal model of the disease. It is possible that similar methodologies could be applied to the *F. tularensis* genome, and the availability of suitable murine models of the disease should facilitate this approach.

An alternative approach to the development of a subunit vaccine against *F. tularensis* that also exploits the availability of the genome sequence has been proposed by Hernychova and his colleagues *(90)*. These workers have compared the proteomic profiles, as determined by two-dimensional electrophoresis, of the attenuated LVS strain of *F. tularensis* and two virulent clinical isolates with the aim of identifying proteins produced only by fully virulent strains, which might serve as vaccine antigens. More than 50 differentially regulated proteins were identified, and preliminary work has identified one form of a 23-kDa protein and two acid phosphatases that are apparently produced only by virulent strains.

5.1.5. Novel Antimicrobial Targets

The availability of genome sequences has fueled a range of projects to devise new antimicrobial compounds that could be active toward individual pathogens or even selected groups of pathogens *(91,92)*. Such antimicrobials would be active against gene products that are essential for bacterial viability or for the bacterium to grow in vivo and cause disease *(91)*. Clearly, to ensure a high therapeutic index, structurally related gene products should not be present in the host. In the near term, it is likely that antimicrobials developed against targets in other pathogens will be screened against *F. tularensis* on the basis of known orthologues identified from the genome sequence. For example, interruption of the shikimate pathway has been shown to attenuate a range of pathogens and drugs that target enzymes in this pathway (such as dehydroquinate synthase) have already been identified as a targets for the development of antimicrobials *(93)*. Dehydroquinate synthase is encoded in the *F. tularensis* genome and compounds targeting this enzyme might be antibacterial. A range of other targets for antibacterial drugs, such as DNA adenine methylase *(94)*, have also been identified in other bacteria and should *F. tularensis* possess an ortholog of this enzyme then inhibitors of this enzyme might be antibacterial.

6. CONCLUSION

In spite of the significance of *F. tularensis* as a cause of disease in naturally exposed individuals and the potential for this pathogen to be used illegitimately as a bioterrorism agent, very little is known about the genetic makeup of this bacterium, virulence factors possessed by this bacterium, or the nature of the immune response that is required for protection against tularemia. These gaps in our knowledge severely limit our attempts to devise improved diagnostic systems, improved vaccines, and improved antimicrobials. Clearly the availability of the genome sequence of *F. tularensis* is likely to underpin much of the future research with this pathogen. These data have already allowed numerous biochemical pathways to be reconstructed *in silico*, and the predicted functionality of these pathways suggest that they would be good targets for disruption and the generation of a rationally attenuated mutant as a live vaccine. In parallel, *in silico* techniques for the prediction of surface-located proteins and virulence determinants might allow a subunit vaccine to be devised. The significance of this work extends beyond the development of vaccines. Candidate virulence determinants might prove to be ideal targets for the development of detection and diagnostic systems capable of discriminating between low- and high-virulence strains of *F. tularensis*. In addition, proteins necessary for the virulence of *F. tularensis* might serve as ideal targets for the development of new antimicrobials. However, the full exploitation of the *F. tularensis* genome sequence will almost certainly be dependent on an ability to construct defined allelic replacement mutants of the bacterium. Therefore, the development of such methods must therefore be considered to be one of the highest priorities for future research with this bacterium.

REFERENCES

1. Mörner, T. and Sandström, G. (1997) Tularemia, in *Manual of Standards for Diagnostic Tests and Vaccines*, 3rd ed. Office International Des Epizooties, Paris, France.
2. Hubalek, Z., Sixl, W., and Halouzka, J. (1998) *Francisella tularensis* in *Dermacentor reticulatus* ticks from the Czech Republic and Austria. *Wien Klin Wochenschr.* **110,** 909, 910.
3. Stewart, S. J. (1996) Tularemia: association with hunting and farming. *FEMS Immunol. Med. Microbiol.* **13,** 197–199.
4. Morner, T. (1992) The ecology of tularemia. *Rev. Sci. Tech. Off. Int. Epiz.* **11,** 1123–1130.
5. Ohara, Y., Sato, T., and Homma, M. (1998) Arthropod-borne tularemia in Japan: clinical analysis of 1374 cases observed between 1924 and 1996. *J. Med. Entomol.* **35,** 471–473.
6. Tarnvik, A., Sandstrom, G., and Sjostedt, A. (1996) Epidemiological analysis of tularemia in Sweden 1931-1993. *FEMS Immunol. Med. Microbiol.* **13,** 201–204.
7. Gill, V. and Cunha, B. A. (1997) Tularemia pneumonia. *Semin. Resp. Infect.* **12,** 61–67.
8. Evans, M. E., Gregory, D. W., Schaffner, W., and McGee, Z. A. (1985) Tularemia: a 30 year experience with 88 cases. *Medicine (Baltimore)* **64,** 251–269.
9. Evans, M. E. (1985) *Francisella tularensis. Infect. Cont.* **6,** 381–383.
10. Eigelsbach, H. T. and Downs, C. M. (1961) Prophylactic effectiveness of live and killed tularemia vaccines. I. Production of vaccine and evaluation in the white mouse and guinea pig. *J. Immunol.* **87,** 415–425.
11. Mangold, T. and Goldberg, J. (1999) *Plague Wars: A True Story of Biological Warfare.* Macmillan, London.
12. Centers for Disease Control. (2001) Basic laboratory protocols for the presumptive identification of *Francisella tularensis*.
13. Forsman, M., Sandstrom, G., and Sjostedt, A. (1994) Analysis of 16S ribosomal DNA sequences of *Francisella* strains and utilisation for determination of the phylogeny of the genus and for identification of strains by PCR. *Int. J. Syst. Bacteriol.* **44,** 38–46.
14. Niebylski, M. L., Peacock, M. G., Fischer, E. R., Porcella, S. F., and Schwan, T. G. (1997) Characterisation of an endosymbiont infecting wood ticks, *Dermacentor andersoni*, as a member of the genus *Francisella. Appl. Environ. Microbiol.* **63,** 3933–3940.
15. Noda, H., Munderloh, U. G., and Kurtti, T. J. (1997) Endosymbionts of ticks and their relationship to *Wolbachia* spp. and tick-borne pathogens of humans and animals. *Appl. Environ. Microbiol.* **63,** 3926–3932.
16. Maidak, B L., Cole, J. R., Lilburn, T. G., et al. (2001) The RDP-II (Ribosomal Database Project). *Nucleic Acids Res.* **29,** 173, 174.
17. Posada, D. and Crandall, K. A. (1998) MODELTEST: testing the model of DNA substitution. *Bioinformatics* **14,** 817, 818.
18. Swofford, D. L. (1999) PAUP*. Phylogenetic Analysis Using Parsimony (*and Other Methods). (Sinauer Associates, Sunderland, Massachusetts). Version 4.
19. Sandstrom, G., Sjostedt, A., Forsman, M., Pavlovich, N. V., and Mishan'kin, B. N. (1992) Characterisation and classification of strains of *Francisella tularensis* isolated in the central Asian focus of the Soviet Union and in Japan. *J. Clin. Microbiol.* **30,** 172–175.

20. Sjöstedt, A. (2002) Family XVII. *Francisellaceae*, genus I. *Francisella*, in *Bergey's Manual of Systematic Bacteriology* (Brenner, D. J., ed.), New York, Springer-Verlag.

21. Jellison, W. L. (1974) Tularemia in North America. 1930–1974. University of Montana.

22. Dienst, J. F. T. (1963) Tularemia—a perusal of three hundred thirty-nine cases. *J. Louisiana State M. So.* **115,** 114–127.

23. Gurycova, D. (1998) First isolation of *Francisella tularensis* subsp. tularensis in Europe. *Eur. J. Epidemiol.* **14,** 797–802.

24. Mitscherlich, E. and Marth, E. H. (1984) *Microbial Survival in the Environment.* Springer-Verlag, Berlin, 741, 742.

25. Parker, R. R., Steinhaus, E. A., Kohls, G. M., and Jellison, W. L. (1951) Contamination of natural waters and mud with *Pasturella tularensis* and Tularemia in beavers and muskrats in the Northwestern United States. *Nat. Inst. Health Bull.* 193.

26. Berdal, B. P., Ting, R. S., Meidell, N. K., Lorentzen-Styr, A. M., and Scheel, O. (1996) Field investigations of tularaemia in Norway. *FEMS Immunol. Med. Micribiol.* **13,** 191–195.

27. Abd, H., Johansson, T., Hägg, K., Golovliov, I., Sandström, G., and Forsman, M. (2003) Survival and growth of *Francisella tularensis* in *Acanthamoeba castellani. Appl. Environ. Microbiol.* **69,** 600–606.

28. Fortier, A. H., Green, S. J., Polsinelli, T., et al. (1994) Life and death of an intracellular pathogen: *Francisella tularensis* and the macrophage. *Immunol. Ser.* 349–361.

29. Gray, C. G., Cowley, S. C., and Nano, F. E. (2002) The identification of five genetic loci of *Francisella novicida* associated with intracellular growth. *FEMS Microbiol. Lett.* **215,** 53–56.

30. Baron, G. S. and Nano, F. E. (1998) MglA and MglB are required for the intramacrophage growth of *Francisella novicida. Mol. Microbiol.* **29,** 247–259.

31. Anthony, L. S. D., Cowley, S. C., Mdluli, K. E., and Nano, F. E. (1994) Isolation of a *Francisella tularensis* mutant that is sensitive to serum and oxidative killing and is avirulent in mice: correlation with the loss of MinD homologue expression. *FEMS Microbiol. Lett.* **124,** 157–166.

32. Sandstrom, G., Lofgren, S., and Tarnvik, A. (1988) A capsule-deficient mutant of *Francisella tularensis* LVS exhibits enhanced sensitivity to killing by serum but diminished sensitivity to killing by polymorphonuclear leukocytes. *Infect. Immun.* **56,** 1194–1202.

33. Sorokin, V. M., Pavlovich, N. V., and Prozorova, L. A. (1996) *Francisella tularensis* resistance to bactericidal action of normal human serum. *FEMS Immunol. Med. Microbiol.* **13,** 249–252.

34. Anthony, L. S. D., Gu, M., Cowley, S. C., Leung, W. W. S., and Nano, F. E. (1991) Transformation and allelic replacement in *Francisella* spp. *J. Gen. Microbiol.* **137,** 2697–2703.

35. Pizza, M., Scarlato, V., Masignani, V., et al. (2000) Identification of vaccine candidates against serogroup B meningococcus by whole-genome sequencing. *Science* **287,** 1816–1820.

36. Karlsson, J., Prior, R. G., Williams, K., et al. (2000) Sequencing of the *Francisella tularensis* strain Schu4 genome reveals the shikimate and purine metabolic pathways, targets for the construction of a rationally attenuated auxotrophic vaccine. *Microb. Comp. Genomics* **5,** 25–39.

37. Pomerantsev, A. P., Obuchi, M., and Ohara, Y. (2001) Nucleotide sequence, structural organization, and functional characterization of the small recombinant plasmid pOM1 that is specific for *Francisella tularensis. Plasmid* **46,** 86–94.

38. Pavlov, V. M., Mokrievich, A. N., and Volkovoy, K. (1996) Cryptic plasmid pFNL10 from *Francisella novicida*-like F6168: the base of plasmids for *Fransicella tularensis. FEMS Immunol. Med. Microbiol.* **13,** 253–256

39. Prior, R. G., Klasson, L., Larsson, P., et al. (2001) Preliminary analysis and annotation of the partial genome sequence of *Francisella tularensis* strain Schu 4. *J. Appl. Microbiol.* **91,** 1–7.

40. Cowley, S. C., Myltseva, S. V., Nano, F. E. (1996) Phase variation in *Francisella tularensis* affecting intracellular growth, lipopolysaccharide antigenicity and nitric oxide production. *Mol. Microbiol.* **20**, 867–874.

41. Koskela, P. and Salminen, A. (1985) Humoral immunity against *Francisella tularensis* after natural infection. *J. Clin. Microbiol.* **22**, 973–979.

42. Pollitzer, R. (1967) History and incidence of tularemia in the Soviet Union. A review. The Institute of Contemporary Russian Studies, Fordham University, New York.

43. Grunow, R., Splettstoesser, W., McDonald, S., et al. (2000) Detection of *Francisella tularensis* in biological specimens using a capture enzyme-linked immunosorbent assay, an immunochromatographic handheld assay, and a PCR. *Clin. Diag. Lab. Immunol.* **7**, 86–90.

44. Forsman, M., Sandstrom, G., and Jaurin, B. (1990) Identification of *Francisella* species and discrimination of type A and type B strains of *F. tularensis* by 16S rRNA analysis. *Appl. Environ. Microbiol.* **56**, 949–955.

45. Forsman, M., Kuoppa, K., Sjöstedt, A., and Tärnvik, A. RNA-hybridisation in a case of ulceroglandular tularemia. *Eur. J. Clin. Microbiol. Infect. Dis.* **9**, 784, 785.

46. Forsman, M., Sandström, G., and Sjöstedt, A. (1994) Analysis of 16S ribosomal DNA sequences of *Francisella* strains and utilization for determination of the phylogeny of the genus and for identification of strains by PCR. *Int. J. Syst. Bacteriol.* **44**, 38–46.

47. Sjostedt, A., Sandstrom, G., Tarnvik, A., and Jaurin, B. (1990) Nucleotide sequence and T cell epitopes of a membrane protein of *Francisella tularensis*. *J. Immunol.* **145**, 311–317.

48. Sjostedt, A., Kuoppa, K., Johansson, T., and Sandstrom, G. (1992) The 17 kDa lipoprotein and encoding gene of *Francisella tularensis* LVS are conserved in strains of *Francisella tularensis*. *Microb. Pathog.* **13**, 243–249.

49. Long, G. W., Oprandy, J. J., Narayanan, R. B., Fortier, A. H., Porter, K. R., and Nacy, C. A. (1993) Detection of *Francisella tularensis* in blood by polymerase chain reaction. *J. Clin. Microbiol.* **31**, 152–154.

50. Sjöstedt, A., Eriksson, U., Berglund, L., and Tärnvik, A. (1997) Detection of *Francisella tularensis* in ulcers of Patients with tularemia by PCR. *J. Clin. Microbiol.* **35**, 1045–1048.

51. Johansson, A., Ibrahim, A., Göransson, I., Eriksson, U., Gurycova, D., Clarridge, III J. E., and Sjöstedt, A. (2000) Evaluation of PCR-based methods for discrimination of species and subspecies of *Francisella tularensis* and the development of a specific PCR that distinguishes the two major subspecies. *J. Clin. Microbiol.* **38**, 4180–4185.

52. Ibrahim, A., Gerner-Smidt, P., and Sjöstedt, A. (1996) Amplification and restriction endonuclease digestion of a large fragment of genes coding for rRNA as a rapid method for discrimination of closely related pathogenic bacteria. *J. Clin. Microbiol.* **34**, 2894–2896.

53. Clarridge, J. E., Raich, T. J., Sjöstedt, A., et al. (1996) Characterization of two unusual clinically significant *Francisella* strains. *J. Clin. Microbiol.* **34**, 1995–2000.

54. de La Puente-Redondo, V. A., del Blanco, N. G., Gutierrez-Martin, C. B., Garcia-Pena, F. J., and Ferri, E. F. (2000) Comparison of different PCR approaches for typing of *Francisella tularensis* strains. *J. Clin. Microbiol.* **38**, 1016–1022.

55. Johansson, A., Göransson, I., Larsson, P., and Sjöstedt, A. (2001) Extensive allelic variation among *Francisella tularensis* strains in a short-sequence tandem repeat region. *J. Clin. Microbiol.* **39**, 3140–3146.

56. Broekhuijsen, M., Larsson, P., Johansson, A., et al. (2003) A genome-wide microarray analysis of *Francisella tularensis* strains demonstrate extensive genetic conservation within the species but identifies regions that are unique to the highly virulent *F. tularensis* subspecies tularensis. *J. Clin. Microbiol.* **41**, 2934–2941.

57. van Belkum, A., Scherer, S., van Alphen, L., and Verbrugh, H. (1998) Short-sequence DNA repeats in prokaryotic genomes. *Microbiol. Mol. Biol. Rev.* **62**, 275–293.

58. Farlow, J., Smith, K. L., Wong, J., Abrams, M., Lytle, M., and Keim, P. *Francisella tularensis* strain typing using multiple-locus variable-number tandem repeat analysis. *J. Clin. Microbiol.* **39**, 3186–3192.

59. Saslaw, S., Eigelsbach, H. T., Prior, J. A., Wilson, H. E., and Carhart, S. (1961) Tularemia vaccine study. II. Respiratory challenge. *Arch. Intern. Med.* **107,** 702–714.

60. Saslaw, S., Eigelsbach, H. T., Wilson, H. E., Prior, J. A., and Carhart, S. (1961) Tularemia vaccine study. I. Intracutaneous challenge. *Arch. Intern. Med.* **107,** 689–701.

61. Eigelsbach, H. T., Hornick, R. B., and Tulis, J. J. (1967) Recent studies on live tularemia vaccine. *Med. Ann. Dist. Columbia* **36,** 282–286.

62. Burke, D. S. (1977) Immunisation against tularemia: analysis of the effectiveness of live *Francisella tularensis* vaccine in prevention of laboratory-acquired tularemia. *J. Infect. Dis.* **135,** 55–60.

63. Elkins, K. L., Rhinehart-Jones, T. R., Culkin, S. J., Yee, D., and Winegar, R. K. (1996) Minimal requirements for murine resistance to infection with *Francisella tularensis* LVS. *Infect. Immun.* **64,** 3288–3293.

64. Dougan, G. (1994) The molecular basis for virulence of bacterial pathogens:implications for oral vaccine development. *Microbiology* **140,** 215–224.

65. Charles, I. and Dougan, G. (1990) Gene expression and the development of live enteric vaccines. *Trends Biotechnol.* **8,** 117–121.

66. Scott, P. C., Markham, J. F., and Whithear, K. G. (1999) Safety and efficacy of two live *Pasteurella multocida aro-A* mutant vaccines in chickens. *Avian Dis.* **3,** 83–88.

67. Cersini, A., Salvia, A. M., and Bernardini, M. L. (1998) Intracellular multiplication and virulence of *Shigella flexneri* auxotrophic mutants. *Infect. Immun.* **6,** 549–557.

68. Marsden, M. J., Vaughan, L. M., Fitzpatrick, R. M., Foster, T. J., and Secombes, C. J. (1998) Potency testing of a live, genetically attenuated vaccine for salmonids. *Vaccine* **16,** 1087–1094.

69. Gunel-Ozcan, A., Brown, K. A., Allen, A. G., and Maskell, D. J. (1997) *Salmonella typhimurium aroB* mutants are attentuated in BALB/c mice. *Microb. Pathog.* **23,** 311–316.

70. Dougan, G., Chatfield, S., Pickard, D., Bester, J., O'Callaghan, D., and Maskell, D. (1988) Construction and characterization of vaccine strains of Salmonella harboring mutations in two different *aro* genes. *J. Infect. Dis.* **158,** 1329–1335.

71. Hone, D. M., Harris, A. M., Chatfield, S., Dougan, G., and Levine, M. M. (1991) Construction of genetically defined double *aro* mutants of *Salmonella typhi. Vaccine* **9,** 810–816.

72. Stocker, B. A. D. (1988) Auxotrophic *Salmonella typhi* as live vaccine. *Vaccine* **6,** 141–145.

73. Hosieth, S. K. and Stocker, B. A. D. (1981) Aromatic-dependent *Salmonella typhimurium* are non-virulent and effective as live vaccines. *Nature* **291,** 238, 239.

74. Andersson, S. G. E., Zomorodipour, A., Andersson, J., et al. (1998) The genome sequence of *Rickettsia prowazekii* and the origin of mitochondria. *Nature* **396,** 133–140.

75. Oyston, P. C. F., Russell, P., Williamson, E. D., and Titball, R. W. (1996) An *aroA* mutant of *Yersinia pestis* is attenuated in the guinea pig, but virulent in mice. *Microbiology* **142,** 1847–1853.

76. Crawford, R. M., Van De Verg, L., Yuan, L., et al. (1996) Deletion of *purE* attenuates *Brucella melitensis* infection in mice. *Infect. Immun.* **64,** 2188–2192.

77. Jackson, M., Phalen, S. W., Lagranderie, M., et al. (1999) Persistence and protective efficacy of a *Mycobacterium tuberculosis* auxotroph vaccine. *Infect. Immun.* **67,** 2867–2873.

78. Brubaker, R. R. (1970) Interconversion of purine mononucleotides in *Pasturella pestis. Infect. Immun.* **1,** 446–454.

79. Ivanovics, G., Marjai, E., and Dobozy, A. (1968) The growth of purine mutants of *Bacillus anthracis* in the body of the mouse. *J. Gen. Microbiol.* **53,** 147–162.

80. McFarland, W. C. and Stocker, B. A. D. (1987) Effect of different purine auxotrophic mutations on mouse-virulence of a Vi-positive strain of *Salmonella dublin* and of two strains of *Salmonella typhimurium. Microb. Pathog.* **3,** 129–141.

81. Neuhard, J. and Nygaard, P. (1987) Purines and pyrimidines, in Escherichia coli *and* Salmonella typhimurium *Cellular and Molecular Biology*, vol. 1. (Neidhardt, F. C., Ingraham,

J. L., Low, K. B., et al., eds.), American Society for Microbiology, Washington, DC, pp. 445–473.

82. Fulop, M., Manchee, R., and Titball, R. (1995) Role of lipopolysaccharide and a major outer membrane protein from *Francisella tularensis* in the induction of immunity against tularemia. *Vaccine* **13,** 1220–1225.

83. Fulop, M., Mastroeni, P., Green, M., and Titball, R. W. (2001) Role of antibody to lipopolysaccharide in protection against low and high-virulence strains of *Francisella tularensis*. *Vaccine* **19,** 4465–4472.

84. Golovliov, I., Ericsson, M., Akerblom, L., Sandström, G., Tärnvik, A., and Sjöstedt, A. (1995) Adjuvanticity of ISCOMs incorporating a T cell-reactive lipoprotein of the facultative intracellular pathogen *Francisella tularensis*. *Vaccine* **13,** 261–267.

85. Sjöstedt, A., Sandström, G., and Tärnvik, A. (1992) Humoral and cell-mediated immunity in mice to a 17-kilodalton lipoprotein of *Francisella tularensis* expressed by *Salmonella typhimurium*. *Infect. Immun.* **60,** 2855–2862.

86. Gomez, M., Johnson, S., and Gennaro, M. L. (2000) Identification of secreted proteins of *Mycobacterium tuberculosis* by a bioinformatic approach. *Infect. Immun.* **68,** 2323–2327.

87. Ross, B. C., Czajkowski, L., Hocking, D., et al. (2001) Identification of vaccine candidate antigens from a genomic analysis of *Porphyromonas gingivalis*. *Vaccine* **9,** 4135–4142.

88. Tettelin, H., Nelson, K. E., Paulsen, I. T., et al. (2001) Complete genome sequence of a virulent isolate of *Streptococcus pneumoniae*. *Science* **293,** 498–506.

89. Rappuoli, R. (2001) Reverse vaccinology, a genome-based approach to vaccine development. *Vaccine* **19,** 2688–2691.

90. Hernychova, L., Stulik, J., Halada, P., Macela, A., Kroca, M., Johansson, T., and Malina, M. (2001) Construction of a *Francisella tularensis* two-dimensional electrophoresis protein database. *Proteomics* **1,** 508–515.

91. Buysse, J. M. (2001) The role of genomics in antibacterial target discovery. *Curr. Med. Chem.* **8,** 1763–1776.

92. McDevitt, D. and Rosenberg, M. (2001) Exploiting genomics to discover new antibiotics. *Trends Microbiol.* **9,** 611–617.

93. Carpenter, E. P., Hawkins, A. R., Frost, J. W., and Brown, K. A. (1998) Structure of dehydroquinate synthase reveals an active site capable of multistep catalysis. *Nature* **394,** 299–302.

94. Heithoff, D. M., Sinsheimer, R. L., Low, D. A., and Mahan, M. J. (1999) An essential role for DNA adenine methylation in bacterial virulence. *Science* **284,** 967–970.

95. Forsman, M. .Henningsson, E., Johansson, T., Larsson, E., and Sandström, G. (2000) The zoonotic bacterium *Francisella tularensis* does not manifest virulence in viable but nonculturable state. *FEMS Microbiol. Ecol.* **31,** 217–224.

96. Higgins, J. A., Hubalek, Z., Halouzka, J., Elkins, K. L., Sjostedt, A., Shipley, M., Ibrahim, M. S. (2000) Detection of *Francisella tularensis* in infected mammals and vectors using a probe-based polymerase chain reaction. *Am. J. Trop. Med. Hyg.* **62,** 310–318.

97. Johansson, A., Berglund, L., Eriksson, U., et al. (2000) A comparative analysis of PCR versus culture for the diagnosis of ulceroglandular tularemia. *J. Clin. Microbiol.* **38,** 22–26.

21

Genetic Fingerprinting of Biodefense Pathogens for Epidemiology and Forensic Investigation

Luther E. Lindler, Xiao-Zhe Huang, May Chu, Ted L. Hadfield,
and Michael Dobson

1. INTRODUCTION

Genotyping of agents of bioterrorism (BT) can provide valuable information from several viewpoints during an incident. First, as was seen in the *Bacillus anthracis* attack, it provides useful epidemiological information. It allows us to determine if the strain being isolated from patients and/or the environment are genetically identical. This information then helps focus the investigation and aids decisions about treatment of the infected individuals. Second, it will impact the response that the United States might mount against the group or country of origin. Specifically, the official policy of deterrence is that the United States will respond to any use of a biological warfare (BW) agent with equal or greater force *(1)*. Obviously, matching the isolate to a database of strains from around the world would help narrow the focus of the investigation as to the origin of a particular strain. Also, once a potential source is identified, genotyping techniques would be used in a forensic manner to allow an unambiguous match to be made between the recovered material and the strains used in the attack. This latter use would be similar to criminal fingerprinting. In fact, the common term for genotyping of microorganisms is genetic "fingerprinting." Third, genotyping can aid infectious disease specialists, as well as intelligence officers in the identification of potentially modified BW agents. This would be analogous to the Centers for Disease Control and Prevention (CDC) program monitoring food-borne pathogens for the emergence of new, more virulent strains of enteric organisms as part of the Pulsenet program *(2)*. A system of laboratories and databases such as this would allow us to identify isolates of BW agents that are "outside the box" of known genotypes and focus attention on characterization of them.

The genotyping of BW agents presents a unique challenge when compared to other infectious disease-causing organisms. The genetic relationship between many infectious bacteria has been determined based on single-nucleotide polymorphisms (SNPs), presence of various known virulence factors, and macrorestriction patterns of the genomic DNA *(3–11)*. Generally, BW agents such as *B. anthracis, Francisella tularensis, Brucella* spp., and *Yersinia pestis* are relatively monomorphic *(12–16)*. However, the term monomorphic refers to a specific locus or technique used to exam-

From: *Infectious Diseases: Biological Weapons Defense: Infectious Diseases and Counterterrorism*
Edited by: L. E. Lindler, F. J. Lebeda, and G. W. Korch © Humana Press Inc., Totowa, NJ

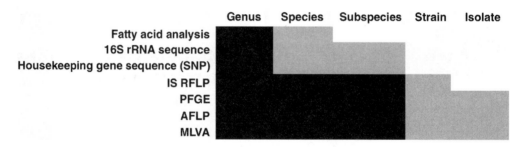

Fig. 1. Approximate sensitivity of various techniques for differentiation of bacterial strains and isolates. The black bars represent techniques that can differentiate between members within the various levels of classification of bacteria *(83)*. The gray bars indicate techniques that can sometimes differentiate between members within the class. For example, the 16S ribosomal RNA (rRNA) sequence can differentiate between various genera of bacteria. However, only in some cases is the 16S rRNA sequence specific for a particular species within a given genera. For the purposes of this diagram, subspecies are exemplified by biotype, serotype, phagetype, and so on. The term strain designates characterized isolates of a particular organism such as the Ames strain of *B. anthracis*. In this context, an isolate is considered as an organism cultured from a patient or the environment. IS RFLP, insertion sequence restriction fragment length polymorphism; AFLP, amplified fragment length polymorphism; MLVA, multi-locus variable number tandem repeat analysis.

ine the genetic material of the organism. Accordingly, the biology of the organism being examined will influence the diversity seen when various techniques are applied to genetic characterization. For example, if the organism does not contain many duplicated or homologous regions within the genome, then the diversity seen by pulsed-field gel electrophoresis (PFGE) will not be very large. Each of the techniques used in genotyping reveals diversity or polymorphism at different levels of the genome. A general outline of the sensitivity of the various common techniques used to determine the relatedness and genetic "fingerprint" of bacterial isolates is presented in Fig. 1. Of course, this is only a general guideline because the specificity of any given technique depends on the loci being examined and the amount of available information obtained from a large group of diverse, as well as homogeneous, strains *(11)*. Therefore, it is critical to understand the basis for the polymorphism and invest in characterization of genomic changes using various techniques applied to the same strains of the organism. In the following sections, we will briefly describe each technique and relate in which level of the genome the technique attempts to identify polymorphisms.

1.1. Pulsed-Field Gel Electrophoresis

The analysis of chromosomal DNA by PFGE requires the restriction digestion of unfragmented (intact) whole-cell DNA with enzymes that cleave the genetic material at relatively few sites *(17)*. The restriction fragments then are separated on agarose gels ran in a rotating electric field that causes the DNA to migrate farther than if a simple electric field were applied. The combination of field switching times, field strength, agarose concentration, and length of time used in the separation all influence the size of fragments that can be resolved by this technique. Conditions can be used that resolve fragments in the size range from kilobase pairs (kb) to megabase pairs (mb) *(17,18)*. Therefore, it is critical to choose PFGE conditions that match the restriction enzyme used for DNA digestion and the range of fragment sizes generated from that cleavage. Once the conditions for digestion of genomic DNA and separation of the fragments have been established for an organism, the technique can be applied repeatedly with as many isolates as is desired and results of the macrorestriction pattern can be compared to determine genetic relatedness.

The difference in PFGE fingerprint between strains of a given organism can arise through several mechanisms. First, single base changes in the DNA can either create new restriction enzyme recognition sites or, if they occur within a site, they can destroy them. Either of these occurrences produces fragments that migrate to a new position on the gel. Second, banding patterns can change because of the activity of mobile genetic elements inserting or deleting material from the genome fragments. Third, changes in the banding pattern can be caused by recombination between segments of the chromosome. Generally, this would be homologous insertion sequences (IS) or possibly duplicated regions of the genome. A fourth possibility is through changes in methylation pattern of the DNA that would influence the ability of the restriction enzyme used in the assay to cleave the genome. This possibility can be negated by the choice of restriction enzymes that are not sensitive to DNA methylation. As indicated earlier, this technique is most useful when the amount of whole genome plasticity is high and large rearrangements in the chromosome occur frequently.

1.2. Restriction Fragment Length Polymorphism

The technique of restriction fragment length polymorphism (RFLP) is similar to PFGE in that it relies on restriction enzyme digestion of the whole genome. However, the chromosomal banding pattern is generated by hybridization of a labeled probe sequence with the digested and separated DNA fragments after they have been transferred to a membrane support *(19)*. Accordingly, this technique analyzes a relatively narrow region of the genome around the regions that are homologous with the probe used. Again, the choice of electrophoresis conditions for the separation of the DNA fragments and the choice of restriction enzyme used are critical to the resolving power of the technique and must be empirically determined. The choice of probe is also critical in that the number of copies of the gene that are present in the genome of the organism will influence the number of hybridizing fragments (bands) and, therefore, the amount of the genome that can be analyzed for diversity. A common and useful probe for this type of fingerprinting is derived from IS sequences. Polymorphisms in the RFLP fingerprint of an organism are generally caused by the same influences described for PFGE.

1.3. Amplified Fragment Length Polymorphism

The technique of amplified fragment length polymorphism (AFLP) combines features of RFLP with the sensitivity and precision of polymerase chain reaction (PCR)-based assays *(20)*. The use of two restriction enzymes greatly increases the potential number of polymorphisms that can be detected. Two rounds of PCR amplification and the use of fluorescent dye-labeled primers during the final round of amplification permits as little as 10 ng of DNA to be assayed. These dyes also permit the use of automated analyzers.

Analyses are performed by digesting total DNA with two restriction enzymes: one that is a frequent cutter and the other that is a rare cutter. Normally, *Eco*R1 and *Mse*1 are employed. However, for cases where these enzymes do not cut the bacterial DNA sufficiently, other pairs can be used. For example, *Hin*dIII and *Taq*I have been used with *Streptococcus pnuenoniae (21)*, *Hin*dII and *Hha*I, *Mse*1, or *Taq*I were used with *Campylobacter (22)*, and *Bgl*II and *Mfe*I were used with *Mycoplasma (23)*. An adapter consisting of a core sequence and a cohesive end for each of the two enzymes used is ligated to the DNA. Next, 20 rounds of PCR amplification are performed using primers complimentary to each adapter sequence but lacking a fluorescent dye. This initial set of fragments is too numerous for analysis so a second set of 30 rounds of PCR amplification is performed using the above primers with 0, 1, or 2 base extensions in various combinations. In all cases, the primer corresponding to the infrequent cutting restriction enzyme is labeled with the fluorescent dye. The goal is to use sets of primers that generate 30–50 bands in the 35- to 500-bp range. The fragments are separated using acrylamide gel or capillary electrophoresis on instruments equipped with fluorescent detectors. By combining the patterns from multiple primer pairs, it is frequently possible to observe strain variation even among highly monomorphic species and genera.

1.4. Variable Number Tandem Repeat Analysis

The technique of variable number tandem repeat analysis is relatively recent in the application to fingerprinting BW agents *(24)*. It is similar to microsatellite genotyping of humans *(25)* and relies on the same basic principle. Genomic DNA contains regions of tandem directly repeated sequences that can undergo deletions or insertions (indel) of any number of the repeat sequence units during DNA replication or possibly recombination. Le Feche et al. *(26)* recently published a database of these sequences for bacterial genomes. The technique is employed by generating PCR primers that flank the tandem repeated sequences. The locus of repeats is amplified and the size is determined by gel electrophoresis. If the repeat is chosen to be of sufficient size and the PCR product is in a size range that can easily resolve differences in the number of repeats, then polymorphisms can be detected between strains. If several tandem repeat loci are examined, then the technique is designated multilocus variable number of tandem repeats (VNTR) analysis (MLVA) and the differentiation power between strains is greatly enhanced. The more loci that are used for the analysis, the more specific the analysis will be. The number of loci used in the analysis is chosen to address the level of resolution needed from the genotyping information and must be determined empirically by examining strains of the organism in question.

1.5. Single Nucleotide Polymorphism

With the advent of high-throughput DNA sequencing augmented by robotics, it has become possible to determine the DNA sequences of large amounts of genomic material in a short period of time. The utility of sequencing variable regions of genes isolated from pathogens to determine the phylogenetic relationship between strains was recognized approx 10 yr ago *(27)*. Briefly, target gene sequences are amplified by PCR and sequenced using internal oligonucleotide primers. The targets for sequencing can be any genes, from 16S ribosomal RNA to housekeeping genes *(4,5,9,12)*. The amount of polymorphism observed in a gene sequence obviously depends on the selective pressure on that gene as well as other factors such as the number of generations of bacterial growth between the isolation of the strains. The method of detecting SNPs described earlier is slow because it depends on the PCR amplification of specific genes. A more useful approach has been made possible through the use of high-throughput whole genome shotgun sequencing where SNPs can be identified relatively quickly. Specific genes can then be targeted for SNP analysis to determine genetic diversity within the strains of the organism.

2. *B. ANTHRACIS*

The causative agent of anthrax has long been a part of the offensive BW programs of nations or groups formerly or currently engaged in developing such weapons and continues to pose a threat *(28,29)*. Several studies on molecular polymorphism of *B. anthracis* have shown relatively little differences at the molecular level *(13,30–32)*. Indeed, it is often not possible to distinguish *B. anthracis* from other *Bacillus* species with some techniques *(33,34)*. However, we hope to show you in the following sections that advances in genotyping technology may now show sufficient variation with some of these methods to permit the tracking of an individual strain used as a BW or BT agent back to its source.

2.1. *PFGE, rRNA Sequencing, and Ribotyping*

Only a limited analysis of *B. anthracis* and near neighbors has been performed with these techniques. Ribotyping was the least successful in demonstrating differences. Sequencing of the 16s rRNA genes of *B. anthracis* and *B. cereus* gave identical sequences *(33)*, whereas 23s rRNA gene sequencing showed a two-nucleotide difference between these species *(34)*. Sequencing of intergenic spacer regions (ISR) was a little better. The ISR between 16s rRNA and 23s rRNA was identical for two strains of *B. anthracis* and differed by only one base from the sequence of *B. cereus* and by 13 bases from *B. mycoides (13)*. Comparing the ISR between *gyrA* and *gyrB* showed only a single base difference when compared to *B. cereus* and *B. mycoides* although the region sequenced was larger than that for the rRNA genes. Using PFGE with three different enzymes, it was possible to distinguish *B. anthracis* from other *Bacillus* species, but this method could not distinguish among three strains of *B. anthracis*. Thus, it is apparent that these methods do not have sufficient sensitivity to be useful at the strain level but may be useful for initial classification of an unknown *Bacillus*.

2.2. *AFLP*

A more comprehensive analysis of *B. anthracis* strains has been performed using AFLP. A total of 79 isolates with a worldwide distribution were analyzed *(31)*. Roughly one-half of the isolates were from the United States or Canada, whereas the remainder ranged from Pakistan to Norway, Africa, and South America. Also included were six closely related *Bacillus* species. Analyses were performed using all 16 possible +1 combinations of the *Eco*R1/*Mse*1 primer pairs. When five of the 79 strains of *B. anthracis* were compared with the other six *Bacillus* species, a total of 357 polymorphic DNA fragments were generated among the 7 species and 12 species tested. AFLP could clearly differentiate among the various species within this set and produced two clusters within the set of five anthrax strains *(31)*. In contrast, when all 79 *B. anthracis* strains used in this study were analyzed by AFLP, a total of 1221 DNA fragments were produced of which 105 fragments were derived from the two plasmids, pXO1 and pXO2. The plasmid fragments were used to confirm the presence or absence of the two plasmids in the strains studied but not otherwise used to discriminate among the strains. Only 31 of the remaining 1106 chromosomal DNA fragments showed polymorphisms, demonstrating the highly monomorphic nature of *B. anthracis*. Despite the small percentage of polymorphic markers, specific clustering patterns emerged. Two major groupings were observed with the majority of the strains, 73 found in one and the remainder in the other. Overall, there were 33 distinct patterns observed *(31)*. Of particular interest was the observation that the majority of the North American isolates were very similar even when separated by distances of over 1000 km and times in excess of 20 yr, suggesting a single source for the ongoing epidemic in the United States and Canada.

These results indicate that AFLP can be used to differentiate among strains of *B. anthracis* as well as to distinguish it from near neighbors. AFLP takes less time and smaller amounts of DNA than other procedures and, therefore, may have a significant advantage for strain comparisons over other techniques. However, there does not appear to be a sufficient number of polymorphic DNA fragments to reliably use AFLP to track strain variation during the relatively short periods of an ongoing epidemic nor does it appear that new polymorphisms arise often enough to permit the positive identification of laboratory variants of the same strain.

2.3. VNTR

VNTR analysis may be the most sensitive method for differentiation among strains of *B. anthracis*. Using a variant of the method termed MLVA, Keim aet al. *(35)* analyzed 426 worldwide isolates. Their analysis used eight different variable repeat regions: six that were found on the bacterial chromosome, and one on each of the two plasmids. A total of 89 different genotypes were identified within the set of 426 strains analyzed *(35)*. These could be grouped into six major clusters that formed two distinct groups. The percent distribution of strains between the two major groups appeared to be about the same as was seen with AFLP *(31,35)*. In addition, the geographical origins associated with these two groups also reflect the distribution seen with AFLP. In both types of analyses, genotypes in the smaller of the two groups were found almost exclusively in South Africa, whereas the genotypes in the larger group had a worldwide distribution.

Looking at the subgroups in the larger group, other clustering patterns were seen. One subgroup, A1, was dominated by isolates from Western North America, whereas the largest subgroup, A3, had an even worldwide representation. The smallest, A2, contained just a single isolate from Pakistan. The final subgroup in this set, A4, was made up of strains similar to strain Vollum. Natural isolates were analyzed from the United States, Europe, Norway, and Asia, but not Africa. One strain in this group differed from the other Vollum strains by a single repeat at one locus and may represent a variation acquired during passage in the laboratory *(35)*. Using this technique, 98 isolates from the Kruger National Park, South Africa were analyzed *(36)*. This is an area known for periodic anthrax outbreaks with two foci of origin. Four genotypes were identified, but the vast majority were either of two genotypes. Combined, these two genotypes totaled 95 of the 98 isolates studied. The dominant genotype contained 74 isolates and was from group A. There were two other group A genotypes represented by three isolates. The remaining 21 isolates were a single genotype from group B. Although group A and group B genotypes were found throughout the park, group A clustered in the central region of the park and group B was in the northern region.

2.4. B. anthracis *Summary*

From the results described here, it is clear that techniques such as PFGE and ribotyping are of limited utility for forensic genotyping of *B. anthracis*. In contrast, AFLP and MLVA can be very useful for tracking an epidemic and determining if more than one strain is involved. However, MLVA may still not be sensitive enough to track strains back to the origin in a BW or BT incident. An analysis of the strain used in the anthrax attacks of September and October 2001 clearly showed it was an Ames strain using the eight loci of the above studies (Subheading 2.3.) but was unable to pinpoint which of the labs known to be studying the Ames strain might have been the source because they were all identical at these eight loci. Thus, MLVA was able to distinguish this isolate to the strain level (*see* Fig. 1). A recently completed comparison of the complete DNA sequence of the attack strain with reference strain sequences has revealed additional regions for comparison *(37)*. The draft genome sequence of the *B. anthracis* Florida strain could not differentiate it from two other laboratory isolates of the Ames strain but easily differentiated the Florida isolate from three diverse Ames-like natural isolates. Thus, random genome sequencing for forensic investigation did not specifically type the Florida strain relative to other Ames strains but did at least suggest that the bioterrorist strain was probably not a natural isolate and likely originated more recently from a laboratory stock of the organism. Future genomic sequencing of diverse *B. anthracis* strains will likely improve our understanding of the genetic diversity of this homogeneous organism and may lead to methods that are specifically targeted to polymorphic sites.

3. *Y. PESTIS*

Y. pestis is the causative agent of bubonic and pneumonic plague. Classically, the organism has been divided into three biovars, Antiqua, Medievalis, and Orientalis, based on biochemical reactions *(38)*. The organism is also a good example of a BW agent that is very monomorphic at the nucleotide sequence level but polymorphic at lower levels of genomic resolution *(15,39–41)*. We will discuss these differences and their utility for genotyping the organism in the next subheadings. Although in many cases, the same strains have not been analyzed by two or more of these techniques, some general conclusions can be drawn from the analysis of the genome by these various techniques.

3.1. SNP

Until recently, *Y. pestis* was thought to be highly monomorphic at the gene sequence level. In 1999, Achtman et al. *(15)* reported that they found no SNPs after partial sequencing of six genes from a diverse group of 36 strains of *Y. pestis* that had been isolated from four continents during a 56 yr timeframe. The total number of nucleotides sequenced in this study was more than 90 kb. We conducted a similar study using a different set of diverse strains and different cellular genes but also did not find any SNPs. Our study included the sequence of approx 65 kb of housekeeping genes from 11 strains isolated from four continents spanning 100 yr in time. These sequences have been deposited in GenBank under accession numbers AF282219, AF282309, AF282311, AF282314, and AF282318. We and others *(15)* have identified SNPs that occur within these genes when *Yersinia pseudotuberculosis* and *Y. pestis* are compared. Accordingly, specific housekeeping gene sequences can differentiate *Yersinia* isolates down to the species level (*see* Fig. 1). Recently, we have found SNPs within the species *Y. pestis* (L. Lindler, Y. Liu, P. Worsham, unpublished). However, these changes are not useful for general typing of *Y. pestis* strains because they occur in a very atypical group of plague isolates referred to as "Pestoides" strains *(42,43)*.

3.2. RFLP

One of the most widely accepted and utilized RFLP methods for *Y. pestis* genotyping is ribotyping *(40,41)*. Both 16S rDNA and 23S rDNA amplified from the *Escherichia coli* or the *Y. pestis* KIM5 chromosome have been used as probes *(39,40)*. The mixture of the two probes is labeled and hybridized with *Eco*RI or *Eco*RV-digested *Y. pestis* chromosomal DNAs. The *Eco*RI and *Eco*RV hybridization patterns are combined for grouping into different types (ribotypes) of *Y. pestis*. Twenty ribotypes designated type A to T have been identified from examination of *Y. pestis* strains isolated on four continents including North America, South America, Africa, and Asia *(40,41,44)*. However, ribotyping showed much less variability when used to analyze isolates obtained from specific local regions. For instance, all 37 strains and isolates of *Y. pestis* from the western United States revealed an identical ribotype pattern, ribotype B *(39)*. This result suggests that ribotyping may be useful for global investigation of *Y. pestis* divergence but is less applicable for epidemiological studies investigating an outbreak in a specific local region. Although a direct comparison of the ability of ribotyping to distinguish *Yersinia* isolates to the species level has not been preformed, this technique is unable to distinguish many individual strains and thus is of limited utility for forensic investigation of an outbreak.

IS elements have been loosely defined as small (<2.5 kb), phenotypically cryptic segments of DNA with a simple genetic organization and capable of inserting at multiple sites in a target molecule *(45)*. Some specific IS elements at defined places in the chromosome are sufficiently stable to allow them to be used as markers in RFLP for species or subspecies identification. Alternatively, unstable IS elements may be useful for epidemiological studies. At least four different IS elements have been found in the chromosome of *Y. pestis (46–51)*. There are 66 complete or partial copies of IS*1541*, 44 of IS*100*, 21 of IS*285*, and 9 of IS*1661*on the chromosome of *Y. pestis* CO92 *(47)*. Thus, some of these IS elements can be used as genetic markers for RFLP typing of *Y. pestis (15,43,46,49)*.

We have used IS*100* as a probe to hybridize with *Hind*III digested *Y. pestis* DNA. Twenty-five *Y. pestis* strains from New Mexico were tested. About 20 distinguishable DNA fragments were found that hybridized with the probe and allowed us to divide the 25 strains into 12 types if a single band change was considered to be a unique type *(52)*. Fourteen of the 25 strains (56%) belonged to type 1, as indicated following analysis with the Bionumeric software package (*see* Fig. 2). The 11 remaining strains had unique

Percent Similarity   **ID Number**   **Strain Origin**

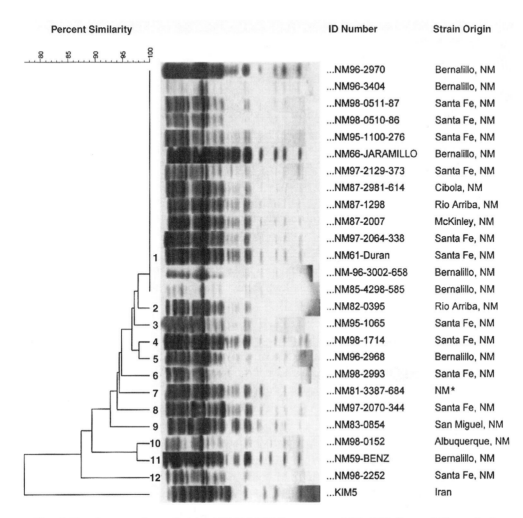

	ID Number	Strain Origin
	...NM96-2970	Bernalillo, NM
	...NM96-3404	Bernalillo, NM
	...NM98-0511-87	Santa Fe, NM
	...NM98-0510-86	Santa Fe, NM
	...NM95-1100-276	Santa Fe, NM
	...NM66-JARAMILLO	Bernalillo, NM
	...NM97-2129-373	Santa Fe, NM
	...NM87-2981-614	Cibola, NM
	...NM87-1298	Rio Arriba, NM
	...NM87-2007	McKinley, NM
	...NM97-2064-338	Santa Fe, NM
1	...NM61-Duran	Santa Fe, NM
	...NM-96-3002-658	Bernalillo, NM
	...NM85-4298-585	Bernalillo, NM
2	...NM82-0395	Rio Arriba, NM
3	...NM95-1065	Santa Fe, NM
4	...NM98-1714	Santa Fe, NM
5	...NM96-2968	Bernalillo, NM
6	...NM98-2993	Santa Fe, NM
7	...NM81-3387-684	NM*
8	...NM97-2070-344	Santa Fe, NM
9	...NM83-0854	San Miguel, NM
10	...NM98-0152	Albuquerque, NM
11	...NM59-BENZ	Bernalillo, NM
12	...NM98-2252	Santa Fe, NM
	...KIM5	Iran

Fig. 2. Dendrogram from digitized IS*100* RFLP patterns of *Hin*dIII-digested *Y. pestis* chromosomal DNA of 25 New Mexico strains hybridized with alkaline phosphatase labeled IS*100* probe. Percentage of similarity is shown above the dendrogram. The Dice coefficient was used for calculating similarities and unweighted pair group method (UPGMA) with average linkages was used for clustering analysis with the BioNumerics software package (Applied Maths, Kortrjk, Belgium). In general, bands were automatically assigned by the computer and corrected manually after checking the original images by eye. Only clearly resolved bands were counted. The IS*100* RFLP types are labeled with numbers. The position tolerance was 1.8%. The ID numbers of the isolates are as listed at the right. The external standard listed was *Y. pestis* KIM5 and was used as an outgroup. Strain KIM5 was also used as the global standard to allow normalization of different gels before analysis. The designation of NM represents state of New Mexico. The number following that represents the year the organism was isolated. The number after the first dash represents the ID number of the patient or animal. A second dash indicates that the isolate was from a flea with the number after the second dash indicating the flea ID number. The locations of strains isolated are labeled on the left of the figure. An asterisk indicates that the strain was isolated from New Mexico but no information for specific location was available.

IS*100* RFLP types but shared more than 87% similarity using dice coefficient analysis. Only one strain, *Y. pestis* KIM5, was significantly different from this group of US isolates. The KIM5 external standard strain had its own IS*100* RFLP pattern and shared much less similarity (77%) with the New Mexico isolates. This result indicates that the genetic variability of *Y. pestis* IS*100* RFLP pattern is greater than that seen with rRNA-based RFLP because all of the strains shown in Fig. 2 belong to a single ribotype. Interestingly, these results also demonstrate that the genome of *Y. pestis* is polymorphic near the sites of IS*100* integration in keeping with the recently reported results of Motin et al. *(43)*. The genome sequence of two different strains of *Y. pestis* has revealed that recombination between repeated IS elements in the genome is very common and is responsible for a large number of inversions and rearrangements *(47,53)*. These facts should be viewed in the light of our results. We have found strains isolated from the same general geographic region and time can have different IS*100* RFLP patterns (Fig. 2 strains isolated from Santa Fe). Taken together, these results suggest that the genomic plasticity seen through recombination between IS elements is most likely independent within a population of endemic *Y. pestis* foci. Furthermore, our results *(39)* as well as others *(43,49)* indicate that IS*100* RFLP analysis can differentiate *Yersinia* isolates at least to the species level and possibly to the strain (*see* Fig. 1).

3.3. PFGE

PFGE, which separates DNA fragments upon digestion of the chromosome with restriction endonucleases that cleave infrequently *(54)*, can facilitate a broad look at the whole genome of the organism. Although the method has been used to estimate the genome size and for detection of the gross chromosome restriction pattern for a limited number of strains *(55)*, it has not previously been used to systematically determine genetic relatedness between *Y. pestis* strains. To investigate the ability of PFGE to discriminate between the origins of *Y. pestis* isolates, a homogeneous group of *Y. pestis* from New Mexico and a heterogeneous group of *Y. pestis* strains from 10 different countries distributed on four continents were analyzed by PFGE. Because *Spe*I can produce a relatively wide range of *Y. pestis* DNA fragments that could easily be resolved using PFGE (*see* Fig. 3), this restriction enzyme was chosen for digestion of the genomic DNA. Figure 3 shows an example of PFGE pattern from a wide range of *Y. pestis* strains. Each international strain had a unique PFGE pattern, whereas the US strains we examined shared a similar major pattern. We could identify minor unique differences among the New Mexico strains we examined if they were obtained from different parents (*see* Fig. 4).

Figure 4 shows the PFGE dendrogram of a homogeneous group of *Y. pestis* strains isolated from seven local areas of New Mexico. Most New Mexico strains shared more than 80% similarity. However, the external standard strain KIM5 (isolated from Iran) shared only 66% similarity with the US strains (*see* Fig. 4). Although there is a high degree of similarity among all US isolates, most PFGE patterns revealed at least one band difference if they were from different parent strains (*see* Fig. 4). We observed 20 pulsotypes if only identical patterns were considered as one type *(56)*. However, four groups of independent isolates were found to be identical. The first group, NM96-2970 with NM96-3002-658, and NM96-3404 revealed identical PFGE patterns. The second group was NM98-1714 and NM61-Duran. The third group was NM66-Jaramillo and NM85-4298-585, and the last group was NM98-0510-86 and NM98-0511-87 (*see* Fig. 4). These independent but identical strains were all obtained from the same local area

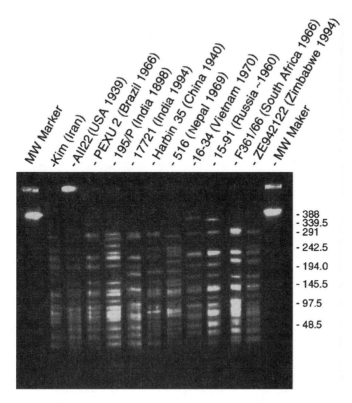

Fig. 3. *Spe*I restriction profiles found in all of our international *Y. pestis* strain collection *(55)*. The left lane is the standard MW marker and the sizes (in kb) are indicated on the left side of the gel. The content of each lane is indicated at the top of the figure. The country of origin is also indicated on the top of the gel. Pulse times were ramped from 10 to 30 s over 24 h at 200 V in 1% agarose.

and the first and the fourth groups of strains were isolated in the same year. Interestingly, the first group of strains shared the exact same PFGE and RFLP patterns and was isolated in the same year and same local area, Bernalillo, NM. These isolates were obtained from a flea pool, rodent and human sources, respectively. Thus, this group may represent a cycle of a plague in an endemic area. Accordingly, it is likely that these three strains were epidemiologically related. In selected studies, isolates recovered from plague patients produced identical patterns with isolates recovered subsequently from related case investigations, thus lending more support for epidemiological understanding of the microevolutionary changes in localized foci. These PFGE data strongly support the concept introduced in Subheading 3.2. that the genomic restriction profile of *Y. pestis* may develop independently within a plague endemic area. These data also indicate that PFGE can generally differentiate *Y. pestis* to the strain level of specificity (*see* Fig. 1) and typically to the level of the individual isolate.

3.4. VNTR

VNTR analysis shows great promise for being able to rapidly and accurately genotype *Y. pestis* isolates. Adair et al. *(42)* first described a CAAA repeat that encoded 9 different alleles in 35 strains of *Y. pestis*. Variability of this single locus was able to

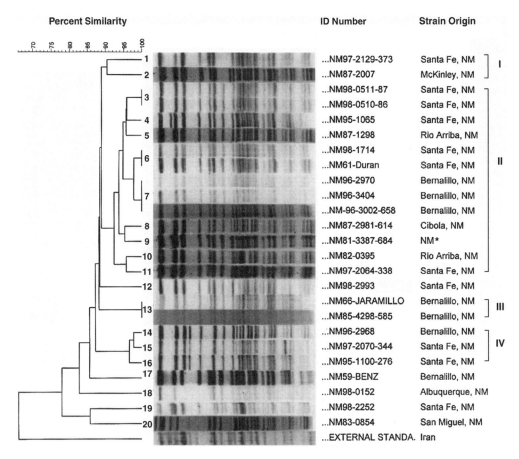

Fig. 4. Dendrogram from digitized PFGE patterns for the 25 New Mexico *Y. pestis* strains and isolates digested with *Spe*I was constructed by similarity and clustering analysis using BioNumerics software as described in the legend of Fig. 2. Percentage of similarity is shown above the dendrogram. The PFGE types are marked with numbers and the clusters with similarity values above 90% are marked with roman numerals. The position tolerance was 1.1%. The ID numbers of the US isolates are as listed on the right side. The strains designation is as in the Fig. 2 legend. The external standard listed was *Y. pestis* KIM5 and was included as an outgroup. An asterisk indicates that a strain was isolated from New Mexico but no information for specific location was available.

differentiate most strains examined. However, alleles H and K were found in eight and six different strains, respectively. The stability of this VNTR locus was found to be highly stable in several different strains representing two different biovars of the organism. Later, this same group performed MLVA on *Y. pestis (57)*. DNA sequence analysis allowed these researchers to identify 77 different possible loci with repeat units (*see* Subheading 1.4.) ranging from 1 to 145 bp in length that might be useful for MLVA. Of these loci, 42 were found to be polymorphic, with between 2 and 11 alleles within the group of 24 strains of *Y. pestis* examined. Analysis of the variability seen in these loci demonstrated that the highest diversity was seen in repeats that ranged from 6 to 9 bp in repeat unit length. Although exact isolate locations were not presented, analysis of the 42 variable loci grouped all of the biovar Orientalis strains together. Most of these strains were from North and South America with the single exception of a strain from Indonesia. The second general group of strains was more diverse, representing both the Medievalis and Antiqua biovars from China, India, Kurdistan, the former Soviet Union, and two countries on the African continent. As expected, a phylogenetic tree prepared using all 42 VNTR loci revealed the largest amount of genetic diversity among this second group of strains. In general, the biovars grouped together in this second clade of strains with the exception of a strain designated Pestoides F, an atypical strain from the former Soviet Union *(58,59)*. Although this strain is of biovar Antiqua, it grouped within other strains of biovar Medievalis. Generally, MLVA was able to differentiate each strain of *Y. pestis* as unique, with the notable exception of strains that would be expected to be genetically similar. Specifically, eight strains isolated in California were homogeneous at the 42 VNTR loci. Taken together *(42,57)*, VNTR has been shown to be able to genotype *Yersinia* to the species level (*see* Fig. 1) and generally to the strain level unless the isolates were related geographically.

3.5. AFLP

We have just begun to analyze *Y. pestis* using AFLP and the preliminary results are promising. We have looked at 10 strains covering all three biovars consisting of seven from Orientalis, three from Medievalis, and one from Antiqua. Eight primer pairs have been identified that show promise for differentiating among these three biovars. In addition, as shown in Fig. 5, variation can be seen within both Orientalis and Medievalis. Using the primer set *Eco*RI-A/*Mse*I-CC, it can be seen that the three Orientalis strains 195/P, PEXU 2, and 15-91 all have a doublet at about 150 bp whereas only a single band is found in the other four Orientalis strains as well as the Medievalis and Antiqua strains. Another interesting feature of the banding pattern with this primer set is the band at 250 bp found only in the two Medievalis strains as well as the doublet at 45 bp shared by the Medievalis strain Harbin from China and the Antiqua strain 516 from Nepal.

Although the sample set is quite small, especially for Medievalis and Antiqua, these preliminary results indicate that AFLP can discriminate between biovars. Initial results do not show clustering by geographic region of origin but only a single primer pair has been evaluated. There is some indication of variation within a biovar and the use of additional primer pairs may show additional variation that may lead to discrimination down to the level of geographic regions or strains.

3.6. Y. pestis *Summary*

Y. pestis is a good example of an organism whose monomorphic nature depends on the technique used to examine the genetic material (*see* Fig. 1). At the gene level, SNPs are of little utility to differentiate the organism even to the resolution of a particular strain. Typing by IS*100* RFLP can distinguish some strains of the organism, but whole genome fingerprinting with PFGE provides a much greater level of resolution most likely caused by chromosomal rearrangements at sites of IS elements. Although PFGE is an older technique that is more labor intensive requiring larger amounts of DNA, it is the only technique to date that has been shown to be useful for epidemiological studies and that can differentiate geographically closely related isolates. An even greater de-

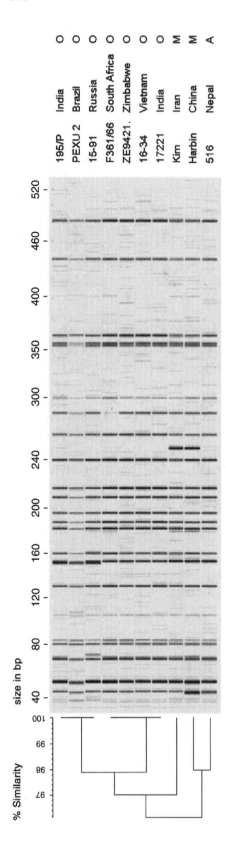

Fig. 5. AFLP dendrogram of *Y. pestis* strains. Binary bandmatching was performed by the Dice coefficient and UPGMA using GelCompar II v 2.5 software (Applied Maths). Percent similarity is an indication of the number of bands in common. The strain designation, isolation location and biovar, respectively, are given to the right of the figure.

gree of specificity may be obtained through a combination of the whole genome approach (PFGE) and microtechniques such as AFLP or MLVA.

4. *B. melitensis*

Brucellosis is a zoonotic disease of domestic and wild animals contracted by humans through ingestion of contaminated food, contact with infected animals. or inhalation of aerosols. Classically, six members of the genus *Brucella* have been recognized: *B. melitensis, B. abortus, B. suis, B. canis, B. ovis,* and *B. neotomae (60)*. However, DNA hybridization studies have shown a high degree of homology among these species *(61)* and led to the conclusion that *Brucella* is a monospecific genus with *B. melitensis* as the only member *(62)*. The previous species are now considered heterotrophs of *B. melitensis* but the original names can be used for nontaxonomic purposes. Here, we will refer to the members in the nontaxonomic form. Recently additional, distinct members of this group have been recovered from marine mammals and have been shown to consist of multiple subtypes *(63,64)*. The name *Brucella maris* has been proposed for this group of organisms *(65)*, but based on polymorphism at the omp2 locus and host specificity, two new species names, *B. pinnipediae* and *B. cetaceae* have also been proposed for the marine *Brucella (64)*. Despite the genetic homogeneity, as will be seen here, various of fingerprinting methods can provide discrimination to the strain level *(see* Fig. 1).

4.1. PFGE

Initial studies using PFGE demonstrated that it was capable of differentiation between subspecies of *B. melitensis* and in some cases could distinguish among biovars of the same subspecies *(16)*. A comprehensive study on *B. abortus* strains isolated from cattle, bison, and elk showed they could clearly be distinguished from the vaccine strains RB51 and strain 19 and the wildtype strain 2308, as well as genetically modified strain 19. Additionally, three distinct but closely related patterns were observed among the eight *B. abortus* biovars *(66,67)*. A similar study was performed with isolates from marine mammals *(67)*. As in the previous study, the *Brucella* formed clear groups by subspecies; however, the marine isolates did not all group together. Those from dolphins were found within a cluster containing *B. canis* and *B. suis,* whereas those from seals and porpoises clustered with *B. ovis (68)*.

4.2. AFLP

Analysis by AFLP produced results similar to PFGE but with greater discrimination among the biotypes of a subspecies. Using 11 primer pairs, we were able to clearly distinguish each biotype strain from the other biotypes within a subspecies. We could also easily distinguish the *B. abortus* vaccine strains from other *B. abortus* strains. Figure 6 shows a binary bandmatching dendrogram for the various *Brucella* type strains including one member of the marine *Brucella* group. Each subspecies forms its own cluster within the overall pattern. Two superclusters were seen, one containing *B. abortus* and *B. melitensis* and the other containing the remaining *Brucella* subspecies. Although unique clusters are seen for each of the species within the genus *Brucella*, the degree of similarity is such that they are all subspecies of a single genomic species according to the criteria proposed by Savelkoul et al. *(69)*.

% Similarity

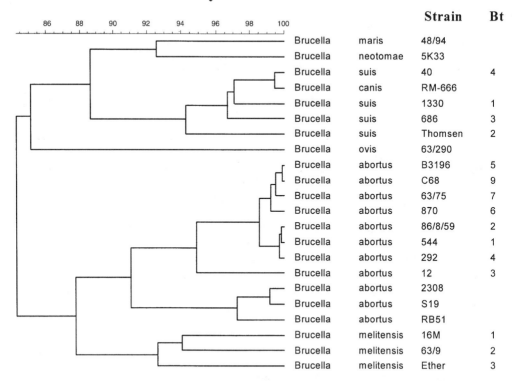

Fig. 6. Composite AFLP dendrogram of *Brucella* type strains. The results from 11 primer pairs were combined for binary bandmatching analysis. The tree was constructed by calculating the Dice coefficient and UPGMA. Percent similarity is an indication of the number of bands in common. The organism that gave rise to each AFLP patterns is labeled to the right of the figure. Bt, biotype.

We have also begun analyzing a large number of strains from each subspecies. In a collection of more than 100 strains of *B. melitensis* from the United States and Mexico, three pattern types were seen. Greater than 80% of these strains had AFLP patterns that were identical or very similar to the pattern of *B. melitensis* 16M (biotype 1). The least common pattern, seen in just two strains, was that for *B. melitensis* Ether (biotype 3). In contrast, all 36 strains from Egypt that were analyzed exhibited patterns most closely resembling those of *B. melitensis* Ether (M. Dobson and T. Hadfield, unpublished). One can speculate that the two patients from the United States with AFLP fingerprints resembling biotype 3 became infected while traveling in or near Egypt. The remainder of the isolates resembled the pattern for *B. melitensis* 63/9 (biotype 2) suggesting the possibility that two genotypes are present in United States and Mexican isolates. In addition, some of the isolates displayed fingerprints that were slightly different from the three type strains that defined each genotype.

Although less extensive analysis has been done to date, results with *B. abortus* and *B. suis* also indicate more than one genotype is present within the United States. Results with the marine *Brucella* support the observation seen with PFGE that those isolated from dolphins form a separate cluster. However, a greater degree of variation was seen within the other isolates tested compared to the results with PFGE (M. Dobson and T. Hadfield, unpublished). In addition, cluster analysis of the AFLP data grouped the marine *Brucella* closer to *B. melitensis* and *neotomae* than to the *B. suis/canis* group seen by PFGE.

4.3. RFLP, IS, and Ribotyping

RFLP, IS, and ribotyping fingerprinting have also been used for genotyping *Brucella,* although primarily for comparison of the marine isolates with the six species. Sequencing of the 16s rRNA gene showed the marine isolates were identical to five of the six *Brucella* species (*B. ovis* differs by a single base) *(70).* However, analysis using the insertion sequence IS*711* showed them to be quite distinct from the biovars of the six species. All of the marine isolates had many more copies of IS*711* than did the other strains except for *B. ovis*. In addition, the IS patterns of the marine isolates could be grouped by host species.

RFLP analysis of the *omp2* locus of *Brucella* also showed that the strains isolated from marine mammals formed a unique group of organisms. A specific marker in the *omp2b* gene was found in all marine isolates but was not found in any isolates from terrestrial animals *(64).* In addition, they formed two distinct groups. Isolates from dolphins, porpoises, and a minke whale had two copies of *omp2b* along with an *omp2a* gene, whereas those from otters or seals carried one *omp2a* and one *omp2b*. This latter pattern is similar to isolates from terrestrial animals with the single exception of one isolate from a seal. There is also one exception to the *omp2* pattern seen in terrestrial isolates, which is for *B. ovis*. This strain has two closely related copies of *omp2a* instead of one copy of *omp2a* and *omp2b* *(71).*

4.4. Brucella *Summary*

For members of the genus *Brucella*, ribotyping can be used to place an unknown isolate within the genus but cannot discriminate among the species. PFGE, RFLP, and IS analysis can discriminate down to the level of subspecies and even biotype, but are complex, time-consuming methods. Furthermore, these methods probably do not provide discrimination between strains (*see* Fig. 1). AFLP can distinguish between biovars within a subspecies and at least in some cases can differentiate between strains within a biovar. Given the results described above, however, even AFLP may not be useful for distinguishing strains within *Brucella* spp. Accordingly, to date no technique has been shown to be able to specifically differentiate between isolates. Further advances will be made possible once the complete genomes of *B. melitensis, B. suis* and *B. abortus* have been completed.

5. F. *tularensis*

Recently, there have been changes in the classification of this genus. The current classification is divided into the species *F. tularensis* and *F. philomirangia* that are both pathogenic for humans to different degrees. The organisms in the genus share 99.2% or greater 16S rRNA sequence similarity. *F. tularensis* is further divided into the subspecies *F. tularensis,* subsp. *tularensis, holarctica* (formally *palaearctica*), *novicida,* and *mediasiatica (72–75).* The subspecies of *F. tularensis* are based on virulence in rabbits and on biochemical characteristics with subspecies *tularensis* being the most virulent. Classically, *Francisella* was divided into biotypes A and B based on the ability to ferment glycerol. *F. tularensis,* subsp. *holarctica* is the sole member of biotype B. Differences in virulence characterize the species: *F. tularensis,* subsp. *tularensis* type A is the most virulent of all the subspecies, with a LD_{50} of 10 cells or fewer for laboratory mice and rabbits, although *F. tularensis,* subsp. *mediaasiatica* and *F. tularensis,* subsp. *novicida,* share the same 16S rRNA signature nucleotide sequence and biochemical properties of type A, they are considered, along with *F. philomiragia,* to be of low virulence. Type B organisms *(F. tularensis,* subsp. *holarctica)* are of intermediate virulence, with LD_{50} of 1000 cells or fewer for laboratory animals *(12).*

Several laboratories have been interested in developing robust methods for typing of *F. tularensis,* particularly in the differentiation of the more virulent subspecies *tularensis* from the other subspecies, and to develop DNA-based subspecies markers. Some advances have been made in the last few years, but the final analysis of the appropriate typing methods will be greatly assisted by the completion of the genomic sequencing of the prototypic type A strain Schu4 *(76,77)* (http://artedi.ebc.uu.se/Projects/Francisella/) and comparison with the prototypic type B, live vaccine strain (E. Garcia, Lawrence Livermore National Laboratory, CA). The genotypic markers generally agree with the phenotypic traits of these agents and those of type B are easily separated from the rest of the subspecies. With some of the genotyping methods, subspecies *tularensis* and subspecies *novicida* are not easily distinguished. Additionally, each isolate of subspecies *novicida* appears to be different genotypically as is *F. philomiragia.* Only limited analysis of subspecies *mediaasiatica* has been carried out; therefore, information pertaining to how this subspecies can be genetically separated remains to be determined.

5.1. SNP

The first SNP reported within the genus *Francisella* was at position 1153 (*E. coli* numbering) of the 16S rRNA *(78).* This study found that an adenosine residue at that position was specific for classic biotype B strains, whereas biotype A strains encoded a guanosine in this position. Later, this same group identified other SNPs within the 16S rRNA following examination of a larger and more diverse group of *Francisella* strains *(12).* The majority of the 26 nucleotide changes were located in two clusters between basepairs 375–526 and basepairs 26–215 (*E. coli* numbering). Although this study did not report the 16S rRNA sequences of the strains according to the current subspecies classification, their results generally support the breakdown on *F. tularensis* into subspecies. Furthermore, the sequences of *F. tularensis,* subsp. *novicida* strains are very closely related to *F. tularensis,* subsp. *tularensis* sequences and cannot be reliably differentiated with SNPs within the 16S rRNA gene region.

We have examined a group of 25 *Francisella* isolates for SNPs in housekeeping genes to determine if the heterogeneity seen in 16S rRNA extends to other loci. The result of our galactose epimerase (*galE*) sequencing is shown in Fig. 7. Although we did not generally categorize these strains into subspecies, the sequences clustered according to the classic definition of the biotypes. All biotype A sequences were identical and all biotype B sequences were identical but formed two distinct clusters. The *F. tularensis galE* sequence is 1020 bp in length and includes five nucleotide differences. All of the differences between the two biotypes occurred in the same positions. Only

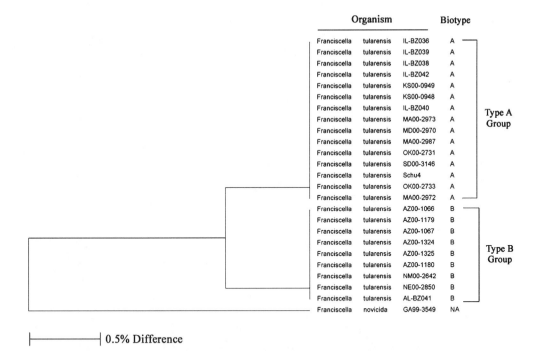

Fig. 7. Phylogenetic tree of *Franciscella* strains based on their *galE* sequence. The gene plus flanking DNA was amplified by PCR and sequenced using oligonucleotide primers based on the *F. tularensis* subspecies *tularensis* Schu4 sequence obtained from the genome sequencing project website http://artedi.ebc.uu.se/Projects/Francisella/blast/. The sequences were assembled and edited using Seqman (Lasergene, Madison, Wisconsin). The sequences were trimmed to include only the GalE coding region before alignment. The predicted protein product from the Schu4 sequence was 63% identical with *Bacillus subtilis* GalE (NP_391765) over the entire length of the protein. The sequences were aligned and the phylogenetic tree prepared using the Bionumerics software package (Applied Maths). The sequences were aligned using the default sequence comparison settings which were pairwise alignment and UPGMA clustering. These sequences along with *asd* and *mdh* have been deposited in GenBank and given accession numbers AF513250 through AF513321. NA, not applicable.

one *F. tularensis,* subsp. *novicida* strain (GA99-3549) was examined, and its sequence differed significantly from either the biotype A or B sequences. The *F. tularensis,* subsp. *novicida* strain *galE* sequence encoded 19 SNPs of which 14 were specific to this subspecies. The GA99-3549 sequence was identical to the classic biotype B sequence in the five SNP positions that were common between biotype A and biotype B (i.e., this *F. tularensis.* subsp. *novicida* sequence was most similar to the biotype B sequence). The results obtained by sequencing of the aspartate semialdehyde dehydrogenase (*asd*) and malate dehydrogenase (*mdh*) genes were similar to those shown in Fig. 7 (data not shown). Taken together, the results of SNP studies clearly suggest that this technique is useful for the characterization of *Francisella* isolates to the subspecies level (e.g., can differentiate *F. tularensis,* subsp. *holartica* and *novicida* from the other subspecies of *F. tularensis*).

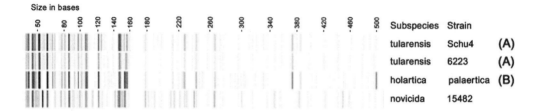

Fig. 8. AFLP pattern using primers EcoR1-T/Mse1-T for three *F. tularensis* subspecies. The subspecies and strain that gave rise to these patterns is indicated on the right portion of the figure. The biotype of the strain is indicated in parenthesis.

5.2. AFLP

AFLP analyses of *Francisella* have just begun. Preliminary studies on strains from three of the subspecies groups (*tularensis, holartica,* and *novicida*) are promising. We have identified eight *Eco*R1/*Mse*1 primer pair combinations that give usable fingerprint patterns. Even with a limited number of strains analyzed to date, some distinct patterns are emerging. The classical biotype A and biotype B strains are readily distinguished from each other. Figure 8 shows the AFLP pattern using *Eco*R1-T/*Mse*1-T primers for two biotype A strains and one biotype B strain. The pattern for the *novicida* subspecies clearly differs from the other strains. Although the patterns for the *tularensis* and *holartica* subspecies are similar, they can be distinguished from each other. Of particular interest is the ability to discriminate between the avirulent strain 6223 and the virulent Schu4 strain within the *tularensis* subspecies group.

Figure 9 presents a composite dendrogram produced from the AFLP banding patterns using four primer pairs. With the exception of the avirulent strain 6223, all the biotype A strains cluster apart from the biotype B strains. Within the biotype B cluster three distinct subclusters are seen that reflect the geographic region that the strains were isolated from. All of the strains isolated in the United States are found in cluster B1. Cluster B2 contains isolates from central or eastern Europe, whereas cluster B3 contains isolates from the southwest of Europe. Of particular interest is the observation that the *F. tularensis,* subsp. *tularensis* and *holartica* have about 90% of their bands in common compared to 73% for subspecies *novicida*. This degree of difference may be justification for promoting the *novicida* subspecies back to species level in the *Francisella* taxonomy. The unique species *F. philomiragia* has less than 25% of its bands in common with *F. tularensis*. These results indicate that AFLP provides solid discrimination at the subspecies level and can be used to distinguish strains originating in one geographic region from those originating in another region (*see* Fig. 1).

5.3. RFLP

The genome sequencing of Schu4 has shown that there are at least four IS-like elements with differences in copy number and molecular characteristics when compared to limited sequences of other *F. tularensis* strains. These IS-like elements are being examined for their utility as tools to discriminate *F. tularensis* strains as molecular typing tools. A 864-bp sequence has been identified as an IS element and has been designated IS*Ftu1 (45)*. We examined a panel of 65 *Francislla* spp. DNAs using this

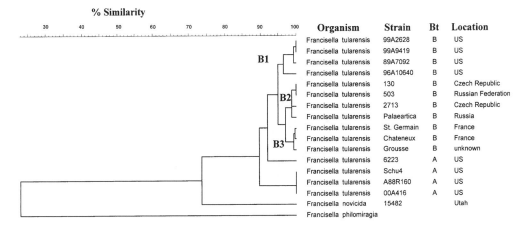

Fig. 9. Composite AFLP dendrogram for *Francisella sp.* This is a binary comparison of bands from four primer pairs. Comparison was by Dice coefficient and UPGMA using GelCompar II software (Applied Maths). Bt, biotype; location, area isolated. Percent similarity is an indication of how many bands were in common.

ISFtu1 probe sequence (Zhou and Chu, unpublished data). This panel of strains specifically focused on North American isolates of type A, type B, and *F. tularensis,* subsp. *novicida* along with *F. philomiragia* and European strains for comparison. *Bgl*II-digested genomic DNAs were hybridized with a ISFtu1 495-bp probe that was internal to the IS element. Clustered patterns of type A strains were noted (*see* Fig. 10, panel A) specifically those of the eastern part of the United States vs those of the western part of the country. Type A strains carry 12–17 copies, whereas type B isolates have 26–30 copies. Each of the *F. tularensis,* subsp. *novicida* were different (*see* Fig. 10, panel B) in profile, whereas only 2 of 15 *F. philomiragia* were blot-positive with 1 and 2 copies of ISFtu1 (*see* Fig. 10, panel B and data not shown). These results suggest that IS profiles are also useful to apply to genotyping of *F. tularensis* and may allow differentiation of the organism down to at least the subspecies level (*see* Fig. 1).

5.4. Francisella *Summary*

Although the available information pertaining to genotyping of *Francisella* isolates is limited, it appears that the genetic diversity of this organism may be higher than the other BW agents discussed earlier. Of course, this may be at least partially caused by nomenclature and taxonomic considerations. However, it is clear that SNP analysis can easily differentiated *F. tularensis,* subsp. *novicida* from any of the other subspecies of *Francisella* and that this technique can distinguish members of *F. tularensis,* subsp. *holartica* from other members of this group. Also, differences have been noted in RFLP patterns and MLVA (discussed in Chapter 24) that may be useful for characterizing isolates. Further development will be necessary to establish which method will be best suited for investigation of any future outbreaks or events.

6. SUMMARY

Genotyping methods are tools for classifying isolates to obtain additional insights into the epidemiology, geographic origin, phenotypic behavior, or any aspects that are

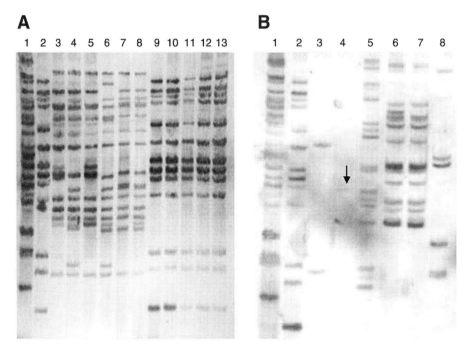

Fig. 10. IS*Ftu1* Southern Blot profiles using *Bgl*II-digested genomic DNA and 495-bp probe. **(A)** Lane 1, type B (LVS); lanes 9 and 13, type A (Schu4); lanes 2–8 type A, Western US (ND, NM, TX, WY, CO, UT, and AZ); lanes 9–12 type A, Eastern US (OH, KS, MO, and AR). **(B)** Lane 1, type B (LVS); lane 2, type A (Schu4); lanes 3 and 4, *F. philomiragia* ATCC 25015 (2 bands) and ATCC 25017 (single faint band, black arrow); lanes 5–8, *F. tularensis,* subsp. *novicida* isolates.

under study. Because the requirements for classifying agents differ and often change depending on study design or purpose, no one method is preferred over another, rather the study goals should dictate the genotyping method to be used. As indicated in Fig. 1, various typing methods can differentiate to various levels of specificity. For instance, if the purpose of the investigation is to study how individual genes are evolving within a genus or species, one would consider SNP analysis. In contrast, if one intends to study how strains evolve and change over time in an endemic area, isolates might be better grouped by IS-element probing that looks more at global, large DNA differences. The IS-based typing would then be extended further by performing MLVA or AFLP to examine the population dynamics within a single group. The diversity observed by a given method obviously depends on the organism under study. For example, the genome of *Y. pestis* encodes many copies of IS*100,* which makes this organism subject to typing using this sequence as a probe. However, the closely related species *Y. pseudotuberculosis* encodes few copies of IS*100,* which limits the utility of this probe in that species. Newer approaches should be examined and evaluated for their ability to discriminate to higher levels or resolution. Some of the methods that would likely be useful aside from genomic sequences *(37)* are mircoarray-based typing *(79),* adaptation of the PFGE approach, further analysis of VNTRs that permit targeted amplification of specific loci, and phenotypic expression patterns of particular strains. Approaches should be developed to produce rapid typing results directly from specimens to allow for shortened response time during an intentional release. The techniques and studies described earlier have already revealed genetic heterogeneity in organisms that were thought to be difficult to differentiate based on phenotypic properties, specifically *Francisella* and *Brucella*. These studies are also revealing new insights into what were once thought to be genetically monomorphic organisms such as *Y. pestis* and *B. anthracis.*

As many new approaches are adapted, the difficulty will be understanding the capability of each method and how that may be appropriately applied. All methods, no matter how appropriate, should be standardized so that results may be readily accessed and compared. To ensure standardization, there two critical needs that must be addressed: (a) develop a robust set of reference strains to which every new method is applied to determine applicability compared to previous methods and, (b) data can be shared on a common software platform so that the results may be compared. This is similar to the PulseNet program established by the CDC for monitoring emerging strains of enteric pathogens *(80,81)* and was recently proposed by Cummings and Relman after the initial publication of the draft *B. anthracis* Florida strain genome sequence *(82)*. As transferring of live cultures becomes more difficult, a set of "gold" reference standards using attenuated strains or purified DNA should be produced and distributed from a reference laboratory to be analyzed and incorporated into every method. Genotyping methods are in many cases complicated, laboratories should commit to keeping up their skills by developing and practicing field evaluation of the methods. For this to happen, agencies given the responsibility to be prepared and respond to biothreat events must pool their resources and ensure the reference program success. Establishment of a PulseNet-like laboratory network and database is a large undertaking, but with the ability to utilize the experience of an already in-place system, the learning curve should not be as long. The above described biothreat genome fingerprint database will link the results from many laboratories and permit ready analysis when reliable and rapid answers are needed during national emergencies.

ACKNOWLEDGMENTS

The authors wish to thank Sydney Lee for genetic analysis using the Bionumeric software package, Ying Liu for DNA sequencing, and Yan Zhou for developing the IS*Ftu1* typing system. Lee Collins is kindly thanked for artwork. All of the members of the Lindler, Chu, Dobson, and Hadfield laboratories are thanked for their diligent work. This work was supported by the US Army Medical Research and Materiel Command and the Centers for Disease Control and Prevention.

REFERENCES

1. Lebeda, F. J. (1997) Deterrence of biological and chemical warfare: a review of policy options. *Mil. Med.* **162,** 156–161.
2. Ransom, G. and Kaplan, B. (1998) USDA uses PulseNet for food safety [news]. *J. Am. Vet. Med. Assoc.* **213,** 1107.
3. Boyd, E. F., Nelson, K., Wang, F. S., Whittam, T. S., and Selander, R. K. (1994) Molecular genetic basis of allelic polymorphism in malate dehydrogenase (mdh) in natural populations of *Escherichia coli* and *Salmonella enterica. Proc. Natl. Acad. Sci. USA* **91,** 1280–1284.
4. Chun, J., Huq, A., and Colwell, R. R. (1999) Analysis of 16S-23S rRNA intergenic spacer regions of *Vibrio cholerae* and *Vibrio mimicus. Appl. Environ. Microbiol.* **65,** 2202–2208.

5. Byun, R., Elbourne, L. D., Lan, R., and Reeves, P. R. (1999) Evolutionary relationships of pathogenic clones of *Vibrio cholerae* by sequence analysis of four housekeeping genes. *Infect. Immun.* **67,** 1116–1124.

6. Garcia-Martinez, J., Martinez-Murcia, A., Anton, A. I., and Rodriguez-Valera, F. (1996) Comparison of the small 16S to 23S intergenic spacer region (ISR) of the rRNA operons of some *Escherichia coli* strains of the ECOR collection and *E. coli* K-12. *J. Bacteriol.* **178,** 6374–6377.

7. Groisillier, A. and Lonvaud-Funel, A. (1999) Comparison of partial malolactic enzyme gene sequences for phylogenetic analysis of some lactic acid bacteria species and relationships with the malic enzyme. *Int. J. Syst. Bacteriol.* **49(Pt 4),** 1417–1428.

8. Karaolis, D. K., Lan, R., and Reeves, P. R. (1995) The sixth and seventh cholera pandemics are due to independent clones separately derived from environmental, nontoxigenic, non-O1 *Vibrio cholerae. J. Bacteriol.* **177,** 3191–3198.

9. Perez Luz, S., Rodriguez-Valera, F., Lan, R., and Reeves, P. R. (1998) Variation of the ribosomal operon 16S-23S gene spacer region in representatives of *Salmonella enterica* subspecies. *J. Bacteriol.* **180,** 2144–2151.

10. Sproer, C., Mendrock, U., Swiderski, J., Lang, E., and Stackebrandt, E. (1999) The phylogenetic position of *Serratia, Buttiauxella* and some other genera of the family *Enterobacteriaceae. Int. J. Syst. Bacteriol.* **49(Pt 4),** 1433–1438.

11. Swaminathan, B. and Matar, G. M. (1993) Molecular typing methods: definition, applications and advantages, in *Diagnostic Molecular Microbiology.* (Persing, D. H., Smith, T. F., Tenover, F. C., et al., eds.), ASM, Washington, DC, pp. 26–50.

12. Forsman, M., Sandstrom, G., and Sjostedt, A. (1994) Analysis of 16S ribosomal DNA sequences of *Francisella* strains and utilization for determination of the phylogeny of the genus and for identification of strains by PCR. *Int. J. Syst. Bacteriol.* **44,** 38–46.

13. Harrell, L. J., Andersen, G. L., and Wilson, K. H. (1995) Genetic variability of *Bacillus anthracis* and related species. *J. Clin. Microbiol.* **33,** 1847–1850.

14. Jackson, P. J., Hill, K. K., Laker, M. T., Ticknor, L. O., and Keim, P. (1999) Genetic comparison of *Bacillus anthracis* and its close relatives using amplified fragment length polymorphism and polymerase chain reaction analysis. *J. Appl. Microbiol.* **87,** 263–269.

15. Achtman, M., Zurth, K., Morelli, G., Torrea, G., Guiyoule, A., and Carniel, E. (1999) *Yersinia pestis,* the cause of plague, is a recently emerged clone of *Yersinia pseudotuberculosis. Proc. Natl. Acad. Sci. USA* **96,** 14,043–14,048.

16. Allardet-Servent, A., Bourg, G., Ramuz, M., Pages, M., Bellis, M., and Roizes, G. (1988) DNA polymorphism in strains of the genus *Brucella. J. Bacteriol.* **170,** 4603–4607.

17. Schwartz, D. C. and Cantor, C. R. (1984) Separation of yeast chromosome-sized DNAs by pulsed field gradient gel electrophoresis. *Cell* **37,** 67–75.

18. Carle, G. F. and Olson, M. V. (1984) Separation of chromosomal DNA molecules from yeast by orthogonal-field- alternation gel electrophoresis. *Nucleic Acids Res.* **12,** 5647–5664.

19. Southern, E. M. (1974) Detection of specific sequences among DNA fragments separated by gel electrophoresis. *J. Mol. Biol.* **98,** 503–517.

20. Vos, P., Hogers, R., Bleeker, M., et al. (1995) AFLP: a new technique for DNA fingerprinting. *Nucleic Acids Res.* **23,** 4407–4414.

21. van Eldere, J., Janssen, P., Hoefnagels-Schuermans, A., van Lierde, S., and Peetermans, W. E. (1999) Amplified-fragment length polymorphism analysis versus macro-restriction fragment analysis for molecular typing of *Streptococcus pneumoniae* isolates. *J. Clin. Microbiol.* **37,** 2053–2057.

22. Duim, B., Wassenaar, T. M., Rigter, A., and Wagenaar, J. (1999) High-resolution genotyping of *Campylobacter* strains isolated from poultry and humans with amplified fragment length polymorphism fingerprinting. *Appl. Environ. Microbiol.* **65,** 2369–2375.

23. Kokotovic, B., Friis, N. F., Jensen, J. S., and Ahrens, P. (1999) Amplified-fragment length polymorphism fingerprinting of *Mycoplasma* species. *J. Clin. Microbiol.* **37,** 3300–3307.

24. Keim, P., Klevytska, A. M., Price, L. B., et al. (1999) Molecular diversity in *Bacillus anthracis*. *J. Appl. Microbiol.* **87,** 215–217.
25. Hubert, R., Weber, J. L., Schmitt, K., Zhang, L., and Arnheim, N. (1992) A new source of polymorphic DNA markers for sperm typing: analysis of microsatellite repeats in single cells. *Am. J. Hum. Genet.* **51,** 985–991.
26. Le Fleche, P., Hauck, Y., Onteniente, L., et al. (2001) A tandem repeats database for bacterial genomes: application to the genotyping of *Yersinia pestis* and *Bacillus anthracis*. *BMC Microbiol.* **1,** 2.
27. Dean, D., Patton, M., and Stephens, R. S. (1991) Direct sequence evaluation of the major outer membrane protein gene variant regions of *Chlamydia trachomatis* subtypes D', I', and L2'. *Infect. Immun.* **59,** 1579–1582.
28. Friedlander, A. M. (1997) Anthrax, in *Medical Aspects of Chemical and Biological Weapons*. (Sidell, F. R., Takafuji, E. T., and Franz, D. R., eds.), Office of the Surgeon General. Department of the Army, Washington, DC, pp. 476–478.
29. Eitzen, E. M. (1997) Use of biological weapons, in *Medical Aspects of Chemical and Biological Weapons*. (Sidell, F. R., Takafuji, E. T., and Franz, D. R., eds.), Office of the Surgeon General. Department of the Army, Washington, DC, pp. 437–450.
30. Jackson, P. J., Walthers, E. A., Kalif, A. S., et al. (1997) Characterization of the variable-number tandem repeats in vrrA from different *Bacillus anthracis* isolates. *Appl. Environ. Microbiol.* **63,** 1400–1405.
31. Keim, P., Kalif, A., Schupp, J., et al. (1997) Molecular evolution and diversity in *Bacillus anthracis* as detected by amplified fragment length polymorphism markers. *J. Bacteriol.* **179,** 818–824.
32. Henderson, I., Yu, D., and Turnbull, P. C. (1995) Differentiation of *Bacillus anthracis* and other 'Bacillus cereus group' bacteria using IS231-derived sequences. *FEMS Microbiol. Lett.* **128,** 113–118.
33. Ash, C., Farrow, J. A., Dorsch, M., Stackebrandt, E., and Collins, M. D. (1991) Comparative analysis of *Bacillus anthracis*, *Bacillus cereus*, and related species on the basis of reverse transcriptase sequencing of 16S rRNA. *Int. J. Syst. Bacteriol.* **41,** 343–346.
34. Ash, C. and Collins, M. D. (1992) Comparative analysis of 23S ribosomal RNA gene sequences of *Bacillus anthracis* and emetic *Bacillus cereus* determined by PCR-direct sequencing. *FEMS Microbiol. Lett.* **73,** 75–80.
35. Keim, P., Price, L. B., Klevytska, A. M., et al. (2000) Multiple-locus variable-number tandem repeat analysis reveals genetic relationships within *Bacillus anthracis*. *J. Bacteriol.* **182,** 2928–2936.
36. Smith, K. L., DeVos, V., Bryden, H., Price, L. B., Hugh-Jones, M. E., and Keim, P. (2000) *Bacillus anthracis* diversity in Kruger National Park. *J. Clin. Microbiol.* **38,** 3780–3784.
37. Read, T. D., Salzberg, S. L., Pop, M., et al. (2002) Comparative Genome Sequencing for Discovery of Novel Polymorphisms in *Bacillus anthracis*. *Science* **9,** 9.
38. Perry, R. D. and Fetherston, J. D. (1997) *Yersinia pestis*—etiologic agent of plague. *Clin. Microbiol. Rev.* **10,** 35–66.
39. Huang, X., Engelthaler, D. M., Chu, M., and Lindler, L. E. (2002) Genotyping of a homogeneous group of *Yersinia pestis* strains isolated in the United States. *J. Clin. Microbiol.* **40,** 1164–1173.
40. Guiyoule, A., Grimont, F., Iteman, I., Grimont, P. A., Lefevre, M., and Carniel, E. (1994) Plague pandemics investigated by ribotyping of *Yersinia pestis* strains. *J. Clin. Microbiol.* **32,** 634–641.
41. Guiyoule, A., Rasoamanana, B., Buchrieser, C., Michel, P., Chanteau, S., and Carniel, E. (1997) Recent emergence of new variants of *Yersinia pestis* in Madagascar. *J. Clin. Microbiol.* **35,** 2826–2833.
42. Adair, D. M., Worsham, P. L., Hill, K. K., et al. (2000) Diversity in a variable-number tandem repeat from *Yersinia pestis*. *J. Clin. Microbiol.* **38,** 1516–1519.

43. Motin, V. L., Georgescu, A. M., Elliott, J. M., et al. (2002) Genetic variability of *Yersinia pestis* isolates as predicted by PCR-based IS*100* genotyping and analysis of structural genes encoding glycerol-3-phosphate dehydrogenase (*glpD*). *J. Bacteriol.* **184,** 1019–1027.

44. Ramalingaswami, V. (1995) Plague in India. *Nat. Med.* **1,** 1237–1239.

45. Mahillon, J. and Chandler, M. (1998) Insertion sequences. *Microbiol. Mol. Biol. Rev.* **62,** 725–774.

46. Bobrov, A. G. and Filippov, A. A. (1997) Prevalence of IS*285* and IS*100* in *Yersinia pestis* and *Yersinia pseudotuberculosis* genomes. *Mol. Gen. Mikrobiol. Virusol.* **2,** 36–40.

47. Parkhill, J., Wren, B. W., Thomson, N. R., et al. (2001) Genome sequence of *Yersinia pestis*, the causative agent of plague. *Nature* **413,** 523–527.

48. Portnoy, D. A. and Falkow, S. (1981) Virulence-associated plasmids from *Yersinia enterocolitica* and *Yersinia pestis*. *J. Bacteriol.* **148,** 877–883.

49. McDonough, K. A. and Hare, J. M. (1997) Homology with a repeated *Yersinia pestis* DNA sequence IS*100* correlates with pesticin sensitivity in *Yersinia pseudotuberculosis*. *J. Bacteriol.* **179,** 2081–2085.

50. Filippov, A. A., Oleinikov, P. V., Motin, V. L., Protsenko, O. A., and Smirnov, G. B. (1995) Sequencing of two *Yersinia pestis* IS elements, IS*285* and IS*100*. *Contrib. Microbiol. Immunol.* **13,** 306–309.

51. Odaert, M., Devalckenaere, A., Trieu-Cuot, P., and Simonet, M. (1998) Molecular characterization of IS*1541* insertions in the genome of *Yersinia pestis*. *J. Bacteriol.* **180,** 178–181.

52. Speijer, H., Savelkoul, P. H., Bonten, M. J., Stobberingh, E. E., and Tjhie, J. H. (1999) Application of different genotyping methods for *Pseudomonas aeruginosa* in a setting of endemicity in an intensive care unit. *J. Clin. Microbiol.* **37,** 3654–3661.

53. Deng, W., Burland, V., Plunkett, G., et al. (2002) Genome sequence of *Yersinia pestis* KIM. *J. Bacteriol.* **184,** 4601–4611.

54. Smith, C. L. and Condemine, G. (1990) New approaches for physical mapping of small genomes. *J. Bacteriol.* **172,** 1167–1172.

55. Lucier, T. S. and Brubaker, R. R. (1992) Determination of genome size, macrorestriction pattern polymorphism, and nonpigmentation-specific deletion in *Yersinia pestis* by pulsed-field gel electrophoresis. *J. Bacteriol.* **174,** 2078–2086.

56. Joo, Y. S., Fox, L. K., Davis, W. C., Bohach, G. A., and Park, Y. H. (2001) *Staphylococcus aureus* associated with mammary glands of cows: genotyping to distinguish different strains among herds. *Vet. Microbiol.* **80,** 131–138.

57. Klevytska, A. M., Price, L. B., Schupp, J. M., Worsham, P. .L, Wong, J., and Keim, P. (2001) Identification and characterization of variable-number tandem repeats in the *Yersinia pestis* genome. *J. Clin. Microbiol.* **39,** 3179–3185.

58. Worsham, P. L. and Hunter, M. (1998) Characterization of pestoides F, an atypical strain of *Yersinia pestis*. *Med. Microbiol.* **6(Suppl. II),** 24–35.

59. Welkos, S. L., Friedlander, A. M., and Davis, K. J. (1997) Studies on the role of plasminogen activator in systemic infection by virulent *Yersinia pestis* strain C092. *Microb. Pathog.* **23,** 211–223.

60. Corbel, M. J. and Brinley-Morgan, W. J. (1984) Genus *Brucella*, in *Bergey's Manual of Systematic Bacteriology*. (Kreig, N. R. and Holt, J. G., eds.), Williams and Wilkins, Baltimore, MD, pp. 377–388.

61. Verger, J. M., Grimont, F., Grimont, P. A. D., and Grayon, M. (1985) *Brucella*, a monospecific genus as shown by deoxyribonucleic acid hybridization. *Int. J. Syst. Bacteriol.* **35,** 292–295.

62. Wayne, L. G., Brenner, D. J., Colwell, R. R., et al. (1987) Report of the ad hoc committee on reconciliation of approaches to bacterial systematics. *Int. J. Syst. Bacteriol.* **37,** 463–464.

63. Bricker, B. J. (2000) Characterization of the three ribosomal RNA operons *rrnA, rrnB*, and *rrnC*, from *Brucella melitensis*. *Gene* **255,** 117–126.

64. Cloeckaert, A., Verger, J. M., Grayon, M., et al. (2001) Classification of *Brucella* spp. isolated from marine mammals by DNA polymorphism at the omp2 locus. *Microb. Infect.* **3,** 729–738.

65. Jahans, K. L., Foster, G., and Broughton, E. S. (1997) The characterisation of *Brucella* strains isolated from marine mammals. *Vet. Microbiol.* **57,** 373–382.

66. Jensen, A. E., Ewalt, D. R., Cheville, N. F., Thoen, C. O., and Payeur, J. B. (1996) Determination of stability of *Brucella abortus* RB51 by use of genomic fingerprint, oxidative metabolism, and colonial morphology and differentiation of strain RB51 from *B. abortus* isolates from bison and elk. *J. Clin. Microbiol.* **34,** 628–633.

67. Jensen, A. E., Cheville, N. F., Ewalt, D. R., Payeur, J. B., and Thoen, C. O. (1995) Application of pulsed-field gel electrophoresis for differentiation of vaccine strain RB51 from field isolates of *Brucella abortus* from cattle, bison, and elk. *Am. J. Vet. Res.* **56,** 308–312.

68. Jensen, A. E., Cheville, N. F., Thoen, C. O., MacMillan, A. P., and Miller, W. G. (1999) Genomic fingerprinting and development of a dendrogram for *Brucella* spp. isolated from seals, porpoises, and dolphins. *J. Vet. Diag. Invest.* **11,** 152–157.

69. Savelkoul, P. H., Aarts, H. J., de Haas, J., et al. (1999) Amplified-fragment length polymorphism analysis: the state of an art. *J. Clin. Microbiol.* **37,** 3083–3091.

70. Bricker, B. J., Ewalt, D. R., MacMillan, A. P., Foster, G., and Brew, S. (2000) Molecular characterization of *Brucella* strains isolated from marine mammals. *J. Clin. Microbiol.* **38,** 1258–1262.

71. Cloeckaert, A., Verger, J. M., Grayon, M., and Grepinet, O. (1995) Restriction site polymorphism of the genes encoding the major 25 kDa and 36 kDa outer-membrane proteins of *Brucella. Microbiology* **141,** 2111–2121.

72. de la Puente-Redondo, V. A., del Blanco, N. G., Gutierrez-Martin, C. B., Garcia-Pena, F. J., and Rodriguez Ferri, E. F. (2000) Comparison of different PCR approaches for typing of *Francisella tularensis* strains. *J. Clin. Microbiol.* **38,** 1016–1022.

73. Johansson, A., Ibrahim, A., Goransson, I., et al. (2000) Evaluation of PCR-based methods for discrimination of *Francisella* species and subspecies and development of a specific PCR that distinguishes the two major subspecies of *Francisella tularensis. J. Clin. Microbiol.* **38,** 4180–4185.

74. Johansson, A., Goransson, I., Larsson, P., and Sjostedt, A. (2001) Extensive Allelic Variation among *Francisella tularensis* Strains in a Short-Sequence Tandem Repeat Region. *J. Clin. Microbiol.* **39,** 3140–3146.

75. Farlow, J., Smith, K. L., Wong, J., Abrams, M., Lytle, M., and Keim, P. (2001) *Francisella tularensis* strain typing using multiple-locus, variable-number tandem repeat analysis. *J. Clin. Microbiol.* **39,** 3186–3192.

76. Prior, R. G., Klasson, L., Larsson, P., et al. (2001) Preliminary analysis and annotation of the partial genome sequence of *Francisella tularensis* strain Schu 4. *J. Appl. Microbiol.* **91,** 614–620.

77. Karlsson, J., Prior, R. G., Williams, K., et al. (2000) Sequencing of the *Francisella tularensis* strain Schu 4 genome reveals the shikimate and purine metabolic pathways, targets for the construction of a rationally attenuated auxotrophic vaccine. *Microb. Comp. Genomics* **5,** 25–39.

78. Forsman, M., Sandstrom, G., and Jaurin, B. (1990) Identification of *Francisella* species and discrimination of type A and type B strains of *F. tularensis* by 16S rRNA analysis. *Appl. Environ. Microbiol.* **56,** 949–955.

79. Hakenbeck, R., Balmelle, N., Weber, B., Gardes, C., Keck, W., and de Saizieu, A. (2001) Mosaic genes and mosaic chromosomes: intra- and interspecies genomic variation of *Streptococcus pneumoniae. Infect. Immun.* **69,** 2477–2486.

80. Swaminathan, B., Barrett, T. J., Hunter, S. B., and Tauxe, R. V. (2001) PulseNet: the molecular subtyping network for foodborne bacterial disease surveillance, United States. *Emerg. Infect. Dis.* **7,** 382–389.

81. Graves, L. M. and Swaminathan, B. (2001) PulseNet standardized protocol for subtyping *Listeria monocytogenes* by macrorestriction and pulsed-field gel electrophoresis. *Int. J. Food Microbiol.* **65,** 55–62.
82. Cummings, C. A. and Relman, D. A. (2002) Microbial forensics—when pathogens are "cross-examined." *Science* **9,** 9.
83. Bergey, D. H. and Holt, J. G. (1994) *Bergey's Manual of Determinative Bacteriology.* 9th ed. Williams & Wilkins, Baltimore, MD.

22

Yersinia pestis as an Emerged Pathogen

What Lessons Can Be Learned?

Luther E. Lindler

1. INTRODUCTION

"The evidence of ongoing genome fluidity, expansion and decay suggests Yersinia pestis is a pathogen that has undergone large-scale genetic flux and provides a unique insight into the ways in which new and highly virulent pathogens evolve." *(1)*

Probably the most difficult potential biological weapon to counter is the genetically engineered threat. Although the bioengineering of microorganisms as weapons has been the subject of fiction in recent years *(2),* unfortunately it has become a reality *(3–5).* Advances in biology, genetic engineering, and microbiology coupled with a willingness to exploit these sciences for nefarious purposes have made this possible. The number and type of genetic manipulations that might be undertaken to circumvent standard, as well as advanced, laboratory identification of a pathogen are almost limitless. However, selective pressure and natural genetic exchange have combined to create many serious pathogens in nature. Therefore, much can be learned about the development of a deadly pathogen by the study of the process through natural selection. This knowledge might then be used to estimate what might be done in the laboratory and then develop countermeasures for an engineered pathogen.

One of the best examples of a pathogen able to cause acute disease that has evolved from a less pathogenic organism can be found in the comparison of the diseases caused by *Yersinia pestis* and *Yersinia pseudotuberculosis*. *Y. pestis* is the bacterium responsible for causing plague, a rapidly fatal disease resulting in dissemination of the organism through the epidermis or lungs into the lymphatic system followed by colonization of the liver and spleen and later release into the blood stream *(6,7).* Infection by the organism can be initiated through the bite of an infected flea (bubonic plague) or by aerosol droplets from an infected host (pneumonic plague). Gastrointestinal exposure may also produce infection *(7).* Death from infection by *Y. pestis* is a result of vascular collapse, multiple organ failure, and disseminated intravascular coagulation precipitated by massive bacterial growth in the host *(8).* The cascade of events is initiated by bacterial endotoxin but is not dependent on persistent insult by this component of the Gram-negative envelope. In contrast, *Y. pseudotuberculosis* causes a mesenteric lym-

From: *Infectious Diseases: Biological Weapons Defense: Infectious Diseases and Counterterrorism*
Edited by: L. E. Lindler, F. J. Lebeda, and G. W. Korch © Humana Press Inc., Totowa, NJ

Table 1
Comparison of Virulence of *Y. pestis* and *Y. pseudotuberculosis* in Animals[a]

Species	Guinea pig			Mouse		
	sc	ip	iv	sc	ip	iv
Y. pestis	<10	<10	<10	<10	<10	<10
Y. pseudotuberculosis	approx 10^4	approx 10^2	approx 10	approx 10^4	approx 10^4	approx 10

[a]Data are taken from Brubaker *(18)*.
sc, subcutaneous; ip, intraperitoneal; iv, intravenous.

phadenitis initiated through the oral route of infection that is usually self-limiting *(9)*. Rarely does the infection penetrate to deeper tissues except in cases where there are other medical complications such as in immunocompromised individuals. Accordingly, the major difference between the pathogenesis of *Y. pseudotuberculosis* and *Y. pestis* infection is the latter's ability to penetrate the host from peripheral routes of infection and establish disease in deep tissues. The data in Table 1 illustrates the fact that the virulence of *Y. pestis* and *Y. pseudotuberculosis* are significantly different when physical barriers within the host must be crossed to cause infection (i.e., the invasiveness of the two species is vastly different).

Three plague pandemics have occurred. The first is thought to have spread from the African continent around 541 AD and is known as the Justinian's plague *(10,11)*. The second pandemic known as the Black Death probably spread from Asia around 1330–1346 and the third pandemic spread from the Yunnan province of China in 1855. The *Y. pestis* strains that caused the first, second, and third pandemics are thought to belong to the three biovars of the organism, Antiqua, Medievalis, and Orientalis, respectively *(12)*. Genotyping of the organism has clustered the biovars together and generally supported the proposed pandemic–biovar relationship *(10,12)*. *Y. pestis* is thought to have arisen from an ancestral *Y. pseudotuberculosis*-like organism approx 1500–20,000 yr ago *(10)*. This latter dateline coupled with the possible origin of the first pandemic suggests that the organism that causes plague may have evolved on the African continent.

The pathogenic potential of these two species is especially striking given the approx 90% DNA homology between *Y. pestis* and *Y. pseudotuberculosis* *(13,14)* and identical rDNA sequences *(15)*. The properties that differentiate the ability of *Y. pseudotuberculosis* and *Y. pestis* to cause disease have been reviewed elsewhere *(16)*. Pertinent virulence and physiological properties that are common or unique to the two species are listed in Table 2. The goal of this chapter is to discuss the genetics and briefly describe the virulence factors that make *Y. pestis* such a deadly pathogen, as well as present new evidence for the emergence of this organism from *Y. pseudotuberculosis*.

2. PLASMIDS

The virulence of *Yersinia* spp. is significantly dependent on the presence of plasmids *(16–19)*. *Y. pestis* typically harbors three plasmids, two of which are species specific. The species-specific plasmids, designated here as pPst and pFra, are approx 9.5 and 100 kilobase pairs (kb), respectively. The third plasmid that is common to the pathogenic species of *Yersinia*, including *Y. pestis* and *Y. pseudotuberculosis*, is approx 70 kb in size and is designated here as pYV (*Yersinia* virulence). It should be pointed

Table 2
Comparison of Y. *pestis* Properties With Y. *pseudotuberculosis*

Characteristic	Yps[a]	Yptb[b]	Function	Ref.
pYV	+	+	YOP production	59
pPst	+	–	Plasminogen activator production	22
pFra	+	–	Murine toxin and capsule synthesis	32
HPI	+	±[c]	Yersiniabactin siderophore production	79,125
pgm loci	+	+[d]	Pigmentation on Congo red agar	87
pH 6 antigen	+	+	Putative adhesin	126
YadA	–	+	Adhesin	71
LPS *O*-antigen	–	+	Cell structure	94
Invasin (Inv)	–	+	M cell translocation	127,128
Ail	±[e]	+	Host cell attachment and serum resistance	129
IS*1541* and IS*100*	++[f]	+	Insertion sequence elements	1,118, 127
Low calcium response (LCR)	++[f]	+	Regulation of YOPs and reduced growth at 37°C in the absence of added Ca^{+2}	18
Motility at 26°C	–	+	Chemotaxis	101
Rhamnose fermentation	–[g]	+	Sugar metabolism	101
Melibiose fermentation	–[g]	+	Sugar metabolism	101
Urease	–[g]	+	Nitrogen assimilation	103

[a]Yps, *Y. pestis.*
[b]Yptb, *Y. pseudotuberculosis.*
[c]Nonpathogenic strains are negative.
[d]The 68-kb *pgm* locus is present in *Y. pseudotuberculosis* but is usually silent *(81,85).*
[e]In some strains of *Y. pestis*, *ail* is interrupted by a copy of IS*285* but in others this locus is intact *(1).*
[f]The ++ and + refers to the higher number of these insertion sequence elements or relative intensity of the LCR seen in *Y. pestis* vs *Y. pseudotuberculosis*, respectively.
[g]Metabolic capability known to undergo reversion.

out that these designations are relatively generic names for these plasmids and that in some cases specific names are associated with plasmids harbored by either a particular strain or species. The following subheadings will discuss each of these molecules and their known contribution to pathogenesis.

2.1. The "Pesticin" Plasmid pPst

The "pesticin" plasmid is a small 9.5-kb molecule that is generally conserved among *Y. pestis* strains *(20)*. The plasmid encodes a bacteriocin (pesticin), pesticin immunity, and plasminogen activator-coagulase activity *(21–23)*. A single protein of 34.6-kDa encodes both the plasminogen activator activity as well as the coagulase activity and has been designated the Pla protease. Although temperature-dependent expression of *pla* has not been observed, the protein does produce higher plasminogen activator activity at 37°C, whereas coagulase activity is enhanced at 26°C. Besides Pla activity toward host proteins, it is also active on the *Yersinia* outer proteins (YOPs) and causes their degradation *(24)*.

Pla is thought to play a role in pathogenesis of plague infection by enhancing the organism's invasiveness possibly impeding fibrin-mediated antibacterial activity. In fact, Pla-negative *Y. pestis* strains KIM and CO92 have been shown to be avirulent in the mouse model *(25,26)*. In contrast, other strains of *Y. pestis* do not appear to need Pla for full virulence of the organism as judged by changes in LD_{50} *(26,27)*. This inconsistency in the requirement of *Y. pestis* for Pla activity to be fully virulent is likely to be strain specific. However, in all studies where *pla+* and *pla–* strains have been compared, a reduced inflammation near the site of injection as well as a more rapid spread of the organism to deeper tissues and reduced mean time to death has been noted in cells able to make the protease. Therefore, it is well-established that Pla enhances the virulence of *Y. pestis* and may at least partially account for the invasiveness of this organism compared with *Y. pseudotuberculosis*. A possible role for Pla in the *Y. pestis*-specific flea portion of the lifecycle has also been suggested *(28)*. The addition of Pla activity to two different strains of *Y. pseudotuberculosis* did not enhance the virulence of this gastrointestinal pathogen by the peripheral route of infection *(29)*. Taken together, these studies demonstrate that other factors along with Pla differentiate the pathogenesis of *Y. pestis* and *Y. pseudotuberculosis*. These studies also suggest that rapid spread of the organism in the host and decreased time until death may be a selective pressure in nature that maintains pPst in the *Y. pestis* population.

2.2. The "Murine Toxin" Plasmid pFra

The largest plasmid that is specific for *Y. pestis* is approx 100 kb in size. The involvement of this plasmid in virulence is controversial because *Y. pestis* strains lacking this plasmid show different effects on virulence depending on the animal model used *(18,30)*. In any case, pFra has been shown to encode two different proteins that may be involved in virulence *(31,32)*. These are the protein capsular antigen designated F1 and the murine toxin.

The F1 capsule is composed of multimers of a 17.6-kDa protein *(33)* that forms aggregates in the kDa to mega-Dalton size range *(34,35)*. Native capsule consists of this protein possibly linked to polysaccharide *(11,36)*. The capsule is only produced when the organism is grown at 37°C and is maximally induced when calcium is omitted from the growth medium *(37)*. The fact that F1 capsule synthesis enhances the resistance of *Y. pestis* to phagocytosis *(38)* suggested that it might protect the organism from nonspecific immune responses during penetration of deeper tissues. Recently, a more in-depth study of the antiphagocytic properties of defined *Y. pestis* F1-negative mutants was reported *(39)*. These studies found that F1-negative strains were partially reduced in their ability to resist phagocytosis by the mouse macrophage cell line J774.1. A greater reduction was seen when mutants also defective in the production of *Yersinia* outer proteins (YOPs, *see* Subheading 2.3.) were tested. These results may help explain why numerous studies have shown that F1-negative mutants of *Y. pestis* are virulent in mice by both the subcutaneous and aerosol routes of infection *(30,37,40–42)*. F1-nega-

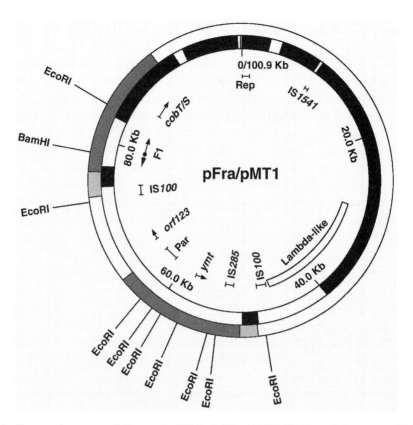

Fig. 1. Composite map of *Y. pestis* KIM pMT1 (AF074611) and *Y. pestis* CO92 pFra (AL117211). Black areas represent DNA sequences within the pMT1 sequence that are at least 90% identical to *S. enterica* serovar Typhi pHCM2 (AL513384). The dark gray regions represent regions of *Y. pestis* KIM pMT1 that are contiguous in the pFra sequence but rearranged, presumably because of IS activity *(53)*. The light gray areas represent DNA sequences encoded by *Y. pestis* KIM pMT1 that have been deleted in the CO92 pFra sequence. Regions that are colored white on the inner circle, therefore, generally represent pMT1/pFra-specific sequences with the exception of IS-associated DNA. The gene encoding Orf123 is labeled specifically because of the association with the *E. coli* virulence plasmid harbored by serotype O:157 *(55)*. Other regions of interest such as the origin of replication, partitioning region, insertion sequences and virulence-associated genes are also labeled.

tive strains are also virulent by aerosol in a monkey model *(43)*. The additional antiphagocytic effect of YOPs may be sufficient to allow the organism to cause death of infected animals in the absence of the ability to produce the F1 capsule. However, although the LD_{50} of noncapsulated mutants is not significantly affected, there is an increase in the mean time to death. In contrast with the virulence studies described above, the evidence for F1 as a protective antigen is substantial *(30,35,44–46)*. It follows then that although F1 is not a critical virulence factor of *Y. pestis* as defined classically, it is protective if an immune response (presumably antibody) can be mounted against the protein. Taken together, these facts suggest that *Y. pestis* produces virulence factors other than F1 that are not encoded by the enteric pathogen *Y. pseudotuberculosis,* which allow it to attack and proliferate within the host in an enhanced manner.

The second characterized protein encoded by *Y. pestis* pFra is the murine toxin (Ymt). Initially, Ymt was proposed to be involved in pathogenicity because it is highly lethal for mice *(47)*. Recently, this protein has been shown to belong to the phospholipase D superfamily of proteins *(48)*. Mutation of the gene encoding Ymt has little impact on the overall virulence of the organism but may enhance the speed at which death occurs in the mouse *(37,49)*. Recently, Ymt has been shown to be involved in survival of *Y. pestis* in the flea midgut *(50)* possibly by protecting the organism from toxic breakdown products of blood plasma. The fact that the gene encoding the toxin is slightly upregulated at 26°C is in keeping with a role for the protein in the insect vector *(37)*.

The complete DNA sequence of *Y. pestis* KIM pFra (designated pMT1) has been independently determined by two groups *(51,52)* as well as for strain CO92 *(53)*. *Y. pestis* KIM and CO92 belong to biovar Medievalis and Orientalis, respectively. The murine toxin plasmid shows the most diverse size distribution of all of the characterized *Y. pestis* plasmids *(20)*. This is at least partially caused by the number of complete or partial insertion sequence (IS) elements encoded by this plasmid (*see* Fig. 1). An illustration of the instability of pFra was obtained upon completion of the *Y. pestis* CO92 plasmid sequence *(53)*. The transposition of a copy of IS*100* near the F1 operon and apparent recombination between that element and a second copy of IS*100* resulted in a 6.7-kb deletion and 37-kb inversion of the *Y. pestis* CO92 plasmid compared to the KIM strain molecule *(52)*. The inversion includes the F1 operon *ymt* as well as the plasmid partitioning region of pFra. After testing 1 Antiqua, 1 Mediaevalis, and 12 Orientalis *Y. pestis* strains, the authors concluded that the 6.7-kb deletion in pFra was biovar-specific *(53)*.

A surprising and intriguing fact discovered by the complete sequencing of pFra from strain CO92 was that more than 50% of the molecule shares significant nucleotide identity (>90%) with a *Salmonella enterica* serovar Typhi cryptic plasmid pHCM2 *(53,54)* as shown in Fig. 1. This is even more striking than the previously noted protein homology between a pFra (pMT1) open reading frame (ORF) and a similar protein encoded on the *Escherichia coli* virulence plasmid pO157 *(55)*. The DNA homology between pFra and pHCM2 is dispersed over the two molecules with the largest continuous block being approx 30-kb. This 30-kb section includes a previously identified low G + C region near an IS*200*-like (IS*1541*) element as well as a group of lambdoid-phage tail proteins *(51)*. In relation to extrachromosomal element evolution and pathogens, the sequence comparison between *Y. pestis* pFra and the *S. enterica* serovar Typhi cryptic plasmid has revealed a common replication mechanism but independent partitioning functions. It is likely that the cointegration of the ancestral plasmids and undefined recombination events that formed these molecules was promoted by recombinational hot spots designated "Chi" sites given the large proportion of these sequences found on pFra and pHCM2 *(53)*. Mobility of these pathogen-associated plasmids and acquisition of DNA from chromosomal material is evidenced by the encoding of typical chromosomal genes (*cobT* and *cobS*) as well as a tRNA gene unique to pHCM2. How pFra might have been formed from ancestors of the *S. enterica* serovar Typhi pHCM2 and another plasmid is obviously a subject for conjecture. However, one possible mechanism would involve genetic transfer between the two gastrointestinal pathogens, *Y. pseudotuberculosis* and *Salmonela,* in a coinfected host. Alternatively, genetic exchange might occur in the flea vector that was coinfected with these two bacteria.

2.3. The "Yersinia" Virulence Plasmid pYV

The third *Y. pestis* plasmid is not species specific (i.e., it is also harbored by *Y. pseudotuberculosis*). pYV is approx 70 kb and is absolutely required for virulence *(17,18)*. The major virulence factors encoded by this plasmid include effector YOPs as well as the type III secretion apparatus to deliver these proteins to the host cell. This aspect of *Yersinia* pathogenesis has been reviewed elsewhere *(56–60)*. The literature pertaining to the function and delivery of YOPs to host cells is quite extensive and, given that this plasmid is common to *Y. pestis* and *Y. pseudotuberculosis*, this subject will not be covered in detail in this chapter. However, it is important to point out that significant differences encoded by the plasmids of these two species are known.

The most significant and well-studied virulence factors encoded by the pYV plasmids are the YOPs and the associated accessory proteins. The major portion of the *Yersinia* YOP virulon is an approx 26-kb contiguous group of genes and encodes the type III secretion apparatus as well as regulatory loci that allows delivery of the effector YOPs (YopE, H, J, M, YpkA) to the host *(61–63)*. The effector YOPs are encoded outside of the 26-kb central type III-encoding region with the exception of LcrV, a protective antigen and significant virulence factor *(16,64,65)*. The effector YOPs are generally involved in precipitating physiological changes within the target host cells in vitro including disruption of intracellular signaling, prevention of phagocytosis, and induction of cytotoxicity *(60)*. Homologs of the type III secretion apparatus are widely disseminated among pathogenic bacteria *(66)*, although, in general, the effector proteins secreted by these systems have a much more narrow distribution among genera. The YOPs encoded by the pathogenic *Yersinia* are highly homologous with only two having less than 92% homology at the protein level *(63)*. Accordingly, it is unlikely that differences in the YOPs or YOP-accessory proteins account for the much higher pathogenic potential of *Y. pestis* as compared to *Y. pseudotuberculosis*.

The pYV plasmid does encode at least one protein that may in part differentiate the pathogenesis of *Y. pestis* from *Y. pseudotuberculosis*. *Y. pseudotuberculosis* pYV encodes an approx 45-kDa protein designated as YadA (*Yersinia* adhesin A) *(59)*. Initially, YadA mutants of *Y. pseudotuberculosis* were thought to be hypervirulent *(67)*. Subsequently, it was shown that the original mutants tested in this study were not isogenic *(68)*. When isogenic mutants of YadA were tested, this protein appears to have little effect on the virulence of *Y. pseudotuberculosis (68)* but *yadA* mutants of the other gastrointestinal pathogenic *Yersinia*, *Yersinia enterocolitica*, are attenuated *(69)*. The involvement of YadA in the pathogenesis of *Y. enterocolitica* is through the adhesive nature of the protein and the requirement for effective YOP delivery by surface attached bacteria *(60)*. The invasin (Inv) protein is at least one of the proteins that performs the function of surface attachment for YOP delivery to host cells in *Y. pseudotuberculosis (70–73)* although *yadA* mutants have not been tested orally. In *Y. pestis,* the *yadA* locus is a pseudogene because of a frame-shift mutation that causes early termination during translation of the gene *(67)*. The fact that *inv* (*see* Table 2) and *yadA* encoded by *Y. pestis* are inactivated leaves open the question of what protein allows the plague bacillus to bind host cells and deliver YOPs in an effective manner.

2.4. Other Plasmids

The plasmids discussed in Subheadings 2.1.–2.3. are the plasmids that are consistently present in *Y. pestis* in general. However, natural isolates of both *Y. pestis* and *Y.*

pseudotuberculosis can harbor other plasmids as well. The genetic nature of these plasmids is generally undefined and, therefore, will not be discussed in this chapter. There are two specific instances where other "nontypical" plasmids of these species are of interest.

First, two different antibiotic resistance plasmids have been identified in strains of *Y. pestis* isolated in Madagascar *(74,75)*. One of the plasmids is 150 kb in size and encodes resistance to ampicillin, kanamycin, sulfonamides, streptomycin, tetracycline and chloramphenicol. This plasmid belongs to the Inc6-C incompatibility group. The second plasmid is 40 kb in size and belongs to the IncP incompatibility group. This plasmid encodes resistance to streptomycin only. Both of these plasmids are self-transmissible and are of broad host range. Beside the concern for public health and the threat that antibiotic resistant plague strains present to it, these isolates give further evidence of the potential evolution of *Y. pestis* from *Y. pseudotuberculosis*. The incompatibility grouping, conjugation characteristics and type of antibiotic resistance genes encoded by these molecules indicate an origin of these R-plasmids from within the *Enterobacteriaceae*. The recent introduction of these resistance transfer plasmids to *Y. pestis* might be considered as "history repeating itself" in view of the extraordinarily high nucleotide homology between pFra and the *S. enterica* serovar Typhi cryptic plasmid *(53)* described above. Again, the question of the opportunity for transfer between *Y. pestis* (or a predecessor in the case of pFra) and another enteric bacterium is raised. Obviously, the circumstances that allowed the creation of pFra were not unique and may be repeated in the future.

Second, a small 6-kb cryptic plasmid isolated from *Y. pestis* has been completely sequenced *(76)*. This plasmid has been emerging from the Yunnan province of China in larger numbers over a wider area since it was first isolated in 1990. The pYC plasmid does not encode any obvious virulence factors. It does encode two putative ORFs with motifs found in the LuxR-family of transcriptional regulators and two other ORFs involved in DNA stability. These latter two ORFs may partially explain the continued dissemination of pYC in *Y. pestis* isolates in this region of China. ORFs and nucleotide sequences encoded by pYC were highly homologous, with sequences found in the genome and plasmids of enteric bacteria, *E. coli*, and *Shigella sonnei (76)*. Again, the relationship between the acquisition of putative and confirmed fitness plasmids by *Y. pestis* and gene exchange with enteric organisms has been identified in a molecule left as "evidence."

3. THE HIGH-PATHOGENICITY ISLAND AND PIGMENTATION PHENOTYPE

The high-pathogenicity island (HPI) and the pigmentation (Pgm) determinant are both involved in iron acquisition by *Y. pestis* *(11)*. At least portions of these two systems are encompassed within a 102-kb region of *Y. pestis* DNA that frequently undergoes spontaneous deletion caused by flanking copies of IS*100* in direct repeat *(77,78)*. The HPI genes involved in iron metabolism are encoded by yersiniabactin (*ybt*) and within the Pgm region the hemin storage (*hms*) genes are necessary for accumulation and storage of iron (*see* Fig. 2). Both of these loci are generally also present in *Y. pseudotuberculosis*. Generally, the HPI and *hms* loci are linked in both *Y. pestis* and *Y.*

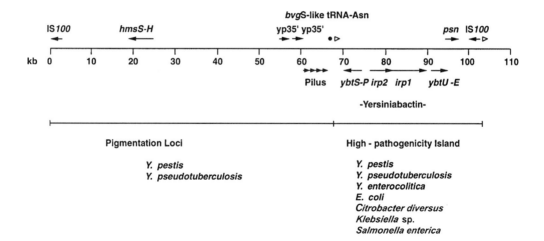

Fig. 2. Map of the *Yersinia* Pgm locus and HPI. The borders of the Pgm locus and HPI are indicated below the map. Arrows indicate the direction of transcription of the genes or elements that are labeled. The arrows indicating ORFs are not drawn to scale. The locations of IS*100* elements that flank the entire region are shown. The closed circle above the map indicates the tRNA-Asn near the HPI insertion site. The position of direct repeats flanking the HPI is represented by open triangles. The organisms where the two major elements are found are indicated at the bottom.

pseudotuberculosis (79,80). However, these two loci are independent and have been shown to be physically located in different positions within the *Y. pseudotuberculosis* chromosome *(81,82)* although this has not been demonstrated for *Y. pestis* to date. Classically, the Pgm locus or Pgm region has been referred to as the complete 102-kb region including the *hms* genes as well as the HPI shown in Fig. 2. Here, we do not follow that nomenclature for two reasons. First, the *hms* genes (and thus the Pgm phenotype) can be lost independent of the HPI in *Y. pestis,* demonstrating that these are independent regions of DNA *(77–79,83).* Second, the HPI has been found in multiple sites within the genome of *Y. pseudotuberculosis (81,82)* and is thus independent from the Pgm locus. Third, DNA sequence analysis reveals a vastly different G + C content for the HPI and the Pgm locus *(80).* Accordingly, here we will refer to the Pgm locus as the approx 68-kb region from the left copy of IS*100* to the asn-tRNA shown in Fig. 2. The HPI then extends from the asn-tRNA to just beyond the second copy of IS*100* on the right. The following sections discuss the phenotypes encoded by these elements and what is known about their functions and compares these elements between the two species.

3.1. The Pgm Phenotype

The Pgm+ phenotype refers to the ability of *Y. pestis* to form red colonies on media containing the planar compound Congo red. Originally, the Pgm locus *(pgm)* was thought to be a 102-kb unstable region within the chromosome of *Y. pestis* as discussed earlier and elsewhere *(78).* This region was later shown to include other genes involved in iron metabolism *(77).* We now know that the 102-kb Pgm determinant located between two copies of IS*100* is actually two regions that encode at least part of different iron acquisition systems (*see* Fig. 2 and the review by Perry and Fetherston in ref. *11*). The actual approx 68-kb Pgm locus has been shown to encode only one group of linked genes, designated as *hmsF, H, R,* and *hmsS* (*see* Fig. 2), involved in hemin storage. Perry et al. *(84)* generated transposon mutants in the *hms* region and showed that these loci were involved in pigmentation. The cloned *hms* genes were able to restore the Pgm phenotype of spontaneous *Y. pestis* Δ*pgm* mutants but did not confer a Pgm phenotype on *E. coli* harboring the construct. More recently, a second locus designated *hmsT* has been identified that is encoded by *Y. pestis* outside of the 102-kb Pgm determinant *(85)*. The above findings have led to the separate designations of the specific *hms* phenotype from the more generic *pgm* phenotype when referring to reactivity on Congo red media.

The genes encoding *hms* are also present within the *Y. pseudotuberculosis* 102-kb region but the Pgm phenotype in this species is variable and may be strain-dependent *(81,86)*. Furthermore, strains of *Y. pseudotuberculosis* that are converted to Pgm$^+$ by transformation with the cloned *hmsHFRS* and *hmsT* loci do not display the same phenotype as *Y. pestis* cells *(85)*. Loci other that *hmsT* outside the 102-kb region may also be involved in the Pgm phenotype. These facts leave open the possibility that some strains of *Y. pseudotuberculosis* may not display the Pgm phenotype because of mutations outside the classic 102-kb Pgm determinant. A systematic study of the genetics of the Pgm phenotype in *Y. pseudotuberculosis* has not been reported.

The involvement of Pgm in the virulence of *Y. pestis* in mammals is unclear (for review, *see* ref. *11*). The fact that *Y. pestis* is only pigmented on Congo red-agar when incubated at 26°C suggested that it might play a role in the flea vector *(87)*. It is now clear that the *hms* loci are necessary for blockage of fleas to allow the organism to be transmitted by that vector *(88,89)*. Although the exact mechanism by which this occurs is unclear, the involvement of the *hms* system in transmission of plague by fleas would explain the variability seen in the Pgm phenotype observed in *Y. pseudotuberculosis*.

Almost nothing is known about the 68-kb Pgm determinant except that it encodes the *hms* genes described earlier. These genes encompass approx 6-kb of the entire Pgm region. Recently, the entire 68-kb Pgm locus and HPI were sequenced from *Y. pestis* strain 6/69 *(80)*. The analysis of the sequence within the 68-kb Pgm determinant has not led to the discovery of any other loci that might obviously be involved in with iron metabolism. However, this region does encode a potential pilus operon that was previously unknown in *Y. pestis* (*see* Fig. 2). The only difference between the *Y. pestis* and *Y. pseudotuberculosis* sequences within the 68-kb Pgm determinant was a single nucleotide change in a gene designated as *yp35*. The mutation introduced a frame shift in this gene, but only in the biovar Orientalis strains. Accordingly, this frame shift is a recent event in the diversification of *Y. pestis* from *Y. pseudotuberculosis*.

3.2. The HPI

The HPI encodes a siderophore iron acquisition system designated as yersiniabactin. The region encoding the Ybt has been designated a pathogenicity island based on the fact that it is inserted near a tRNA gene, includes 17 bp direct repeat sequences that flank the region that are related to the bacteriophage P4 attachment site, and encodes within this region a bacteriophage P4-like integrase gene *(80,90,91)*. This element has been found in all three species of pathogenic *Yersinia,* as well as other pathogenic enteric pathogens *(92,93)* as indicated in Fig. 2. Interestingly, the HPI harbored by pathogenic *E. coli* is more related to the island found in the *Y. pestis*-linage of the element underscoring the relationship between evolution of the plague bacillus and enteropathogenic organisms *(92).* Various forms of the HPI are more widely disseminated among pathogenic enterics than the Pgm locus described earlier.

The HPI of *Y. pestis* and *Y. pseudotuberculosis* are almost identical in DNA sequence. The only difference described to date is the fact that the *Y. pseudotuberculosis* HPI has been found inserted near one of three copies of the asn-tRNA *(81,82)* whereas the *Y. pestis* element has only been shown to be associated with the same location as the Pgm locus. The conservation in the HPI sequences derived from *Y. pestis* and *Y. pseudotuberculosis* shows a recent common evolutionary link between the two organisms. The mechanism that has resulted in the various locations of the element in *Y. pseudotuberculosis* remains unclear. The observations pertaining to the location of the HPI in these two species are consistent with the acquisition of the Pgm locus by a particular strain of *Y. pseudotuberculosis* that then later emerged as what we now know as *Y. pestis.*

4. PHYSIOLOGY

Y. pestis and *Y. pseudotuberculosis* have several notable differences in their physiology that may be related to their pathogenesis. Although this is not intended to be an exhaustive review of these differences, we will point out the significant differences where they relate to the emergence of plague from the enteropathogenic species.

4.1. Lipopolysaccharide Structure

Y. pestis lipopolysaccharide (LPS) does not contain the typical somatic or *O*-sugar sidechains present on other *Enterobacteriaceae* when cultivated at either 26°C or 37°C *(16,94).* Similarly, *Y. pseudotuberculosis* does not produce *O*-antigen sugars when grown at 37°C but does produce type-specific somatic antigen when grown at 28°C in vitro *(16,95).* Thus, *Y. pseudotuberculosis* displays temperature-dependent regulation of LPS *O*-side chains not shown by *Y. pestis.* This may reflect the contaminated water or food-borne aspect of infections caused by *Y. pseudotuberculosis* where *O*-polysaccharide may afford a survival advantage for the organism. Keeping with the idea that longer *O*-antigen sidechains might aide in the foodborne portion of *Y. pseudotuberculosis* infection is the fact that the other gastrointestinal *Yersinia* pathogen, *Y. enterocolitica,* also upregulates *O*-antigen synthesis at lower growth temperature *(96).* However, unlike other enteric Gram-negative pathogens, *Y. pestis* and *Y. pseudotuberculosis* are both resistant to complement killing that would occur following infection of a mammalian host in the absence of *O*-polysaccharides *(97).* The inability of *Y. pestis* to make LPS *O*-side-chains has been found to be due to frame-shift mutations in five genes within a putative LPS biosynthetic cluster *(94,98).* These frame-shift mutations are not present in the same region of the *Y. pseudotuberculosis* genome. The LPS *O*-antigen genes of *Y. pseudotuberculosis* serotype O:1b were found to be the most closely related to those encoded by *Y. pestis (98)* following restriction endonuclease digestion and DNA sequence analysis. Recently, several genes involved in LPS core as well as *O*-antigen biosynthesis have been found to be necessary for *Y. pseudotubercu-*

losis to survive in mice following intravenous injection *(99)*. These results indicate that the regulation of *O*-antigen synthesis may be different in vivo compared to in vitro observations. More interestingly, given the mutations present in the *Y. pestis* LPS gene cluster, it suggests that other mechanisms to avoid host defenses have evolved in this organism yielding a much more virulent pathogen.

Besides the protection that LPS provides from complement fixation, this molecule is also involved in the endotoxic reaction seen in most Gram-negative infections. The action of LPS on host cells results in complement fixation as well as the release of proinflammatory cytokines that recruit immune cells including granulocytes to the point of infection. The bioactive portion of LPS generally resides within the lipid A portion of the molecule. Given the high degree of septicemia caused by *Y. pestis* infection, it is important to note that the LPS of this organism has been shown to possess far less endotoxic properties than does the LPS of *E. coli* (100). It follows then that the envelope structure of *Y. pestis* is atypical compared to most Gram-negative pathogens and most likely has evolved such that it enhances the pathogenesis of this organism.

4.2. Motility

One of the basic distinguishing characteristics between *Y. pestis* and the entero-pathogenic *Yersinia* is the lack of motility displayed by the former (*see* Table 2). However, recently upon completion of the genome sequence of *Y. pestis* CO92 two sets of genes involved in flagella biosynthesis were identified *(1)*. One of these encodes a frame-shift in *flhA* whose product is involved in flagella subunit transport and assembly. The second flagella gene cluster did not encode any obvious mutations and is, therefore, potentially functional. Either these genes are nonfunctional owing to uncharacterized interactions in flagella synthesis or they may be expressed under as yet undefined conditions.

4.3. Biochemical Reactions

Y. pseudotuberculosis is generally able to ferment the sugars melibiose and rhamnose, whereas *Y. pestis* cannot (*see* Table 2). However, this is not universally true as would be expected in light of the fact that *Y. pestis* has been found to ferment these sugars when selective pressure for reversion is present *(101)*. This would suggest that single-point mutations are responsible for the inability of *Y. pestis* to utilize these sugars. Similarly, some natural isolates of *Y. pseudotuberculosis* have been found that lack the ability to ferment melibiose *(102)*. Unlike *Y. pestis*, pathogenicity of these strains was generally low because of the absence of the HPI and/or pYV. Given that *Y. pestis* is highly pathogenic and encodes these virulence factors, this suggests the possibility that plague arose from one of these low pathogenic strains of *Y. pseudotuberculosis*. Alternatively, *Y. pestis* may have arisen from a melibiose-positive ancestor that has since lost the ability to ferment this sugar.

Another metabolic capability that differentiates *Y. pestis* from *Y. pseudotuberculosis* is urease activity, with the former being urease-negative. However, as with melibiose and rhamnose fermentation, this characteristic has been shown to undergo reversion. The point mutation in *ureD* that renders *Y. pestis* urease-negative has been characterized *(103)*. Loss of urease activity in *Y. pestis* is presumably caused by slipped-strand replication errors at a string of guanine residues that introduces a non-sense codon early in *ureD*. The presence or absence of urease activity apparently has no effect on virulence of *Y. pestis*.

4.4. Growth Restriction

Growth restriction refers to the inability of pathogenic *Yersinia* to grow at 37°C in the absence of added millimolar concentrations of calcium *(18)*. One of the well-documented consequences of growth restriction is the maximal production of at least the pYV-encoded virulence factors (YOPs) *(56,57)*. The upregulation of virulence factors and the cessation of growth were very paradoxical and suggested that some other environmental cues might be responsible for in vivo regulation of these genes. Recently, this has been shown to be the case for *Y. enterocolitica (104)* and most likely is also true for the other pathogenic *Yersinia*.

Although growth of *Y. pseudotuberculosis* is slowed upon shift from growth at 26°C to 37 °C in the absence of added calcium, the organism does continue to divide during the period from 4 to 16 h after temperature increase of the culture *(18)*. In comparison, the division of *Y. pestis* completely stops during the same time period (*see* Table 2). *Y. pestis* continues to make mRNA at a normal rate during restriction, but stable RNA synthesis is reduced. There is a concomitant moderate decrease in protein synthesis during this physiological state. However, the synthesis of DNA is dramatically reduced and is blocked at the stage after completion of chromosome replication but before cell division. Obviously, these are observations made on cells growing in vitro, and as indicated above, the regulation of restriction and virulence factor production by calcium is an artifact of these growth conditions. The use of calcium to study virulence regulation in vitro has led to the discovery and characterization of what we now know to be a common theme of pathogenesis used by many organisms, specifically, the type III secretion of virulence factors. Although the relationship of tighter virulence regulation (enhanced growth restriction) with the difference in pathogenesis of *Y. pestis* compared to *Y. pseudotuberculosis* is unknown, it seems likely that there may be a correlation that is worthy of further investigation.

5. GENOME AND GENETIC RELATEDNESS

We have pointed out known genetic differences between *Y. pestis* and *Y. pseudotuberculosis* in relation to whole plasmid content, pathogenicity islands, the Pgm locus, and individual gene sequences in the preceding sections. However, given the recent completed genome sequence of two different strains of *Y. pestis (1,105)* and the ongoing genome sequencing project of *Y. pseudotuberculosis* IP32953 at Lawrence Livermore National Laboratory (http://bbrp.llnl.gov/bbrp/html/microbe.html), we felt it important to discuss important findings that relate to the genomes of these two pathogenic *Yersinia*. In the following sections, we will describe well-known differences in the two genomes such as the difference in IS content and similarity in rDNA sequences. We will also discuss information that is newly available after analysis of the genome sequences and finally add new results that apply to the emergence of *Y. pestis* from *Y. pseudotuberculosis*.

5.1. The Complete Genome Sequence

The complete genome sequence of *Y. pestis* CO92 not only revealed the presence of a possible functional flagellar operon discussed earlier but also the possible presence of an additional type III secretion operon located on the chromosome *(1)*. The putative chromosomal type III system is similar in sequence and gene order to the *Salmonella enterica* serovar *Typhimurium* pathogenicity island 2 (SPI-2) *(106,107)*. There is a surprising degree of conservation between the gene order of the structural and regulatory ORFs located at the right and left extremities of SPI-2. However, the effector molecules and chaperones associated with them encoded by the central region of SPI-2 are absent from the putative *Y. pestis* element. This suggests that the "core" genes encoding structural and regulatory components of the type III system can be inherited generally as a block. This may also be true of the 26-kb region of type III secretion genes encoded on pYV as discussed in Subheading 2.3. The fact that there are no obvious effector molecules associated with the putative *Y. pestis* element is probably a result of different mechanisms of pathogenesis compared with *Salmonella*. This possibility is supported by the fact that a SPI-2 gene product SpiC has been shown to be involved in blocking phago–lysosomal fusion in infected macrophages *(108)*. However, fusion of the phagosome containing *Y. pestis* to macrophage lysosomes is not disrupted *(109)* therefore, the putative type III system would not be expected to encode a SpiC-like activity. SPI-2 is so far unique in that the type III secretion system it encodes functions from within the host cell instead of delivering virulence factors through the host-cell surface. This fact may suggest some location for the function for this putative *Y. pestis* type III system given that no phenotype has been identified for the element. Although the data is not complete, a search of the unfinished *Y. pseudotuberculosis* genome sequence reveals that at least some of the DNA sequences are present in that genome, suggesting that this element may not be unique to *Y. pestis*. A more careful comparison will be possible once that genome is finished.

A second finding that may be relevant to *Yersinia* pathogenesis was the finding of six possibly functional adhesin associated chaperone-usher systems in the *Y. pestis* CO92 genome sequences *(1)*. Another two systems encoded mutations in the usher component of the secretion apparatus. Similar findings were also made in the more ancient Medievalis biovar strain KIM *(105)*. The potential identification of so many possible adhesins is of great importance given the fact that the molecule employed by *Y. pestis* to deliver YOPs in an effective manner to host cells is still unknown *(110,111)*.

A third group of putative proteins that emerged following the complete genome sequence were proteins involved in interaction with pathogens and insects *(1)*. At least some of the insecticidal toxins identified may be nonfunctional because of frameshift mutations in one of the protein subunits. One particularly interesting protein showed 25% identity with a baculovirus protein that might be involved in penetration of the flea gut by *Y. pestis*. This ORF was most likely acquired by horizontal gene transfer given the nature of nearby genes. Oddly, the gene is also present in *Y. pseudotuberculosis* suggesting an association between this species and insects before the emergence of *Y. pestis*.

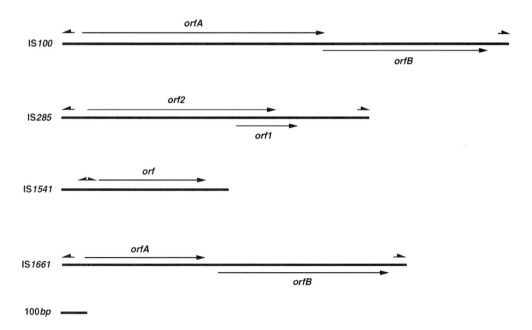

Fig. 3. General map of known or hypothetical IS elements found in the *Y. pestis* genome. ORFs are labeled as indicated in the references and are depicted by complete arrows. Half arrows indicate the position of inverted repeats. Each element is drawn to scale.

5.2. Insertion Sequences

Both *Y. pestis* and *Y. pseudotuberculosis* harbor three characterized IS elements. IS285 is an approx 1.3-kb element with an 8-bp target sequence that is directly duplicated at each end *(112)*. IS100 encompasses approx 1.9-kb and is flanked by a 7-bp directly duplicated target sequence. Both IS100 and IS285 include terminal inverted repeats and potentially encode two proteins as shown in Fig. 3. The third element is only approx 708 bp and has been designated IS1541 *(113–115)*. This element does not include terminal repeats nor does it appear that there is a target site duplication as with other members of the IS200 family of mobile elements *(116)*. These elements are thought to encode a single polypeptide of approx 150 amino acids. A fourth recently discovered IS in the *Y. pestis* genome has been designated IS1661 *(1)*. This putative element is approx 1.4 kb in length and is related to IS1397 previously described in *E. coli (117)*.

The chromosomal restriction fragment length polymorphism (RFLP) observed with these IS as probe is significant enough to allow the identification of unique patterns associated with each of these elements. Both IS100 and IS1541 have been used to evaluate the RFLP patterns of *Y. pestis* and *Y. pseudotuberculosis (113,115,118)*. *Y. pestis* encodes the largest number of copies of these IS elements compared to *Y. pseudotuberculosis*. This is in agreement with the concept that *Y. pestis* harbors a larger number of IS elements than the enterpathogenic *Yersinia (119)* and agrees with the finding that the genome of *Y. enterocolitica* is the most stable of the three species *(120)*. The relationship that the genomic flux has to the possible pathogenesis or to the pathogenic potential of *Y. pestis* is uncertain. However, it is clear that the genomic plasticity of this organism is high and correlates with pathogenic potential of the species. The completion of the *Y. pestis* genome sequence has determined exactly the number and location of these IS in the chromosome *(1)*. This work has confirmed that the relative number of these elements is IS*1541*>IS*100*>IS*285*>IS*1661*. It has also provided direct evidence for recombination between IS elements as a mechanism for large chromosomal rearrangements that result in rapid macrorestriction pattern changes or genomic instability near copies of IS*100* in *Y. pestis (12,121)*.

5.3. Ribosomal RNA and Housekeeping Gene Sequencing

As discussed earlier, *Y. pestis* and *Y. pseudotuberculosis* are highly related at the DNA level *(13,122)*. In fact, it has been suggested that they be considered varieties of one species based on DNA–DNA hybridization studies and 16S rDNA sequencing. Trebesius et al. *(15)* determined the 16S rDNA sequence from nine strains of *Y. pestis* that included representatives of all three biovars and compared those sequences obtained from nineteen strains of *Y. pseudotuberculosis* and found them to be identical. For historical and public health reporting reasons the individual species names have been retained.

The first described single nucleotide polymorphism (SNP) described in a *Y. pestis* compared to a *Y. pseudotuberculosis* gene was found in the Pgm region as discussed in Subheading 3.1. In a more extensive study, Achtman et al. *(10)* determined the DNA sequence of six housekeeping genes from a diverse group of *Y. pestis* strains. These strains included representatives of all three biotypes and spanned 56 yr of collection from 11 countries on four continents. The results indicated that the housekeeping gene sequences of this group of *Y. pestis* strains did not encode any SNPs after completing the sequences of mor than 90 kb of DNA. This study also included 12 strains of *Y. pseudotuberculosis* representing five serotypes. Comparison of the *Y. pestis* sequences with the *Y. pseudotuberculosis* sequences of the same genes revealed diversity that ranged from 0 to 4.4%, depending on the strain examined. This provided direct genetic evidence that *Y. pseudotuberculosis* was the older of the two species and allowed the authors to determine that the organism may have emerged around 1500–20,000 yr ago.

We have performed similar housekeeping gene-sequencing experiments on a different group of genes and strains. Altogether, we have determined the DNA sequences of more than 200 kb of housekeeping genes encoded by these two *Yersinia* spp. We have found that the sequences derived from a "typical" group of *Y. pestis* strains were absolutely identical although this group of strains originated from four continents spanning over 100 yr in time (GenBank accession numbers AF282306-AF282318). These results are in full agreement with those discussed above *(10)*. "Typical" strains are defined as being rhamnose and melibiose negative. However, we have recently examined an "atypical" group of *Y. pestis* strains that can ferment these two sugars *(121,123,124)* and compared these housekeeping gene sequences to ones obtained from a more diverse group of *Y. pseudotuberculosis* strains. The "atypical" *Y. pestis* strains show SNPs at synonymous sites compared to some of the *Y. pseudotuberculosis* strains (unpublished data). The results from galactose epimerase (*galE*) sequencing clearly demon-

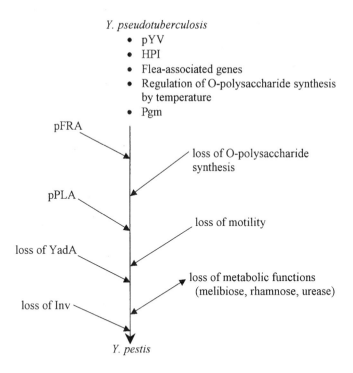

Y. pseudotuberculosis
- pYV
- HPI
- Flea-associated genes
- Regulation of O-polysaccharide synthesis by temperature
- Pgm

pFRA

loss of O-polysaccharide synthesis

pPLA

loss of motility

loss of YadA

loss of metabolic functions (melibiose, rhamnose, urease)

loss of Inv

Y. pestis

Fig. 4. Possible events involved in the emergence of *Y. pestis*. The diagram is intended to show the observed traits known to differentiate *Y. pseudotuberculosis* from *Y. pestis*. The order of addition of traits is not intended to suggest any particular order during the emergence of *Y. pestis*. The ancestral *Y. pseudotuberculosis* may have encoded the pYV plasmid, HPI, temperature-dependent regulation of *O*-polysaccharide and genes that promoted an association with insects possibly including the Pgm region.

strates that the "atypical" *Y. pestis* (generally referred to as pestoides strains) are a separate cluster from the "typical" strains that are even more related to *Y. pseudotuberculosis* (Lindler and Worsham, unpublished data). This conclusion drawn from *galE* sequencing results is consistent with the results of IS*100* genotyping *(121)*. Accordingly, the "atypical" pestoides group of *Y. pestis* strains may represent a more ancient form of the organism that is genetically closer to the link between the organism that causes plague and *Y. pseudotuberculosis*.

6. CONCLUSIONS

What can be learned about possible engineering of biological agents and emerging threats from this comparison? One thing is clear, although we have identified many unique properties of *Y. pestis,* the factors that make the disease what it is compared to gastroenteritis caused by *Y. pseudotuberculosis* are yet to be defined. A diagrammatic outline of the observed differences between the two organisms is shown in Fig. 4. Much of the information that might allow a more complete answer to this question is only on the horizon. The complete genome sequence of two strains of *Y. pestis* and of a single strain of *Y. pseudotuberculosis* will allow researchers to target specific areas and genes to determine what effect they have on virulence. However, the results from functional genomic studies are still years and perhaps decades away. From the genomic sequences, it is clear that the ancestors of these organisms have been associated with insects for a long period of time. It is also clear that genes involved in the enteropathogeic route of infection such as *inv* have mostly been lost in *Y. pestis*. Whether this provides a selective advantage to the systemic route of infection or simply reflects the lack of need for this protein remains to be determined. As is usual with the information gained from genome sequencing projects, the number of questions raised by the information is vast compared to the number of answers gained. Specific areas of interest are the newly identified type III secretion system encoded on the chromosome, the putative iron transport genes and the large number of previously unknown potential adhesins encoded by the chromosome *(1,105)*.

The addition of pPla encoding the plasminogen activator to a *Y. pseudotuberculosis*-like organism was undoubtedly an important genetic event in the emergence of plague. Interestingly, several "atypical" strains of *Y. pestis* lack this plasmid, and at least one of these is known to be virulent *(26)*. The addition of pFra encoding the murine toxin and F1 capsule antigen obviously must be important given that this plasmid is maintained in nature although the results from animal testing with mutants is conflicting. Interestingly, both F1 and Ymt encoded by pFra have been shown to be involved in more rapid death of infected animals. This fact coupled with the high degree of inheritance of pFra in natural strains of *Y. pestis* suggests that more rapid killing affords a selective advantage to the organism. The fact that pFra appears to be the least stable in terms of size, especially in "atypical" strains of *Y. pestis,* suggests that it is a recently acquired plasmid and is still in the process of reductive evolution. The Pgm locus is present in *Y. pseudotuberculosis* strains but appears to be silent in many of them. The requirement of a locus within the Pgm region for blockage of fleas and the presence of this locus in *Y. pseudotuberculosis* underscores the acquisition of genes involved in the insect stage of plague infection by an ancestral organism. This information taken together with genome sequencing data suggests that the evolution of *Y. pestis* was a multistep process and that the movement away from being an enteropathogen occurred partially in great leaps by the acquisition of blocks of genetic material through horizontal transfer. The Pgm region-associated HPI is clearly involved in pathogenesis of both species and in *Yersinia* as a whole. Of these virulence-associated proteins, the only protein that clearly promotes *Y. pestis* pathogenesis and differentiates it from *Y. pseudotuberculosis* is Pla. However, characteristics such as LPS structure coupled with capsule synthesis as well as other factors surely promote plague systemic invasion.

The evolution of a pathogen is a combination of selective pressure and environment. The combination of elements that have come together to create *Y. pestis* are certainly a function of environment. The fact that genetic material was passed from enteric bacteria to create pFra and is still being transferred to create new antibiotic resistant strains points to the environmental source of the characteristics that were involved in emergence of *Y. pestis*. The form of the organism (which is still evolving) that we see today is a combination of gene acquisition, gene loss, and backbone mutation that has coalesced into *Y. pestis*. How might we use this information? Monitoring of genetic changes within nonpathogenic environmental neighbors of pathogens is an obvious need but a tremendous undertaking. The most efficient way to perform this might be through rapid genome sequencing to identify near relatives to known virulence factors. Development of diagnostic probes based on known and newly identified virulence factor orthologs will also be beneficial. Databases to store and process this information are also critical if we are to gain any possibility of spotting potentially modified agents. If we do not begin to develop these tools now, then we will be left with our historical response that has been to react rather than be prepared. Hopefully this will not be the case.

ACKNOWLEDGMENTS

We thank all of the members of the Lindler Laboratories for their diligent work. We thank Sara Cohen for helpful discussions. Robert Brubaker and Mark Achtman are thanked for review of the manuscript. Lee Collins is kindly thanked for artwork. This work was supported by the US Army Medical Research and Materiel Command as part of the Biodefense Research Program.

REFERENCES

1. Parkhill, J., Wren, B. W., Thomson, N. R., et al. (2001) Genome sequence of *Yersinia pestis*, the causative agent of plague. *Nature* **413**, 523–527.
2. Preston, R. (1997) *The Cobra Event: A Novel.* 1st ed. Random House, New York.
3. Borzenkov, V. M., Pomerantsev, A. P., and Ashmarin, I. P. (1993) The additive synthesis of a regulatory peptide in vivo: the administration of a vaccinal *Francisella tularensis* strain that produces beta-endorphin. *Biull. Eksp. Biol. Med.* **116**, 151–153.
4. Pomerantsev, A. P., Staritsin, N. A., Mockov Yu, V., and Marinin, L. I. (1997) Expression of cereolysine AB genes in *Bacillus anthracis* vaccine strain ensures protection against experimental hemolytic anthrax infection. *Vaccine* **15**, 1846–1850.
5. Alibek, K. and Handelman, S. (1999) *Biohazard: The Chilling True Story of the Largest Covert Biological Weapons Program in the World, Told From the Inside by the Man Who Ran It.* 1st ed. Random House, New York.
6. Pollitzer, R. (1954) *Plague.* World Health Organization, Geneva.
7. Butler, T. (1983) *Plague and Other Yersinia Infections.* Plenum Medical Book, New York.
8. Beran, G. W. (1994) *Handbook of Zoonoses.* 2nd ed. CRC, Boca Raton, FL.
9. Murray, P. R. and American Society for Microbiology. (1999) *Manual of Clinical Microbiology.* 7th ed. ASM Press, Washington, DC.
10. Achtman, M., Zurth, K., Morelli, G., Torrea, G., Guiyoule, A., and Carniel, E. (1999) *Yersinia pestis*, the cause of plague, is a recently emerged clone of *Yersinia pseudotuberculosis. Proc. Natl. Acad. Sci. USA* **96**, 14,043–14,048.
11. Perry, R. D. and Fetherston, J. D. (1997) *Yersinia pestis*—etiologic agent of plague. *Clin. Microbiol. Rev.* **10**, 35–66.
12. Guiyoule, A., Grimont, F., Iteman, I., Grimont, P. A., Lefevre, M., and Carniel, E. (1994) Plague pandemics investigated by ribotyping of *Yersinia pestis* strains. *J. Clin. Microbiol.* **32**, 634–641.
13. Moore, R. L. and Brubaker, R. R. (1975) Hybridization and deoxyribonucleotide sequences of *Yersinia enterocolitica* and other selected members of *Enterobacteriaceae. Inter. J. Syst. Bacteriol.* **25**, 336–339.
14. Bercovier, H., Mollaret, H. H., Alsonso, J. M., et al. (1980) Intra- and interspecies relatedness of *Yersinia pestis* by DNA hybridization and its relationship to *Yersinia pseudotuberculosis. Curr. Microbiol.* **4**, 225–229.
15. Trebesius, K., Harmsen, D., Rakin, A., Schmelz, J., and Heesemann, J. (1998) Development of rRNA-targeted PCR and in situ hybridization with fluorescently labelled oligonucleotides for detection of *Yersinia* species. *J. Clin. Microbiol.* **36**, 2557–2564.

16. Brubaker, R. R. (1991) Factors promoting acute and chronic diseases caused by yersiniae. *Clin. Microbiol. Rev.* **4,** 309–324.

17. Ben-Gurion, R. and Shafferman, A. (1981) Essential virulence determinants of different *Yersinia* species are carried on a common plasmid. *Plasmid* **5,** 183–187.

18. Brubaker, R. R. (1983) The Vwa+ virulence factor of yersiniae: the molecular basis of the attendant nutritional requirement for Ca++. *Rev. Infect. Dis.* **5(Suppl. 4),** S748–758.

19. Portnoy, D. A. and Martinez, R. J. (1985) Role of a plasmid in the pathogenicity of *Yersinia* species. *Curr. Top. Microbiol. Immunol.* **118,** 29–51.

20. Filippov, A. A., Solodovnikov, N. S., Kookleva, L. M., and Protsenko, O. A. (1990) Plasmid content in *Yersinia pestis* strains of different origin. *FEMS Microbiol. Lett.* **55,** 45–48.

21. Beesley, E. D., Brubaker, R. R., Janssen, W. A., and Surgalla, M. J. (1967) Pesticins. 3. Expression of coagulase and mechanism of fibrinolysis. *J. Bacteriol.* **94,** 19–26.

22. Sodeinde, O. A. and Goguen, J. D. (1988) Genetic analysis of the 9.5-kilobase virulence plasmid of *Yersinia pestis. Infect. Immun.* **56,** 2743–2748.

23. Sodeinde, O. A. and Goguen, J. D. (1989) Nucleotide sequence of the plasminogen activator gene of *Yersinia pestis*: relationship to ompT of *Escherichia coli* and gene E of *Salmonella typhimurium. Infect. Immun.* **57,** 1517–1523.

24. Sodeinde, O. A., Sample, A. K., Brubaker, R. R., and Goguen, J. D. (1988) Plasminogen activator/coagulase gene of *Yersinia pestis* is responsible for degradation of plasmid-encoded outer membrane proteins. *Infect. Immun.* **56,** 2749–2752.

25. Sodeinde, O. A., Subrahmanyam, Y. V., Stark, K., Quan, T., Bao, Y., and Goguen, J. D. (1992) A surface protease and the invasive character of plague. *Science* **258,** 1004–1007.

26. Welkos, S. L., Friedlander, A. M., and Davis, K. J. (1997) Studies on the role of plasminogen activator in systemic infection by virulent *Yersinia pestis* strain C092. *Microb. Pathog.* **23,** 211–223.

27. Samoilova, S. V., Samoilova, L. V., Yezhov, I. N., Drozdov, I. G., and Anisimov, A. P. (1996) Virulence of pPst+ and pPst- strains of *Yersinia pestis* for guinea-pigs. *J. Med. Microbiol.* **45,** 440–444.

28. McDonough, K. A., Barnes, A. M., Quan, T. J., Montenieri, J., and Falkow, S. (1993) Mutation in the pla gene of *Yersinia pestis* alters the course of the plague bacillus-flea (*Siphonaptera: Ceratophyllidae*) interaction. *J. Med. Entomol.* **30,** 772–780.

29. Kutyrev, V., Mehigh, R. J., Motin, V. L., Pokrovskaya, M. S., Smirnov, G. B., and Brubaker, R. R. (1999) Expression of the plague plasminogen activator in *Yersinia pseudotuberculosis* and *Escherichia coli. Infect. Immun.* **67,** 1359–1367.

30. Friedlander, A. M., Welkos, S. L., Worsham, P. L., et al. (1995) Relationship between virulence and immunity as revealed in recent studies of the F1 capsule of *Yersinia pestis. Clin. Infect. Dis.* **21(Suppl. 2),** S178–181.

31. Cherepanov, P. A., Mikhailova, T. G., Karimova, G. A., Zakharova, N. M., Ershov, I. V., and Volkovoi, K. I. (1991) Cloning and detailed mapping of the fra-ymt region of the *Yersinia pestis* pFra plasmid. *Mol. Gen. Mikrobiol. Virusol.* 19–26.

32. Protsenko, O. A., Anisimov, P. I., Mozharov, O. T., Konnov, N. P., and Popov, I. A. (1983) Detection and characterization of the plasmids of the plague microbe which determine the synthesis of pesticin I, fraction I antigen and "mouse" toxin exotoxin. *Genetika* **19,** 1081–1090.

33. Galyov, E. E., Smirnov, O., Karlishev, A. V., et al. (1990) Nucleotide sequence of the *Yersinia pestis* gene encoding F1 antigen and the primary structure of the protein. Putative T and B cell epitopes. *FEBS Lett.* **277,** 230–232.

34. Bennett, L. G. and Tornabene, T. G. (1974) Characterization of the antigenic subunits of the envelope protein of *Yersinia pestis. J. Bacteriol.* **117,** 48–55.

35. Andrews, G. P., Heath, D. G., Anderson, G. W., Jr., Welkos, S. L., and Friedlander, A. M. (1996) Fraction 1 capsular antigen (F1) purification from *Yersinia pestis* CO92 and

from an *Escherichia coli* recombinant strain and efficacy against lethal plague challenge. *Infect. Immun.* **64,** 2180–2187.

36. Glosnicka, R. and Gruszkiewicz, E. (1980) Chemical composition and biological activity of the *Yersinia pestis* envelope substance. *Infect. Immun.* **30,** 506–512.

37. Du, Y., Galyov, E., and Forsberg, A. (1995) Genetic analysis of virulence determinants unique to *Yersinia pestis. Contrib. Microbiol. Immunol.* **13,** 321–324.

38. Cavanaugh, D. C. and Randall, R. (1959) The role of multiplication of *Pasturella pestis* in mononuclear phagocytes in the pathogenesis of flea-borne plague. *J. Immunol.* **83,** 348–363.

39. Du, Y., Rosqvist, R., and Forsberg, A. (2002) Role of fraction 1 antigen of *Yersinia pestis* in inhibition of phagocytosis. *Infect. Immun.* **70,** 1453–1460.

40. Worsham, P. L., Stein, M. P., and Welkos, S. L. (1995) Construction of defined F1 negative mutants of virulent *Yersinia pestis. Contrib. Microbiol. Immunol.* **13,** 325–328.

41. Welkos, S. L., Davis, K. M., Pitt, L. M., Worsham, P. L., and Freidlander, A. M. (1995) Studies on the contribution of the F1 capsule-associated plasmid pFra to the virulence of *Yersinia pestis. Contrib. Microbiol. Immunol.* **13,** 299–305.

42. Drozdov, I. G., Anisimov, A. P., Samoilova, S. V., et al. (1995) Virulent non-capsulate *Yersinia pestis* variants constructed by insertion mutagenesis. *J. Med. Microbiol.* **42,** 264–268.

43. Davis, K. J., Fritz, D. L., Pitt, M. L., Welkos, S. L., Worsham, P. L., and Friedlander, A. M. (1996) Pathology of experimental pneumonic plague produced by fraction 1- positive and fraction 1-negative *Yersinia pestis* in African green monkeys (*Cercopithecus aethiops*). *Arch. Pathol. Lab. Med.* **120,** 156–163.

44. Titball, R. W., Howells, A. M., Oyston, P. C., and Williamson, E. D. (1997) Expression of the *Yersinia pestis* capsular antigen (F1 antigen) on the surface of an *aroA* mutant of *Salmonella typhimurium* induces high levels of protection against plague. *Infect. Immun.* **65,** 1926–1930.

45. Anderson, G. W., Jr., Worsham, P. L., Bolt, C. R., et al. (1997) Protection of mice from fatal bubonic and pneumonic plague by passive immunization with monoclonal antibodies against the F1 protein of *Yersinia pestis. Am. J. Trop. Med. Hyg.* **56,** 471–473.

46. Simpson, W. J., Thomas, R. E., and Schwan, T. G. (1990) Recombinant capsular antigen (fraction 1) from *Yersinia pestis* induces a protective antibody response in BALB/c mice. *Am. J. Trop. Med. Hyg.* **43,** 389–396.

47. Montie, T. C. (1981) Properties and pharmacological action of plague murine toxin. *Pharmacol. Ther.* **12,** 491–499.

48. Rudolph, A. E., Stuckey, J. A., Zhao, Y., et al. (1999) Expression, characterization, and mutagenesis of the *Yersinia pestis* murine toxin, a phospholipase D superfamily member. *J. Biol. Chem.* **274,** 11,824–11,831.

49. Hinnebusch, J., Cherepanov, P., Du, Y., et al. (2000) Murine toxin of *Yersinia pestis* shows phospholipase D activity but is not required for virulence in mice. *Int. J. Med. Microbiol.* **290,** 483–487.

50. Hinnebusch, B. J., Rudolph, A. E., Cherepanov, P., Dixon, J. E., Schwan, T. G., and Forsberg, A. (2002) Role of *Yersinia* murine toxin in survival of *Yersinia pestis* in the midgut of the flea vector. *Science* **296,** 733–735.

51. Lindler, L. E., Plano, G. V., Burland, V., Mayhew, G. F., and Blattner, F. R. (1998) Complete DNA sequence and detailed analysis of the *Yersinia pestis* KIM5 plasmid encoding murine toxin and capsular antigen. *Infect. Immun.* **66,** 5731–5742.

52. Hu, P., Elliott, J., McCready, P., et al. (1998) Structural organization of virulence-associated plasmids of *Yersinia pestis. J. Bacteriol.* **180,** 5192–5202.

53. Prentice, M. B., James, K. D., Parkhill, J., et al. (2001) *Yersinia pestis* pFra shows biovar-specific differences and recent common ancestry with a *Salmonella enterica* serovar Typhi plasmid. *J. Bacteriol.* **183,** 2586–2594.

54. Parkhill, J., Dougan, G., James, K. D., et al. (2001) Complete genome sequence of a multiple drug resistant *Salmonella enterica* serovar Typhi CT18. *Nature* **413,** 848–852.

55. Burland, V., Shao, Y., Perna, N. T., Plunkett, G., Sofia, H. J., and Blattner, F. R. (1998) The complete DNA sequence and analysis of the large virulence plasmid of *Escherichia coli* O157:H7. *Nucleic Acids Res.* **26,** 4196–4204.

56. Straley, S. C. (1988) The plasmid-encoded outer-membrane proteins of *Yersinia pestis*. *Rev. Infect. Dis.* **10(Suppl. 2),** S323–326.

57. Straley, S. C., Skrzypek, E., Plano, G. V., and Bliska, J. B. (1993) Yops of *Yersinia* spp. pathogenic for humans. *Infect. Immun.* **61,** 3105–3110.

58. Cornelis, G. R. and Wolf-Watz, H. (1997) The *Yersinia* Yop virulon: a bacterial system for subverting eukaryotic cells. *Mol. Microbiol.* **23,** 861–867.

59. Cornelis, G. R., Boland, A., Boyd, A. P., et al. (1998) The virulence plasmid of *Yersinia*, an antihost genome. *Microbiol. Mol. Biol. Rev.* **62,** 1315–1352.

60. Cornelis, G. R. (1998) The *Yersinia* deadly kiss. *J. Bacteriol.* **180,** 5495–5504.

61. Iriarte, M. and Cornelis, G. R. (1999) The 70-kilobase virulence plasmid of yersiniae in *Pathogenicity Islands and Other Mobile Virulence Elements*. (Kaper, J. B. and Hacker, J., eds.), ASM, Washington, DC, pp. 91–126.

62. Perry, R. D., Straley, S. C., Fetherston, J. D., Rose, D. J., Gregor, J., and Blattner, F. R. (1998) DNA sequencing and analysis of the low-Ca2+-response plasmid pCD1 of *Yersinia pestis* KIM5. *Infect. Immun.* **66,** 4611–4623.

63. Snellings, N. J., Popek, M., and Lindler, L. E. (2001) Complete DNA sequence of *Yersinia enterocolitica* serotype 0:8 low- calcium-response plasmid reveals a new virulence plasmid-associated replicon. *Infect. Immun.* **69,** 4627–4638.

64. Leary, S. E., Griffin, K. F., Galyov, E. E., et al. (1999) *Yersinia* outer proteins (YOPS) E, K and N are antigenic but non- protective compared to V antigen, in a murine model of bubonic plague. *Microb. Pathog.* **26,** 159–169.

65. Roggenkamp, A., Geiger, A. M., Leitritz, L., Kessler, A., and Heesemann, J. (1997) Passive immunity to infection with *Yersinia* spp. mediated by anti- recombinant V antigen is dependent on polymorphism of V antigen. *Infect. Immun.* **65,** 446–451.

66. Cornelis, G. R. and Van Gijsegem, F. (2000) Assembly and function of type III secretory systems. *Annu. Rev. Microbiol.* **54,** 735–774.

67. Rosqvist, R., Skurnik, M., and Wolf-Watz, H. (1988) Increased virulence of *Yersinia pseudotuberculosis* by two independent mutations. *Nature* **334,** 522–524.

68. Han, Y. W. and Miller, V. L. (1997) Reevaluation of the virulence phenotype of the *inv yadA* double mutants of *Yersinia pseudotuberculosis*. *Infect. Immun.* **65,** 327–330.

69. Pepe, J. C., Wachtel, M. R., Wagar, E., and Miller, V. L. (1995) Pathogenesis of defined invasion mutants of *Yersinia enterocolitica* in a BALB/c mouse model of infection. *Infect. Immun.* **63,** 4837–4848.

70. Rosqvist, R., Forsberg, A., Rimpilainen, M., Bergman, T., and Wolf-Watz, H. (1990) The cytotoxic protein YopE of *Yersinia* obstructs the primary host defence. *Mol. Microbiol.* **4,** 657–667.

71. Bliska, J. B., Copass, M. C., and Falkow, S. (1993) The *Yersinia pseudotuberculosis* adhesin YadA mediates intimate bacterial attachment to and entry into HEp-2 cells. *Infect. Immun.* **61,** 3914–3921.

72. Andersson, K., Carballeira, N., Magnusson, K. E., et al. (1996) YopH of *Yersinia pseudotuberculosis* interrupts early phosphotyrosine signalling associated with phagocytosis. *Mol. Microbiol.* **20,** 1057–1069.

73. Monack, D. M., Mecsas, J., Ghori, N., and Falkow, S. (1997) *Yersinia* signals macrophages to undergo apoptosis and YopJ is necessary for this cell death. *Proc. Natl. Acad. Sci. USA* **94,** 10,385–10,390.

74. Guiyoule, A., Gerbaud, G., Buchrieser, C., et al. (2001) Transferable plasmid-mediated resistance to streptomycin in a clinical isolate of *Yersinia pestis*. *Emerg. Infect. Dis.* **7,** 43–48.

75. Galimand, M., Guiyoule, A., Gerbaud, G., et al. (1997) Multidrug resistance in *Yersinia pestis* mediated by a transferable plasmid. *N. Engl. J. Med.* **337,** 677–680.

76. Dong, X. Q., Lindler, L. E., and Chu, M. C. (2000) Complete DNA sequence and analysis of an emerging cryptic plasmid isolated from *Yersinia pestis. Plasmid* **43,** 144–148.

77. Fetherston, J. D. and Perry, R. D.(1994) The pigmentation locus of *Yersinia pestis* KIM6+ is flanked by an insertion sequence and includes the structural genes for pesticin sensitivity and HMWP2. *Mol. Microbiol.* **13,** 697–708.

78. Fetherston, J. D., Schuetze, P., and Perry, R. D. (1992) Loss of the pigmentation phenotype in *Yersinia pestis* is due to the spontaneous deletion of 102 kb of chromosomal DNA which is flanked by a repetitive element. *Mol. Microbiol.* **6,** 2693–2704.

79. Buchrieser, C., Prentice, M., and Carniel, E. (1998) The 102-kilobase unstable region of *Yersinia pestis* comprises a high- pathogenicity island linked to a pigmentation segment which undergoes internal rearrangement. *J. Bacteriol.* **180,** 2321–2329.

80. Buchrieser, C., Rusniok, C., Frangeul, L., et al. (1999) The 102-kilobase pgm locus of *Yersinia pestis*: sequence analysis and comparison of selected regions among different *Yersinia pestis* and *Yersinia pseudotuberculosis* strains. *Infect. Immun.* **67,** 4851–4861.

81. Buchrieser, C., Brosch, R., Bach, S., Guiyoule, A., and Carniel, E. (1998) The high-pathogenicity island of *Yersinia pseudotuberculosis* can be inserted into any of the three chromosomal asn tRNA genes. *Mol. Microbiol.* **30,** 965–978.

82. Hare, J. M., Wagner, A. K., and McDonough, K. A. (1999) Independent acquisition and insertion into different chromosomal locations of the same pathogenicity island in *Yersinia pestis* and *Yersinia pseudotuberculosis. Mol. Microbiol.* **31,** 291–303.

83. Iteman, I., Guiyoule, A., de Almeida, A. M., Guilvout, I., Baranton, G., and Carniel, E. (1993) Relationship between loss of pigmentation and deletion of the chromosomal iron-regulated irp2 gene in *Yersinia pestis*: evidence for separate but related events. *Infect. Immun.* **61,** 2717–2722.

84. Perry, R. D., Pendrak, M. L., and Schuetze, P. (1990) Identification and cloning of a hemin storage locus involved in the pigmentation phenotype of *Yersinia pestis. J. Bacteriol.* **172,** 5929–5937.

85. Hare, J. M. and McDonough, K. A. (1999) High-frequency RecA-dependent and -independent mechanisms of Congo red binding mutations in *Yersinia pestis. J. Bacteriol.* **181,** 4896–4904.

86. Burrows, T. W. (1973) Observations on the pigmentation of *Yersinia pseudotuberculosis. Contrib. Microbiol. Immunol.* **2,** 184–189.

87. Jackson, S. and Burrows, T. W. (1956) The pigmentation of *Pasturella pestis* on a defined medium containing haemin. *Br. J. Exp. Pathol.* **37,** 570–576.

88. Kutyrev, V. V., Filippov, A. A., Oparina, O. S., and Protsenko, O. A. (1992) Analysis of *Yersinia pestis* chromosomal determinants Pgm+ and Psts associated with virulence. *Microb. Pathog.* **12,** 177–186.

89. Hinnebusch, B. J., Perry, R. D., and Schwan, T. G. (1996) Role of the Yersinia *pestis* hemin storage (hms) locus in the transmission of plague by fleas. *Science* **273,** 367–370.

90. Schubert, S., Rakin, A., Karch, H., Carniel, E., and Heesemann, J. (1998) Prevalence of the "high-pathogenicity island" of *Yersinia* species among *Escherichia coli* strains that are pathogenic to humans. *Infect. Immun.* **66,** 480–485.

91. Carniel, E., Guilvout, I., and Prentice, M. (1996) Characterization of a large chromosomal "high-pathogenicity island" in biotype 1B *Yersinia enterocolitica. J. Bacteriol.* **178,** 6743–6751.

92. Carniel, E. (2001) The *Yersinia* high-pathogenicity island: an iron-uptake island. *Microbes. Infect.* **3,** 561–569.

93. Karch, H., Schubert, S., Zhang, D., et al. (1999) A genomic island, termed high-pathogenicity island, is present in certain non-O157 Shiga toxin-producing *Escherichia coli* clonal lineages. *Infect. Immun.* **67,** 5994–6001.

94. Prior, J. L., Parkhill, J., Hitchen, P. G., et al. (2001) The failure of different strains of *Yersinia pestis* to produce lipopolysaccharide O-antigen under different growth conditions is due to mutations in the O-antigen gene cluster. *FEMS Microbiol. Lett.* **197,** 229–233.

95. Samuelson, K., Lindberg, B., and Brubaker, R. R. (1974) Structure of O-specific side chains of lipopolysaccharides from *Yersinia pseudotuberculosis*. *J. Bacteriol.* **117,** 1010–1016.

96. al-Hendy, A., Toivanen, P., and Skurnik, M. (1991) The effect of growth temperature on the biosynthesis of *Yersinia enterocolitica* O:3 lipopolysaccharide: temperature regulates the transcription of the *rfb* but not of the *rfa* region. *Microb. Pathog.* **10,** 81–86.

97. Porat, R., McCabe, W. R., and Brubaker, R. R. (1995) Lipopolysaccharide-associated resistance to killing of yersiniae by complement. *J. Endotoxin. Res.* **2,** 91–97.

98. Skurnik, M., Peippo, A., and Ervela, E. (2000) Characterization of the O-antigen gene clusters of *Yersinia pseudotuberculosis* and the cryptic O-antigen gene cluster of *Yersinia pestis* shows that the plague bacillus is most closely related to and has evolved from *Y. pseudotuberculosis* serotype O:1b. *Mol. Microbiol.* **37,** 316–330.

99. Karlyshev, A. V., Oyston, P. C., Williams, K., et al. (2001) Application of high-density array-based signature-tagged mutagenesis to discover novel *Yersinia* virulence-associated genes. *Infect. Immun.* **69,** 7810–7819.

100. Prior, J. L., Hitchen, P. G., Williamson, D. E., et al. (2001) Characterization of the lipopolysaccharide of *Yersinia pestis*. *Microb. Pathog.* **30,** 49–57.

101. Brubaker, R. R. (1972) The genus *Yersinia*: biochemistry and genetics of virulence. *Curr. Top. Microbiol. Immunol.* **57,** 111–158.

102. Fukushima, H., Matsuda, Y., Seki, R., et al. (2001) Geographical heterogeneity between far eastern and western countries in prevalence of the virulence plasmid, the superantigen *Yersinia pseudotuberculosis*-derived mitogen, and the high-pathogenicity island among *Yersinia pseudotuberculosis* strains. *J. Clin. Microbiol.* **39,** 3541–3547.

103. Sebbane, F., Devalckenaere, A., Foulon, J., Carniel, E., and Simonet, M. (2001) Silencing and reactivation of urease in *Yersinia pestis* is determined by one G residue at a specific position in the *ureD* gene. *Infect. Immun.* **69,** 170–176.

104. Lee, V. T., Mazmanian, S. K., and Schneewind, O. (2001) A program of *Yersinia enterocolitica* type III secretion reactions is activated by specific signals. *J. Bacteriol.* **183,** 4970–4978.

105. Deng, W., Burland, V., Plunkett, G., et al. (2002) Genome sequence of *Yersinia pestis* KIM. *J. Bacteriol.* **184,** 4601–4611.

106. Hensel, M., Shea, J. E., Waterman, S. R., et al. (1998) Genes encoding putative effector proteins of the type III secretion system of *Salmonella* pathogenicity island 2 are required for bacterial virulence and proliferation in macrophages. *Mol. Microbiol.* **30,** 163–174.

107. Cirillo, D. M., Valdivia, R. H., Monack, D. M., and Falkow, S. (1998) Macrophage-dependent induction of the *Salmonella* pathogenicity island 2 type III secretion system and its role in intracellular survival. *Mol. Microbiol.* **30,** 175–188.

108. Uchiya, K., Barbieri, M. A., Funato, K., Shah, A. H., Stahl, P. D., and Groisman, E. A. (1999) A *Salmonella* virulence protein that inhibits cellular trafficking. *EMBO J.* **18,** 3924–3933.

109. Straley, S. C. and Harmon, P. A. (1984) *Yersinia pestis* grows within phagolysosomes in mouse peritoneal macrophages. *Infect. Immun.* **45,** 655–659.

110. Cowan, C., Jones, H. A., Kaya, Y. H., Perry, R. D., and Straley, S. C. (2000) Invasion of epithelial cells by *Yersinia pestis*: evidence for a *Y. pestis*-specific invasin. *Infect. Immun.* **68,** 4523–4530.

111. Straley, S. C. (1993) Adhesins in *Yersinia pestis*. *Trends Microbiol.* **1,** 285, 286.

112. Filippov, A. A., Oleinikov, P. N., Motin, V. L., Protsenko, O. A., and Smirnov, G. B. (1993) Sequencing of two *Yersinia pestis* IS elements, IS*285* and IS*100*. *Contrib. Microbiol. Immunol.* **13,** 306–309.

113. Odaert, M., Devalckenaere, A., Trieu-cuot, P., and Simonet, M. (1998) Molecular charac-terization of IS*1541*insertions in the genome of *Yersinia pestis. J. Bacteriol.* **180,** 178–181.

114. Devalckenaere, A., Odaert, M., Trieu-cuot, P., and Simonet ,M. (1999) Characterization of IS*1541*-like elements in *Yersinia enterocolitica* and *Yersinia pseudotuberculosis. FEMS Microbiol. Lett.* **176,** 229--233.

115. Odaert, M., Berche, P., and Simonet, M. (1996) Molecular typing of *Yersinia pseudotu-berculosis* by using an IS*200*-like element. *J. Clin. Microbiol.* **34,** 2231–2235.

116. Beuzon, C. R. and Casadesus, J. (1997) Conserved structure of IS*200* elements in *Salmo-nella. Nucleic Acids Res.* **25,** 1355–1361.

117. Clement, J. M., Wilde, C., Bachellier, S., Lambert, P., and Hofnung, M. (1999) IS*1397* is active for transposition into the chromosome of *Escherichia coli* K-12 and inserts spe-cifically into palindromic units of bacterial interspersed mosaic elements. *J. Bacteriol.* **181,** 6929–6936.

118. McDonough, K. A. and Hare, J. M. (1997) Homology with a repeated *Yersinia pestis* DNA sequence IS*100* correlates with pesticin sensitivity in *Yersinia pseudotuberculosis. J. Bacteriol.* **179,** 2081–2085.

119. Bobrov, A. G. and Filippov, A. A. (1997) Prevalence of IS*285* and IS*100* in *Yersinia pestis* and *Yersinia pseudotuberculosis* genomes. *Mol. Gen. Mikrobiol. Virusol.* **2,** 36–40.

120. Najdenski, H., Iteman, I., and Carniel, E. (1995) The genome of *Yersinia enterocolitica* is the most stable of the three pathogenic species. *Contrib. Microbiol. Immunol.* **13,** 281–284.

121. Motin, V. L., Georgescu, A. M., Elliott, J. M., et al. (2002) Genetic variability of *Yersinia pestis* isolates as predicted by PCR-based IS*100* genotyping and analysis of structural genes encoding glycerol-3-phosphate dehydrogenase (*glpD*). *J. Bacteriol.* **184,** 1019–1027.

122. Ibrahim, A., Goebel, B. M., Liesack, W., Griffiths, M., and Stackebrandt, E. (1993) The phylogeny of the genus *Yersinia* based on 16S rDNA sequences. *FEMS Microbiol. Lett.* **114,** 173–177.

123. Klevytska, A. M., Price, L. B., Schupp, J. M., Worsham, P. L., Wong, J., and Keim, P. (2001) Identification and characterization of variable-number tandem repeats in the *Yersinia pestis* genome. *J. Clin. Microbiol.* **39,** 3179–3185.

124. Adair, D. M., Worsham, P. L., Hill, K. K., et al. (2000) Diversity in a variable-number tandem repeat from *Yersinia pestis. J. Clin. Microbiol.* **38,** 1516–1519.

125. Bearden, S. W., Fetherston, J. D., and Perry, R. D. (1997) Genetic organization of the yersiniabactin biosynthetic region and construction of avirulent mutants in *Yersinia pes-tis. Infect. Immun.* **65,** 1659–1668.

126. Lindler, L. E. and Tall, B. D. (1993) *Yersinia pestis* pH 6 antigen forms fimbriae and is induced by intracellular association with macrophages. *Mol. Microbiol.* **8,** 311–324.

127. Simonet, M., Riot, B., Fortineau, N., and Berche, P. (1996) Invasin production by *Yersinia pestis* is abolished by insertion of an IS*200*-like element within the *inv* gene. *Infect. Immun.* **64,** 375–379.

128. Isberg, R. R. and Falkow, S. (1985) A single genetic locus encoded by *Yersinia pseudotu-berculosis* permits invasion of cultured animal cells by *Escherichia coli* K-12. *Nature* **317,** 262–264.

129. Miller, V. L. and Falkow, S. (1988) Evidence for two genetic loci in *Yersinia enterocolitica* that can promote invasion of epithelial cells. *Infect. Immun.* **56,** 1242–1248.

PART IV

DIAGNOSTIC DEVELOPMENT FOR BIOWARFARE AGENTS

23

Requirements for Biological Threat Identification Systems

Erik A. Henchal and George V. Ludwig

1. INTRODUCTION

Rapid identification of bioterrorism or biological warfare agents is most urgent within the first 24 h after an attack *(1–3)*. After that period, the ability to affect the prognosis of patients that have been infected with a highly virulent organism, such as *Bacillus anthracis*, sharply declines *(2)*. For less virulent organisms, identification during the pre-symptomatic stage is critical because the clinical picture is often confusing. Some patients may present with "flu-like" symptoms, rash or unusual skin lesions, respiratory or gastrointestinal illness *(1,4–5)*. Definitive identification of biological threats requires an integrated approach *(see* Fig. 1). No single identification technology is sufficient to definitively identify biological threats because of the microbial diversity, an often confusing clinical presentation, the close antigenic and genetic relatedness of some biological agents *(see* Table 1) and the consequences of misidentification *(1,4–8)*. A system of overlapping technologies and approaches are required to achieve the highest level of confidence and decrease the number of "false alarms" *(9)*. The Food and Drug Administration (FDA) has not reviewed the performance of many technologies proposed for the rapid identification of biological threat agents. All identifications must be confirmed by using "gold standard" or FDA-approved methods, such as bacterial culture. In the future, first responders, medical care providers, and laboratories will need a combination of overlapping diagnostic approaches tied together by a robust information management system when responding to a bioterrorism attack *(9)*.

Previously, we described a role for the clinical laboratory as part of a national response to biological terrorism and outlined laboratory methods for biological threat agent identification *(9,10)*. Recent bioterrorism events in the United States encourage a reassessment of the nation's preparedness *(4)*. Although the Center for Disease Control and Prevention (CDC) Laboratory Response Network for Bioterrorism (LRN) was prepared to detect the first incidences of clinical cases of anthrax *(10–12)*, it was unprepared to evaluate the larger number of environmental samples that came to the laboratories as a result of hoaxes and consequence management activities. More comprehensive analytical guidance for processing the wide variety of environmental samples, including air filters, suspicious powders, and surface swipes, were absent *(12–*

From: *Infectious Diseases: Biological Weapons Defense: Infectious Diseases and Counterterrorism*
Edited by: L. E. Lindler, F. J. Lebeda, and G. W. Korch © Humana Press Inc., Totowa, NJ

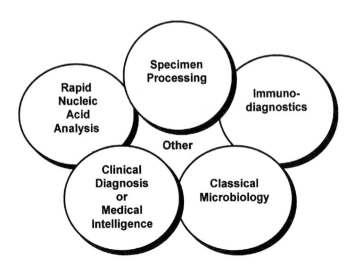

Fig. 1. Proposed Integrated Diagnostic System. Venn diagram represents the requirement for overlapping technologies with interactive information systems to obtain laboratory results with the highest level of confidence. No single approach or technology is sufficient by itself to definitively identify biological threat agents.

14). Between September 11, 2001 and December 14, 2001, Department of Defense (DOD) clinical and reference laboratories received more than 5151 clinical specimens and 11,747 environmental samples suspected of contamination by biological threat agents (US Army Medical Command, San Antonio, TX, unpublished data). CDC and civilian LRN laboratories processed an even greater number of samples (70,000–100,000; Dr. Richard Kellogg, CDC, Atlanta, GA, personal communication). Considering that this effort was the result of a limited threat through the postal service, and not because of a weapon of mass destruction (WMD), it is imperative to prepare our laboratory responses for larger incidences in the near future. Our survival after the next attack may depend on new or emerging technology and more aggressive agent identification strategies. This chapter reviews future requirements for the rapid identification of biological threats in civilian and military settings.

2. CIVILIAN REQUIREMENTS

Civilian requirements for biological threat agent identification can be placed into three different categories: first responder, clinical laboratory, and environmental screening and consequence management (*see* Table 2). No single approach can satisfy the requirements of every user category. When choosing a diagnostic approach, the user must balance cost, sensitivity, specificity, and speed. Classical clinical microbiological methods have evolved as the most cost-effective (less than $100 per standard bacteriological screening, including labor and materials) but may take more than 24 h to obtain results. Inexpensive immunodiagnostic assays can be performed in less than 15 min but are among the least sensitive. Emerging gene-detection systems may be rapid, sensitive, and specific but are among the most expensive, from $100 to $1000 per assay, including labor, materials, and equipment *(9)*.

Table 1
Characteristics of Selected Bioterrorism Agents

Biological agent • Disease	Initial clinical presentation	Clinical diagnosis "rule out"	Genetic nearest neighbors	Laboratory "rule out" methods
Bacillus anthracis				
• Inhalation anthrax	Fever, cough, malaise, and headache	• Bacterial pneumonia • Influenza • Glanders/melioidosis	• *Bacillus cereus* • *Bacillus thuringiensis* • *B. cereus*, subsp. *mycoides*	• Culture • Gammaphage-sensitivity • DFA

• Cutaneous anthrax	Pruritic macule or papule; ulcer; black eschar	• Brown recluse spider bite
		• Staphylococcal or
		  streptococcal cellulitis
		• Scrub typhus
			• Attenuated *B. anthracis*
			• Antigen-specific immuno-
			  assays
				• PCR

Yersinia pestis				
• Pneumonic Plague	Fever, cough, malaise, headache, and bloody sputum	• Pneumonia • Glanders	• *Y. enterocolitica* • *Y. pseudotuberculosis* • *Y. kristensenii* • *Y. frederiksenii*	• Phage sensitivity • Culture • PCR • DFA • Antigen-specific immunoassays
Variola major				
• Smallpox	High fever, malaise, and prostration with headache and backache	• Chicken pox • Monkeypox • Smallpox vaccine postimm unization complication	• Monkeypox virus • Cowpox virus • Vaccinia virus	• PCR • DNA sequencing
Botulinum Toxin				

• Inhalation botulism	Blurred vision and generalized weakness	• Polyradiculoneuropathy
		• Myasthenia gravis
		• Foodborne botulism
		• Chemical neurotoxins
			• *C. butyricum*
			• *C. baratii*
			• *C. perfringens*
				• Mouse neutralization
				  assay
				• Toxin-specific
				  immunoassays

(continued)

Table 1 (continued)

Biological agent • Disease	Initial clinical presentation	Clinical diagnosis "rule out"	Genetic nearest neighbors	Laboratory "rule out" methods
Francisella tularensis • Tularemia	Fever, cough, malaise, and headache	• Bubonic plague • Q fever • Brucellosis • Pneumonia • Bacterial meningitis	• *F. tularensis*, subsp. *novicida* • *F. tularensis*, subsp. *mediaasiatica* • *F. tularensis*, subsp. *holarctica* • *F. philomiragia*	• Slide agglutination • Culture • PCR • DFA
Brucella sp. • Brucellosis	Fever, cough, malaise, and headache	• Q fever • Typhoid fever • Osteomyelitis/sacroiliitis • Malaria • Bacterial meningitis	• *Acinetobacter spp.* • *Psychrobacter phenylpyruvicus* • *Haemophilus influenzae* • *Bordetella bronchiseptica* • *Ochrabacterium anthropi* • *Oligella ureolytica*	• Culture • DFA • PCR • Slide agglutination

The first-responder community, including hazardous material teams, police, fire and emergency medical service personnel, is responsible for protecting public safety and providing life-saving support in case of an overt WMD attack. The first responder needs inexpensive agent-screening methods that are easy to use and are robust for field applications (*see* Table 2). First responders use these tools to quickly differentiate between credible threats and hoaxes but not to make therapeutic decisions. Because definitive genus and species identification is not required for the immediate response, it is not necessary that frontline-screening tools have high specificity (>95%), and tests with specificities as low as 85% could be tolerated. However, it is essential that first-responder tools routinely be able to detect true positives or have high sensitivity, otherwise false-negatives might be missed and public safety threatened (*see* Table 2). Future devices that combine gene- and antigen-detection methods would improve the reliability of first responder data. Many identification tools are being developed for future first-responder applications, but only a limited number of options are available now. Commercial hand-held assays (HHAs) or lateral flow assays, similar to common pregnancy tests for home use, are available for specific environmental detection applications *(15)*. If used inappropriately, these devices may provide incorrect results, especially with test materials containing chromatic substances or cross-reacting, closely related biological agents (unpublished data). HHAs are not approved for medical use, and the CDC did not recommend them for the LRN. The DOD first developed these devices for environmental surveillance of aerosolized threats, especially using high-volume air samplers. Because of limits of detection in the range 10,000–100,000 colony-forming unit (CFU) per test aliquot (as reported by the manufacturers, unpublished data), currently available assays would be ineffective for evaluating low levels of contamination that can still cause infection *(9)*.

Consequence management teams, which respond after a bioterrorism attack and assist in decontamination, have requirements similar to the first-responder community (*see* Table 2). Inexpensive agent-screening methods that are easy to use and are robust for field use would enhance estimation of the extent of contamination and document the success of decontamination. However, the assays used must have very high sensitivity and specificity. Our experience with teams responding to the contamination of Senate office buildings in Washington, DC, and our own laboratory suggest that low levels of contamination (less than 100 CFUs) would never be tolerated by the public. Assays that document the presence of antigens and nucleic acids cannot be used by themselves to estimate infection risk of living agents. In our hands, only bacterial culture was sensitive and specific enough to establish the risk of entering contaminated areas.

For the public health laboratories, the CDC continues to implement a strategic plan that was first formulated in 2000 *(12)*. Currently, laboratories participating in the CDC LRN have the capacity to screen for *Bacillus anthracis* (anthrax), *Yersinia pestis* (plague), *Francisella tularensis* (tularemia), *Brucella* species (brucellosis), *Clostridium botulinum* toxin, and *Variola major* (smallpox) *(10–12)*. Laboratories in the LRN are expected to use assays of the highest sensitivity and specificity (*see* Table 2). However, some Sentinel (Level A) laboratories cannot perform "high complexity" testing, as defined in the Clinical Laboratory Improvement Act of 1988 (CLIA 88) or Title 42 of the Code of Federal Regulations, section 493 *(16)*. CLIA 88 regulates the operation of laboratories that support clinical diagnosis of disease. Since 1999, the FDA is respon-

Table 2
Characteristics of Identification Approaches for Different Civilian Scenarios

Response scenario	Complexity[a]	Ruggedness[b]	Speed	Throughput[c]	Cost[d]	Sensitivity[e]	Specificity[e]	Sample
First responder	Waived	High	<15 min	1–20 samples per hour	<$1.00	>95%	>85%	Environmental and clinical
Clinical laboratory	Medium to high	Low	1–24 h	20–100 samples per 24 h	$1 to $100	>98%	>98%	Clinical
Environmental screening and consequence management	Waived	High	<15 min	1–20 samples per h	<$1.00	>95%	>95%	Environmental

[a]Complexity is defined in 42 CFR 493.16 Laboratories performing "high-complexity" tests must satisfy the maximum personnel, quality control, and proficiency testing requirements specified in the regulation. Personnel performing "waived" tests require little or no oversight.

[b]Ruggedness refers to the ability of a test to be performed with acceptable result variation (Correlate of Variation of less than 15%) under the conditions of use. Tests intended by First Responder and Consequence Management Teams must be able to perform in extremes of environmental conditions by personnel with limited training.

[c]Throughput requirements were estimated based on criteria at the US Army Medical Research Institute for Infectious Diseases (Fort Detrick, MD) set during October to December 2001.

[d]Costs are estimated and depend on the price and cost tolerance of the user.

[e]Sensitivity is defined as the analytical ability to detect a true positive. Specificity is defined as the ability to detect a true negative.

sible for placing clinical assays into categories of complexity: low (waived), moderate, and high. Extensive lists of clinical tests and kits by category are available (*see* http://www.fda.gov/cdrh/clia/). Laboratories certified under the CLIA 88 inspection program to perform "high-complexity" tests must satisfy the maximum personnel, quality control, and proficiency testing requirements specified in the regulation. All unassigned tests or tests not approved by FDA are automatically assigned to the "high-complexity" category. Thus, Sentinel laboratories screen samples by using classical microbiology methods and forward suspicious cultures and samples to Reference laboratories at the state or county level. Reference laboratories were first equipped with procedures for six biological threats and specialized reagents, including fluorescently labeled reference antibodies and anthrax-specific gammaphage. Recently, the CDC began to equip select Reference laboratories with polymerase chain reaction gene amplification assays, which were previously available only at the CDC and DOD reference laboratories. In the future, the CDC will push new diagnostic technologies to the Reference laboratories and broaden the scope of etiological agents that can be identified. The CDC is focusing future development on the validation of assays for the rapid identification of the filoviruses (Ebola and Marburg), arenaviruses (Lassa fever and Junin viruses), alphaviruses (Venezuelan equine encephalitis virus, eastern equine encephalitis virus, and western equine encephalitis virus), *Coxiella burnetii* (Q fever), ricin toxin, *Burkholderia mallei* (glanders), and staphylococcal enterotoxin B. Among the new identification tools being introduced are time-resolved fluorescence assays for the sensitive detection of agent-specific antigens and toxins *(17)*.

A weakness of the CDC LRN is the limited identification capabilities that are available to Sentinel clinical laboratories, which are closest to the patient and the physician. The CDC LRN currently places its most sophisticated capabilities at the level of the state public health laboratory or higher in the network, which may be far removed from the patient bedside. In reality, Sentinel laboratories are at the "frontline" of our bioterrorism response *(10,11)*. Sentinel laboratories can "rule out" other pathogens but must refer out more complex testing that is essential for definitive threat agent identification. The time required to perform Sentinel procedures, transport specimens to another LRN member laboratory and begin "rule in" analysis (*see* Table 3) may result in an increase in morbidity and mortality during a WMD event *(3,18)*. During investigation of a recent bioterrorism incident in Florida, the hospital clinical laboratory identified suspicious bacilli in the cerebrospinal fluid and blood of the first fatal case of bioterrorism-related inhalation anthrax within hours. However, the LRN state public health laboratory did not report the definitive identification until 48 h later *(4)*. If this had been a WMD event, this delay might have resulted in hundreds or thousands of additional deaths and increased hospitalization costs *(3,18)*. Because of the short duration of illness and rapid onset of some classical biological warfare agents, such as *B. anthracis*, *Y. pestis*, or botulinum toxin, the window for therapeutic intervention is exceedingly short (*see* Table 3). After the destruction of the World Trade Center towers, air transportation of specimens across the country was shut down for several days (September 11–18, 2001). If the September–October 2001 anthrax attacks had occurred at the same time as the interruption of air travel, the national response would have been severely handicapped. Because Sentinel laboratories do not have methods and reagents for identifying toxins, the detection of botulinum neurotoxin, staphylococcus entero-

Table 3
CDC LRN Sentinel Laboratory Turn-Around Times for Selected Biological Threats

Biological agent	Level A procedures Minimum turn around time[a]	Projected % fatalities (untreated cases)[c]	Incubation period[c]	Disease duration (after onset)[c]
B. anthracis	18–24 h	>80%	1–6 d	3–5 d
Y. pestis	2 d	90%	2–3 d	1–6 d
V. major (smallpox)	NA	30%	7–17 d	4 wk
Botulinum toxin[b]	NA	30%	24–36 h	1–3 d
F. tularensis	3 d	5–20%	1–21 d	>2 wk
Brucella sp.	2–7 d	<5%	5–60 d	Weeks to months
Viral hemorrhagic fevers	NA	>75%	4–21 d	7–16 d

[a]Direct staining of clinical and environmental specimens is possible for *B. anthracis, Y. pestis, Brucella* spp., and *F. tularensis*; however, some culture-based "rule out" is required. "NA" means that suspect specimens must be forwarded to the nearest Reference laboratory or directly to the CDC (e.g., *Variola major*).

[b]Sentinel laboratory procedures are available for detection of classical *Clostridium* infections but not for purified toxin. Sentinel laboratories can only identify *Clostridium* bacteria to the genus level. Result turn around times for *Clostridium sp.* will range from 3 to 5 d.

[c]See refs. *19–25.*

toxin, and ricin toxin, which can be delivered in cell-free preparations, must wait until there are suspicious casualties. Moreover, the CDC LRN emphasizes the identification of the etiological agents, but neglects providing assays for identifying agent-specific IgM and IgG antibodies, which are important tools for confirming clinical diagnosis of other diseases. Level B protocols only describe simple agglutination assays for detecting patient antibodies to *Brucella* sp. and *Francisella*. However, more sophisticated tools could be made available by using microplate enzyme-linked immunoassays, electrochemiluminescence, or time-resolved immunoassays for all of the highest priority biological threats *(9)*. Scientists at the US Army Medical Research Institute of Infectious Diseases (Fort Detrick, MD) and the Navy Medical Research Center (Silver Spring, MD) have developed microplate enzyme-linked immunoassays for detecting agent-specific IgG or IgM antibodies for 84 etiological agents, including classical biological warfare, endemic, and enzootic diseases (unpublished data). Immunoassays that can sensitively detect agent-specific antibodies might be a reasonable substitute for agent-detection assays for bacteria or viruses that cannot be cultured safely outside of federal reference centers. For example, the culture of variola virus would be a safety hazard for a hospital clinical virology laboratory; however, protocols could be developed to inactivate sera and safely screen for the presence of diagnostic antibodies for smallpox that appear by the sixth day of rash *(21)*.

The response of the front-line clinical laboratory can be improved by the development of rapid identification systems with limited test complexity. The best systems would be compatible with raw clinical specimens, have high sensitivity and specificity, and can be performed rapidly while the patient is still in the examining room. Some automated and self-contained identification systems may qualify for a waiver of FDA regulation *(26)*. CLIA 88 allowed the waiver of regulatory oversight if the tests employ methodologies that are so simple and accurate as to render the likelihood of erroneous results negligible or pose no reasonable risk of harm to the patient if the test is performed incorrectly *(16,26)*. Assay systems that are self-contained and require little user manipulation or interpretation would fulfill this requirement. However, future systems must be compatible with high-throughput laboratory systems available in hospital clinical laboratories, not only for agents of bioterrorism but also for endemic infectious diseases. Separate systems for endemic infectious diseases and bioterrorism agents would not be tolerated by most laboratory managers attempting to contain costs.

By far the largest number of samples processed since the first bioterrorism attacks of September 2001 were from environmental sources. More than 9000 samples were taken during remediation efforts in Senate office buildings. The CDC LRN was not designed to process environmental samples. Although the Environmental Protection Agency, the National Institutes of Occupational Safety and Health, and the DOD organized environmental sampling teams, few civilian federal or state partners were prepared to provide laboratory or analytical support to bioterrorism consequence management and remediation efforts. Response teams and laboratories initially used various of analytical approaches, including immunodiagnostic assays, rapid gene amplification systems, and HHAs. The CDC cautioned against the sole use of experimental and unvalidated methods to assess contamination *(14)*. Because of its sensitivity even at the lowest levels of contamination, only bacterial culture provided the analytical performance necessary to protect health and safety *(9)*. To clear buildings after an attack and provide a rapid evaluation of decontamination efforts, consequence management teams require rapid, low complexity identification assays of the highest sensitivity (see Table 2). Assays of higher specificity and cost would not be required once the contaminating agent has been identified.

3. MILITARY REQUIREMENTS

Military service members receive most of their care through medical troop clinics or primary care facilities (27). These limited-care clinics depend on larger medical treatment facilities or hospitals to provide comprehensive laboratory support. In the near future, rapid identification of biological threats in military patient populations may depend on the availability of identification tools that can be used in the equivalent of a doctor's office or an emergency room. Tests would have to meet the criteria for waived or low complexity assays to be run outside of an accredited laboratory (16,26). On the battlefield, the combat medic or the Navy corpsman's role is to provide immediate life-saving care. It is doubtful whether adding additional diagnostic capability to the medic's supply chest would improve the response to the first use of a biological war agent. However, lightweight, rapid, and sensitive devices, similar to those intended for use in emergency rooms, would be appropriate for the first level of definitive medical care on the battlefield.

DOD medical treatment facilities within the continental United States (CONUS) have the same standards of healthcare and laboratory requirements as civilian hospitals. Military clinical laboratories, especially in CONUS, are linked to the CDC LRN through the joint armed services Center for Clinical Laboratory Medicine (Armed Forces Institute of Pathology, Washington, DC), which acts as a "gatekeeper" to the civilian response network. All participating military clinical laboratories (over 113 laboratories currently) adhere to guidelines of the LRN. However, practices in overseas laboratories may be modified based on unique military requirements. The military laboratories enrolled in the LRN as Reference laboratories may be able to respond to incidences of bioterrorism more quickly than public health LRN laboratories. Although the DOD has many stand-alone laboratories supporting epidemiology and medical research, many military Reference laboratories are located at DOD regional medical centers. Because military medical treatment facilities are more closely linked than civilian centers, reference laboratory services and high-complex testing are located closer to the point of care. Front-line laboratories are backed by military national laboratory centers at the US Army Medical Research Institute of Infectious Diseases (Fort Detrick, MD), the Navy Medical Research Center (Silver Spring, MD), Institute for Environmental Safety and Occupational Health Risk Analysis (Brooks Air Force Base, TX), and the Armed Forces Institute of Pathology (Washington, DC).

Military laboratories and medical treatment facilities located overseas (OCONUS) may have different testing responsibilities than domestic US facilities. OCONUS laboratories, especially field laboratories serving war-fighting commands, support field preventive medicine activities, and provide confirmatory services for various environmental biological warfare agent detectors. These laboratories, such as the Army's 520th Theater Army Medical Laboratory, US Air Force Biological Assessment Teams (or Biological Warfare Defense Laboratories), Theater Medical Surveillance Teams, Navy Environmental Preventive Medicine Units, and other activities, play a critical role to protect the health of service members worldwide. Because CONUS reference centers may be far removed from theaters of operation, these military laboratories require the same capabilities as the CDC Level B public health laboratories but in a lightweight and robust form. Few civilian clinical laboratories could provide analytical services in the limited confines of a military field laboratory.

4. THE FUTURE

The most significant deficiency of the nation's bioterrorism response during Fall 2001 was the lack of effective communication networks. For the most part, CDC LRN and DOD laboratories were prepared scientifically and technically to identify the etiological cause of anthrax. However, the nation lacked information management and communication systems to exchange information between different agencies and transmit results rapidly to senior leaders. The laboratories, which were processing hundreds of samples per day as a result of hoaxes or credible threats, were unable to transmit information or to report results in a timely manner. Often during the height of the crisis, multiple teleconferences, briefings, or frequent electronic mailings were needed to transmit preliminary and confirmed results to the senior managers of the national response to bioterrorism. There are several electronic networks being developed to resolve this problem. Soon, the CDC plans to create or enhance a secure LRN website to support secure communications, Web-based laboratory reporting, and sentinel surveillance. The CDC's Health Alert Network is a nationwide, integrated information and communications system for distributing health alerts, prevention guidelines, and other information, as well as distance learning, national disease surveillance, and electronic laboratory reporting. The Health Alert Network now connects the public health departments of all 50 states and some US territories. Additionally, the CDC is developing real-time surveillance and analytical methods as part of the CDC Enhanced Surveillance Project (ESP). During special events, CDC ESP will monitor sentinel hospital emergency department visit data to establish syndrome baseline and threshold. The ESP was tested at national and international conferences and meetings, including the World Trade Organization Ministerial in Seattle (1999), the Republican and Democratic National Conventions (2000), and the Super Bowl/Gasparilla Festival in Tampa, FL (2001). To align and integrate the large number of state and federal disease reporting systems, the CDC is setting up the National Electronic Disease Surveillance System, which will permit more accurate and timely reporting of disease information. For more information, *see* www.bt.cdc.gov (valid January 18, 2002).

Since 1819, the US Army has actively collected wound, disease, and injury information in military units, camps, and posts *(28)*. Presidential Decision Directive NTSC-7 established national policy and implementing actions to address the threat of emerging infectious diseases by improving surveillance, prevention, and response measures *(29)*. In 1997 the DOD established the Global Emerging Infections Surveillance and Response System (DOD-GEIS) *(30)*. GEIS provides an early-warning system for emerging infections by building on an established network of worldwide DOD medical research units and the global DOD military health system. The research units monitor the incidence of selected infections and report on new threats, endemic diseases, and epidemics. Although efforts focus on identifying new strains of drug-resistant malaria, drug-resistant diarrhea, influenza, and other febrile illnesses including dengue, infections caused by agents of bioterrorism may also be detected.

The Lightweight Epidemiological Advanced Detection and Emergency Response System (LEADERS) is a comprehensive set of Web-based software tools and data storage capabilities *(31)*. LEADERS, which emerged from research supported by the Defense Advanced Research Projects Agency with commercial partners and the US Air Force, will support the collection, storage, analysis, and distribution of critical sets of medical data to aid with rapid, effective response to natural disease outbreak or over/ covert biological attacks to the civilian populations and military forces. In 2001, information systems based on LEADERS were transferred to the commercial sector as a source of medical surveillance data for subscribers. The DOD will continue to seek approaches to improve real-time disease surveillance, which will require the development of comprehensive, high-throughput laboratory support systems to be effective.

The Department of Defense is developing the Joint Biological Agent Identification and Diagnostic System (JBAIDS). JBAIDS, which will be fielded by 2004, will be a comprehensive integrated diagnostic capable of reliably identifying multiple biological threat agents and endemic infectious diseases (*see* Fig. 1). Systems will include gene and antigen-detection systems and other emerging technologies linked to an interactive information management framework. JBAIDS will support reliable, fast, and specific identification of biological agents from various clinical and environmental sources and samples. JBAIDS will enhance healthcare by guiding the choice of appropriate treatments, effective preventive measures, and prophylaxis at the earliest stage of disease. JBAIDS will identify and quantify biological agents that could effect military readiness and effectiveness. Technologies included in JBAIDS will be selected based on their reliability, technological maturity, and supportability.

5. VALIDATION REQUIREMENTS

Diagnostic assays using culture, animals models, immunodiagnostic assays, and gene amplification assays for many classical biological warfare threats have existed in DOD reference laboratories for more than 10 yr *(9)*. Beginning in 1999, identification protocols for *B. anthracis* (anthrax), *Y. pestis* (plague), *F. tularensis* (tularemia), *Brucella* species (brucellosis), *C. botulinum* toxin, and *V. major* virus (smallpox); reagents; and diagnostic approaches were shared with the CDC to enhance the domestic LRN. Since 1999, the CDC and its partners identified and developed improved gene and antigen detection assays by using emerging diagnostic technologies *(9,10,12)*. The identification assays and approaches currently available can be used for medical research, forensic analysis, epidemiological studies, and environmental surveillance without restriction from the FDA, as long as the results do not have a bearing on the clinical diagnosis or treatment of patients *(16,26)*. Although the testing of environmental samples or forensic samples is unregulated, the FDA may wish to review the performance data of tests not intended for clinical use if populations will be treated prophylactically after a bioterrorism attack. It would be a mistake to set a lower standard for the performance of tests on environmental samples when the consequences of a misidentification are so great.

As discussed previously, most of the assays would be classified as having "high complexity." Clinical use of these assays would require FDA approval and validation studies to determine accuracy, precision, analytical sensitivity, analytical specificity (with and without interfering substances), reportable range of patient test results, reference range, and any other performance characteristics as described in 42 CRF 493.1213 *(16)*. Because infections with threat agents occur rarely, and clinical populations of sufficient size are unavailable, validation and approval of new medical diagnostic assays for many bioterrorism agents will be difficult.

Medical devices, which are regulated through the FDA Center for Devices and Radiological Health (Rockville, MD), are placed into three classes (I, II, and III) according to the increasing risk *(26)*. The FDA has general and special controls for class I and II devices, respectively. Class I devices are exempt from premarket notification and are used as adjuncts to the clinical diagnosis or with gold standard diagnostic assays. Special controls for class II devices include labeling requirements, mandatory performance standards, and postmarket surveillance. Both class I and II devices must undergo premarket review and clearance by the FDA in accordance with section 510 (k) of the Food, Drug and Cosmetic Act *(26,32)*. Class III is the most stringent regulatory category for devices for which insufficient information exists to assure safety and effectiveness solely through general or special controls. Premarket approval is the required process of scientific review to ensure the safety and effectiveness of Class III devices. Many older identification assays currently employed in the CDC LRN, such as the gammaphage sensitivity test and immunofluorescence assays, were developed before 1976 and were used in federal reference laboratories in conjunction with standard culture methods. These approaches, if classified as class II devices, may be able to be distributed in the future to CDC LRN members after a FDA-cleared 510 (k) Premarket Notification *(26)*. Other assays developed for use on rapid gene-amplification systems, such as the RAPID (Idaho Technologies, Salt Lake City, UT) or SmartCycler instruments (Cepheid, Sunnyvale, CA), which that can identify agents in less than 40 min after specimen processing, will require approval as class III devices, until review and approval by the FDA and the CDC. Both the CDC and the DOD are planning qualifying and validation studies of emerging gene- and antigen-detection methods for future FDA review.

6. SUMMARY

Recent bioterrorism incidents have underscored the need for vigilant preparation for a more dangerous future. Although many new bioterrorism response programs have begun, the first responders, clinical laboratories, and others still require better diagnostic systems to rapidly identify biological threats. A comprehensive system with smart information management and overlapping technologies will improve the reliability of our test results in the future. We can expect the development of some systems, such as the JBAIDS, to be fast tracked to enhance military and domestic preparedness. Significant challenges still remain in completing validation studies and clearance of proposed methods by the FDA. Accomplishing this effort may require a consortium of partners from industry, federal reference, and national laboratories, and state and local public health laboratories.

ACKNOWLEDGMENTS

We acknowledge the contributions of Melanie Dautle, Randy Schoepp, Leonard Wasieloski, and William Nauschuetz for reviewing the manuscript. Jon Woods, Jeffrey Teska, and Gerry Howe reviewed rule-out diagnosis and agent identification information. We acknowledge the professionalism and dedication of the Diagnostic Systems Division staff and contractor employees who provided continuous 24/7 counter-bioterrorism support for Operation Noble Eagle from September 11, 2001 to May 15, 2002.

REFERENCES

1. Franz, D. R., Jahrling, P. B., Friedlander, A. M., et al. (1997) Clinical recognition and management of patients exposed to biological warfare agents. *JAMA* **278,** 399–411.
2. Friedlander, A. M., Welkos, S. L., Pitt, M. L., et al. (1993) Postexposure prophylaxis against experimental inhalation anthrax. *J. Infect. Dis.* **167,** 1239–1241.
3. Giovachino, M. and Carey, N. (2000) Modeling the consequences of bioterrorism response. *Mil. Med.* **166,** 925–930.
4. Jernigan, J. A., Stephens, D. S., Ashford, D. A., et al. (2001) Bioterrorism-related inhalational anthrax: the first 10 cases reported in the United States. *Emerg. Infect. Dis.* **7,** 933–944.
5. Cieslak, T. J., Rowe, J. R., Kortepeter, M. G., et al. (2000) A field-expedient algorithmic approach to the clinical management of chemical and biological casualties. *Mil. Med.* **165,** 659–662.
6. Finlay, B. J. and Esteban, G. F. (2001) Exploring Leeuwenhoek's legacy: the abundance and diversity of protozoa. *Int. Microbiol.* **4,** 125–133.
7. Logan, N. A. and Turnbull, P. C. B. (1999) Bacillus and recently derived genera, in *Manual of Clinical Microbiology*, 7th ed., (Murray, P. R., Baron, E. J., Pfaller, M. A., Tenover, F. C., and Yolken, R. H., eds.), American Society for Microbiology, Washington, DC, pp. 357–369.
8. Keim, P., Kalif, A., Schupp, J., et al. (1997) Molecular evolution and diversity in *Bacillus anthracis* as detected by amplified fragment length polymorphism markers. *J. Bacteriol.* **179,** 818–824.
9. Henchal, E. A., Teska, J. D., Ludwig, G. V., Shoemaker, D. R., and Ezzell, J. W. (2001) Current laboratory methods for biological threat agent identification, in *Laboratory Aspects of Biowarfare*, Vol. 21. (Marty, A. M., ed.), W.B. Sanders, Philadelphia, PA, pp. 661–678.
10. Henchal, E. A., Teska, J., and Ezzell, J. W. (2000) Bioterrorism response: a role for the clinical laboratory. *Clin. Lab. News* **26,** 14–18.
11. Gilchrist, M. J. R. (2000) A national laboratory network for bioterrorism: evolution from a prototype network of laboratories performing routine surveillance. *Mil. Med.* **156(Suppl.),** 28–34.
12. (2000) Biological and chemical terrorism: strategic plan for preparedness and response. *MMWR Morb. Mortal. Wkly. Rep.* **49,** 1–14.
13. (2001) Notice to Readers: Interim guidelines for investigation of and response to *Bacillus anthracis* exposures. *MMWR Morb. Mortal. Wkly. Rep.* **50,** 987–990.
14. (2001) Use of onsite technologies for rapidly assessing environmental *Bacillus anthracis* contamination on surfaces in buildings. *MMWR Morb. Mortal. Wkly. Rep.* **50,** 1087.
15. Burans, J., Keleher, A., O'Brien, T., Hager, J., Plummer, A., and Morgan, C. (1996) Rapid method for the diagnosis of *Bacillus anthracis* infection in clinical samples using a hand-held assay. *Salisbury Med. Bull.* **87,** 36, 37.
16. Title 42, Code of Federal Regulations, section 493.
17. Smith, D. R., Rossi, C. A., Kijek, T. M., Henchal, E. A., and Ludwig, G. V. (2001) Comparison of dissociation-enhanced lanthanide fluorescent immunoassays to enzyme-linked immunosorbent assays for detection of staphylococcal enterotoxin *B, Yersinia pestis*-specific F1 antigen, and Venezuelan equine encephalitis virus. *Clin. Diag. Lab. Immunol.* **8,** 1070–1075.

18. Kaufmann, A. F., Meltzer, M. I., and Schmid, G. P. (1997) The economic impact of a bioterrorist attack: are prevention and postattack intervention programs justifiable? *Emerg. Infect. Dis.* **3,** 83–94.
19. Inglesby, T. V., Henderson, D. A., Bartlett, J. G., et al. (1999) Anthrax as a biological weapon: medical and public health management. Working Group on Civilian Biodefense. *JAMA* **281,** 1735–1745.
20. Inglesby, T. V., Dennis, D. T., Henderson, D. A., et al. (2000) Plague as a biological weapon: medical and public health management. Working Group on Civilian Biodefense. *JAMA* **283,** 2281–2290.
21. Henderson, D. A., Inglesby, T. V., Bartlett, J. G., et al. (1999) Smallpox as a biological weapon: medical and public health management. Working Group on Civilian Biodefense. *JAMA* **281,** 2127–2137.
22. Arnon, S. S., Schechter, R. , Inglesby, T. V., et al. (2001) Working group on civilian biodefense. botulinum toxin as a biological weapon: medical and public health management. *JAMA* **285,** 1059–1070.
23. Dennis, D. T., Inglesby, T. V., Henderson, D. A., et al. (2001) Working group on civilian biodefense. Tularemia as a biological weapon: medical and public health management. *JAMA* **285,** 2763–2773.
24. Hoover, D. L. and Friedlander, A. M. Brucellosis, in *Medical Aspects of Chemical and Biological Warfare.* (Zajchuk, R., ed.), Borden Institute, Washington, DC, pp. 513–522.
25. Isaacson, M. (2001) Viral hemorrhagic fever hazards for travelers in Africa. *Clin. Infect. Dis.* **33,** 1707–1712.
26. Gutman, S., Richter, K., and Alpert, S. (1998) Update on FDA regulation of in vitro diagnostic devices. *JAMA* **280,** 190–192.
27. Department of the Army. (1991) *FM 8-10. Health Service Support in a Theater of Operations.* Washington, DC.
28. Bayne-Jones, S. (1968) *The Evolution of Preventive Medicine in the United States Army, 1607–1939.* US Government Printing Office, Washington, DC.
29. Presidential Decision Directive, NTSC-7, Addressing the threat of Emerging Infectious Diseases, June 12, 1996.
30. Brachman, P. S., O'Maonaigh, H. C., and Miller, R. N. (2001) *Perspectives on the Department of Defense Global Emerging Infections Surveillance and Response System: A Program Review.* National Academy Press, Washington, DC.
31. Lightweight Epidemiological Advanced Detection and Emergency Response System (LEADERS). http://www.eyt.com\pdf\Leaders_Med_Readiness.ppt (valid February 1, 2002).
32. The Medical Device Amendments of 1976. Public Law No. 94-295, 90 Stat 539.

24

DNA-Based Diagnostic Tests for Detection and Identification of Biological Weapons

Luther E. Lindler, David Norwood, Michael Dobson, and Ted L. Hadfield

1. INTRODUCTION

Classically, microorganisms have been identified by bacteriological means *(1)*. Typically, this would involve plating of the specimen on suitable growth media, incubation at least overnight to allow growth, streak purification of individual suspect colonies followed by another overnight incubation and inoculation of specific biochemical reactions that are useful for differentiation of the organism from other genera or species possibly followed by a third overnight incubation. Thus, the "gold standard" for the identification of bacteria that might be used to identify an organism included in a bioweapon is cultivation followed by differential testing to specifically identify the agent. In the best case, the amount of time needed to identify these organisms could be reduced if specific antiserum was available that could be used after the initial specimen has been plated and incubated to obtain individual bacterial colonies (*see* Chapter 25). Thus, a presumptive identification using antibody-based methods would be available after approx 24 h. Beside being time consuming, this process produces a large burden in terms of logistics to get the reagents and equipment to the site of testing. The above scenario is for a bacterial agent and the logistical burden is even heavier for viral agents given the specialized reagents and equipment needed for their identification. This is simply not acceptable because therapy for infections caused by these agents generally must begin within the first few hours after exposure if the patient is to survive *(2)*.

There are several possible end users for new diagnostic technologies. The number of programs aimed at the development of these new identification technologies is far to numerous to be covered in this chapter. Each user will have a unique set of requirements such that not all technologies will be suitable for a particular application. This aspect of biological agent identification is covered in Chapter 23. However, DNA-based methods will likely play a large part in any of these future technologies. The assays described in the following sections are examples of current tests either being used or developed by the US Army, US Air Force, and US Navy laboratories to identify biological warfare (BW) agents. Generally, the assays described in the following sections are similar to the assays used during Fall 2001 in response to the anthrax attack in the United States. These assays have been developed with military applica-

From: *Infectious Diseases: Biological Weapons Defense: Infectious Diseases and Counterterrorism*
Edited by: L. E. Lindler, F. J. Lebeda, and G. W. Korch © Humana Press Inc., Totowa, NJ

tions in mind but are readily adaptable to civilian usage. Furthermore, these tests and platforms likely represent the first generation of technology in the DNA-based identification of infectious agents with many improvements to come in the future. The intention here is to present to the reader the current state of this particular application of laboratory diagnostics to the problem of identification of agents of BW. It should be mentioned that the primer/probe sequences have not been included intentionally for security reasons.

2. METHODS AND HARDWARE

For years, we have known that the detection of infectious agents by identification of their DNA offers significant advantages of speed and sensitivity over more classical techniques such as culturing followed by biochemical or antibody-based assays. This is especially true of the BW agents because several of them grow slowly, taking days to form visible colonies. Although the promise of DNA-based identification of microorganisms has been known for some time, very few of these assays have actually been used in a clinical setting. This trend has not been followed by the military in the case of the development of identification assays for the agents of BW. This trend-breaking attitude has been at least partially precipitated by the need to be able to rapidly move the testing capability and to process large numbers of samples once "on station." There are numerous possible chemistries employed to detect amplification of DNA. This section covers the various modern fluorescent chemistries used in detection of DNA by fluorescence as well as the platforms capable of sensing those products. We limit our discussion to the modern techniques employed by the Department of Defense (DOD) laboratories and do not discuss chemistries such as enzyme-linked detection of polymerase chain reaction (PCR) amplification.

2.1. Polymerase Chain Reaction

The ability to amplify DNA specifically has been employed to develop many assays that can detect various genes *(3–5)*. However, most of the detection methods utilized gel electrophoresis and staining to visualize the PCR product to analyze the reaction. Recently, Molecular Probes, Inc. (Eugene, OR) developed a dye, designated as SYBR green, that emits fluorescent light when intercalated into double-stranded DNA *(6–8)*. Although the dye does not differentiate specific from nonspecific amplification, it can allow the detection of amplification of agent DNA without the need for cultivation *(6,7)*. If the oligonucleotide primers are specific, SYBR green can be a cost effective and rapid means of qualitative and quantitative analysis of PCR amplification. The production of product can be assayed in real time as an increase in fluorescence with increasing reaction time. Alternatively, melting curve analysis can be performed where the DNA product is subjected to increasing temperature, and a decrease in fluorescence is seen when the double-stranded product denatures. The latter method produces a melting peak temperature that is characteristic according to the size and guanine plus cytosine content of the PCR product. Accordingly, SYBR green reactions can be a good method of preliminary screening of samples for the presence of pathogen DNA.

2.2. Probe Degradation-Based Assay

The degradation of a fluorescent DNA probe can be used to detect the specific amplification of a PCR product *(9)*. During the amplification of DNA, the polymerase

5'- to 3'-nuclease activity hydrolyzes the probe annealed to the PCR product into individual mononucleotides as shown in Fig. 1A. This in turn allows the fluorescence from the 5'-label to increase because of decreased quenching by the label at the 3'-end of the probe *(10)*. This amplification product detection chemistry has been commonly referred to as a hydrolysis reaction, 5'-nuclease assay, degradation probe reaction or TaqMan (Roche Molecular Systems, Indianapolis, IN). The number of applications of this chemistry are numerous and beyond the scope of this chapter.

2.3. Hybridization Probe Assay

A second method for the detection of the specific amplification of a PCR product is the Hybridization Probe reaction (Roche Molecular Diagnostics) shown in Fig. 1B. This method *(11)* relies on fluorescence resonance energy transfer (FRET) where the interacting light-absorbing and -emitting molecules must be in close proximity to one another. Also, their absorption and emission spectra must be compatible. The two light-sensitive molecules interact most effectively when they bind in close proximity on an amplified fragment of DNA and position the photoactive molecules next to each other such that light is emitted and can be detected by the instrumentation (*see* Fig. 1B). Binding of the labeled probes to the amplified product can be analyzed during the reaction (real-time) to detect the production of the specific DNA fragment. Alternatively, after the reaction is completed, a melting curve can be performed to characterize the thermal interaction of the probes with the product and detect single nucleotide polymorphisms. Both of these types of data analysis have been used to develop assays based on Hybridization Probe chemistry *(12)*.

2.4. Detection Platforms

The platforms for real-time PCR detection are listed in Table 1. Although there are other machines available, we have limited our discussion to the instruments that are commonly used in the military diagnostics programs. Each of these instruments has advantages and disadvantages. In this section, we discuss each of the platforms. The right cycler for an individual need depends on the specific application and requirements.

2.4.1. The Ruggedized Advanced Pathogen Identification System and the Roche LightCycler

The Ruggedized Advanced Pathogen Identification System (RAPID) was developed by Idaho Technologies, Inc. as a modification of the LC-32 LightCycler (Roche Diagnostics, Mannheim, Germany). The instrument was funded by the US Air Force to be hardened for field use. The RAPID is basically a ruggedized version of the LightCycler. The RAPID instrument uses 110, 220, or 12 V electrical sources. Sample capacity is 32 cuvets. The reaction volume is 20 µL, but as little as 5 µL can be used for PCR. The reaction vessel is a glass capillary which intensifies the fluorescent signal above the fluorometer. Each sample is surveyed for fluorescent signal by rotating the capillaries over the fluorometer lens at a prescribed time depending on the type of assay. The instruments heats and cools using air. This results in very fast changes in temperature adding to the specificity of the reaction. The device reads three colors allowing three reactions to be detected in a single tube. Additionally, several modifications of the software compared to the LightCycler were designed to make the device user friendly. A simplified start-up screen allows selection of batch assays or screening assays. Batch assays offer the greatest number of tests per set of controls (30 tests, 1 positive control,

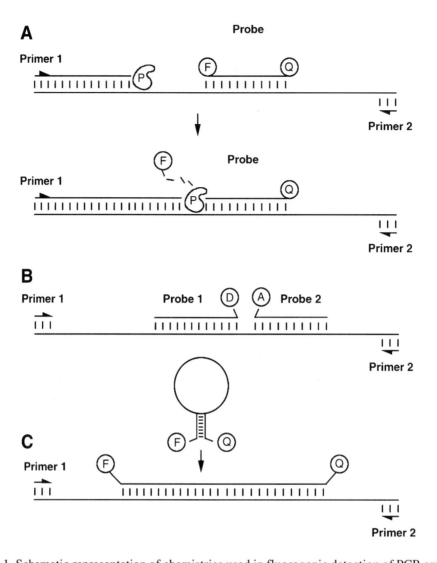

Fig. 1. Schematic representation of chemistries used in fluorogenic detection of PCR amplification reactions. **(A)** shows the general properties of a 5'-nuclease reaction. The probe is labeled with a fluorescent dye on the 5'-(designated F) and 3'-(designated Q) ends. During the reaction when PCR product is produced, the probe hybridizes with the product. During DNA synthesis, the polymerase (designated P) 5'-nuclease activity cleaves the probe releasing the fluorescent dyes and causing the fluorescence emitted by the dye labeled F to increase. **(B)** shows a probe-PCR product interaction during the hybridization probe reaction. The donor probe (designated D) binds next to the acceptor-labeled probe (designated A) and excites the emission of fluorescence. As more probes bind to the accumulating PCR product during the reaction, the amount of fluorescence increases. Alternatively, if melting peak analysis is performed, the probes melt off of the PCR product and fluorescence decreases with increasing temperature. **(C)** shows the probe used in the "molecular beacons" fluorescence-based DNA detection assay. Before PCR product is produced, the inverted repeats at the ends of the probe bring the fluorescent dye (designated F) and the quenching dye (labeled Q) into close proximity. As PCR product is produced, the probe binds and the F and Q labels are moved apart, thus, resulting in increased fluorescence as PCR product accumulates. As with the hybridization probe reaction, melting peak analysis can be performed to determine when the probe melts from the PCR product. Because this chemistry is not currently used by any of the DOD laboratories in assay development, it is not discussed in the text. The reader is referred to the Internet site http://www.molecular-beacons.org/ for further information.

Table 1
Detection Platforms Commonly Used in Various Diagnostics Programs to Identify Agents of Biowarfare/Bioterrorism

Instrument	Manufacturer	Internet address
RAPID	Idaho Technologies, Inc.	www.idahotech.com
LightCycler	Roche Diagnostics	www.lightcycler-online.com
Smart Cycler	Cepheid	www.cepheid.com
iCycler	Bio-Rad Laboratories, Inc.	www.biorad.com
7700 Sequence Detector	Applied Biosystems, Inc.	www.appliedbiosystems.com
7900 Sequence Detector	Applied Biosystems, Inc.	www.appliedbiosystems.com

and 1 negative control). The screening selection offers a series of screening tests, i.e., on one run you could test for *Bacillus anthracis, Yersinia pestis, Francisella tularensis, Brucella, Coxiella,* and *Burkholderia mallei* (glanders). This requires 12 wells for positive and negative controls, 18 of the remaining 20 wells are used to test three samples for each of the organisms. Both "screening" and "batch" screens allow the user to enter specimen identification data. The instrument can be preprogrammed for various of tests so the end user only has to select the test they want to use. Alternatively, the user can program the cycling parameters for each assay he is going to perform. This device has the advantage of a lot of flexibility for the skilled user while offering a user-friendly platform for nonskilled users. Further, for the nonskilled user, the instrument can interpret the results of the thermal cycling and provide a report.

2.4.2. The Cepheid Smart Cycler

The Cepheid Smart Cycler *(13,14)* is a device similar to the Idaho Technologies Light Cycler but developed through US Army contracts. The device comes in two configurations, a laboratory model and a field model *(14,15)*. This device consists of 16 independent thermal cyclers (I-CORE®, intelligent cooling/heating optical reaction module) employing a microelectronic design with control through a computer. Because each thermal cycler is independently controlled, one can perform PCR with assays using primers with different Tms in the same run, or you can perform PCR and reverse transcription-PCR (RT-PCR) in the same run. The instrument reads four colors allowing four-color real-time fluorometric detection. The excitation and emission range is 450 to 800 nM. To date, it has not been widely used to support FRET as described by the LightCycler groups *(11)*. However, it can do thermal melt analysis using SYBer green real-time reactions. There is a laboratory version (110 or 220 V) as well as a field version that uses batteries. The cuvet is a plastic polymer with a diamond designed. The diamond-shaped cell can hold 25 or 100 µL of reaction mix. The sides of the cuvet allow excitation light to enter from the lower right side of the cuvet and the excitation light to be read from the lower left side of the cuvet. This provides the longest light path, resulting in maximization of signal in the reaction vessel. Heating and cooling of the reaction mixture is accomplished in a "mini" thermal heater cell. Cooling occurs by turning off the heater and allowing a fan to "air cool" the reaction mixture. The software requires a skilled user to operate the device. Each set of reactions has to be programmed or recalled from memory by entering a program file. Data entry is done before cycling can begin. Currently, there are no supporting interpretation screens with this software. Each assay has to be interpreted by the user at the completion of the cycling. The Smart Cycler allows 16 tests to be done at a time. Positive and negative controls plus 14 tests in a batch mode or one sample can be tested for five different organisms (single plex assays). The user can "daisy chain" the thermal cycling units together to allow greater capacity of testing but this increases the footprint of the system.

2.4.3. The Applied Biosystems 7700

The Applied Biosystems 7700 DNA Sequence Detection System is a laboratory-based system only. It uses a 96-well format for the samples. The dynamic range for testing is at least five orders of magnitude in starting copy number. The 7700 uses an Apple computer operating system and requires 200/208 V power to run the laser. The footprint is large (37" × 24" × 28.5") and it weighs 286 lbs. The device does not show real-time data while the instrument is cycling but displays the results on completion of the cycling. It has a built in thermal cycler, a laser to induce fluorescence, a charge coupled device detector, and real-time sequence detection (but not reporting) software. It is capable of continuous wavelength detection from 500- to 660-nM, allowing use of multiple fluorophores in a single reaction. The software is only moderately user friendly and requires toggling between screens to set up and read results. This system was designed to use 5'-nuclease reagents. Only PCR or RT-PCR can be done on the device but they cannot be done simultaneously. This is a high-throughput system with excellent math functions. The device uses an aluminum block for heating and cooling of the samples and is slower than the other devices for heating and cooling. Time from beginning to end of cycling is around 2 h on this device.

2.4.4. The iCycler

The Bio-Rad Laboratories (Richmond, CA) iCycler is similar to the 7700 DNA Sequence Detector in that it uses a 96-well format and 200-μL tubes for the samples. That is where the similarities end. The iCycler extends its capability by also being able to use a 384-well plate. Interchangeable sample blocks, including a dual-block configuration allows independent protocols to be run simultaneously (i.e., PCR in one block and RT-PCR in the other block). The software is fairly user friendly with menu-driven screens and ready-made templates for easy viewing, editing, and running. The device provides summary run reports and detailed validation reports. It is the only device with US National Institute of Standards and Technology traceable temperature performance. The footprint is also small. The device comes as a standard thermal cycler or with an add-on to upgrade the system to real-time PCR. The range of fluorophores excitation and emission is from 400 to 700 nM. The device is a four-color instrument, allowing four dyes to be tracked per reaction. The device allows real-time tracking of 96 samples simultaneously. It is not a hardened instrument and, therefore, is more suited as a laboratory-based system. However, its small size and high-throughput format make it an attractive device for field use.

3. IDENTIFICATION OF SPECIFIC AGENTS

Specific assays for bacteria with potential for use in weapons of mass destruction are being developed by several of groups around the country. At present, the Mayo Clinic and Roche have partnered to get a hybridization assay for *B. anthracis* approved by the US Food and Drug Administration (FDA). It is the only FDA approved test currently available for PCR platforms. However, the US Army, the US Air Force and US Navy have numerous of 5'-nuclease tests, as well as hybridization probe-based assays developed. The major hurdle to overcome in assay development begins with the availability of sequence information. GenBank and other sites such as the institute for Genomic Research and the Sanger Center have sequence information available but it often is from one or a few isolates of the organism of interest and there may be no sequence information for other species within the genus. This is being remedied with each passing month as more sequences of the biothreat agents are entered into these databases through government-funded projects. One also has to consider if the assay is to be used for detection or identification. This will drive the design to either be highly sensitive or highly specific. Considerations such as the sample source (culture, direct environmental test, direct clinical test) will influence design. The "end user" must determine what level of false-positives or false-negatives they are willing to have for the test to be useful. Selection of gene target is also of primary interest. Selection of gene sequence unique for the organism of interest may be acceptable even if the gene function is unknown. Of equal interest, selection of virulence factors generally prevents genetic engineering of the target sequence because engineering may alter the function of the gene and reduce the virulence of the organism. Development of numerous of assays for each target ensures a battery of assays available for use in the event that an aggressor does try to engineer a DNA sequence to defeat an assay currently in use. Most teams developing reagents for these organisms have targeted the major virulence factors. Ideally, chromosomal markers unique to each of these organisms will be identified and used in assay development. Two or three such markers based on virulence factors and chromosomal genes would potentially allow confirmation of the organism's presence in the absence of culture.

3.1. Assays to Identify B. anthracis

Identification of *B. anthracis* generally targets the pX01 and pX02 plasmid genes. There are numerous papers suggesting other chromosomal gene targets, but they appear to have homologous sequence in at least a portion of the other *Bacillus* species *(16–18)*. Selection of a particular gene requires a lot of sequence information on the near neighbor relatives of the target organism to reduce the possibility of generating primers and probes that are crossreactive with species other than the target organism. The pX01 plasmid contains three genes associated with virulence, lethal factor (LF), edema factor (EF), and protective antigen (PA). These genes are frequently used for primer and probe development for *B. anthracis*. Likewise, pX02 also contains a gene group associated with virulence. These genes code for the capsular antigen (Cap) and are called *capA* and *capB*. There are numerous other genes on pX01 and pX02, but many of them have unknown functions *(19,20)*. The search is still on for good chromosomal markers for use in DNA-based diagnostic testing, but there is no doubt it is required. Plasmids can, and likely do, pass among other species of *Bacillus*. Real-time assays for pX01 and pX02 are numerous. These assays were recently shown to have excellent sensitivity and specificity for environmental samples (Hadfield and Dobson, unpublished). The assays based on the gene sequences that encode LF, EF, PA, Cap, and a recently identified chromosomal marker used at the Armed Forces Institute of Pathology all have sensitivities to the 0.1-pg level. Sensitivity of these assays is based on reactions that give a positive signal in greater than 58 out of 60 tests. Generally, the testing of these assays employed Brain Heart Infusion cultures of environmental samples including swab collections, HEPA vacuum collections and powders, and other samples submitted for examination. Sample preparation consisted of centrifugation of 1 mL of broth culture and suspension of the cells in 0.5 mL of water. The preparation was lysed by boiling for 10 min. The suspension was centrifuged to pellet the cell debris and 5 µL of supernatant was used as PCR template.

3.1.1. Multiplex 5'-Nuclease Assay for Detection of B. anthracis

As described in the previous section, an ideal diagnostic assay would be able to identify the presence of *B. anthracis* by using information from at least three DNA targets (pX01, pX02, and the chromosome). Here, we describe the ability to look at multiple targets by performing one reaction for several targets, specifically pX01 and pX02. The ability to assay multiple targets in a single reaction provides several advantages for diagnostic systems, specifically the number of assays to be run will be reduced and uniform conditions will be encountered for multiplexed targets *(21–23)*. Multiplexing assays may require extensive optimization and evaluation to ensure that end point detection and specificity is not compromised by the cocktails of primers and probes used. Furthermore, one of the limitations of multiplexing is the ability of the real-time hardware to detect multiple dyes simultaneously. The available dyes for multiplexing of reactions have overlapping emission spectra, and these areas of overlap must be addressed by instrument software. At the US Army Research Institute of Infectious Disease, we are currently using the Stratagene MX4000 (Stratagene, La Jolla, CA) to optimize multiplex reactions. This platform is being used because it has the ability to distinguish various of dyes, up to four in any one reaction.

The use of internal controls for fluorogenic 5'-nuclease assay primers and probes is a necessary component of any diagnostic assay to be implemented in the field *(24)*. Any good internal control must be able to distinguish whether a negative result is caused by the absence of target DNA (true-negative) or the inability to amplify the target DNA that exists in the reaction (false-negative). An internal positive control must consist of target sequences that do not cross-react with the assay-specific sequences. Building on this idea, we decided to construct a universal internal positive control by mutating the primer and probe sites of a pre-existing *B. anthracis* assay. The amplification product was cloned into a plasmid and the primer and probe site sequences were modified by oligonucleotide-directed mutagenesis. The mutated sequences had identical nucleotide content to the original sites but were randomized to produce a sequence that had no known homology to any published nucleotide sequences. The product of this construction is a clone that has unique primer and probe sites that should not crossreact with any known assay sequences. The construct concentration was titrated to prevent competition with assays of interest and to be sensitive to inhibitors of PCR. This construct is spiked in the reactions described here as the internal positive control (IPC).

Currently, we have developed a triplex assay for *B. anthracis* consisting of an assay for pXO1, pXO2, and the IPC. The pXO1 probe was labeled with VIC dye, the pXO2 probe was labeled with FAM dye, and the IPC was labeled with ROX dye (Perkin Elmer Biosystems, Foster City, CA). The multiplex assay was on the Stratagene MX4000 because of its excellent capability to differentiate multiple dye assays (*see* Table 2). Although not as quick as some of the rapid cyclers, truncated two-step cycling (45 cycles) allowed the assay to be complete in 55 min. Our initial testing revealed that the pXO1 assay had the highest PCR efficiency, indicating that it was competing for assay components at the expense of the pX02 assay. The primer concentrations for pXO1 were limited to ensure optimal efficiency of the assays for the other two targets without loss of pX01 sensitivity. We have found that the key to a successful multiplex DNA-based assay is to prevent the most efficient primer pair from outcompeting less efficient pairs for reaction components. In our experience, limiting the most efficient assay does not alter limits of detection but rather simply limits the amount of product that can be produced. The net effect is that components are then available for other assays to work efficiently within the multiplex mixture. Eight replicates were tested to determine the limit of detection for each component of the multiplex assay. The multiplex assay is sensitive to 100 fg (100% detection) for both plasmid targets, which is equivalent to limits of detection for the assays run individually. At 10 fg of target input the pX01 assay detected seven of the eight replicates whereas the pXO2 assay detected six of the eight replicates. Based on genome size, the assay can detect about 20 genome copies of *B. anthracis* DNA (assuming plasmid and chromosome copy numbers are equivalent). The IPC was positive at all concentrations tested with virtually identical crossing threshold (Ct) values. There was no statistical difference among Ct values for the IPC regardless of the amount of *B. anthracis* DNA input. Separate experimentation has shown that the IPC concentration used is sensitive to inhibitors of PCR, such as ethylenediamine tetraacetic acid (data not shown).

The multiplex assay described here allows for the simultaneous detection of three important components for the identification of *B. anthracis*-containing samples. The assay can detect both plasmids at clinically significant levels, allowing for the distinction between pathogenic and vaccine strains of the organism. Furthermore, inhibitors of PCR in a sample can be detected, allowing for the elimination of potential false-negatives. Current work involves extending this approach to multiple agent detection in a single tube. Whereas rapid cyclers such as the Cepheid Smart Cycler™ and the Idaho Technologies RAPID can run similar assays in under 30 min, currently only one assay (single-plex assay) per tube is being performed on these instruments. Therefore, the 55-min total assay time for the multiplex assay is competitive because it requires fewer total assay tubes and less labor. However, the Cepheid Smart Cycler™ currently has multiple dye (four-channel) capability and assay transfer to this machine is underway and may greatly reduce total assay time. As multiplexing capability and platforms for detection mature, the total number of tests required for the analysis of samples will decrease. The future of real-time PCR testing may allow for the analysis of dozens of biological agents with a handful of multiplex assays.

Table 2
Results of Multiplex DNA-Assay for the Specific Identification of *B. anthracis*[a]

	pXO1 (VIC)		pXO2 (FAM)		IPC (ROX)	
Template	Ct[b]	No. of positives	Ct	No. of positives	Ct	No. of positives
1 pg	28.5	8	29.76	8	30.27	8
100 fg	33.02	8	33.37	8	30.29	8
10 fg	40.65	7	37.86	6	30.38	8
1 fg	—	0	—	0	30.57	8
NTC[c]	—	0	—	0	30.84	8

[a]Serial dilutions of purified *B. anthracis* genomic DNA (Ames strain) analyzed by a multiplex 5'-nuclease assay. Eight replicates at each template concentration were performed. The multiplex consists of a pXO1 assay containing a VIC-labeled probe, a pXO2 assay containing a FAM labeled probe, and an internal positive control (IPC) containing a ROX labeled. Both plasmid targets had similar limits of detection. The IPC was highly consistent among samples regardless of agent template input. The assay allows for the detection of both plasmids required for virulence and can identify true negatives by the presence of a positive IPC reaction.

[b]Ct is defined as the cycle at which fluorescence crosses threshold. The threshold is calculated by the instrument (MX4000) and is equivalent to one standard deviation above background fluorescence. Background fluorescence is the average fluorescence from cycles 5–10.

[c]NTC, no template control.

3.2. Identification of Y. pestis

Y. pestis is a member of the *Enterobacteriaceae,* which makes design and development of species specific PCR assays more difficult. The number of near neighbors (*Yersinia* species) is great and the other *Enterobacteriaceae* are also related to *Y. pestis* genetically. The nearest neighbor is *Yersinia pseudotuberculosis* (83%) by DNA–DNA homology studies *(25,26).* As with *B. anthracis,* selection of appropriate gene sequences and showing they do not exist in other species of *Yersinia* or the *Enterobacteriaceae* is important for sensitivity and specificity. *Y. pestis* contains three plasmids, each of which contains virulence genes. The three plasmids vary in size *(27–30);* pMT1 is approx 100,000 bp, pCD1 is 70,504 bp, and pBCP1 is 9610 bp. pMT1 contains the genes for F1 capsular antigen and anchoring protein and murine toxin (*ymt*) among numerous of other genes with putative or unknown functions. pCD1 consists of the genes modulating low calcium response and includes genes for the *Yersinia* outer proteins and accessory proteins. These genes are conserved among the pathogenic *Yersinia* species (*Y. pestis, Y. pseudotuberculosis,* and *Yersinia enterocolitica*). The smallest plasmid, pCP1, contains the sequences for plasminogen activator (*pla*), pesticin, pesticin immunity protein, and ColE1-like replicon. Searches for chromosomal sequences unique to *Y. pestis* are in progress. Assays for detection of *Y. pestis* in fleas were very successful *(31,32).* Fluorescent based probe detection methods for identification of *Y. pestis* have excellent sensitivity achieving detection of as few as three copies of target gene in genomic DNA preparations. Engelthaler et al. *(33)* demonstrated PCR to be equally or more sensitive than mouse inoculation for identifying *Y. pestis.* We have also developed *Y. pestis*-specific assays in our laboratory. An example of the *Y. pestis* assay is shown in Fig. 2.

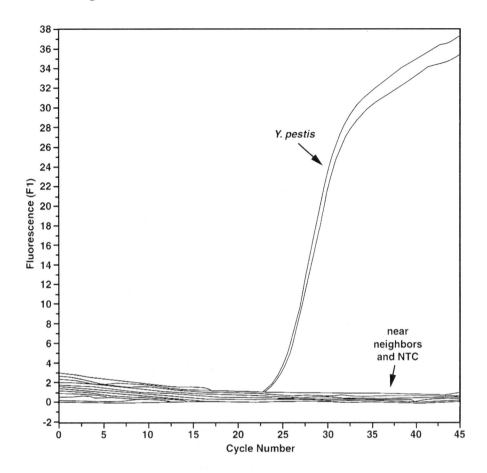

Fig. 2. *Y. pestis* specificity test. Eleven samples of *Y. pestis* were included in a panel of 84 near neighbors. The near neighbors included 12 strains of *Y. pseudotuberculosis* and 9 strains of *Y. enterocolitica*. Two samples containing *Y. pestis* DNA are positive in the test run shown in the above graph. NTC, no template control.

3.3. Identification of Brucella

Brucella organisms are small, difficult to grow, Gram-negative rods that frequently infect cattle, sheep, and pigs in many countries. In the United States, approx 100 cases of *Brucella* are reported each year, usually as a result of ingestion of contaminated food products such as nonpasteurized cheese from foreign countries or from consumption of *Brucella* infected animal tissues, usually swine or wild game. *Brucella* can be difficult to identify and may be even more difficult to speciate because of cross-reacting antigens and variance in their biochemical reactions. Genetic identification of *Brucella* is faster and more reliable than phenotypic identification. However, DNA-based identification of *Brucella* species directly from specimens has not been shown to be reliable. The types of specimens and specimen preparation is critical to quality performance of PCR assays for *Brucella*. Zerva et al. *(34)* identified *Brucella* in whole blood or serum of infected patients in their study of 31 patients with brucellosis over a 4-mo period. They used primers reported by Leal-Klevezas for detection of *Brucella* from blood and milk of infected animals *(35)*. The search for genes with sufficient polymorphisms to allow distinction between the different *Brucella* species has not been fruitful. Although some genes appear to be unique, they often do not identify all the serogroups within the species or they crossreact with other species of *Brucella*. This supports the claim of homogeneity of the genus *(36)*. Other PCR-based methods of genetic analysis such as amplified fragment length polymorphism are able to discriminate the various species of *Brucella* (*see* Chapter 21).

3.4. Identification of F. tularensis

F. tularensis is an uncommon but well-recognized pathogen of humans. Most often contracted by handling or eating infected rabbits, the infection can be transmitted by biting insects, contact with contaminated mud or waters, or by inhalation of aerosols of *F. tularensis*. Recognition of this infection can be difficult if the patient does not have a history of handling rabbits or insect bites. *Francisella* grows in blood culture bottles but may not subculture to primary plating media because of a requirement for elevated cysteine in the media. It will grow readily on media typically used for growth of *Neisseria gonorrhea* or *Legionella pneumophilia*. Gram stains of the culture may not show the presence of the organism because *Francisella* is very small and easily overlooked when scanning smears. PCR can be done directly from the blood culture bottle with appropriate blood sample protocols or from cultures. Direct testing of blood or organ tissue generally yields positive tests but does not reflect the actual amount of *Francisella* present. Low levels of *Francisella* present a diagnostic problem even with PCR. An outer membrane protein (OMP) eliciting a major antibody response is FopA and appears to be unique to *Francisella*. PCR assays for this gene are very sensitive and appear to be specific with the samples tested reported by Fulop et al. *(37)* and Higgins et al. *(38)*. Outbreaks of tularemia rarely occur in the United States but do occur in Sweden and Norway. Swedish investigators tested wound specimens for *Francisella* using primers for the 16S rRNA gene and a 17-kDa lipoprotein *(39,40)*. In both studies, approx 25% of the patients had PCR-negative results, but some of the patients were diagnosed based on serology. Those patients may not have had any *Francisella* organisms or DNA in the lesion site when tested. Experimental results suggest a much better performance of PCR for identification of *Francisella* from blood and cultures *(41)*. Detection levels were in the range of one organism per microliter of sample being tested (5–10 µL/reaction). Junhui et al. *(42)* also found PCR to be more sensitive than culture when working with infected animals. They were detecting approx 15 colony-forming units (CFU) of *Francisella* in blood and tissues from infected mice. Researchers in Norway evaluated environmental testing *(43)*. They reported PCR worked best on water samples, whereas enzyme-linked immunosorbent assay rapid immuno-chromatography worked best with tissue samples. PCR testing at the Armed Forces Institute of Pathology includes three PCR assays for *Francisella*. Genes targeted for PCR include *tul4, fopA* and one encoding super oxide dismutase. A PCR assay for *fopA* is shown in Fig. 3. This assay reliably detects 15–20 copies of the target in a PCR 95% of the time. None of the PCR assays reported distinguish between the biotype A and biotype B strains of *F. tularensis (44)*. The *fopA*-based assay is also positive when DNA isolated from the low virulence organism *Francisella novicida* is used as template.

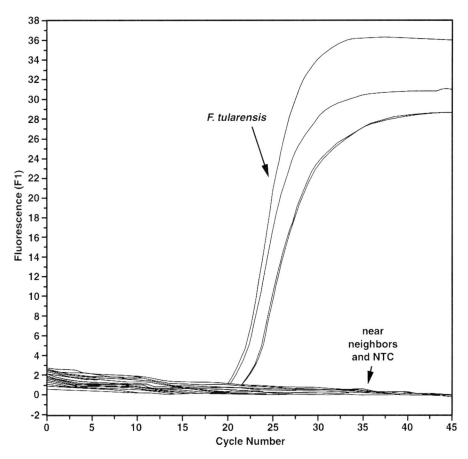

Fig. 3. *F. tularensis* specificity test: The panel consisted of 56 near neighbors including *Francisella philomirangia* and 4 isolates of *F. tularensis* biotypes A and B as well as *F. novicida*. *F. novicida* is positive as are 3 isolates of *F. tularensis* type A and B in the graph shown above. NTC, no template control.

3.5. Viral Agents

Detection of viral agents using DNA-based techniques has lagged behind that of the bacterial agents mainly because of the technical aspects inherent in laboratory manipulation of these organisms. One major technical difficulty is the intrinsic genetic variability of these viruses. However, as with the bacterial agents, gene selection and alignment of multiple sequences allows one to pick a region of sequence for development of a PCR. These assays will typically focus on the RNA viruses such as the equine encephalitis viruses, Hanta viruses, and arboviruses as examples necessitating the use of RT-PCR in the detection assay. Growth of the viruses in cell culture or hosts also adds some new dimensions to assay development. Extraction of RNA yields both the target RNA and host RNA. This may be overcome by purification of the target organism before isolating the RNA but this is often not practical for operational use.

3.5.1. West Nile Virus

Prior to 1999, West Nile Virus (WNV) did not occur in the United States. At some point prior to the recognition of WNV in the United States, it is assumed infected mosquitoes were transported to the United States in cargo ships and escaped into the environment and began feeding on native domestic animals and wildlife. Humans, horses, and domestic are usually incidental hosts. When the epidemic of WNV was recognized, scientists sequenced the virus to identify it as WNV and began making PCR assays to identify it. To develop a DNA-based assay for WNV, we selected a region in the noncoding portion of the genome because it appeared to be common for all strains of the virus. WNV was grown in cell culture and in mosquitoes. Preparations were harvested and split into two samples. One sample was used to isolate the virus for quantitation; the other was used to harvest RNA in Trizole. One tube of PCR was used for assay development. Initially, primers and probes must be shown not to react with the sample type (uninfected mosquito pools or the human genome). rt-PCR assays were highly sensitive, detecting as few as 5 PFU in mosquito preparations *(45)*. One infected mosquito could be detected in a pool of 50 mosquitoes. In some instances, pools of 500 mosquitoes were screened and positives were detected. RT-PCR is now the standard for epidemiological monitoring of WNV in the Eastern states of the United States.

3.5.2. Equine Encephalitis Virus

Venezuelan, eastern, and western equine encephalitis viruses (VEE, EEE, and WEE, respectively) are zoonotic RNA viruses in the alphavirus genus. Members of each of the species have been sequenced *(46–51)*. These viruses are transmitted to equines and humans by mosquitoes. Like WNV, they are maintained in their zoonotic cycle by certain mosquito species and in either rodents or birds, which serve as the natural hosts. Linssen et al. *(52)* reported development of several assays to identify these viruses. The sensitivity of the assays ranged from 20 to 3000 copies. The test was used to diagnose several human cases of VEE in the Amazon River Basin in Peru, South America. The VEE assay was designed to identify the medically important VEE strains in VEE-IAB, -IC, -ID, and -II. VEE exhibits a high degree of polymorphism and specific assays may not detect all VEE strains especially in enzootic foci *(48)*. However, development of specific assays for a particular strain of VEE would be useful for elucidating the occurrence, spread and epidemiology of the strain. This becomes particularly useful for following medically important equine encephalitis viruses.

4. ANTIBIOTIC-RESISTANT GENE DETECTION

Generally, it is assumed that any BW agent that might be used in an act of terrorism or on the battlefield will be antibiotic-resistant *(53)*. It is relatively simple to construct such strains and could significantly enhance their impact. The ability to identify strains of BW agents resistant to the drugs of choice for their treatment would enhance our ability to give timely and effective treatment to infected individuals. This might aid in one of two ways. First, it might be possible to detect the resistant organisms in the blood of infected individuals. This would obviously depend on the pathogenesis of the organism in question. Second, once the organism is isolated, it could be identified as an antibiotic resistant strain more rapidly than by standard culture techniques that generally require an extra day of incubation before resistance profiles can be determined.

The following two sections present our current assays developed to identify antibiotic-resistant BW agents.

4.1. Ciprofloxacin Resistance

Ciprofloxacin (Cp) is a quinolone antibiotic that inhibits DNA replication by inhibiting enzymes involved in supercoiling. Cp resistance is generally caused by single-point mutations in cellular topoisomerases such as *gyrA, gyrB,* or *parC (54,55)* rendering their gene products insensitive to the drug. The region of these genes where the point mutations occur has been designated the quinolone resistance determining region (QRDR) *(56–58)* and is confined to an approx 120-bp area. The identification of Cp resistant bacteria presents a unique problem in that a specific gene need not be detected but rather a specific mutation within a cellular "housekeeping" gene must be identified.

To compare the results obtained with other bacteria to the mechanism of Cp resistance in a BW agent and to develop a DNA-based assay to rapidly identify resistant organisms, we isolated and characterized Cp resistant mutants of *Y. pestis (59).* After isolation and characterization of 65 Cp-resistant strains, we found that all of the mutations occurred within a 10-bp region of *gyrA.* All of these mutations resulted in amino acid substitutions that had previously been identified in other Cp-resistant organisms and were confined to two specific amino acid residues. Furthermore, we determined the DNA sequence of *gyrB* and *parC* from the wildtype strain, as well as randomly selected Cp-resistant mutants and did not detect any secondary mutations in these genes. This was necessary because double mutations in combinations of these genes have been shown to confer high-level resistance to Cp *(56,60,61).* From these studies, it appears that the mechanism and position of mutations resulting in Cp-resistant *Y. pestis* is similar to those previously described.

4.1.1. Fluorogenic PCR to Identify Cp-Resistant Y. pestis

We used the data collected on *Y. pestis* Cp resistance described in Subheading 4.1. to develop a single hybridization probe assay that could identify all of the point mutations described earlier *(59).* Our development of this assay was facilitated because all of the mutations were clustered within a narrow region of *gyrA.* We designed a pair of FRET probes such that all of the mutations were encompassed by a labeled-oligonucleotide similar to the depiction of Probe 1 in Fig. 1B. The probe was 100% homologous with the wildtype *Y. pestis gyrA* sequence. We reasoned that the DNA amplified from Cp resistant *Y. pestis* would produce a melting curve that would be significantly less than the melting peak produced following amplification of the wildtype allele because the single basepair mismatch between the PCR product of the mutant compared to the wildtype sequence of Probe 1. The melting peak produced by the mutants ranged from 4–11°C less than the melting peak produced by the wildtype sequence as shown in Fig. 4 and elsewhere *(59).* The melting temperature (T_m) detected by changes in fluorescence with increasing temperature was consistent within one degree centigrade between experiments. The single hybridization probe assay was also able to detect cultures of mixed mutants that individually yielded a melting peak with a unique T_m as shown in Fig. 4.

One of the significant considerations during the development of any assay is the sensitivity and specificity of the method. Initially, the hybridization probe assay was

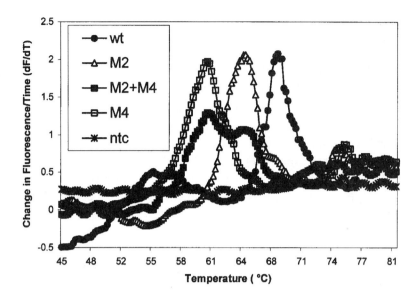

Fig. 4. Melting peak analysis of wildtype (Cp-sensitive) and mutant (Cp-resistant) *Y. pestis*. *Y. pestis* Cp-resistant mutants M2 and M4 encode different point mutations within *gyrA (59)*. The sample used to generate the curve labeled M2+M4 contained a mixture of both mutants. The melting curve of the wildtype (wt) Cp-sensitive strain displayed a T_m of approx 69°C compared to the M2 and M4 Cp-resistant mutant's T_m of 64 and 60°C, respectively. Ntc, no template control. The experimental samples each contained the equivalent of approx 10^5 CFU of bacteria per reaction prepared as a crude cell lysate. The reactions and analysis were as described elsewhere *(59)* using the LightCycler (Roche).

sensitive to 10 pg of purified DNA template. However, we desired to develop the assay so that it might be used in a diagnostic setting where purification of DNA would not be practical or timely. We needed to develop the assay for use on crude bacterial lysates. The most amenable method would begin this process after the isolation of the organism on solid medium. Our initial attempts used single colonies suspended in sterile water followed by dilution and boiling for 5 min. We found this method to be undesirable because of decreased sensitivity of the assay. The decreased sensitivity was undesirable because the window of positive reactions was narrow and might cause false-negatives in a field environment where different personnel would be performing the evaluation. Next, we tested short growth periods in liquid medium before the culture was washed in sterile water, diluted, and boiled before analysis. After only 2 h of growth of a single colony in 100 µL of complex media, we could detect from 10^5 to less than 10 CFU Cp-resistant *Y. pestis (59)*. The difference in the sensitivity of the assay between direct suspension of bacteria from agar plates and a short growth period in liquid medium illustrates the physiological details that must be considered when developing assays that might be employed in the field.

To compare and contrast different fluorogenic chemistries used in DNA-based detection methods, a degradation probe (5′-nuclease, Fig. 1A) assay was developed to identify Cp-resistant *Y. pestis*. Although the development of a probe hydrolysis assay to detect single point mutations is more difficult, it is possible, as shown in Fig. 5. This figure shows the use of a labeled probe that is homologous to the wildtype sequence of

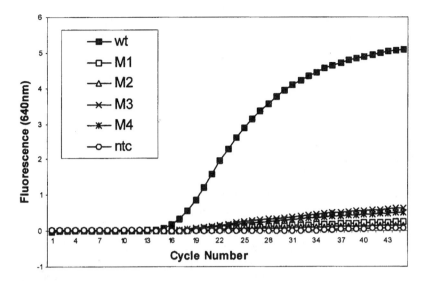

Fig. 5. Hydrolysis probe (5'-nuclease) assay to screen *Y. pestis* isolates for Cp resistance. A single probe homologous to the wild type (labeled wt) *Y. pestis gyrA* sequence was used in all reactions. Mutants M1 through M4 are described elsewhere *(59)*. Each reaction contained 10 ng of purified genomic DNA, except the no template control (designated ntc) that contained water. Numbers after the mutant allele designation (M1–M4) indicate the *Y. pestis* Cp-resistant genotype. Reaction conditions were 45 cycles of 94°C for 0 s followed by 69°C for 20 s using the Hybridization Probe Master Mix (Roche) buffer.

Y. pestis gyrA used to screen five different colonies for Cp resistance. The probe binds to the region of *gyrA* that encoded all of the point mutations found to confer resistance to Cp *(59)*. Given the proper reaction conditions, the single basepair mismatch between the probe and PCR product present in the hybrids formed with the mutants is sufficient to prevent binding of the probe and thus result in a negative signal from those samples. We found that the annealing temperature of the reaction is critical for the success of use of this chemistry for the detection of single basepair changes. Generally, an annealing temperature for the reaction close to the probe T_m results in a specific reaction where the probe homology with the PCR product is 100%. The confirmatory test utilizes probes that match the point mutations and would thus contain a mismatch with the wildtype sequence. However, the single wildtype probe reaction is useful for screening purposes. The sensitivity of the probe hydrolysis assay to detect Cp resistance was approx 1 CFU in the PCR, which is similar to the sensitivity seen with the hybridization probe assay described earlier.

4.1.2. DHPLC Identification of Cp-Resistant Y. pestis

The major problem with identification of Cp-resistant bacteria as described earlier is the large number of probes that must be developed to identify all possible mutations that give rise to antibiotic resistance. With this in mind, we have begun to develop technology that can detect any point mutations within a defined region of the genome. This technique is denaturing high-performance liquid chromatography (DHPLC). DHPLC has been employed in a wide range of applications, including nucleotide polymorphism analysis *(62)*, gene mapping *(63)*, analysis of genes *(64)*, screening for mutations *(65)*, analysis of primer extension products *(66)*, and quantification of gene expression *(67)*. DHPLC identifies mutations by detecting sequence variation in reannealed DNA strands (heteroduplexes). Sequence variation creates a mixed population of heteroduplexes and homoduplexes during reannealing of wildtype and mutant DNA. When this mixed population is analyzed by DHPLC under partially denaturing temperatures, the heteroduplexes elute from the column earlier than the homoduplexes because of their reduced melting temperature. The technique can efficiently detect single nucleotide and insertion/deletion variation in crude PCR products directly without DNA sequencing.

DHPLC chemistry consists of stationary and mobile phases. A DNASep column, consisting of a polystyrene-divinylbenzene copolymer, is the stationary phase. The mobile phase consists of an ion-pairing reagent of triethylammonium acetate (TEAA). The TEAA mediates binding of DNA to the stationary phase (column). Acetonitrile (ACN) is the organic agent that subsequently achieves separation of the DNA from the column. Application of a linear gradient of ACN allows separation of fragments based on size and/or presence of heteroduplexes. We are currently using the Transgenomic Wave (Omaha, NE) instrument to perform DHPLC on genes of interest. DHPLC methodology consists of four parts: amplification by the PCR, quantification, hybridization, and analysis of hybridized product. After PCR, heteroduplexes between wildtype and experimental amplification products are formed during the hybridization step. Mismatches between wildtype and mutant DNA sequences disrupt the structure of the heteroduplex, and DHPLC is capable of resolving these differences.

We have used DHPLC to detect and characterize Cp-resistant strains of *Y. pestis*. Primers were designed to span the QRDR of the *gyrA* in *Y. pestis*. A blinded collection of eight Cp-resistant strains of *Y. pestis* were *(59)* analyzed. The resultant 460 bp amplification products were hybridized to a *Y. pestis* strain containing the wildtype *gyrA* and DHPLC was performed (*see* Fig. 6). DHPLC identified the four previously characterized mutants *(59)* and elucidated a fifth mutation from the collection of eight strains. DNA sequence analysis confirmed the presence of the previously characterized mutations in the QRDR of *Y. pestis gyrA (59)* as well as a cytosine-to-guanosine transversion that defined the fifth mutation (designated M5, GenBank accession AF487466). DHPLC was capable of distinguishing all mutations from one another and chromatograms were 100% consistent with confirmatory sequencing. The illustrated example demonstrates that DHPLC can be as powerful as DNA sequencing in elucidating molecular mutations.

Although DHPLC will not replace DNA sequencing in the molecular laboratory, the technique can be used to screen a large number of samples (96 per run) in a relatively short period of time (5 min per sample). Additional work has shown that amplification across areas of genetic variability followed by DHPLC may provide the identification of organisms to the species level (D. Norwood, unpublished data). DHPLC assays may become an important diagnostic tool in reference laboratories, providing a means to survey the genetic variability in biological threat agents.

4.2. Tetracycline Resistance Gene Detection

Resistance to tetracycline (Tc) occurs by two basic mechanisms *(68)*. Unlike the genetic mechanism of Cp resistance described in Subheading 4.1., both of these mecha-

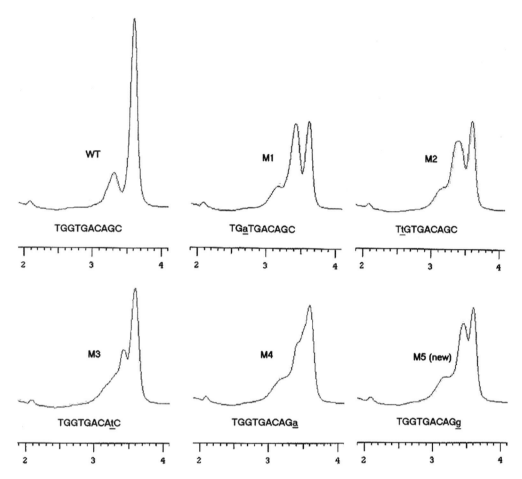

Fig. 6. DHPLC chromatograms of the gyrase A QRDR region of wildtype (wt) and ciprofloxacin resistant strains (M1, M2, M3, M4, and M5) of *Y. pestis*. Following amplification, equimolar amounts of wildtype and mutant DNA were combined, heated to 95°C, and slowly cooled to allow heteroduplexes to form. Heteroduplexes were melted and analyzed on a Transgenomic Wave instrument (Omaha, NE). The resultant chromatograms illustrate the ability of the DHPLC to distinguish subtle changes (base substitutions) in DNA sequence.

nisms require the addition of a new gene to a sensitive organism. There are currently 31 different known classes of Tc resistance determinants based on hybridization studies and sequence homology *(69)*. However, several assays based on PCR have been developed to identify various Tc resistance gene classes *(70–73)* all require gel electrophoresis.

We began our systematic development of fluorogenic PCR tests to identify Tc-resistant bacteria with the common classes found in Gram-negative organisms *(74)*. Initially, we felt it desirable to develop assays that can be easily multiplexed to screen organisms for Tc resistance genes. We reasoned that a SYBR green assay could be developed that would allow the preliminary identification of Tc-resistant organisms. If the PCR products are of different T_m, then melting peak analysis can be used to differentiate the classes of determinants amplified in the reaction. Figure 7 shows a multi-

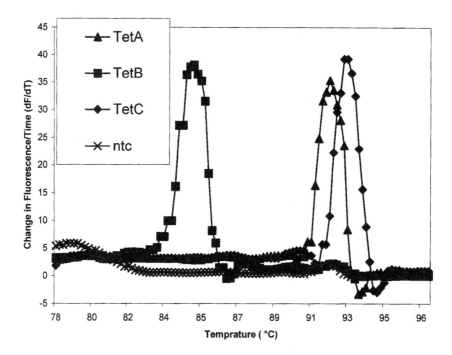

Fig. 7. Melting peak analysis of SYBR green reaction identification of Tc-resistance determinants. The reaction contained primers that recognize Tc resistance gene classes A, B, and C described elsewhere *(70)*. Each reaction contained 10 ng of purified genomic DNA prepared from bacteria encoding the Tc-resistance gene class as shown in the inset. NTC, no template control. The thermocycling conditions were 45 cycles of 95°C for 0 s, 58°C for 10 s, and 72°C for 20 s using a Roche LightCycler followed by melting peak analysis over the range of 45–95°C. The buffer used was the SYBR Green I Master Mix (Roche).

plex SYBR green-based assay using primers *(70)* to amplify Tc resistance classes A, B, and C in the same reaction. The T_m of each product is sufficiently different such that when the proper controls are used, an initial determination can be made as to the class of Tc resistance determinant. The predicted T_ms (Primer Express software, Applied Biosystems, Foster City, CA) for the class A, B, and C amplicons were 85, 42, and 84°C, respectively, which closely resembles the observed melting peaks *(see* Fig. 7). The multiplex reaction is specific although the highest level of sequence identity was 83% between the Tc resistance class B and C genes.

To confirm the classification of the Tc-resistance determinants indicated by the SYBR green reactions discussed earlier, we developed probe hydrolysis assays *(see* Fig. 1A) that are specific for each gene. Examples of these reactions are shown in Fig. 8. For development of the probe hydrolysis assays, we aligned the sequences of the class A, B, and C genes then chose specific primers and probes using Primer Express (Applied Biosystems). The amplicons were 90, 65, and 121 bp for Tc class A, B, and C reactions, respectively. The higher T_m for the class A-specific probe required the annealing/elongation step of the reaction to be run at a slightly higher temperature *(see* Fig. 8 legend). We have been successful in using crude lysates prepared from bacteria freshly isolated from agar plates to perform the Tc-resistance detection and classification reactions. Taken together, the combination of rapid screening and specific confir-

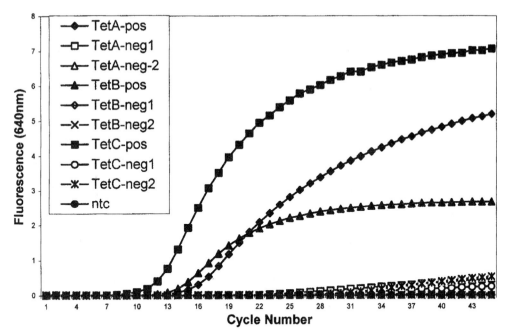

Fig. 8. Probe hydrolysis assay for the specific identification of class A, B, and C Tc-resistance determinants. Each reaction contained 10 ng of purified DNA or water (designated ntc) as indicated in the inset. The TetA and TetB samples were prepared from *Shigella flexneri* clinical samples known to encode the appropriate class of Tc resistance determinant. The TetC sample was purified pBR322 plasmid DNA. Samples designated with the "pos" suffix indicate reactions that contained predicted homologous probe and template. Samples labeled with the suffix "neg1" or "neg2" contained DNA prepared from strains encoding different nonhomologous Tc resistance determinants. The assay thermocycling conditions were 45 cycles of 94°C 0 s followed by 50°C (55°C for class A) for 20 s on the LightCycler (Roche).

mation of the presence of Tc-resistance determinants can be accomplished through a combination of fluorogenic PCR-based chemistries.

5. CONCLUDING REMARKS

The use of nucleic acid technologies to identify infectious agents is well-established for both DNA- and RNA-based pathogens. These technologies generally have excellent detection capabilities provided the source of DNA is free of inhibitors. Furthermore, the design of the assays can result in very high specificity but adequate validation of the assay using actual specimens is a stringent requirement before putting the test into general use. Real-time PCR simplifies nucleic acid amplification and reduces the potential for contamination because of release of amplicons during post-PCR analysis. As laboratories become more familiar with the use of nucleic acid, amplification methods, and real-time PCR, it will become the method of choice for the difficult to grow pathogens and the exceptionally dangerous pathogens. PCR will save time, money, and effort when identifying selected infectious diseases and will simplify the efforts of epidemiological tracking but it will never replace standard microbiological practices. Too often microbes make subtle changes or new diseases emerge into a human population. PCR will not detect or identify newly emerging strains of the classic threats if the gene sequences used to develop these assays are not of sufficient diversity. Additionally, these assays will likely fail to identify previously unidentified pathogens. Cultures of new or divergent organisms will always be required to generate new sequence data and to track the evolution of organisms. PCR applications can be used to monitor changes throughout the genome using methods such as amplified fragment length polymorphism. This latter point exemplifies the link between genotyping of these organisms and development of robust diagnostics.

Currently, we have the capability for both laboratory-based and field-deployed identification of biothreats. Of course, new technologies are being developed in the wake of the bioterrorism incident perpetrated on the United States in Fall 2001. However, these may be years in development and there are several areas where our current capabilities are in need of improvement. Most notably is the development of DNA-based tests for the classic platforms that might be used in an attack. These include specific chromosomal gene markers for most of the classic bacterial and viral agents. Furthermore, our depth of assays for particular organisms needs attention. Regulatory validation of these assays is also a large area of concern for the future. These shortcomings along with the knowledge gap of sequence diversity will best be addressed by collaborations between government agencies with laboratories involved in applied as well as basic research. The bioterrorism attack of 2001 was carried out with a well-defined classic agent of BW that all of the laboratories involved in diagnostics development were well-prepared to identify and characterize. Attention must be paid to other agents on the threat list to develop similar levels of capabilities and confidence.

ACKNOWLEDGMENTS

We would like to thank Dr. Antoinette Hartman for supplying Tc-resistant *Shigella* isolates. Wei Fan is gratefully acknowledged for antibiotic-resistance gene detection assay development. We also thank Nazma Jahan for isolation of the Cp-resistant *Y. pestis*. Lee Collins is acknowledged for his excellent graphic artwork. This work was supported by the US Army Medical Research and Materiel Command as part of the Biodefense Research Program.

REFERENCES

1. Murray, P. R. and American Society for Microbiology. (1999) *Manual of Clinical Microbiology*. 7th ed. ASM, Washington, DC.
2. Franz, D. R., Jahrling, P. B., Friedlander, A. M., et al. (1997) Clinical recognition and management of patients exposed to biological warfare agents. *JAMA* **278,** 399–411.
3. Tenover, F. C. and Unger, E. R. (1993) Nucleic acid probes for detection and identification of infectious agents, in *Diagnostic Molecular Microbiology: Principles and Applications.* (Persing, D. H., Smith, T. F., Tenover, F. C., and White, T. J., eds.), American Society for Microbiology, Washington, DC, pp. 3–25.
4. Whitcombe, D., Newton, C. R., and Little, S. (1998) Advances in approaches to DNA-based diagnostics. *Curr. Opin. Biotechnol.* **9,** 602–608.
5. Pfeffer, M., Wiedmann, M., and Batt, C. A. (1995) Applications of DNA amplification techniques in veterinary diagnostics. *Vet. Res. Commun.* **19,** 375–407.
6. Jung, M., Muche, J. M., Lukowsky, A., Jung, K., and Loening, S. A. (2001) Dimethyl sulfoxide as additive in ready-to-use reaction mixtures for real-time polymerase chain reaction analysis with SYBR Green I dye. *Anal. Biochem.* **289,** 292–295.

7. Dhar, A. K., Roux, M. M., and Klimpel, K. R. (2001) Detection and quantification of infectious hypodermal and hematopoietic necrosis virus and white spot virus in shrimp using real-time quantitative pcr and sybr green chemistry. *J. Clin. Microbiol.* **39,** 2835–2845.

8. Skeidsvoll, J. and Ueland, P. M. (1995) Analysis of double-stranded DNA by capillary electrophoresis with laser- induced fluorescence detection using the monomeric dye SYBR green I. *Anal. Biochem.* **231,** 359–365.

9. Livak, K. J., Flood, S. J., Marmaro, J., Giusti, W., and Deetz, K. (1995) Oligonucleotides with fluorescent dyes at opposite ends provide a quenched probe system useful for detecting PCR product and nucleic acid hybridization. *PCR Methods Appl.* **4,** 357–362.

10. Lakowicz, J. R. (1999) *Principles of Fluorescent Spectroscopy.* 2nd ed. Plenum, New York.

11. Caplin, B. E., Rasmussen, R. P., Bernard, P. S., and Wittwer, C. T. (1999) LightCycler hybridization probes: the most direct way to monitor PCR amplification for quantitation and mutation detection. *Biochemica* **1,** 5–9.

12. Meuer, S., Wittwer, C., and Nakagawara, K. (2001) *Rapid Cycle Real-Time PCR.* Springer Verlag, Berlin, Germany.

13. Northrup, M. A., Christel, L., McMillan, W. A., et al. (1998) A new generation of PCR instruments and nucleic acid concentration systems in *PCR Protocols.* (Gelfand, I. and Sninsky, J. J., eds.), Academic, San Diego, CA.

14. Belgrader, P., Benett, W., Hadley, D., et al. (1999) PCR detection of bacteria in seven minutes. *Science* **284,** 449, 450.

15. Belgrader, P., Young, S., Yuan, B., et al. (2001) A battery-powered notebook thermal cycler for rapid multiplex real-time PCR analysis. *Anal. Chem.* **73,** 286–289.

16. Etienne-Toumelin, I., Sirard, J. C., Duflot, E., Mock, M., and Fouet, A. (1995) Characterization of the *Bacillus anthracis* S-layer: cloning and sequencing of the structural gene. *J. Bacteriol.* **177,** 614–620.

17. Patra, G., Sylvestre, P., Ramisse, V., Therasse, J., and Guesdon, J. L. (1996) Isolation of a specific chromosomic DNA sequence of *Bacillus anthracis* and its possible use in diagnosis. *FEMS Immunol. Med. Microbiol.* **15,** 223–231.

18. Qi, Y., Patra, G., Liang, X., et al. (2001) Utilization of the *rpoB* gene as a specific chromosomal marker for real- time PCR detection of *Bacillus anthracis. Appl. Environ. Microbiol.* **67,** 3720–3727.

19. Okinaka, R. T., Cloud, K., Hampton, O., et al. (1999) Sequence and organization of pXO1, the large *Bacillus anthracis* plasmid harboring the anthrax toxin genes. *J. Bacteriol.* **181,** 6509–6515.

20. Okinaka, R., Cloud, K., Hampton, O., et al. (1999) Sequence, assembly and analysis of pX01 and pX02. *J. Appl. Microbiol.* **87,** 261, 262.

21. Sen, K. and Asher, D. M. (2001) Multiplex PCR for detection of *Enterobacteriaceae* in blood. *Transfusion* **41,** 1356–1364.

22. Corless, C. E., Guiver, M., Borrow, R., Edwards-Jones, V., Fox, A. J., and Kaczmarski, E. B. (2001) Simultaneous detection of Neisseria meningitidis, Haemophilus influenzae, and Streptococcus pneumoniae in suspected cases of meningitis and septicemia using real-time PCR. *J. Clin. Microbiol.* **39,** 1553–1558.

23. Boyapalle, S., Wesley, I. V., Hurd, H. S., and Reddy, P. G. (2001) Comparison of culture, multiplex, and 5' nuclease polymerase chain reaction assays for the rapid detection of *Yersinia enterocolitica* in swine and pork products. *J. Food Prot.* **64,** 1352–1361.

24. Courtney, B. C., Smith, M. M., and Henchal, E. A. (1999) Development of internal controls for probe-based nucleic acid diagnostic assays. *Anal. Biochem.* **270,** 249–256.

25. Achtman, M., Zurth, K., Morelli, G., Torrea, G., Guiyoule, A., and Carniel, E. (1999) *Yersinia pestis,* the cause of plague, is a recently emerged clone of *Yersinia pseudotuberculosis. Proc. Natl. Acad. Sci. USA* **96,** 14,043–14,048.

26. Moore, R. L. and Brubaker, R. R. (1975) Hybridization and deoxyribonucleotide sequences of *Yersinia enterocolitica* and other selected members of *Enterobacteriaceae. Inter. J. Syst. Bacteriol.* **25,** 336–339.

27. Lindler, L. E., Plano, G. V., Burland, V., Mayhew, G. F., and Blattner, F. R. (1998) Complete DNA sequence and detailed analysis of the *Yersinia pestis* KIM5 plasmid encoding murine toxin and capsular antigen. *Infect. Immun.* **66,** 5731–5742.

28. Perry, R. D., Straley, S. C., Fetherston, J. D., Rose, D. J., Gregor, J., and Blattner, F. R. (1998) DNA sequencing and analysis of the low-Ca2+-response plasmid pCD1 of *Yersinia pestis* KIM5. *Infect. Immun.* **66,** 4611–4623.

29. Hu, P., Elliott, J., McCready, P., et al. (1998) Structural organization of virulence-associated plasmids of *Yersinia pestis. J. Bacteriol.* **180,** 5192–5202.

30. Prentice, M. B., James, K. D., Parkhill, J., et al. (2001) *Yersinia pestis* pFra shows biovar-specific differences and recent common ancestry with a *Salmonella enterica* serovar Typhi plasmid. *J. Bacteriol.* **183,** 2586–2594.

31. Hinnebusch, J. and Schwan, T. G. (1993) New method for plague surveillance using polymerase chain reaction to detect *Yersinia pestis* in fleas. *J. Clin. Microbiol.* **31,** 1511–1514.

32. Higgins, J. A., Ezzell, J., Hinnebusch, B. J., Shipley, M., Henchal, E. A., Ibrahim, M. S. (1998) 5' nuclease PCR assay to detect *Yersinia pestis. J. Clin. Microbiol.* 36, 2284–2288.

33. Engelthaler, D. M., Gage, K. L., Montenieri, J. A., Chu, M., and Carter, L. G. (1999) PCR detection of *Yersinia pestis* in fleas: comparison with mouse inoculation. *J. Clin. Microbiol.* **37,** 1980–1984.

34. Zerva, L., Bourantas, K., Mitka, S., Kansouzidou, A., and Legakis, N. J. (2001) Serum is the preferred clinical specimen for diagnosis of human brucellosis by PCR. *J. Clin. Microbiol.* **39,** 1661–1664.

35. Leal-Klevezas, D. S., Martinez-Vazquez, I. O., Lopez-Merino, A., and Martinez-Soriano, J. P. (1995) Single-step PCR for detection of *Brucella* spp. from blood and milk of infected animals. *J. Clin. Microbiol.* **33,** 3087–3090.

36. Weisburg, W. G., Barns, S. M., Pelletier, D. A., and Lane, D. J. (1991) 16S ribosomal DNA amplification for phylogenetic study. *J. Bacteriol.* **173,** 697–703.

37. Fulop, M., Leslie, D., and Titball, R. (1996) A rapid, highly sensitive method for the detection of *Francisella tularensis* in clinical samples using the polymerase chain reaction. *Am. J. Trop. Med. Hyg.* **54,** 364–366.

38. Higgins, J. A., Hubalek, Z., Halouzka, J., et al. (2000) Detection of *Francisella tularensis* in infected mammals and vectors using a probe-based polymerase chain reaction. *Am. J. Trop. Med. Hyg.* **62,** 310–318.

39. Johansson, A., Berglund, L., Eriksson, U., et al. (2000) Comparative analysis of PCR versus culture for diagnosis of ulceroglandular tularemia. *J. Clin. Microbiol.* **38,** 22–26.

40. Sjostedt, A., Eriksson, U., Berglund, L., and Tarnvik, A. (1997) Detection of *Francisella tularensis* in ulcers of patients with tularemia by PCR. *J. Clin. Microbiol.* **35,** 1045–1048.

41. Long, G. W., Oprandy, J. J., Narayanan, R. B., Fortier, A. H., Porter, K. R., and Nacy, C. A. (1993) Detection of *Francisella tularensis* in blood by polymerase chain reaction. *J. Clin. Microbiol.* **31,** 152–154.

42. Junhui, Z., Ruifu, Y., Jianchun, L., et al. (1996) Detection of *Francisella tularensis* by the polymerase chain reaction. *J. Med. Microbiol.* **45,** 477–482.

43. Berdal, B. P., Mehl, R., Haaheim, H., et al. (2000) Field detection of *Francisella tularensis. Scand. J. Infect. Dis.* **32,** 287–291.

44. Forsman, M., Sandstrom, G., and Sjostedt, A. (1994) Analysis of 16S ribosomal DNA sequences of *Francisella* strains and utilization for determination of the phylogeny of the genus and for identification of strains by PCR. *Int. J. Syst. Bacteriol.* **44,** 38–46.

45. Hadfield, T. L., Turell, M., Dempsey, M. P., David, J., and Park, E. J. (2001) Detection of West Nile virus in mosquitoes by RT-PCR. *Mol. Cell. Probes* **15,** 147–150.

46. Weaver, S. C., Hagenbaugh, A., Bellew, L. A., et al. (1993) A comparison of the nucleotide sequences of eastern and western equine encephalomyelitis viruses with those of other alphaviruses and related RNA viruses. *Virology* **197,** 375–390.

47. Weaver, S. C., Hagenbaugh, A., Bellew, L. A., et al. (1994) A comparison of the nucleotide sequences of eastern and western equine encephalomyelitis viruses with those of other alphaviruses and related RNA viruses. *Virology* **202,** 1083.

48. Brault, A. C., Powers, A. M., Chavez, C. L., et al. (1999) Genetic and antigenic diversity among eastern equine encephalitis viruses from North, Central, and South America. *Am. J. Trop. Med. Hyg.* **61,** 579–586.

49. Meissner, J. D., Huang, C. Y., Pfeffer, M., and Kinney, R. M. (1999) Sequencing of prototype viruses in the Venezuelan equine encephalitis antigenic complex. *Virus Res.* **64,** 43–59.

50. Netolitzky, D. J., Schmaltz, F. L., Parker, M. D., et al. (2000) Complete genomic RNA sequence of western equine encephalitis virus and expression of the structural genes. *J. Gen. Virol.* **81,** 151–159.

51. Kramer, L. D. and Fallah, H. M. (1999) Genetic variation among isolates of western equine encephalomyelitis virus from California. *Am. J. Trop. Med. Hyg.* **60,** 708–713.

52. Linssen, B., Kinney, R. M., Aguilar, P., et al. (2000) Development of reverse transcription-PCR assays specific for detection of equine encephalitis viruses. *J. Clin. Microbiol.* **38,** 1527–1535.

53. Koshland, D. E., Jr. (1994) The biological warfare of the future [editorial]. *Science* **264,** 327.

54. Wiedemann, B. and Heisig, P. (1994) Mechanisms of quinolone resistance. *Infection* **22,** S73–79.

55. Piddock, L. J. (1999) Mechanisms of fluoroquinolone resistance: an update 1994–1998. *Drugs* **58,** 11–18.

56. Deguchi, T., Fukuoka, A., Yasuda, M., et al. (1997) Alterations in the GyrA subunit of DNA gyrase and the ParC subunit of topoisomerase IV in quinolone-resistant clinical isolates of *Klebsiella pneumoniae. Antimicrob. Agents. Chemother.* **41,** 699–701.

57. Yoshida, H., Bogaki, M., Nakamura, M., and Nakamura, S. (1990) Quinolone resistance-determining region in the DNA gyrase gyrA gene of *Escherichia coli. Antimicrob. Agents. Chemother.* **34,** 1271, 1272.

58. Yoshida, H., Bogaki, M., Nakamura, M., Yamanaka, L. M., and Nakamura, S. (1991) Quinolone resistance-determining region in the DNA gyrase gyrB gene of *Escherichia coli. Antimicrob. Agents. Chemother.* **35,** 1647–1650.

59. Lindler, L. E., Fan, W., and Jahan, N. (2001) Detection of ciprofloxacin-resistant *Yersinia pestis* by fluorogenic PCR using the lightcycler. *J. Clinical. Microbiol.* **39,** 3649–3655.

60. Heisig, P. (1993) High-level fluoroquinolone resistance in a *Salmonella typhimurium* isolate due to alterations in both gyrA and gyrB genes. *J. Antimicrob. Chemother.* **32,** 367–377.

61. Heisig, P. (1996) Genetic evidence for a role of parC mutations in development of high-level fluoroquinolone resistance in *Escherichia coli. Antimicrob. Agents. Chemother.* **40,** 879–885.

62. Cargill, M., Altshuler, D., Ireland, J., et al. (1999) Characterization of single-nucleotide polymorphisms in coding regions of human genes. *Nat. Genet.* **22,** 231–238.

63. Schriml, L. M., Peterson, R. J., Gerrard, B., and Dean, M. (2000) Use of denaturing HPLC to map human and murine genes and to validate single-nucleotide polymorphisms. *Biotechniques* **28,** 740–745.

64. Liu, W. O., Oefner, P. J., Qian, C,. Odom, R. S., and Francke, U. (1997) Denaturing HPLC-identified novel FBN1 mutations, polymorphisms, and sequence variants in Marfan syndrome and related connective tissue disorders. *Genet. Test.* **1,** 237–242.

65. McCallum, C. M., Comai, L., Greene, E. A., and Henikoff, S. (2000) Targeted screening for induced mutations. *Nat. Biotechnol.* **18,** 455–457.

66. Hoogendoorn, B., Owen, M. J., Oefner, P. J., Williams, N., Austin, .J, and O'Donovan, M. C. (1999) Genotyping single nucleotide polymorphisms by primer extension and high performance liquid chromatography. *Hum. Genet.* **104,** 89–93.

67. Hayward-Lester, A., Oefner, P. J., and Doris, P. A. (1996) Rapid quantification of gene expression by competitive RT-PCR and ion- pair reversed-phase HPLC. *Biotechniques* **20,** 250–257.

68. Roberts, M. C. (1996) Tetracycline resistance determinants: mechanisms of action, regulation of expression, genetic mobility, and distribution. *FEMS Microbiol. Rev.* **19,** 1–24.

69. Levy, S. B., McMurry, L. M., Barbosa, T. M., et al. (1999) Nomenclature for new tetracycline resistance determinants. *Antimicrob. Agents. Chemother.* **43,** 1523, 1524.

70. Ng, L. K., Martin, I., Alfa, M., and Mulvey, M. (2001) Multiplex PCR for the detection of tetracycline resistant genes. *Mol. Cell. Probes.* **15,** 209–215.

71. Aminov, R. I., Garrigues-Jeanjean, N., and Mackie, R. I. (2001) Molecular ecology of tetracycline resistance: development and validation of primers for detection of tetracycline resistance genes encoding ribosomal protection proteins. *Appl. Environ. Microbiol.* **67,** 22–32.

72. Carlson, S. A., Bolton, L. F., Briggs, C. E., et al. (1999) Detection of multiresistant *Salmonella typhimurium* DT104 using multiplex and fluorogenic PCR. *Mol. Cell. Probes.* **13,** 213–222.

73. Roberts, M. C., Pang, Y., Riley, D. E., Hillier, S. L., Berger, R. C., and Krieger, J. N. (1993) Detection of Tet M and Tet O tetracycline resistance genes by polymerase chain reaction. *Mol. Cell. Probes.* **7,** 387–393.

74. Roberts, M. C. (1994) Epidemiology of tetracycline-resistance determinants. *Trends. Microbiol.* **2,** 353–357.

25

Concepts for the Development of Immunodiagnostic Assays for Detection and Diagnosis of Biothreat Agents

George V. Ludwig, Cynthia A. Rossi, and Robert L. Bull

1. INTRODUCTION

An integrated approach to agent detection and identification provides the most reliable laboratory data and is essential to a complete and accurate disease diagnosis. To achieve more rapid biological agent identification with a high level of confidence, a combination of state-of-the-art antigen and nucleic acid analysis methods is required. The most significant problem associated with the development of an integrated diagnostic system has been the inability of antigen-detection technologies to detect agents with sensitivities approaching those of nucleic acid-detection technologies. These differences in assay sensitivity increase the probability of obtaining disparate results, thus complicating medical decisions. However, advances in immunodiagnostic technologies provide the basis for developing antigen-detection platforms capable of meeting stringent requirements for sensitivity, specificity, assay speed, robustness, and simplicity. Such advances must be exploited to increase the confidence of immunodiagnostic testing and to ensure the success of the integrated approach toward diagnosis of disease caused by biological warfare (BW) agents.

Detection of specific protein antigens and host-produced antibodies directed against such antigens constitutes one of the most widely used and successful methods for identifying biological agents and for diagnosing the diseases they cause. Nearly all methods for detecting antigens and antibodies rely on the production of complexes made of one or more receptor molecules and the entity being detected (antigen, antibody, or other molecule) (*see* Fig. 1). At the most fundamental level, the efficacy of any given immunologically based detection system is dependent on two major factors: the effectiveness and consistency of complex formation and the ability to detect these complexes. The nature of the complex and the method for detecting the complex vary and depend on the goals of the test and what is being detected. The purpose of this chapter is to survey methods for forming complexes and to describe some of the more promising technologies for immunodetection that offer accurate, robust, and timely identification of biological agents and/or disease diagnoses.

Traditionally, assays for detecting proteins and other nonnucleic acid targets, including antigens, antibodies, carbohydrates, and other organic molecules, were con-

From: *Infectious Diseases: Biological Weapons Defense: Infectious Diseases and Counterterrorism*
Edited by: L. E. Lindler, F. J. Lebeda, and G. W. Korch © Humana Press Inc., Totowa, NJ

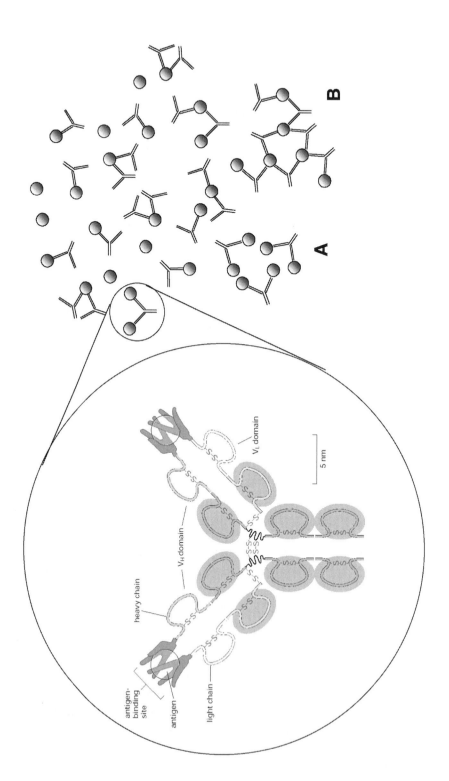

Fig. 1. A schematic of antigen-antibody complexes with a detail of antibody structure. In antigen excess, complex formation favors saturation of antigen-binding sites and little crosslinking of antigen molecules (**A**). In antibody excess, the formation of complexes involving multiple antigen and antibody molecules is favored (**B**). (Antibody detail copyright 1998 from Molecular Biology of the Cell by Alberts, Bray, Johnson, Lewis, Raff, Roberts, Walter. Reproduced by permission of Routledge, Inc., part of The Taylor & Francis Group.)

ducted using antibodies produced in appropriate host animals. As a result, these assays were generically referred to as immunodiagnostic or immunodetection methods. In reality, numerous other nonantibody molecules are now being used to develop these assays (*see* Subheading 4.3.) so affinity-based methods may be more appropriate terminology. However, for the sake of consistency, immunodiagnostic or immunodetection will be used to describe the affinity-based technologies.

The first step of any immunodiagnostic method is the formation of complexes consisting of the assay reagents and the agent being detected. The ability to produce and maintain these complexes is probably the single most important factor to consider when developing antigen- and antibody-detection assays. To form an effective complex, receptors and their ligands must bind efficiently. The central principle behind the formation of the complex is the fundamental interaction between two or more molecules. The nature of these interactions governs the overall sensitivity and specificity of detection assays. Receptor–ligand interactions are dependent on specific elements that dictate the strength of the interaction. The interactions that cause receptors to bind to their respective targets include electrostatic forces, hydrogen bonding, hydrophobic forces, and Van der Waals forces. Like bonds between any molecules, the bonds holding a receptor to its respective ligand are reversible and the complex may readily dissociate depending on the strength of bonds holding them together. The strength of receptor–ligand interactions is usually described in terms of the affinity of the ligand for its specific receptor and can be determined using the law of mass action. The equilibrium dissociation constant (K_d) for a specific interaction is the concentration of receptor–ligand complexes divided by the concentration of free receptor times the concentration of free ligand. In its simplest terms, K_d is expressed as the concentration of ligand required to saturate one-half of the available receptors. If the receptors have a high affinity for the ligand, then the K_d will be low, because it will take a lower concentration of ligand to bind one-half the available receptors. In terms of antigen and antibody detection, receptors with higher affinity are desirable because they are capable of detecting lower concentrations of ligand. Identifying the most useful antibodies to include in immunodiagnostic assays can be automated by using technologies like surface plasmon resonance *(1)*. However, comparing the specific activity (assay activity per unit mass) of different antibodies against a standard antigen preparation yields similar results. The latter procedure requires only the ability to purify antibody preparations and complete standard assays.

Although complex formation is critical to development of effective diagnostic assays, it is the process of assay optimization and detection of complexes that is ultimately responsible for the success or failure of immunodiagnostic assays for detecting biological agents. The methods for optimizing assays and detecting complexes are diverse and the reason for using one method over another depends on the goals and requirements of the test.

2. IMMUNODETECTION OF BIOLOGICAL AGENTS FOR DIAGNOSIS OF DISEASE

Immunodetection of disease-causing agents in biological samples is a multistep process involving formation of multiple complexes, all bound to a solid substrate. This process, or cascade of reactions, is like making a sandwich where detecting the biologi-

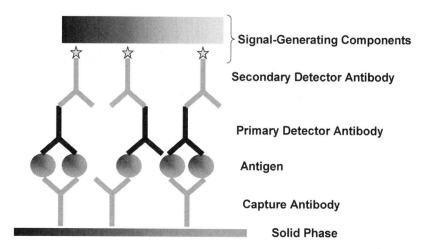

Fig. 2. Components of a typical sandwich immunoassay in which the generation of detectable signal is dependent on the presence of all of the components of the sandwich and their ability to appropriately interact with each other.

cal agent itself depends on forming the entire sandwich and generating a detectable signal by one or more of the assay components (*see* Fig. 2). The primary components of most immunoassays are polyclonal or monoclonal antibodies or antibody fragments. Advanced technology options such as peptides and aptamers (discussed later) have not found their way into common usage and are currently under evaluation by several research laboratories.

Binding one or more of the antibodies onto a solid substrate (*see* Table 1) is usually the first event of the assay reaction cascade. Immunoassays can generally be termed as either heterogeneous or homogeneous depending on the nature of the solid substrate. A heterogeneous assay requires physical separation of bound from unbound reactants by using techniques such as washing or centrifugation. These types of assays can remove interfering substances and, therefore, are, usually more specific. However, heterogeneous assays require more steps and increased manipulation that cumulatively affect assay precision. A homogeneous assay requires no physical separation but may require pretreatment steps to remove interfering substances. Homologous assays are usually faster and more conducive to automation because of their simplicity. However, the cost of these assays is usually greater because of the types of reagents and equipment required.

The final step in any immunoassay is the detection of a signal generated by one or more assay components. This detection step is typically accomplished by using antibodies bound to (or labeled with) inorganic or organic molecules that produce a detectable signal under specific chemical or environmental conditions (*see* Table 2). The earliest labels used were molecules containing radioactive isotopes. Such labels are still used today, and a wide range of commonly available laboratory instruments can detect the presence of these labels with a high degree of sensitivity. However, using radioisotopes presents specific safety hazards; the radioisotopes are closely regulated, and the equipment required to detect the isotopes is expensive, not readily portable, and requires specialized training to operate. As a result, radioisotope labels have gener-

Table 1
Common Solid Substrates Used in the Development of Immunodiagnostic Assays

Plastic	Beads	Membranes	Glass	Cells	Other
Polypropylene well plates	Latex	Nitrocellulose	Slides	Red blood cells	Protein G
"Credit cards"	Gold	Nylon	Capillary tubes	Permissive cell lines	Protein A
	Magnetic			Monoclonal cell lines	Sephadex
	Paramagnetic				Silicon microarrays

Table 2
List of Commonly Used Labels for the Detection Step in the Development of Immunoassays

Enzymes	Particles	Radioisotopes	Fluorochromes	Other
Peroxidase	Gold	^{14}C	Fluorescein	Biotin
Alkaline phosphatase	Latex	^{32}P	Ruthenium	
β-Galactosidase	Paramagnetic	^{3}H	Rhodamine	
Urease		^{35}S	Texas Red	
Glucose oxidase		^{125}I	Bodipy	
		Alexa		
		Europium		

ally been replaced with less cumbersome labels such as enzymes. Enzymes are effective labels because they catalyze chemical reactions, which can produce a signal. Depending on the nature of the signal, the reactants may be detected visually, electronically, chemically, or physically. Because a single enzyme molecule can catalyze many chemical reactions without being consumed in the reaction, these labels are effective at amplifying assay signals. Most common enzyme–substrate reactions used in immunodiagnostics produce a visual signal that can be detected with the naked eye or by a spectrophotometer. Like all organic molecules, enzymes are relatively unstable and require refrigeration or other specialized preservation techniques to maintain activity over time.

Fluorescent dyes and other organic and inorganic molecules capable of generating luminescent signals are also commonly used labels in immunoassays. Assays using these molecules are often more sensitive than enzyme immunoassays but require specialized instrumentation and often suffer from high background contamination as a result of the intrinsic fluorescent and luminescent qualities of some proteins and light-scattering effects. Signals in assays using these types of labels are amplified by integrating light signals over time and cyclic generation of photons. Other commonly used labels include gold, latex, and magnetic or paramagnetic particles. Each can be visualized by the naked eye or by instruments and are quite stable under various environmental conditions. However, these labels are essentially inert and, therefore, do not produce an amplified signal. Signal amplification is useful and desirable because it results in increased assay sensitivity. Increased signal strength can be attained by using amplifiable labels as described earlier or by using molecules capable of forming multiple bonds. These molecules can produce more complex sandwiches containing lattices of signal-generating compounds or molecules. Biotin and avidin are examples of molecules exhibiting these characteristics. They have very high affinities for each other, developing almost irreversible bonds ($K_d = 10^{-15}$ M). Additionally, avidin can bind as many as four biotin molecules, increasing the size of the complex. If biotin is bound to a signal-generating molecule or compound, then the strength of the signal increases proportionally.

3. IMMUNOASSAY DEVELOPMENT

Five important parameters affecting the performance of all immunoassays are temperature, time, reagent concentration, kinetics, and quality of reagents. Optimizing each of the parameters is essential to successful immunoassay development. The most common method used for optimizing most of these parameters is an empiric approach where one or two parameters are varied between experiments using a matrix format (*see* Table 3). Depending on the number of steps involved with an assay, the optimization process can be time consuming and complicated. However, for a given assay platform, many of the parameters such as time and temperature need only be optimized for a single assay. All subsequent assays will probably function well within the specification identified for the first assay.

For many immunodiagnostic assays, particularly heterogeneous assays, diffusion of molecules within an assay matrix is the rate-limiting step. Increasing the assay temperature generally increases the rate of diffusion, thus increasing the opportunity for two assay components to interact. However, antibody affinity decreases as temperature increases, so assay speed and sensitivity must be balanced to meet assay requirements. Again, because diffusion is a rate-limiting step, increasing the incubation time for critical assay steps often results in greater assay sensitivity. The duration of critical assays steps is more critical for nonequilibrium techniques where background or assay noise can have a detrimental effect on assay performance if allowed to continue too long. With some assays, this effect can be minimized by adding compounds that inhibit enzymatic reactions or inactivate the reactants (e.g., stop solution). Reagent concentration is a major concern, especially in development of homogeneous assays, where too little or too much antibody can lead to pro-zone effects where signals are artificially low because of the stoichiometry of the reactions (*see* Fig. 3). Generally, reagent concentration drives the sensitivity of the assay, but it can also affect the rates of false-positive and false-negative results and requires careful optimization.

The efficiency of each step of the assay cascade is governed in part by the assay environment. This environment includes pH, ionic strength, and the presence or absence of additives such as carrier proteins, detergents, enzyme inhibitors, and preservatives in the assay buffers. Because diffusion is a major rate-limiting step, assays generally require less time if reaction volumes are kept small. Each of these parameters must be carefully examined and optimized and may vary significantly for different

Table 3
Example of an Optimization Experiment Designed to Identify
the Most Efficient Dilution of Enzyme-Conjugated Antibody
in an ELISA Test

		Capture antibody dilution					
		1:200	1:400	1:800	1:1600	1:3200	1:6400
Enzyme-conjugated antibody dilution	1:2000	2.11	2.54	2.62	2.65	2.13	1.53
	1:4000	2.12	2.01	2.12	1.72	1.15	0.70
	1:8000	1.34	1.02	1.10	0.83	0.57	0.27
	1:16000	0.41	0.57	0.55	0.33	0.21	0.04
	1:32000	0.13	0.24	0.16	0.03	−0.04	−0.05
	1:64000	0.06	0.02	0.00	−0.03	−0.09	−0.05
	1:128000	0.08	0.01	−0.02	−0.07	−0.05	−0.05
	1:256000	−0.03	0.02	−0.03	−0.06	−0.09	−0.04

Dilutions of capture antibody are made across a multiwell plate while dilutions of conjugate are made down the plate. The optimal dilution of conjugate was determined to be 1:8000 because it produced positive results against the capture antibody across its entire expected dilution range. Darker shades indicate more intense signals.

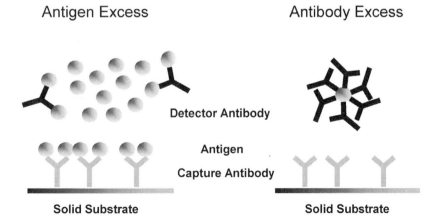

Fig. 3. Effect of reagent concentration on assay performance. Low concentrations of antibody in relationship to the quantity of specific antigen present saturates the binding sites at the level of the capture antibody and divalent binding of detector antibody to free antigen. This results from the failure of complete sandwich formation and a false-negative result. High concentrations of detector antibody in relationship to available antigen concentration may also produce false-negative results if complex formation favors saturation of antigen binding sites by detector antibody. This phenomenon is less common than the antigen excess phenomenon but still should be considered during assay optimization.

assay types and for different detection platforms. Optimizing the environmental variables must be carefully balanced with other assay requirements such as assay speed, sensitivity, specificity, simplicity, and so on to meet the appropriate diagnostic requirements for the assay.

4. IMMUNODIAGNOSTIC LIGANDS

4.1. Antibodies

A principle requirement for immunodiagnostic assays is the availability of organic molecules that can bind to specific domains present on infectious and noninfectious disease agents. Traditionally, antibodies have served as the primary component of immunodiagnostic assays because they are relatively easy to produce and can be selected to possess the desired affinity characteristics.

An organism's response to infection is collectively referred to as an immune response, and depending on the complexity of the organism, the immune response may take various forms. Mammals and birds have evolved adaptive or acquired immune responses, which provide a much more flexible and specific barrier to a broader range of infection-causing organisms. It is this adaptive immune response, more specifically the development and production of antibodies, which provides the basis for immuno-logical-based identification of biological agents. The strength of the bonds between a clonal population of antibodies and their receptors is referred to as affinity (as described earlier), whereas the collective affinities of a mixed population of antibodies are re-ferred to as antibody avidity. Antibodies are globulin proteins formed by a specific class of white blood cell in response to foreign antigens (*see* Fig. 1). The antibodies bind to the antigen, thus supporting agent removal from the host. One important char-acteristic of the host-immune response is the phenomenon of response maturity that occurs over time and after multiple exposures to a given antigen. Hypermutation and rearrangement of genes encoding the antigen-binding portion of the antibody molecule that occur during repeated exposure to antigen results in selection of antibodies of higher affinity *(2–4)*.

4.1.1. Polyclonal Antibody

Selecting high-quality antibodies by hyperimmunizing host animals has been a stan-dard method for producing reagents for immunologically based detection systems. This process is simple, it can produce antibodies with very high avidity, it produces antibod-ies directed against multiple epitopes present on an antigen (polyclonal response), and the antibodies are relatively easy to purify from animal serum or ascites fluid.

The use of polyclonal antibody in diagnostic assays also has some important disad-vantages. It requires use of laboratory animals. Such animals (particularly rabbits, goats, and other larger animals) are genetically outbred and, therefore, vary consider-ably in their ability to respond to vaccination with different antigens. This results in significant variation among lots of antibodies produced. Another important problem is that the antibody response to a given antigen tends to be broad, covering both specific and cross-reactive epitopes. Diagnostic assays that include only polyclonal antibodies can be highly sensitive but are typically not very specific.

The specificity of assays that include polyclonal antibodies can usually be increased by selectively removing crossreactive and less desirable antibodies from the mixture. Most often, this is accomplished by affinity–purifying specific antibody by using an immobilized antigen or by selective absorption of crossreacting antibodies in an extract containing undesirable antigens. Affinity purification of polyclonal antibodies has the added advantage of selecting antibody populations with high avidity by adjusting elu-tion conditions such that lower avidity antibodies are removed from the column before eluting the more-desirable, high-avidity antibodies. Conditions for affinity purification must always be appropriately balanced between selection of the most useful antibodies and loss of antibody activity as a result of the severity of the elution conditions and decreasing antibody yields resulting from an increasing number of manipulations.

4.1.2. Monoclonal Antibody

With the advent of technologies to produce monoclonal antibodies (MAbs), it became possible to develop diagnostic assays that were specific and more reproducible. The process for immortalizing mouse B lymphocytes by fusing them with myeloma cells followed by cloning of individual hybridomas secreting antibody of predefined specificity was developed in the mid-1970s *(5)*. Development of MAbs allowed for production of large quantities of antibodies with little variation between lots. Adapting MAbs to growth in large-scale cultures has also decreased our dependency on mice and other animals. The ability to produce MAbs has had a tremendous impact on diagnostic assay development by allowing custom-designed reagents for specific needs. Selecting antibodies directed against specific molecular targets has led to development of assays that are much more specific than was previously possible with polyclonal antibodies. Conversely, choosing MAbs directed against more common antigens can make an assay less specific. The availability of these reagents has allowed for a level of flexibility in assay development that was never available before the development of MAbs. A common disadvantage with the use of MAbs or any monospecific reagent used in diagnostics is that there is always the possibility for agents to evade detection if the antibodies are no longer capable of binding to their respective biological agents. Such events are known to occur in nature through phenomena known as antigenic drift or shift. These events occur when small or large mutations in the protein-encoding genes become incorporated into agent genomes such that important epitopes are altered and are no longer capable of binding to antibodies with previous known activity. Similarly, antigens could be purposefully modified by genetic engineering or through active selection processes resulting in agents that may be capable of evading detection systems *(6–8)*. To avoid this problem, cocktails of MAbs that are directed against multiple epitopes should be used in diagnostic and detection assays. Another disadvantage with MAbs is that these antibodies rarely possess affinities that match the avidities of good polyclonal antibodies. Therefore, diagnostic assays made with only one MAb are often less sensitive than similar assays with polyclonal antibodies.

4.2. Phage Display

In some instances, development of MAbs by traditional techniques and immunization of animals to obtain polyclonal antisera are unsuccessful in producing reagents with the desired biological characteristics. Phage display is a technology with the potential to overcome some of these problems and to exploit the nearly limitless binding capability of the mammalian immune system *(9–11)*. Phage display is a recombinant DNA technique that couples the speed of bacterial growth and the ability to generate and display fusion proteins on filamentous phages. Genes encoding phage protein (gIII or gVIII) are fused to the antigen-binding segment of antibodies. The antibody segment may encode either a fragment of an antibody molecule, consisting of the light chain disulfide bonded to the amino-terminus of the heavy chain (Fab) or to a synthetic peptide consisting of the amino-terminus of the Fab light (*VL*) chain joined to the carboxy-terminus of the Fab heavy (*VH*) chain (scFVs) *(12,13)*. An advantage of phage display is that identification of antigen-binding sequences can be identified faster than by classical methods of antibody production *(10)*. Phage display of Fab fragments or scFv provides a rapid and specific tool for identifying antibody sequences that can bind biological agents. An added advantage of developing recombinant Fab fragments is that they can be produced in large quantities with little lot-to-lot variation through standard fermentation processes. Another key advantage of using phage display technology is that antibody variable domains can be more easily engineered with desired affinity characteristics. Many methods for making such modifications have been developed. These include (a) site-specific mutagenesis based on the crystal structure or primary or secondary structure of the antibody–antigen complex; (b) V_H and V_L chain shuffling; (c) screening of libraries in which one or more hypervariable domains are subjected to combinatorial mutagenesis; (d) extension of the heavy-chain hypervariable domain 3 loop to introduce additional contacts between the antibody and the antigen; (e) random mutagenesis over the entire V-gene; and (f) recombination of beneficial mutations isolated from a to e *(14,15)*. This customization of antibodies increases the flexibility associated with development of diagnostic reagents by allowing one to tailor reagents with specific biological characteristics.

Although antibodies made by recombinant DNA technology offer several distinct advantages for the development of immunodiagnostic reagents over more traditional methods, they also have some limitations. Fabs and scFvs are less stable in vivo than complete antibodies *(16)*, are unable to crosslink antigens, and may lack critical domains necessary for certain biological functions. The Fabs/scFvs as part of a fully functional antibody has been expressed in a nonlymphocyte cell line *(17)*. Additionally, molecular techniques for homologous recombination in hybridomas have become available *(18–20)*. Theoretically, Fab or scFv variable domain sequences can be cloned into a hybridoma line, from any species, allowing production of fully functional MAbs.

The combination of traditionally based polyclonal and monoclonal antibody development and phage display combined with genetic engineering offer tremendous flexibility in reagent production. However, new technologies hold additional promise for even greater development speed and assay flexibility than can currently be realized.

4.3. Advanced Ligand Formats

Although polyclonal antibodies and MAbs (both classically produced and phage display) continue to be the most commonly used reagents for traditional immunoassays, additional immunodiagnostic affinity matrices are being developed that offer significant promise for improved diagnostic assay development. These antibody "mimics" include random peptides and oligonucleotides whose tertiary structure produce binding sites that are capable of forming noncovalent linkages to proteins and other potentially important receptors.

4.3.1. Peptides

All proteins have a structure that is defined by their amino acid sequence and by folding caused by interamino acid interactions between adjoining and distant amino acids. This structure forms the basis for most biological functions including antibody and antigen binding. Although the importance of protein structure and the structural relationship to function is well-understood, the ability to rationally design proteins to perform specific biological functions is still largely unrealized. However, it is possible to select random peptides produced from cDNA libraries that possess desired traits including ligand-binding characteristics.

Several systems for selecting short peptides with defined biological binding activity have shown some promise for selecting reagents that might be useful for diagnostic purposes. One system was originally designed for probing protein–protein interactions by displaying random peptide libraries on the surface of *Escherichia coli* flagella. This system makes use of a fusion protein made with the entire coding sequence of *E. coli* thioredoxin (trxA) gene and the dispensable region of the gene for flagellin (fliC), the major structural component of the *E. coli* flagellum *(21)*. This fusion protein is efficiently exported and assembled into partially functional flagella on the bacterial cell surface. A library containing more than 10^8 random dodecapeptides can be displayed on the exterior of *E. coli*. These peptides become conformationally constrained by being inserted into the thioredoxin active-site loop. A panning technique is used to isolate bacteria displaying peptides with affinity to immobilized antibodies or antigens. This technique has been used to map linear antibody epitopes *(21)* and has some potential for rapidly selecting peptides that could serve as useful ligands in antigen-detection assays. Although extremely useful, this in vivo procedure often produces proteins that may be toxic to cells, thus limiting the size of the library that can be screened. A modification of this approach has been designed to produce large libraries of peptides fused to their encoding DNA. Peptides made using this procedure do not require living cells and can be made totally in vitro, thus eliminating the lethal negative effect toxic proteins have on host cells during large-scale production. In this process, referred to as PROfusion, peptides with a specific biological function are selected through an iterative process by using large cDNA libraries that produce covalent cDNA-protein fusions for protein display applications. Briefly, a branched mRNA template is developed that is photoligated to a peptidyl acceptor containing a reverse transcription primer at the 3'-end. Translation in vitro followed by reverse transcription produces a protein covalently bonded to its encoding cDNA. Useful peptide-cDNA fusion products are selected by panning against the ligand(s) of interest. The nucleic acid from selected protein-cDNA partners is amplified and transfected into host cells to form a new library. Multiple rounds of selection and in vitro transcription, translation, and reverse transcription results in selection of peptides with desired biological characteristics accompanied by their encoding cDNAs. Their ease of preparation and their inherent stability should make cDNA–protein fusions a useful tool for the in vitro selection and evolution of high-affinity ligands from large libraries of polypeptides *(22–24)*. By eliminating the need for protein production in actively growing prokaryotic cells, the size of the cDNA libraries that can be screened is limited only by the upper limit on peptide size.

4.3.2. Aptamers

Peptide ligands are not the only molecules that may serve as antibody mimics in diagnostic assays. Nucleic acids are also known to form tertiary structures that may bind specifically or nonspecifically to proteins or other nucleic acids. Aptamers are single-stranded nucleic acids that are evolved in vitro to perform some specific biological function that may include therapeutic or diagnostic uses. The most common method for producing aptamers is systematic evolution of ligands by exponential enrichment (SELEX) *(25)*. In this procedure, a large population of single-stranded nucleic acid molecules (RNA or DNA) is screened against an antigen of interest. Antigen–nucleic acid complexes that form are separated from free nucleic acid by one of several different techniques, including affinity chromatography, size exclusion chromatography, electrophoresis, or binding to filters. The selected oligonucleotides are then amplified. Aptamers with the desired biological characteristics are acquired after several rounds of sequential selection and amplification. These enriched oligonucleotides may have K_d equal to or less than 1 nM, representing binding affinities equivalent to or better than many antibodies *(26)*.

Typically, monofunctional aptamer affinities are compared directly to those observed with bifunctional antibody molecules, which may not produce a fair representation of aptamer performance. In at least one study, dimerization of a single aptamer led to significant increases in binding strength resulting from decrease in the dissociation rate constant of the dimerized aptamer for its specific protein target. In this particular case, dimerization of the aptamer produced binding kinetics that rivaled a traditionally produced MAb *(27)*. A recently described modification to the SELEX technique could be used to further enhance the binding efficiency of evolved oligonucleotides (photo-selex). In this procedure, 5-bromo or 5-iodo dUTP or UTP are substituted for the natural triphosphate molecules. During aptamer amplification, these triphosphates are incorporated during DNA or RNA polymerization. Although this substitution has no effect on the evolution of aptamers with low K_d, it does allow for photoinduced crosslinking to the targeted protein. However, the ability of aptamers to photocrosslink to the targeted protein depends on the distance of the substituted triphosphates to specific targets on the protein and, therefore, is under control of a second geometric constraint. If evolution of such aptamers is carried out under conditions in which both initial protein binding and photocrosslinking are constrained, then a single aptamer may provide improvements to diagnostic assay performance equivalent to that realized by using two independent antibody molecules in an equivalent assay *(28–30)*. In addition, the covalent bond formed during crosslinking should also improve assay sensitivity as a result of irreversible attachment of receptor and ligand molecules.

The most important concern associated with aptamers for use in diagnostic testing is related to stability. Free nucleic acids, particularly RNA, are subject to digestion by nucleases found in essentially all common biological and environmental samples. It has been shown that aptamers can be stabilized by modifying sugars on the nucleoside triphosphates *(31,32)*, use of appropriate production phosphoramidites, and by methylation of the 2'OH groups on purine nucleosides *(33)*. Large-scale manufacturing of aptamers is possible at costs that are similar to those associated with antibody production, making these reagents viable candidates for diagnostic and therapeutic reagents.

5. IMMUNODIAGNOSTIC PLATFORMS

The increasing demand for immunodiagnostic assays possessing greater sensitivity, speed, and ease of use is reflected in the number and variety of new assay systems that are continually being developed. Advances in the fields of biomedical engineering, chemistry, physics, and biology have led to an explosion of new diagnostic platforms and assays systems that offer great promise for improving diagnostic capabilities.

Because of the speed with which new diagnostic technologies are being developed, a detailed overview of all new technologies will quickly be out of date. Here, we provide an overview of standard technologies and those that show great promise for near-term use.

5.1. Enzyme-Linked Immunosorbent Assay

Since the 1970s, the enzyme-linked immunosorbent assay (ELISA) has been the standard against which performance of new diagnostic technologies is measured. ELISA is perhaps the most widely used and best understood immunoassay. ELISAs have been developed in many formats and can be designed to detect either antibodies produced by a host in response to agent infection or antigens associated with individual biological agents. ELISAs that detect biological agents are heterogeneous assays in which an agent or an agent-specific antigen is captured onto a plastic multiwell plate by an antibody previously bound to the plate surface (capture antibody). Bound antigen is then detected using a secondary antibody (detector antibody). The detector antibody can be directly labeled with a signal-generating molecule or it can be detected with another antibody that is labeled with an enzyme (*see* Fig. 4). These enzymes catalyze a chemical reaction with substrate that results in a colorimetric change. The intensity of this color can be measured by a modified spectrophotometer that determines the optical density of the reaction using a specific wavelength of light. Many different enzymes are suited for this application (*see* Table 2). Certain enzyme-substrate combinations offer specific advantages because of the wavelength of light absorbed by the reactants. Horseradish peroxidase (HRP) in the presence of 2,2'-azinobis(3-ethylbenz-thiazoline-6-sulphonic acid; ABTS) absorbs light at 410 nm, producing a deep green color. This produces a particularly sensitive assay that can be interpreted without a spectrophotometer if necessary. The format shown in Fig. 2 requires antibody from two different species of animals so there is no direct interaction between sandwich layers. If the detector antibody were directly labeled with enzyme, then antibodies from the same species could be used as both capture and detector reagents.

One of the major advantages of ELISA is that it can be configured for various uses and applications. Equipment requirements can range from very simple, manually operated devices to rapid, automated, high-throughput systems. In every ELISA format, a technician must be able to add reagents during each assay step, wash between steps, and measure the optical density of the final reaction products. As a result, ELISA equipment typically consists of an assay washer, an assay spectrophotometer otherwise known as a reader, a personal computer that assists with assay interpretation, and various liquid handling devices for handling reagents.

In a typical agent-detection ELISA, plastic multiwell plates are coated with a capture antibody. This step can require overnight incubation while the antibody adsorbs onto the well surface or can be as short as 1 h or less if avidin-coated wells and biotin-labeled capture antibodies are used. Specialized plates can also be used that are capable of covalently binding capture antibody on the well surface. These antibody-coated plates can be dried and stored for long periods of time (1–6 mo) at 4°C until used.

After plate coating, samples that may contain biological agents are then added to the antibody-coated wells, and after some previously optimized period of time (typically 1 h), the plates are thoroughly washed and then the detector antibody is added. After another incubation period, plates are again washed and an enzyme-labeled secondary

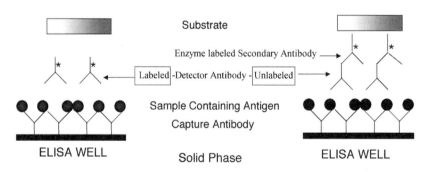

Fig. 4. Typical sandwich formats for antigen detection enzyme-linked immunosorbent assays (ELISAs) commonly used for biological agent detection and diagnoses.

antibody is added. After this next incubation period, the chemical substrate is added and allowed to incubate until the chemical reaction has proceeded for the optimal period of time. Then the results can be measured using an ELISA reader (spectrophotometer) equipped with an optical filter of the appropriate wavelength. Critical assay performance characteristics and assay limits of detection from three typical ELISAs with HRP-based enzyme/substrate systems are shown in Table 4. The major advantages of the ELISAs are that they are commonly used and understood by clinical laboratories and physicians, are amenable to high-throughput laboratory use and automation, do not require highly purified antibodies, and are relatively inexpensive to perform. The major disadvantages are that they are labor-intensive, temperature-dependent, have a narrow antigen concentration dynamic range that makes quantitation difficult, and are relatively slow.

We successfully developed antigen-detection ELISAs for nearly 40 different biological agents and antibody-detection ELISAs for nearly 90 different agents. All of these assays were developed by using the same solid phase, buffers and other reagents, incubation periods, incubation temperatures, and general procedures (*see* Table 4). This was done to maximize the versatility of the assay system while minimizing the supporting logistical burden. The only variables of this particular system are the antibody preparations used during each of the assay steps and their concentrations. Although there is significant variation in assay limits of detection, ELISAs typically are capable of detecting as little as 1 ng of antigen per milliliter of sample. The major variables associated with this system include affinity of the capture and detector antibodies and the sensitivity of the detection system. In our hands, the HRP/ABTS enzyme substrate system provided the best combination of sensitivity and versatility in a field environment.

5.2. Electrochemiluminescence

Among the most promising new technologies is one based on electrochemiluminescence (ECL) detection. One such system, developed by BioVeris, Inc. (Gaithersburg, MD) makes use of antigen-capture assays and a chemiluminescent label (ruthenium, Ru) and includes magnetic beads to concentrate target agents. These beads are coated with capture antibody, and in the presence of biological agent, immune complexes are formed between the agent and the labeled detector antibody. Because of its small size (1057 kDa), Ru can be easily conjugated to any protein ligand using standard chemis-

Table 4
Critical Assay Parameters and Performance Characteristics for Four Immunodiagnostic Technologies

	ELISA	DELFIA-TRF	ECL	Luminex	HHA
Antibody requirements					
Purity	None	Required	Required	Required	Required
Labeling	None	Europium	Biotin/Ruthenium	Biotin/Beads	Beads
Assay parameter					
Coating time	12 h	12 h	0	0	0
Incubation time	3.5 h	2.2 h	15 min	30 min	15 min
Read time	1 s/well	2 s/well	1 min/tube	20–120 s/well	30 s
No. of steps	5	4	1	1	1
No. of buffers required	3	3	1	1	1
Specialized reagents	Conjugate	Decontam. buffer	Assay buffer	Sheath fluid	Sample buffer
	Substrate	Enhancement sol.	Cell cleaner		
Solid phase used	Microtiter well	Microtiter well	Magnetic bead	Colored latex bead	Nitrocellulose
Reaction	Bound	Bound	In solution	In solution	Bound
Detector label used	HRP	Eu	Ru	PE	Gold
Detection method	Colorimetric	Fluorescence	Chemiluminescence	Fluorescence	Visual
Amount of sample per test	100 µL	100 µL	50 µL	50 µL	200 µL
Prozone	No	No	Yes	Yes	No

(continued)

Table 4 (*continued*)

Antibody requirements	ELISA	DELFIA-TRF	ECL	Luminex	HHA
Sample matrix effects	No	No	Yes	Yes	Yes
Multiplexing	No	Potential	No	Yes	Potential
Intraassay variation (%)	15–20%	20–50%	2–12%	10–25%	Undetermined
Potential for PCR analysis	Yes	Yes	Yes	Yes	Yes

Limits of detection were determined from assays developed with identical antibodies and antigen preparations. These values do not necessarily represent maximum limits of detection for the technologies.

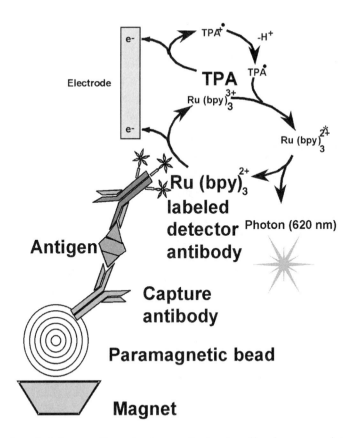

Fig. 5. Typical sandwich assay format using an electrochemiluminescence detection system. An electric current supplies the energy necessary to complete the reduction of ruthinium using H+ donated by tripropylamine (TPA). Ru is recycled to its ground state after emission of a photon of light at 620 nm.

tries without affecting immunoreactivity or solubility of the protein. The heart of the ECL analyzer is an electrochemical flow cell with a photomultiplier tube (PMT) placed just above the electrode. A magnet positioned just below the electrode captures the magnetic bead-Ru-tagged immune complex and holds it against the electrode. The application of an electric field results in a rapid electron transfer reaction between the substrate (tripropylamine) and the Ru. Excitation with as little as 1.5 V results in light emission, which in turn is detected by the PMT. The measurement of a single sample can be repeated numerous times in the analyzer because the electron-transfer, photon-release reaction regenerates the ruthenium (*see* Fig. 5). This results in an amplified signal and requires only a small volume of reagent per test. The magnetic beads provide a greater surface area than conventional surface-binding assays like the ELISA. The reaction does not suffer the surface steric and diffusion limitations encountered in solid-phase immunoassays; instead it occurs in a turbulent bead suspension, thus allowing for rapid reaction kinetics and short incubation time. Detection limits as low as 200 fmol/L with a linear dynamic range that can span six orders of magnitude is possible *(34,35)*. Compared to colorimetric assays like the ELISA, this technology is more sensitive and the instrumentation is simpler. Compared to fluorescence, chemilumines-cence produces no light-scattering effects, and background signal resulting from the presence of impurities is reduced or eliminated. ECL technology has been incorporated into Boehringer Mannheim's Elecsys™ system, Organon Teknika's NASBA™ RNA amplification technology, and Perkin-Elmer-Wallac's QPCR System 5000™ for PCR amplification of DNA sequences.

A typical ECL system (Origen, BioVeris, Inc.) consists of an analyzer and a per-sonal computer with software. The system's strength comes from its speed, sensitivity, accuracy, and precision over a wide dynamic range. Both immunoassays and nucleic acid-based detection assays are compatible with this platform. In a typical agent-detec-tion assay, sample is added to reagents consisting of capture antibody-coated paramag-netic beads and a Ru-conjugated detector antibody. Reagents can be lyophilized. After a short, 15-min incubation period on the vortexing carousel, the analyzer draws the sample into the flow cell, captures and washes the magnetic beads, and measures the ECL signal (up to 1 min per sample cleaning and reading time).

The ECL system has been demonstrated to be effective for detecting staphylococcal enterotoxin B *(36)* ricin toxin, botulinum toxin, *Francisella tularensis*, *Yersinia pestis* F1 antigen, *Bacillus anthracis* protective antigen, and Venezuelan equine encephalitis virus *(37)*. The technology could potentially be used with any biological agent and is limited only by the availability of high-quality, high-affinity antibodies or other ligands that can be used in the assay. Critical assay performance characteristics and detectionlimits from three typical ECL agent-detection assays are shown in Table 4. Although in general, the ECL assays are simple, rapid, and sensitive, assay sensitivities may vary significantly depending on the sample matrices encountered. Because of this, matrix-specific positive- and negative-control samples are used to establish standard curves and cutoff values. The major limitations of these assays are associated with the instrumentation itself including its size and weight and the time required to analyze each assay tube.

5.3. Time-Resolved Fluorescence (DELFIA)

Time-resolved fluorescence (TRF) is an immunodiagnostic technology actively being developed by Perkin-Elmer-Wallac. Applications include detection of agent-specific antibodies, microorganisms, drugs, and therapeutic agents *(38–40)*. In prac-tice, TRF-based assays are sandwich-type assays similar to those used for ELISA. The solid phase is a microwell plate coated in some manner with specific capture antibody, not unlike that used with colorimetric ELISA platforms. However, instead of being labeled with enzymes, detector antibodies are labeled with lanthanide chelates. The technology takes advantage of the differential fluorescence life span of lanthanide che-late labels compared to background fluorescence. The labels have an intense long-lived fluorescence signal and a large Stokes shift (*see* Fig. 6). This results in an assay that has a very high signal-to-noise ratio with high sensitivity *(41)*. Unlike ECL, TRF produces detectable fluorescence through the excitation of the lanthanide chelate by a specific wavelength of light. Fluorescence is initiated in TRF with a pulse of excitation energy, repeatedly and reproducibly. In 1 s, the fluorescent material can be pulse-excited 1000 times with an accumulation of the generated signal. One TRF format is dissociation-enhanced lanthanide fluorescence immunoassay (DELFIA), in which dis-

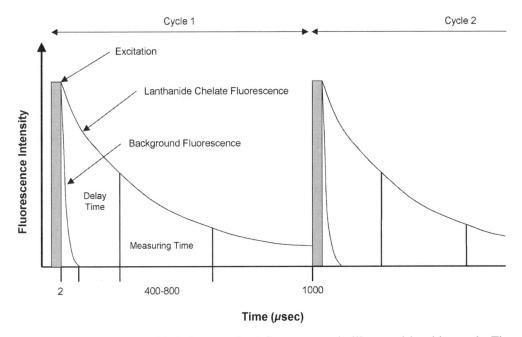

Fig. 6. The concept behind time-resolved fluorescence is illustrated by this graph. The europium chelate is excited by light with a wavelength of 340 nm. A Stokes shift of 273 nm separates the excitation wavelength from the emissions wavelength of 613 nm. By delaying the measurement of emitted light for 400 μs, short-lived background fluorescence is not included in the final measurement.

sociation of the complex-bound chelate caused by adding a low-pH enhancement solution forms long-lasting fluorescent micelles. The manufacturer claims detection limits as low as 10^{-17} moles of europium per well with a dynamic range of at least four logs (lanthanide labeling for time-resolved fluorometry By EG&G WALLAC).

DELFIA equipment includes the 1420 Victor^2 multilabel counter, a personal computer with menu-driven Victor software, dedicated pipetors, a specialized washer (Tecan's OEM M12\2R Columbus plus), and a plate shaker. The assay's strengths come from its sensitivity, similarity with the commonly used ELISA techniques, and the potential for multiplexing. There are four different lanthanides available (europium, samarium, terbium, and dysprosium) each with its own unique narrow emission spectra *(42)*. Both immunoassays and nucleic acid detection assays are compatible with this platform. Like the ECL assays, purified high-quality antibodies are required for this platform. In a typical agent-detection assay, sample is added to plates coated with capture antibody. After a 1-h incubation, plates are thoroughly washed and then Eu-labeled detector antibody is added. After another 1-h incubation, plates are again washed, and then enhancement solution is added. After a final 15-min incubation period, plates are read on the Victor^2 instrument. Because the detector antibody is directly labeled and the signal generated is so strong, the assay can be completed in less time than a colorimetric assay (2.2 vs 3.5 h). ELISA kinetic studies lead us to believe that the DELFIA can be completed in less than 100 min. Critical assay performance characteristics, and assay limits of detection from three typical DELFIA agent detection assays are shown in Table 4. Future improvements in this technology should simplify this platform and may ultimately lead to better overall system performance.

5.4. Flow Cytometry (Luminex)

Flow cytometry, the measurement of physical and chemical characteristics of small particles, has many current applications in the areas of research and health care and are commonplace in most large clinical laboratories. Applications include cytokine detection, cell differentiation, chromosome analysis, cell sorting and typing, bacterial counting, hematology, DNA content, and drug discovery. The technique works by placing biological samples (e.g., cells or other particles) into a liquid suspension. A fluorescent dye, the choice of which is based on its ability to bind to the particles of interest, is added to the solution. The suspension is made to flow in a stream past a laser beam. The light is scattered and the distribution and intensity of scattered light is characteristic of the sample passing through. The wavelength of the light is selected such that it causes the dye, bound to the particle of interest, to fluoresce. A computer counts and/or analyzes the fluorescent sample as it passes through the laser beam (*see* Fig. 7). Using the same excitation source, the fluorescence may be split into different color components so that several different fluorophores can be measured simultaneously and signals interpreted by specialized software. Numerous multiplexed flow cytometry assays have been demonstrated *(43)*. Particles can also be sorted from the stream and diverted into separate containers by applying a charge to the particles of interest.

The Luminex[100] Analysis System (Luminex, Inc.) is a rapid assay system that reportedly can simultaneously perform up to 100 tests on a single sample. It incorporates three familiar technologies; bioassays, microspheres, and fluorescence. The system consists of a flow cytometer with a specific digital signal processing board and control software. Assays occur in solution, thus allowing for rapid reaction kinetics and shorter incubation times. Capture antibodies or ligands are bound to microspheres labeled with two spectrally distinct fluorochromes. By adjusting the ratio of each fluorochrome, microspheres can be distinguished based on their spectral address. Luminex currently offers 100 different microsphere sets, each of which can be used for the simultaneous measurement of a different antigen. Bioassays are conducted on the surfaces of these microspheres. Detector antibodies are labeled with any of a number of different green fluorescent dyes. This detector-bound fluorochrome measures the extent of interaction that occurs at the microsphere surface (i.e., detects antigen in a typical antigen-detection assay). The instrument employs two lasers, one for the detection of the microsphere itself, and the other for the detector. Microspheres are analyzed individually as they pass by two separate laser beams and are classified based on their spectral address and are measured in real time. Thousands (20,000) of microspheres are processed per second, resulting in an assay system theoretically capable of analyzing up to 100 different reactions on a single sample in just seconds. The manufacturer reports assay sensitivities in the femtomole level, dynamic range of 3–4 logs, and claim results are highly consistent and reproducible *(44)*. Because the intensity of the fluorescent label is read only at the surface of each microsphere, any unbound reporter molecules remaining in solution do not affect the assay making homogeneous assay formats possible. The system can employ tubes as well as 96- and 384-well plates and can be automated. Many

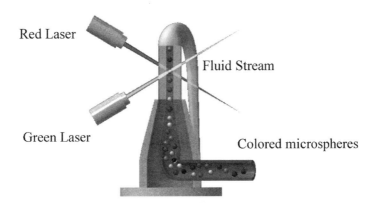

Fig. 7. A representation of the flow cytometry particle stream produced by the Luminex system showing the use of two lasers emitting light at different wavelengths to concurrently detect bead color and the presence or absence of fluorescent antibody.

multiplexed assay kits are commercially available from numerous of different manufacturers for various cytokines, phosphoproteins, and hormones.

In addition to the Luminex instrument, a plate shaker and liquid handling devices are required to complete assays. As with most technologies, several of different formats can be used. In a typical antigen-detection homologous assay format, sample is added to a mixture of reagents consisting of capture antibody-coated, fluorescent polystyrene microspheres, biotinylated detector antibodies, and a green fluorescent-labeled streptavidin. After 30 min incubation on a plate shaker, the microwell plate is loaded onto the XY platform of the Luminex[100], beads are gated (establishes the characteristics of the bead populations in the sample matrix with no analyte or green fluorescent label), and samples are read. The Luminex[100] works by drawing up all but 25 µL of the sample, measuring the green fluorescence on the surface of a particular number of beads (usually 100 beads per type), and then washing the sample input probe (SIP) and associated tubing. This process can take from 20 to 120 s per sample, depending on the sample matrix and its effect on the bead population (i.e., clumping). Critical assay performance characteristics and assay limits of detection from three typical DELFIA agent-detection assays are shown in Table 4. This platform typically lacks the sensitivity seen with platforms like the ECL and TRF. In addition, assay optimization may be difficult because of extensive sample matrix and pro-zone effects. The system requires extensive training and expertise to operate and there are many user-definable parameters that must be optimized individually such as sheath fluid, gating of beads, frequent realignment of SIP, and removal of unbound antibody from latex beads. The major strength of this technology is its ability to multiplex extensively with little or no loss of sensitivity. The number of potential fluorophores that can be used with this system is not as broad as it could be because of the use of a single wavelength 532 nm YAG laser. The total number of bead sets is limited to those the instrument can actually distinguish above matrix noise. Although three different fluorochromes are commonly available (Alexa 532, Bodipy, and Phycoerythrin [PE]), only PE provides reasonable signal intensities and sensitivities. Many other fluorescent labels are relatively short-lived, have specific storage requirements, and are very susceptible to changes in pH, making them unreliable for many applications. Serum and blood samples matrices are particularly problematic for this platform and often result in bead clumping. Despite these problems, the ability to multiplex and the observations that flow cytometry systems are commonplace in most large clinical laboratories and that the FDA has approved numerous human diagnostic assays for flow cytometry makes this a very desirable platform option. Both immunoassays and nucleic acid detection assays are compatible with this platform. Recently Becton Dickensen Biosciences (San Diego, CA) introduced the cytometric bead array system that includes standard flow cytometers and multiple sizes and fluorescent intensities of particles. Several companies now market fluorescent, derivatized bead sets, and other companies continue to expand their repertoire of assay kits available for these systems.

5.5. Fluorescent Polarization

Fluorescence polarization (FP) is an optical property seen when polarized light excites a fluorescent dye causing photons to be emitted in the same plane as the exciting light. The phenomenon was first described in 1926 by F. Perrin *(45)*. FP operates as long as the fluorescent molecule does not change its relative position between excitation and photon emission. By using these properties, it is possible to measure the binding of a fluorescent probe to an antigen in solution. When such a probe binds to an antigen molecule, there is a decrease in the rotation of the probe in solution. The decrease in rotation causes an increase in the FP value of the sample. Commonly available instruments are capable of measuring and reporting FP values. Commercial FP assays for a wide variety of cellular biology applications including those for studying receptor–ligand interactions and for detecting many important cellular proteins. Large molecules labeled with fluorescent tags are problematic because they are more likely to emit polarized light in solution then are small molecules and are also more likely to move in solution. As a result, the size of the probe is one of the key variables for assay development. Smaller probes produce greater FP values than do larger probes because of the loss of orbital rotation that occurs upon binding *(46)* *(see* Fig. 8).

FP assays are one of the simplest types of assay to perform. A fluorescent tag-labeled probe (antibody or other ligand) is mixed with an unknown sample. If the fluorescent probe binds to material in the sample, there will be a detectible change in polarized light emitted from the sample. A positive binding event results in an increase in the FP value caused by a decrease in orbital rotation. FP assays that measure some biological characteristic of an agent can also be developed. Typically, such assays measure enzymatic activity of a molecule. In this case, the assay is designed to measure cleavage of a substrate containing a fluorescent tag-labeled peptide by agent present in a sample. Cleavage causes a decrease in FP value resulting from an increase in orbital rotation. The equipment that is necessary to perform these assays must be able to excite the probe with polarized light and to detect the polarized light that is emitted. Physical characteristics of a given sample such as temperature and viscosity have a direct effect the FP readings of a given assay. These and other physical characteristics of the sample matrix will affect how long it takes for reactants within a sample to come to an equilibrium binding state but do not affect the relative sensitivity of an assay in any given sample matrix.

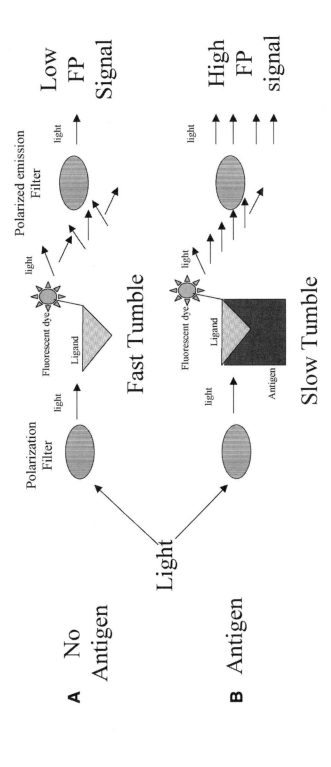

Fig. 8. The effect of ligand binding to an antigen on the FP value. Fluorescently polarized light emitted from a probe that is bound to a large target antigen is greater then that of unbound probe.

In a typical assay, each sample is blanked first then monitored during the time that the reaction is allowed to come to equilibrium. Therefore, the time that it takes to analyze a sample is variable, depending on the sample matrix. Generally, reactions can be read at 15 min. In most cases, a positive, qualitative judgment can be made before the sample reaches equilibrium.

As with any technology, there are advantages and disadvantages to FP. An advantage with FP is that the assay can be carried out in any matrix in which the probe and antigen can be allowed to interact. Therefore, FP assays require minimal sample preparation. There are examples of FP analyses being carried out in phosphate-buffered saline, sera, milk, and other solvents without pretreating or processing of the sample *(47,48)*. There are more than 50 FP assays commercially available for detecting various sample types including protein *(46,49)*, DNA (50), and measurements of enzyme activity *(51)*. FP has also been used to detect serum antibodies *(47)*. Assays for the detection of serum antibodies use a fluorescent-labeled probe that is small, offering limited polarizing effect until it is bound by antibodies. These antibody detection assays are very effective for high-throughput screening because of the lack of a requirement for sample processing. FP can also be used to monitor enzymatic reactions *(52,53)*. In these types of assays, a substrate is labeled with a fluorescent dye such that enzyme activity produces smaller probe fragments and a concomitant decrease in FP value for the sample.

The limiting factor in the development of FP assays is the availability of small molecules suitable as probes. These small probes can be fragments of antibody or any other molecule that will selectively bind with high affinity to the target antigen. Potential probes previously discussed in this chapter such as peptides, products from phage display libraries, and aptamers may someday provide a source of probes needed to expand the array of assays that could be performed using FP technology.

5.6. Lateral Flow Assays

Lateral flow assays have been available on the commercial market for many years. These assays are simple to use and interpret and, therefore, require minimal training. In most cases, the manufacturer provides simple instructions that include pictures of what a positive or negative result should look like. Lateral flow assays typically have shelf lives of more than 2 yr and do not require special storage conditions. However, high humidity and excessive heat degrade assay performance. The most commonly available lateral flow assays are those that screen for abused drugs and those for detecting human chorionic gonadotropin, the presence of which indicates pregnancy. Most lateral flow assays currently in production are performed and read by the user and are interpreted qualitatively. However, there are several instruments that are available or are in development for reading these assays. These readers are being developed with the goal of increasing assay sensitivity and eliminating or reducing the subjectivity associated with assay interpretation, thus making them more quantitative.

Lateral flow assays are typically designed on nitrocellulose or nylon membranes that are contained within a plastic or cardboard housing. A capture antibody is bound to the membrane and a second antibody labeled with some visible marker element is placed on a sample application pad. As the sample moves down the membrane because of capillary action, antigen present in the sample binds to the labeled antibody and is

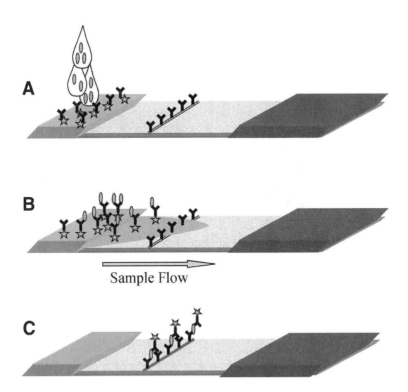

Fig. 9. Antigen capture lateral flow assay. Sample containing the antigen of interest is applied to the sample application pad (**A**). Antigen in the sample binds to antibody conjugated to a visible label found in the sample application pad. Antigen/antibody complexes flow past the capture zone (**B**) and are concentrated there through their interaction with the capture antibody (**C**). A positive assay is indicated by the presence of a visible line in the capture zone.

captured as the complex passes the bound antibody (*see* Fig. 9). Colloidal gold, carbon, paramagnetic, or colored latex beads are commonly used particles that create a visible line in the capture zone of the assay membrane. The method used for determining if an assay is positive depends on if it is a competitive or an antigen capture assay. In the competitive format, antigen in the sample competes with a labeled antigen for binding sites on the capture antibody (*see* Fig. 10). If a line fails to appear, then the test is interpreted as positive for the antigen. The competitive lateral flow format is frequently used to analyze small molecules with a limited number of epitopes. Typical tests in this format include those for small toxins, drugs and drug metabolites, and hormones. The competitive lateral flow assays are often multiplexed and allow the user to test for several antigens simultaneously.

Lateral flow assays are most frequently read visually. Several technologies are being developed to make these assays more quantitative as well as to increase their sensitivity. Methods for analyzing lateral flow assays range from simply scanning the strip and analyzing the digital image to more sophisticated methods that use particles that have energetic properties.

Fluorescent-based readers rely on detection of fluorescent microspheres that are incorporated into the lateral flow assays. One such reader, produced by Response Bio-

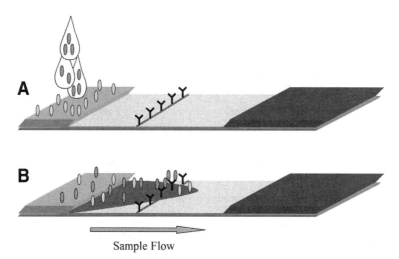

Fig. 10. Competitive lateral flow assay. Sample containing the antigen of interest is applied to the sample application pad (**A**). This sample along with antigen bound to a visible label flows past a capture antibody. Competition between labeled and unlabeled antigen prevents the labeled antigen from binding to the test capture zone. The lack of a visible line in this assay indicates a positive test.

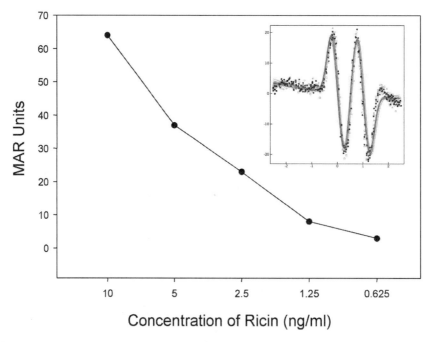

Fig. 11. Results from magnetic lateral flow assays for detecting ricin. The insert in the graph is a representative scan of a line 10 times using the MAR 4 reader developed by Quantum Design.

medical Corporation, allows for quantitative interpretation of the lateral flow assay *(54)*. The incorporation of upconverting phosphors has also been used as a method to make the lateral flow assay quantitative and attempt to increase its sensitivity *(55,56)*. In addition to the development of assays that employ light-producing particles, there are also efforts to use paramagnetic particles and read the assays through changes in magnetic flux within the capture zone (Quantum Design, San Diego, CA). This approach has been successful in improving sensitivity by as much as several orders of magnitude over more traditional lateral flow assays. Based on the method of sample detection, this platform makes accurate quantitative measurement of antigen possible (*see* Fig. 11).

REFERENCES

1. Malmqvist, M. (1993) Surface plasmon resonance for detection and measurement of antibody-antigen affinity and kinetics. *Curr. Opin. Immunol.* **5,** 282–286.
2. Wabl, M., Cascalho, M., and Steinberg, C. (1999) Hypermutation in antibody affinity maturation. *Curr. Opin. Immunol.* **11,** 186–189.
3. Neuberger, M. S., Ehrenstein, M. R., Rada, C., et al. (2000) Memory in the B-cell compartment: antibody affinity maturation. *Philos. Trans. R. Soc. Lond. B. Biol. Sci.* **355,** 357–360.
4. Rudin, C. M. and Thompson, C. B. (1998) B-cell development and maturation. *Semin. Oncol.* **25,** 435–446.
5. Kohler, G. and Milstein, C. (1975) Continuous cultures of fused cells secreting antibody of predefined specificity. *Nature (London)* **256,** 495–497.
6. Allison, L. M. C., Salter, M. W. A. P., Kiguwa, S., and Howard, C. R. (1991) Analysis of the glycoprotein gene of Tacaribe virus and neutralization-resistant variants. *J. Gen. Virol.* **72,** 2025–2029.
7. Agapov, Y. V., Lebedeva, S. D., Razumov, I. A., et al. (1992) Models of Venezuelan equine encephalomyelitis virus resistant to neutralization effect of monoclonal antibodies. *Doklady Akademii Nauk SSSR* **320,** 24–26.
8. Ketterlinus, R., Wiegers, K., and Dernick, R. (1993) Revertants of poliovirus escape mutants: new insights into antigenic structures. *Virology* **192,** 525–533.
9. Smith, G. P. (1985) Filamentous fusion phage: novel expression vectors that display cloned antigens on the virion surface. *Science* **228,** 1315–1317.
10. Huse, W. D., Sastry, L., Iverson, S. A., et al. (1989) Generation of a large combinatorial library of the immunoglobulin repertoire in phage lambda. *Science* **246,** 1275–1281.
11. Persson, M. A., Caothien, R. H., and Burton, D. R. (1991) Generation of diverse high-affinity human monoclonal antibodies by repertoire cloning. *Proc. Natl. Acad. Sci. USA* **88,** 2432–2436.
12. Burton, D. R., Barbas, C. F., III, Persson, M. A., Koenig, S., Chanock, R. M., and Lerner, R. A. (1991) A large array of human monoclonal antibodies to type 1 human immunodeficiency virus from combinatorial libraries of asymptomatic seropositive individuals. *Proc. Natl. Acad. Sci. USA* **88,** 10,134–10,137.
13. Nakayama, G. R., Valkirs, G., McGrath, D., and Huse, W. D. (1996) Improving the copy numbers of antibody fragments expressed on the major coat protein of bacteriophage M13. *Immunotechnology* **2,** 197–207.
14. Maynard, J. and Georgiou, G. (2000) Antibody engineering. *Annu. Rev. Biomed. Eng.* **2,** 339–376.
15. Maynard, J. A., Maassen, C. B., Leppla, S. H., et al. (2002) Protection against anthrax toxin by recombinant antibody fragments correlates with antigen affinity. *Nat. Biotechnol.* **20,** 597–601.
16. Crowe, J. E., Jr., Murphy, B. R., Chanock, R. M., Williamson, R. A., Barbas, C. F., III, and Burton, D. R. (1994) Recombinant human respiratory syncytial virus (RSV) monoclonal antibody Fab is effective therapeutically when introduced directly into the lungs of RSV-infected mice. *Proc. Natl. Acad. Sci. USA* **91,** 1386–1390.

17. Samuelsson, A., Yari, F., Hinkula, J., Ersoy, O., Norrby, E., and Persson, M. A. (1996) Human antibodies from phage libraries: neutralizing activity against human immunodeficiency virus type 1 equally improved after expression as Fab and IgG in mammalian cells. *Eur. J. Immunol.* **26,** 3029–3034.

18. Sun, W., Xiong, J., and Shulman, M. J. (1994) Production of mouse V/human C chimeric kappa genes by homologous recombination in hybridoma cells. Analysis of vector design and recombinant gene expression. *J. Immunol.* **152,** 695–704.

19. Kanda, H., Mori, K., Koga, H., et al. (1994) Construction and expression of chimeric antibodies by a simple replacement of heavy and light chain V genes into a single cassette vector. *Hybridoma* **13,** 359–366.

20. Song, Z., Cai, Y., Song, D., et al. (1997) Primary structure and functional expression of heavy- and light-chain variable region genes of a monoclonal antibody specific for human fibrin. *Hybridoma* **16,** 235–241.

21. Lu, Z., Murray, K. S., Van, C. V., LaVallie, E. R., Stahl, M. L., and McCoy, J. M. (1995) Expression of thioredoxin random peptide libraries on the *Escherichia coli* cell surface as functional fusions to flagellin: a system designed for exploring protein-protein interactions. *Biotechnology (NY)* **13,** 366–372.

22. Kurz, M., Gu, K., Al Gawari, A., and Lohse, P. A. (2001) cDNA - protein fusions: covalent protein–gene conjugates for the in vitro selection of peptides and proteins. *Chembiochemistry* **2,** 666–672.

23. Kurz, M., Gu, K., and Lohse, P. A. (2000) Psoralen photo-crosslinked mRNA-puromycin conjugates: a novel template for the rapid and facile preparation of mRNA-protein fusions. *Nucleic Acids Res.* **28,** E83.

24. Kreider, B. L. (2000) PROfusion: genetically tagged proteins for functional proteomics and beyond. *Med. Res. Rev.* **20,** 212–215.

25. Tuerk, C. and Gold, L. (1990) Systematic evolution of ligands by exponential enrichment: RNA ligands to bacteriophage T4 DNA polymerase. *Science* **249,** 505–510.

26. Brody, E. N. and Gold, L. (2000) Aptamers as therapeutic and diagnostic agents. *Rev. Mol. Biotechnol.* **74,** 5–13.

27. Ringquist, S. and Parma, D. (1998) Anti-L-selectin oligonucleotide ligands recognize CD62L-positive leukocytes: binding affinity and specificity of univalent and bivalent ligands. *Cytometry* **33,** 394–405.

28. Willis, M. C., LeCuyer, K. A., Meisenheimer, K. M., Uhlenbeck, O. C., and Koch, T. H. (1994) An RNA-protein contact determined by 5-bromouridine substitution, photocrosslinking and sequencing. *Nucleic Acids Res.* **22,** 4947–4952.

29. Meisenheimer, K. M., Meisenheimer, P. L., Willis, M. C., and Koch, T. H. (1996) High yield photocrosslinking of a 5-iodocytidine (IC) substituted RNA to its associated protein. *Nucleic Acids Res.* **24,** 981, 982.

30. Golden, M. C., Collins, B. D., Willis, M. C., and Koch, T. H. (2000) Diagnostic potential of PhotoSELEX-evolved ssDNA aptamers. *J. Biotechnol.* **81,** 167–178.

31. Eaton, B. E. and Pieken, W. A. (1995) Ribonucleosides and RNA. *Annu. Rev. Biochem.* **64,** 837–863.

32. Jellinek, D., Green, L. S., Bell, C., et al. (1995) Potent 2'-amino-2'-deoxypyrimidine RNA inhibitors of basic fibroblast growth factor. *BCH* **34,** 11,363–11,372.

33. Ruckman, J., Green, L. S., Beeson, J., et al. (1998) 2'-Fluoropyrimidine RNA-based aptamers to the 165-amino acid form of vascular endothelial growth factor (VEGF165). Inhibition of receptor binding and VEGF-induced vascular permeability through interactions requiring the exon 7-encoded domain. *J. Biol. Chem.* **273,** 20,556–20,567.

34. Yang, H., Leland, J. K., Yost, D., and Massey, R. J. (1994) Electrochemiluminescence: a new diagnostic and research tool. ECL detection technology promises scientists new "yardsticks" for quantification. *Biotechnology (NY)* **12,** 193, 194.

35. Carlowicz, M. (1995) Electrochemiluminescence could spark an assay revolution. *Clin. Lab. News* **21**, 1–3.
36. Kijek, T. M., Rossi, C. A., Moss, D., Parker, R. W., and Henchal, E. A. (2000) Rapid and sensitive immunomagnetic-electrochemiluminescent detection of staphylococcal enterotoxin B. *J. Immunol. Methods* **236**, 9–17.
37. Higgins, J. A., Ibrahim, M. S., Knauert, F. K., et al. (1999) Sensitive and rapid identification of biological threat agents. *Ann. NY Acad. Sci.* **894**, 130–148.
38. Barnard, G., Helmick, B., Madden, S., Gilbourne, C., and Patel, R. (2000) The measurement of prion protein in bovine brain tissue using differential extraction and DELFIA as a diagnostic test for BSE. *Luminescence* **15**, 357–362.
39. Crooks, S. R., Ross, P., Thompson, C. S., Haggan, S. A., and Elliott, C. T. (2000) Detection of unwanted residues of ivermectin in bovine milk by dissociation-enhanced lanthanide fluoroimmunoassay. *Luminescence* **15**, 371–376.
40. Hierholzer, J. C., Johansson, K. H., Anderson, L. J., Tsou, C. J., and Halonen, P. E. (1987) Comparison of monoclonal time-resolved fluoroimmunoassay with monoclonal capture-biotinylated detector enzyme immunoassay for adenovirus antigen detection. *J. Clin. Microbiol.* **25**, 1662–1667.
41. Hemmila, I., Dakubu, S., Mukkala, V. M., Siitari, H., and Lovgren, T. (1984) Europium as a label in time-resolved immunofluorometric assays. *Anal. Biochem.* **137**, 335–343.
42. Merio, L., Pettersson, K., and Lovgren, T. (1996) Monoclonal antibody-based dual-label time-resolved fluorometric assays in a simplified one-step format. *Clin. Chem.* **42**, 1513–1517.
43. Carson, R. T. and Vignali, D. A. (1999) Simultaneous quantitation of 15 cytokines using a multiplexed flow cytometric assay. *J. Immunol. Methods* **227**, 41–52.
44. Fulton, R. J., McDade, R. L., Smith, P. L., Kienker, L. J., and Kettman, J. R., Jr. (1997) Advanced multiplexed analysis with the FlowMetrix system. *Clin. Chem.* **43**, 1749–1756.
45. Perrin, F. (1926) Radium. *J. Phys.* **7**, 390–401.
46. Checovich, W. J., Bolger, R. E., and Burke, T. (1995) Fluorescence polarization—a new tool for cell and molecular biology. *Nature (London)* **375**, 254–256.
47. Nielsen, K., Gall, D., Jolley, M., et al. (1996) A homogeneous fluorescence polarization assay for detection of antibody to *Brucella abortus*. *J. Immunol. Methods* **195**, 161–168.
48. Urios, P. and Cittanova, N. (1990) Adaptation of fluorescence polarization immunoassay to the assay of macromolecules. *Anal. Biochem.* **185**, 308–312.
49. Tencza, S. B., Islam, K. R., Kalia, V., Nasir, M. S., Jolley, M. E., and Montelaro, R. C. (2000) Development of a fluorescence polarization-based diagnostic assay for equine infectious anemia virus. *J. Clin. Microbiol.* **38**, 1854–1859.
50. LeTilly, V. and Royer, C. A. (1993) Fluorescence anisotropy assays implicate protein-protein interactions in regulating trp repressor DNA binding. *BCH* **32**, 7753–7758.
51. Singh, K. K., Rucker, T., Hanne, A., Parwaresch, R., and Krupp, G. (2000) Fluorescence polarization for monitoring ribozyme reactions in real time. *BT* **29**, 344–341.
52. Bolger, R., Lenoch, F., Allen, E., Meiklejohn, B., and Burke T. (1997) Fluorescent dye assay for detection of DNA in recombinant protein products. *BT* **23**, 532–537.
53. Maeda, H. (1979) Assay of proteolytic enzymes by the fluorescence polarization technique. *Anal. Biochem.* **92**, 222–227.
54. Harris, P. and Stephenson, J. (2000) Automating POC instrumentation: a systems view. *IVD Technol.* **6**, 45–49.
55. Niedbala, R. S., Feindt, H., Kardos, K., et al. (2001) Detection of analytes by immunoassay using up-converting phosphor technology. *Anal. Biochem.* **293**, 22–30.
56. Corstjens, P., Zuiderwijk, M., Brink, A., et al. (2001) Use of up-converting phosphor reporters in lateral-flow assays to detect specific nucleic acid sequences: a rapid, sensitive DNA test to identify human papillomavirus type 16 infection. *Clin. Chem.* **47**, 1885–1893.

Index